AF478211

The Segmental Motor System

THE SEGMENTAL MOTOR SYSTEM

Edited by

MARC D. BINDER
University of Washington School of Medicine

LORNE M. MENDELL
State University of New York at Stony Brook

New York   Oxford
OXFORD UNIVERSITY PRESS
1990

Oxford University Press

Oxford   New York   Toronto
Delhi   Bombay   Calcutta   Madras   Karachi
Petaling Jaya   Singapore   Hong Kong   Tokyo
Nairobi   Dar es Salaam   Cape Town
Melbourne   Auckland

and associated companies in
Berlin   Ibadan

Copyright © 1990 by Oxford University Press, Inc.

Published by Oxford University Press, Inc.,
200 Madison Avenue, New York, New York 10016

Oxford is a registered trademark of Oxford University Press

Library of Congress Cataloging-in-Publication Data
The segmental motor system / edited by Marc D. Binder,
Lorne M. Mendell.
p.   cm.
ISBN 0-19-505484-9
1. Motor neurons.   2. Locomotion.   3. Myoneural junction.
I. Binder, Marc D.   II. Mendell, Lorne M.
QP369.S44   1990   599'.01852—dc20   89-32565   CIP

9 8 7 6 5 4 3 2 1

Printed in the United States of America
on acid-free paper

Preface

This volume presents much of the current state of our knowledge on the functional organization of the segmental motor apparatus of mammals. Our purpose in assembling the various chapters that follow was twofold: to provide a systematic attack on some of the fundamental contemporary issues in motor control and to acknowledge the seminal contributions that Professor Elwood Henneman has made both to this area of research and to neuroscience in general.

We have asked the authors to address one of the following interrelated issues: the intrinsic properties of motoneurons and muscle fibers; the phenomenon of orderly motor unit recruitment and its underlying mechanisms; the neural-mechanical correlations between motoneurons and the muscle units they innervate; and the analysis of synaptic inputs to motoneuron pools. In focusing on these issues, we not only emerge with comprehensive coverage of the functional organization of the motoneuron pool and its target tissue, skeletal muscle, but further illuminate the extensive ramifications that research in this area has had on neurobiology.

Over the past 30 years, the mammalian segmental motor system has served as a template for research on neural trophism, synaptic function and connectivity, neuronal recognition, and neuronal modelling, as well as providing the definitive neural aggregation, the motoneuron pool. In addition, a number of important experimental and analytical techniques, including intracellular recording, signal averaging, linear systems analysis, conditioning-testing, spatial facilitation and occlusion, and excitability testing, have emerged from this area of research to become important components of the experimental armamentarium of biologists working throughout the nervous system.

Professor Elwood Henneman has stood at the forefront of this work, providing the conceptual framework on which much of it has been based. Remarkably he has also been instrumental in developing a number of the techniques that have helped fuel progress in this area. Although but few of the authors have actually worked in Professor Henneman's laboratory, it is clear that all of us have been profoundly influenced by his experimental work and insights. The chapters that follow are evidence of that influence and reflect his wide-ranging contributions to neuroscience.

Comments on the Logical Basis
of Muscle Control

ELWOOD HENNEMAN

The essays in this volume will, I am sure, illustrate better than any disquisition how rapidly research on spinal motor function has progressed in the last decades. It is a good time, nevertheless, to be reminded that outsiders looking at our field are often nonplussed by the absence of theories, rules, laws, and principles that lend meaning and dimension to experimental findings. Admittedly, we are data rich and theory poor, as some have charged. Better that than the reverse, however. In an attempt to prop up our empiricism, and at the risk of going over familiar ground, I would like to discuss briefly certain aspects of muscle control, with an emphasis on the logical imperatives that gave rise to the system our research is revealing. In view of the honor they are doing me, I trust that my friends and former colleagues will understand my reluctance to do more on this occasion than look back reflectively at a few of the findings and ideas we shared in the past.

One of the notable advances in recent years has been a growing appreciation of the necessity for large populations of neurons to handle complex functions such as controlling a muscle. Thinking characterized by circuit diagrams in which a single cell represented an entire pool with hundreds of motoneurons, for example, has been replaced by more holistic concepts emphasizing the importance of populations and the well-ordered heterogeneity of their members. Although the motoneurons in such populations all control the actions of a single muscle, their contributions may vary widely. Because of systematic differences in their size and excitability, and corresponding variations in the speed, power, delicacy, and endurance of the motor units they supply, each provides a unique set of attributes. This, of course, is the *raison d' être* of a pool—to supply, through its motor units, the properties without which a muscle would be unable to meet the demands of ordinary activity. Imagine a muscle composed of motor units that did not vary, units all responding at the same time and with equal force to volleys of similar commands like a corps of cadets!

Another logical necessity for the considerable number of motoneurons needed to provide adequate control of single muscles is that, regardless of their particular roles, all muscles must be capable of developing a wide range of tensions quickly and exactly. To do so, a muscle must have available a large assortment of contractile units of different sizes from which suitable combinations can be selected to yield the necessary total forces. Innervating this large set of contractile units is a population of motoneurons finely graded in size. The smallest cells in each pool supply groups of muscle fibers that conduct impulses slowly, fatigue very little, and develop small tensions. Progressively larger motoneurons innervate stronger motor units that conduct impulses more rapidly and fatigue more quickly (Henneman and Mendell, 1981). It is clear that when motor units of different sizes are activated, the contractions accompanying their use may differ in several respects. What internal logic guides the nervous system to take advantage of the different properties of the motor units available to it? It appears that the necessity to develop any required tension precisely is usually, but not invariably, the overriding factor.

The sizable populations of motoneurons that supply skeletal muscles and the varying properties of their motor units present an intriguing problem in motor control. The problem is not difficult to define. How can the different tensions that individual motor units develop be combined by activating appropriate motoneurons to produce any total force that is required with the necessary precision and speed? Simple as it may appear, this is a problem in neural logic that would daunt any control engineer who was not already familiar with nature's solution. This puzzling aspect of motor control has been badly neglected. In fact, judging from the lack of attention it has received in print over the years, it has scarcely been recognized as a key to the organization of input as well as output at the motoneuron level.

A good way to appreciate the nature of this problem is to imagine how an engineer who was introduced to it, but was not aware of a solution, would tend to approach it. His first inclination would be to assume that the inputs to a pool activate individual motoneurons selectively, like the keys on a typewriter. There are, in fact, special circumstances in which differential control has been demonstrated. Our expert would soon realize, however, that if precision was essential, it was simply not feasible to discharge selectively motoneurons of different sizes that would yield the right total tension without testing their combined effects in some way. Such testing would require considerable additional circuitry and lead to unacceptable neural delays. With hundreds of motoneurons in some pools, selection of the right combinations for discharge would necessarily include a time-consuming neural computation preceding each output from the pool. Moreover, for each new set of motoneuronal outputs, a different combination of inputs would be needed, again involving selection and delay. Differential discharge not being feasible as a general rule, our engineer would realize that a highly automatic process not requiring selective inputs and outputs was the only solution. He might also appreciate that such a process would necessarily involve simultaneous summation of all inputs to the pool, both excitatory and inhibitory. Faced with these requirements, our expert would probably throw up his hands.

It is obvious that the output of a pool must be a function of the sum of the inputs (excitatory minus inhibitory) converging on it. Nature, of course, is more ingenious than we are and has developed a logical way of relating output to input that is most precise and flexible. A simple rule governs the discharges of motoneurons in most circumstances. According to this rule, cells are fired monosynaptically, internuncially, repetitively, or in simultaneous combinations, as determined by their excitabilities, i.e., their size-related susceptibilities to discharge. The intensities of the total inputs impinging on cells with different excitabilities automatically determine which ones are fired and what combinations result. Since susceptibilities to discharge are relatively fixed, being closely related to cell size, combinations are formed in a relatively invariant manner. They consist of orderly sequences of motoneurons that include the smallest cell in the pool. A very weak excitatory input fires only this cell, causing contraction of the weakest motor unit in the muscle. Progressively stronger inputs discharge successively bigger motoneurons, adding increasingly large increments of tension to the total force the muscle is exerting. Inputs of different sizes or intensities elicit discharges from every motoneuron in a pool up to a certain size, but from no larger cells. Accordingly, the monosynaptic output from a motoneuron pool may be expressed in the form of a simple equation (Henneman et al., 1974) as follows:

$$O_{\mathrm{T}} = O_1 + O_2 + O_3 + \ldots + O_x$$

where O_{T} = total monosynaptic output of the pool; $O_1 + O_2 + O_3$ = outputs of motoneurons of increasing sizes; and O_x = output of the highest-ranking cell discharged. This equation is a concise formulation of a basic law of combination. It specifies how motoneurons are combined with each other in monosynaptic reflexes and limits the possible number of combinations to the number of cells in the pool minus one. A particular cell in this fixed hierarchy fires only if all the lower-ranking cells in the pool discharge with it. It is clear that an analogous law applies to motoneurons firing repetitively, but it would make a cumbersome equation.

Although we still do not know what is under the hood to make all this possible, the elegance and simplicity of the rank-ordered pool testify to the logic of the neural design. Since the advantages of a law of combination are not all immediately obvious, it is worthwhile to enumerate some of them. (1) The size and composition of output are determined automatically by the total size and intensity of all inputs. (2) Excitatory and inhibitory inputs sum algebraically (Clamann et al., 1974). Addition of inhibition causes effects similar to those of a reduction in excitation. (3) When different inputs are mixed, there is no displacement of rank orders. (4) Delays are minimal because special circuits are not needed to calculate the combined effects of different inputs. (5) Total muscle tensions are controlled with maximum precision. In this process, precision is a function of the largest increment of tension included in any combination, and sequential combination minimizes the size of that increment. (6) The capacity to sustain strong contractions is retained longer and at a higher level because of the greater fatigue resistance of the smaller motor units in the active population. (7) Major differences in the frequency of use of motor units of different size permit significant adaptations in the energy metabolism of their muscle fibers. (8) In emergencies or special circumstances, the usual rank-ordered control process can be overridden. (9) Lastly, the problem of how to combine active units does not arise. To estimate the degree of simplification this represents, consider the alternative, in which all possible combinations (N) of active units might occur. For a pool of 100 motoneurons, N is calculated as follows:

$$N = \sum_{k=1}^{100} \frac{100!}{k!(100 - k)!}$$

With free, unsequenced selection from a pool of this size, there would be 10^{30} possible combinations, constituting an impossible control problem.

There were two particular reasons for reviewing the material in this brief essay in spite of misgivings about its familiarity: (1) it reminds one of the logical inevitability of the system that evolution has bequeathed us and the indispensability of its main features; (2) it reveals why other methods of controlling muscles would be unsatisfactory in general use. If the foregoing account has not been unduly biased in favor of a rank-ordered control system, it follows that deviations from that mode would necessarily occur at the sacrifice of the advantages just outlined, notably precision. It is obvious, of course, that in a few special types of activity, such as very rapid alternating movements in paw shaking, precision is less important than some other parameter. When it is necessary to override the usual control processes, as when a disturbance in equilibrium causes a sudden powerful input from the vestibular system, a very rapid correction must take precedence over all other inputs. We do not yet know how to reconcile occasional departures from rank-ordered activity with the process that prevails most of the time. As in psychiatry, understanding of so-called deviant behavior must await a better knowledge of the mechanisms underlying the usual patterns.

REFERENCES

Clamann, H. P., Gillies, J. D., and Henneman, E. (1974). Effects of inhibitory inputs on critical firing level and rank order of motoneurons, *J. Neurophysiol.* 37, 1350–1360.

Henneman, E., Clamann, H. P., Gillies, J. D., and Skinner, R. D. (1974). Rank order of motoneurons within a pool: Law of combination. *J. Neurophysiol.* 37, 1338–1349.

Henneman, E., and Mendell, L. M. (1981). Functional organization of the motoneuron pool and its inputs. In *Handbook of Physiology* (ed. Vernon B. Brooks), Section 1: *The Nervous System*, Vol. 1, Part 1. American Physiological Society, Bethesda, Md., pp. 423–507.

Contents

Contributors

V. C. ABRAHAMS
Department of Physiology
Queen's University
Kingston, Ontario K7L 3N6
Canada

PARVEEN BAWA
Department of Kinesiology
Simon Fraser University
Burnaby, British Columbia V5A 1S6
Canada

ALBERT J. BERGER
Department of Physiology and Biophys-
    ics, SJ-40
University of Washington
School of Medicine
Seattle, Washington 98195

MARC D. BINDER
Department of Physiology and Biophysics
University of Washington, SJ-40
Seattle, Washington 98195

R. E. BURKE
Laboratory of Neural Control
National Institute of Neurological and
    Communicative Disorders and Stroke
National Institutes of Health
Building 36, Room 5A29
Bethesda, Maryland 20892

BLAIR CALANCIE
Department of Physiology
University of Alberta
Edmonton, Alberta T6G 2H7
Canada

G. R. CHALMERS
Kinesiology and Brain Research Institute
University of California, Los Angeles
Los Angeles, California 90024

P. D. CHENEY
Department of Physiology
University of Kansas
Kansas City, Kansas 66103

H. PETER CLAMANN
Department of Physiology
Medical College of Virginia
Richmond, Virginia 23298

WILLIAM F. COLLINS III
Department of Neurobiology and
    Behavior
State University of New York
Stony Brook, New York 11794

V. R. EDGERTON
Kinesiology and Brain Research Institute
University of California, Los Angeles
Los Angeles, California 90024

ROGER M. ENOKA
Departments of Physiology and Exercise
    and Sport Sciences
University of Arizona
College of Medicine
Tucson, Arizona 85724

E. E. FETZ
Department of Physiology and Biophysics
University of Washington
Seattle, Washington 98195

STEPHEN J. GOLDBERG
Department of Anatomy
Medical College of Virginia
Virginia Commonwealth University
Richmond, Virginia 23298

TESSA GORDON
Division of Neuroscience
Heritage Medical Research Center
University of Alberta
Edmonton, Alberta T6G 2S2
Canada

C. J. HECKMAN
Department of Physiology and Biophysics
University of Washington, SJ-40
Seattle, Washington 98195

ELWOOD HENNEMAN
Department of Physiology
Harvard Medical School
Boston, Massachussets 02115

DANIEL KERNELL
Department of Neurophysiology
University of Amsterdam
Academisch Medisch Centrum
Meibergdreff 15
1105 AZ Amsterdam
The Netherlands

H. RICHARD KOERBER
Department of Neurobiology and
    Behavior
State University of New York
Stony Brook, New York 11794

GERALD E. LOEB
Department of Biomedical Engineering
Queen's University
Kingston, Ontario K7L 3N6
Canada

HANS-R. LÜSCHER
Department of Physiology
University of Bern
Bühlplatz 5
CH-3012 Bern, Switzerland

LORNE M. MENDELL
Department of Neurobiology and
    Behavior
State University of New York
Stony Brook, New York 11794

JOHN B. MUNSON
Department of Neuroscience
College of Medicine
University of Florida
Gainesville, Florida 32610

PATTI M. NEMETH
Department of Neurology
Washington University
St. Louis, Missouri 63110

MARTIN J. PINTER
Department of Anatomy
Medical College of Pennsylvania
3200 Henry Avenue
Philadelphia, Pennsylvania 19129

WILFRID RALL
Mathematical Research Branch
NIDDK
National Institutes of Health
Building 31, Room 4B-54
Bethesda, Maryland 20892

F. J. R. RICHMOND
Department of Physiology
Queen's University
Kingston, Ontario K7L 3N6
Canada

P. K. ROSE
Department of Physiology
Queen's University
Kingston, Ontario K7L 3N6
Canada

R. R. ROY
Kinesiology Department and Brain Re-
    search Institute
University of California, Los Angeles
Los Angeles, California 90024

P. RUDOMIN
Department of Physiology, Biophysics, and
    Neurosciences

Centro de Investigación y de Estudios
     Avanzados del IPN
Ap 14-740
Mexico 14, DF
Mexico

RICHARD B. STEIN
Division of Neuroscience
Heritage Medical Research Center
University of Alberta
Edmonton, Alberta T6G 2S2
Canada

DOUGLAS G. STUART
Department of Physiology
College of Medicine
University of Arizona
Tucson, Arizona 85724

JOANNE TOTOSY DE ZEPETNEK
Division of Neuroscience
Heritage Medical Research Center
University of Alberta
Edmonton, Alberta T6G 2S2
Canada

FELIX E. ZAJAC
Mechanical Engineering Department
Stanford University
Stanford, California 94305-3030
and
Rehabilitation Research and Development
     Center (153)
Veterans Administration Center
Palo Alto, California 94304

The Segmental Motor System

Overview
Henneman's Contributions in Historical Perspective

DOUGLAS G. STUART AND ROGER M. ENOKA

In discourse on the neural control of mammalian posture and movement, it is usually instructive to consider the integrated activity of the "segmental motor system." This term is a convenient rubric for spinal (or brain stem) motor circuitry, motor units, muscle receptors, and the segmental connections of muscle, joint, and cutaneous afferents. Even in the days before electronic stimulation and recording techniques were used, study of the segmental motor system figured prominently in neuroscientific research, probably because it afforded easy experimental entry into the central nervous system (CNS). Early on, emphasis was on reflexes, with work from the Sherrington school being particularly influential (Creed et al., 1932; Liddell, 1960; Granit 1966). With the advent of spinal cord intracellular recording techniques in the late 1940s, the focus switched to the motoneuron, which, as evidenced by many of the contributions to this volume, remains the most popular cell in the CNS for the study of intrinsic biophysical properties, extrinsic synaptic mechanisms, and mathematical modeling. In this brief tribute to Professor Henneman, we provide a historical perspective on his substantial and influential contribution to the study of the segmental motor system.

At the systems level of investigation of the segmental motor system, three integrative areas of study have proven particularly fruitful during the last 30 years. First, work chiefly by the Lundberg school has shown that descending command signals to the segmental motor system are mediated mostly by interneurons on which the majority of the descending and sensory afferent inputs converge (for review, see Baldissera et al., 1981). These investigators (Jankowska and Lundberg, 1981)* have argued that "It seems much more sensible that different receptors which can give useful information combine in the feedback control and this is best achieved by convergence on interneurons in the common reflex pathway." Unfortunately, this idea, which is based on technically virtuosic work (e.g., Jankowska and Roberts, 1972; Brink et al., 1983),

*Reprinted by permission of the Elsevier Science Publishers B.V.

rarely appears in medical and graduate training (see, however, Burke, 1985). Textbooks still emphasize stereotyped rather than alternative (phase-dependent) spinal reflex pathways and motoneurons rather than interneurons as the sites of major convergence. The flexibility inherent in interneurons offers a great challenge to future students of motor control, because it requires delineation of the role of patterns of interneuronal convergence in the control of ongoing movements.

The second area of emphasis has also been slow to reach the classroom. It involves analysis of the brain stem and spinal pattern generation of relatively stereotyped movements—breathing, chewing, walking, swimming. Experimental work has been undertaken on a wide variety of animal models (from insects to humans), sometimes with neuronal activity studied during natural movements and sometimes with the animal paralyzed and the CNS elaborating a "fictive" movement. From the 1970s on, this area has brought together small- and large-systems investigators (e.g., Stein et al., 1973; Herman et al., 1976; Stein, 1985; Grillner et al., 1987) and has helped to create an "interphyletic awareness" (Stuart, 1985) in modern neuroscience. Recently, workers in pattern generation have advocated comparing the neural apparatus and control mechanisms of different movements, such as breathing versus locomotion (von Euler, 1981; Feldman and Grillner, 1983) and speech versus more innate automatic movements (Grillner, 1982). Such comparisons enhance interdisciplinary training in motor control; they foster intellectual growth in the respective areas, and they underscore the integrative nature of the segmental motor system.

The third area of research is emphasized in this volume. It addresses efferent aspects of the segmental motor system (particularly motoneurons and motor units), although interneurons and sensory feedback figure in several chapters. The key issues are (1) the phenomenon of orderly motor unit recruitment; (2) the association between firing threshold properties of motoneurons and the anatomical, biochemical, and physiological properties of the muscle fibers innervated; and (3) the relation between firing threshold and the intrinsic biophysical and extrinsic synaptic input properties of the motoneuron.

Experimental possibilities for the study of motor unit recruitment were abruptly augmented shortly after the advent of "action potential" electromyography (Forbes and Thatcher, 1920; see also Adrian, 1925). It then became possible to record the activity of single motor units in both conscious humans (Adrian and Bronk, 1929) and experimental animals (Denny-Brown, 1949). Initially, the human work was fruitful (e.g., Smith, 1934; Lindsley, 1935), and in less than a decade, it was possible for Denny-Brown and Pennybacker 1938)* to seed the field with an observation that has become known as the "phenomenon of orderly recruitment":

> . . . a particular voluntary movement appears to begin always with discharge of the same motor unit. More intense contraction is secured by the addition of more and more units added in a particular sequence. . . . This "recruitment" of motor units into willed contraction is identical with that occurring in certain re-

*Reprinted by permission of The Macmillan Press Ltd.

> flexes. . . . The early motor units in normal gradual voluntary contraction are always in our experience small ones. . . . The larger and more powerful motor units, each controlling many more muscle fibres, enter contraction late. (p. 324)

Over approximately the same span of time, human electromyographic (EMG) studies from several laboratories had brought forth an idea that is currently in vogue. It was reviewed a decade later by Denny-Brown (1949):†

> . . . individual muscles are used in different ways in different movements. . . . the fixity of the first set of units to come into discharge in a willed contraction is related only to that particular contraction. . . . there are separate pools of units first activated in biceps brachii for flexion of the elbow and supination, but that in a combined movement yet a third set is first used. . . . the set of units in the flexor profounds digitorum first to begin discharge in the contraction of grasping is different from those beginning discharge in the same muscle in flexion of the wrist. (p. 120)

Thus, from the outset, unitary EMG studies in conscious humans revealed that while orderly motor unit recruitment was evident in select circumstances, the rules were altered in others. Interestingly, half a century later, this issue remains controversial (Burke, 1981b; Stuart and Enoka, 1983; chapters 1 and 4, this volume), despite advances in EMG technology and instrumentation (Loeb and Gans, 1986), experimental effort in recording from muscles of the conscious human during high-force voluntary contractions (e.g., Gydikov and Kosarov, 1974; DeLuca et al., 1982; Bigland-Ritchie et al., 1983; Enoka et al., 1988), and elucidation of the motor axon firing patterns in freely moving animals (Hoffer et al., 1981).

Although Denny-Brown had great impact on neurophysiology and clinical neurology (Gilliat, 1981), early work on orderly motor unit recruitment languished throughout the 1950s and early 1960s, due possibly to the seductive appeal of the intracellular recording pipette. The reemergence of some of these ideas and their subsequent development have been profoundly influenced by Henneman. In tribute to him, it is fitting to comment on several areas in which his contributions have been seminal. We have done so previously (Stuart and Enoka, 1983; Enoka and Stuart, 1984), but the field is so dynamic that an update is appropriate, especially for this volume.

THE ORDERLY RECRUITMENT OF MOTOR UNITS

Henneman's contribution to current understanding of the orderly recruitment of motor units began over 30 years ago, when he proposed a "size principle" to explain the phenomenon (Henneman, 1957). Although the precise wording of his hypothesis has been modified over the years, it is sufficient to quote the version published two decades after the original presentation (Henneman, 1977):

---

†Reprinted by permission of the American Medical Association.

The amount of excitatory input required to discharge a motorneuron, the energy it transmits as impulses, the number of fibers it supplies, the contractile properties of the motor unit it innervates, its main rate of firing and even its rate of protein synthesis are all closely correlated with its size. This set of experimental facts and interrelations has been called the "size principle." (p. 50)

This hypothesis should not be considered simply as an encapsulation and extension of Denny-Brown's earlier summary views (see also Kruger, 1952), nor is it an extension of preceding work on the concept of tonic and phasic (kinetic) motoneurons as elaborated in the laboratories of Granit (Granit, 1956; et al., 1956, 1957) and Tokizane (Tokizane, 1955; Tokizane and Shimazu, 1964; for review of these earlier ideas on tonic and phasic motor systems, see Burke, 1981b). Rather, the size principle should be viewed as a new beginning. By the late 1960s, Henneman's initial work on motor unit recruitment, the size principle, and allied issues (Henneman, 1980, 1981; Henneman and Mendell, 1981) led to an intense international research effort that gathered momentum throughout the 1970s and 1980s. Indeed, chapters in this volume provide documentation that work in this area will continue at a rapid pace for the foreseeable future. With due recognition of the earlier contributions of others, Henneman deserves major credit for this sudden increase in interest in motor unit recruitment and allied issues.

Descriptions of orderly motor unit recruitment began to appear in college curricula and clinical neuroscience training programs (McComas, 1977) at least a decade earlier than issues related to the interneuronal focus, probably because the size principle hypothesis provided such a straightforward and systems-oriented framework for relating simultaneously occurring advances in neuronal biophysics and muscle biochemistry and physiology. The experimental results also provided a construct for work undertaken on a variety of animal species, including conscious humans, and for the integration of CNS function with the active musculature.

Although orderly motor unit recruitment is prevalent throughout the animal kingdom (Henneman and Mendell, 1981), this commonality has not created the excitement engendered by interphyletic work on pattern generation over a comparable time period (Herman et al., 1976; Grillner, 1981). This discrepancy is probably attributable more to textbook emphases and individual preferences among scientists than to any difference in merit of the two areas of comparative neurophysiology. For the other comparison, work on interactions between the CNS and muscle function is more advanced for size principle issues than for limb biomechanics (Hasan, et al., 1985; Hasan and Stuart, 1988). In retrospect, this inequity need not have occurred, given the remarkable groundwork in biomechanics provided by Marey in the late nineteenth century (Marey, 1874, 1901) and by Bernstein in the 1920s (Bernstein, 1926). Possibly the Sherringtonian influence is evident here (see, e.g., Wetzel and Stuart, 1976, p. 43), together with fashions in interdisciplinary scientific discourse and training (Loeb, 1987). These asides are made simply to emphasize that the comparative and interdisciplinary aspects of orderly motor unit recruitment and the size principle should not go unrecognized in this brief tribute to Henneman.

Orderly Recruitment

With one exception (Henneman et al., 1976), Henneman's experimental work on orderly recruitment has been done on unanesthetized, decerebrate cat preparations. Comparisons were made between the recruitment order of two or more motoneurons, as detected from the firing patterns of either their muscle units (i.e., EMG spike trains) or their ventral root axons (for review, see Henneman, 1979, 1980, 1981; Henneman and Mendell, 1981). Prior to this work, the ventral root axon technique had been popular in studies comparing the thresholds and firing patterns of alpha and gamma motoneurons (e.g., Hunt, 1951, Figs. 1 and 6B). The ventral (and dorsal) root axon approach was pioneered in Kuffler's laboratory (Kuffler and Hunt, 1949, 1952), adapted by Henneman for the study of motor unit recruitment in experimental animals, and recently extended by Zajac and Faden (1985; Chapter 5, this volume), who simultaneously measured the firing thresholds of axon pairs and the mechanical properties of the muscle fibers (units) supplied by the axons.

There are many unresolved questions concerning motor unit recruitment (Stuart and Enoka, 1983; Enoka and Stuart, 1984). In addition to the key issue of its precision, these questions include its presence or absence during strong isometric contractions, shortening and lengthening contractions, and muscle contributions to force in different directions (e.g., abduction versus flexion). Moreover, much must be learned about the modifications of orderly recruitment by descending command signals and sensory feedback. Given these problems, the study of motor unit recruitment must be regarded as still in its infancy. A major limitation has been the technical difficulty of recording from single motor units under other than low-force, isometric conditions. Our limited knowledge, however, is not completely attributable to technical limits; much remains to be done even in studying isometric movements of limited forcefulness. For example, the complicating effects of ongoing (Miles and Turker, 1986) and prior (Dubose et al., 1987) muscle activity, including fatigue (Kossev et al., 1987), are only just beginning to be explored.

Several recent observations on fatiguing muscle in conscious humans have shown an association between the relaxation rate of whole muscle and the rate of motor unit discharge necessary to optimize force output (e.g., Bigland-Ritchie et al., 1983). This finding and some subsequent work led Bigland-Ritchie and colleagues (1986) to hypothesize that "during fatigue, motoneurone firing rates may be regulated by a peripheral reflex originating in response to fatigue-induced changes within the muscle." However, two recent reports on fatigue-induced changes in cat motor unit behavior (Dubose et al., 1987; Stuart et al., 1988) suggest that fatigue-induced changes within the muscle must occur largely in the higher-force (threshold) motor units and that slowing of motoneuron firing rates should not be anticipated during fatiguing low-force contractions. Furthermore, there is recent evidence that the absolute threshold for motor unit discharge during sustained low-force contractions is altered as fatigue sets in, thereby implying that a change in recruitment order must have taken place (Kossev et al., 1987). These recent findings on muscle fatigue are presented here for three reasons

First, the Bigland-Ritchie hypothesis has the simplicity and elegance of Henneman's original 1957 formulation of the size principle. Second, we anticipate that the fatigue hypothesis must coexist with orderly recruitment and the size principle. Finally, many recent developments in the study of motor unit fatigue appear to have been stimulated, at least in part, by Henneman's contributions (Chapter 13, this volume).

Motoneuron Size

The "size" in Henneman's hypothesis refers to the surface area of the soma and dendrites of the motoneuron. Henneman's approach to this measurement of motoneuron size has been indirect and essentially electrophysiological. If recording is limited to a small group of ventral root filaments, the spike amplitude gives a relatively accurate indication of axon diameter, which, in turn, correlates strongly with the conduction velocity along the peripheral axon. Henneman's laboratory has made major technical and analytical contributions to these various measurements (e.g., Clamann et al., 1974a, 1974b; Henneman et al., 1974; Harris and Henneman, 1979; Bawa et al., 1984). Although the strength of the various correlations with cell size is somewhat problematical, there can be little doubt that the formulation and testing of the size principle were the stimulus for much subsequent valuable work combining structural and functional approaches to size principle issues (for a selected review, see Cullheim, 1978; Kernell and Zwaagstra, 1981; Burke et al., 1982; Stuart and Enoka, 1983; Zajac and Faden, 1985).

Progress in this area is epitomized at the segmental level by the recent successful reconstruction of a Renshaw cell and a motoneuron to which it connects, both cells labeled intracellularly with horseradish peroxidase (Fyffe, 1986), and by direct measurements of motor unit force and the surface area of the soma and dendrites of the innervating motoneuron (Burke et al., 1982). However, the stimulus to develop methodologies to measure motoneuron size cannot be attributed exclusively to the emergence of the size principle. For example, there was also the drive to expand Rall's theoretical 1967 report, in which he provided predictions on the association between the profile of a motoneuron's intracellularly recorded excitatory postsynaptic potential (EPSP) and the spatial and temporal properties of the synaptic input producing the response. Such theoretical work has a separate lineage from that of the size principle, but it is remarkable how closely interwined they have become.

MOTONEURON–MUSCLE UNIT INTERRELATIONS

With few exceptions (e.g., Burke et al., 1982; Kernell and Monster, 1982; Zajac and Faden, 1985), motoneuron–muscle unit interrelations have been explored by comparing work on motoneuron discharge properties to work on a wide variety of muscle unit properties (anatomical, biochemcial, physiological, etc.). Based on these relationships, investigators have drawn inferences on the functional significance of the various associations for the graded development of muscle force. (Nerve–muscle trophism is not considered here, although this interplay, too, is closely related to the size principle.)

Henneman's contribution in the area began after his 1957 report on ventral root axon recording with a sequence of studies on the mechanical properties of motor units (Henneman and Olson, 1965; McPhedran et al., 1965; Wuerker et al., 1965; Olson and Swett, 1966, 1971). It had particular significance for two reasons: population analysis was used to make inferences about whole-muscle function, and the foundation was laid for experiments in other laboratories that led eventually to the widespread use of a quadripartite motor unit classification scheme (Chapter 11, this volume).

Population Analysis

Henneman's laboratory was the first to describe the graded development of muscle force in terms of the integrated activity of the muscle unit population and the distinctive features of a pair of synergistic muscles (Henneman and Olson, 1965). This population analysis approach has since been used in several laboratories to perform similar studies (e.g., McDonagh et al., 1980; Sypert and Munson, 1981) on interactions between motor units and muscle receptors (Houk et al., 1971; Binder et al., 1977), as well as theoretical studies on the association between motor unit recruitment and fatigability (Hatze, 1977a, 1977b, 1979; Hatze and Buys, 1977; Adolf et al., 1982; Harrison, 1983; Valentini and Nelson, 1985). Furthermore, the approach has been extended to the field of comparative morphology (Van de Graaff et al., 1977), where the possibilities are ever increasing (e.g., potential extension of Hermanson et al., 1986; Callister et al., 1987).

In another form, population analysis is a feature of Henneman's law of combination, which states that "There is, then, *a basic law of combination* that specifies how the activities of motoneurons are combined" (Henneman, 1979). An intriguing feature of his argument is that for a spinal motor nucleus containing 300 motoneurons, the alternative arrangement in which all possible combinations (N) of active units might occur would result in an N value of 10^{90}, a logistically impossible task for the mammalian CNS (see also Henneman et al., 1974).

Muscle Unit Classification

It is unnecessary to reiterate our previous evaluation of Henneman's contributions to the present use of various muscle unit classification schemes (Stuart and Enoka, 1983; Stuart et al., 1984), particularly since the relative merits of these schemes have been reviewed exhaustively for over two decades (see, in particular, Close, 1972; Burke and Edgerton, 1975; Burke, 1981a). One point, however, is intriguing for this update. In our 1983 report, we cited a personal communication from Henneman expressing his belief that motor unit typing is potentially misleading to the extent that it detracts attention from the possibility that the properties of motor units, particularly biochemical ones, lie along a continuum. While our opinion remains that typing facilitates analysis of the plastic and comparative properties of muscle design and performance (Stuart et al., 1984), we must concede that further work on typing is necessary. Fortunately, three new developments will facilitate the eventual resolution of this issue.

First, it is now possible to make quantitative biochemical measurements on the fibers of a single muscle unit (Chapter 14, this volume). Second, the techniques of molecular biology can now be applied to single motor units in the mature animal (Gauthier et al., 1983) and in developing muscle fibers (Miller and Stockdale, 1987). Finally, quantitative measurements of motoneuron properties are now being subjected to objective statistical procedures, such as cluster and discriminant analysis (e.g., Zengel et al., 1985; Hamm et al., 1988), to refute or verify classification schemes. As this work proceeds, the seminal contributions from Henneman's laboratory will be ever evident.

INTRINSIC PROPERTIES OF MOTONEURONS AND THEIR SYNAPTIC INPUTS

Chapters 2 and 10 of this volume evaluate facets of Burke's (1981) multifactor model of the mechanisms that regulate the firing threshold and recruitment order of a motoneuron. Henneman's contribution to this line of inquiry has largely involved the study of the organization of synaptic input to motoneurons from functionally identifiable afferent input systems. His work has featured the development of the spike-triggered averaging technique and the formulation of an "afferent" and a "branch point failure" hypothesis.

Spike-Triggered Averaging

For unitary analysis of monosynaptic EPSP connections between the spindle Ia afferents and their homonymous motoneurons, Mendell and Henneman introduced the spike-triggered averaging technique in the late 1960s (Mendell and Henneman, 1968, 1971). We reviewed subsequent developments in 1983 (see also Fetz et al., 1979; Kirkwood and Sears, 1980), and many of them appear in this volume (Chapters 16, 17, 18, and 20). Such prominence emphasizes the significance of this technique, as do recent examples of its application to other problems concerning intraspinal circuitry (e.g., Jankowska and Roberts, 1972; Watt et al., 1976; Brink et al., 1981; Hamm et al., 1987). Spike-triggered averaging has been extended to the analysis of other CNS circuits, including eye movement (e.g., Nakao and Sasaki, 1980), vestibular-neck (e.g., Rapoport et al., 1977) and somatosensory systems (e.g., Meyers and Snow, 1986), and the central projections of vagal pulmonary afferents (e.g., Berger and Averill, 1983). There can be little doubt that this powerful method of Mendell and Henneman has furthered the analysis of spinal circuitry and has limitless possibilites for the study of brain circuitry.

Afferent Aspects of the Size Principle

Early on, Henneman addressed afferent aspects of the size principle (Carpenter and Henneman, 1966). This interest finds current expression in studies on the spinal motoneuronal projections of spindle Ia and group II afferents with the argument that "the size of a sensory neuron not only determines the magnitude of the effect its impulses produce, but may also influence the locations where these effects are exerted postsynaptically" (Luscher et al., 1979). Although this hypothesis attracted almost immediate attention in Munson's laboratory (Sypert et al., 1980; Munson et al., 1982; Chapter 16, this volume), it has remained for Henneman and Luscher to undertake most of the subsequent work on their afferent hypothesis (Chapter 18, this volume). This is puzzling because it seems opportune for testing throughout many central systems. For example, the somatosensory system is amenable to this consideration, particularly in view of the dorsal column and horn projections of the same afferent systems studied by Henneman and Luscher, and the possible extension of the hypothesis to accommodate cutaneous (namely, Meyers and Snow, 1986) and joint afferents.

Branch Point Failure

A corollary of the afferent hypothesis is the argument that "the larger a motoneurone is, the more extensive are the terminal arborizations on it" (Luscher et al., 1979). Henneman and colleagues proposed that since axonal branch points are susceptible to blockage both centrally (arguments of Iles, 1976) and peripherally (Krnjevic and Miledi, 1958; Spira et al., 1976; Stalberg and Trontelj, 1979), more conduction failure will occur along the central projections of Ia axons to large than to small motoneurons. Subsequently, they suggestd that tetanizing the Ia afferent pathway to motoneurons induces a reduction in branch point failure that is differentially manifested among the motoneurons in an order proportional to the number of Ia axonal branch points (Luscher et al., 1983a, 1983b). These various arguments engendered an immediate controversy (Hirst et al., 1981; Jack et al., 1981; Lev-Tov et al., 1983) equivalent to that generated by efferent aspects of the size principle in the late 1960s, and this excitement will likely continue. We must admit a personal excitement here, because branch point failure is another point of convergence for work on the size principle and muscle fatigue, both in the CNS and the peripheral neuromuscular system.

One of Henneman's greatest contributions is unfortunately not documentable. For almost 30 years, national and international meetings on the segmental motor system have featured lively discussions on motor unit recruitment and the size principle. Henneman has participated vigorously in this dialogue, and probably all contributors to the present volume, their collaborators, and students have derived inspiration from their scholarly and personal interactions with him.

Acknowledgments

We are indebted to Professor Jay B. Angevine, a long-time colleague, and Dr. Grant A. Robinson, a postdoctoral fellow in our laboratories, for their criticisms of a draft of this chapter.

Professor Angevine was a faculty colleague of Professor Henneman at Harvard Medical School from 1956 to 1967, during which period they helped to design one of the first interdisciplinary medical neuroscience courses and worked closely together in teaching medical students. Work in our own laboratories on the segmental motor system is supported by NIH grants HL 07249 (a Departmental Training Grant), NS 07309 (a University-wide Motor-Control Training Grant), NS 25077 (to D.G.S), and NS 20544 (a Javits Award to D.G.S. and R.M.E.).

REFERENCES

Adolf, A., Nelson, P. P., and Valentini, F. A. (1982). Mathematical model of muscular fatigue. I. Metabolite level changes during exercise of different intensities. *Int. J. Bio- Medical Computing* 13, 311–327.

Adrian, E. D. (1925). Interpretation of the electromyogram. *Lancet* 1, 1230–1233.

Adrian, E. D., and Bronk, D. W. (1929). The discharge of impulses in motor nerve fibres. Part II. The frequency of discharge in reflex and voluntary contractions. *J. Physiol. (Lond.)* 67, 119–151.

Baldissera, F., Hultborn. H., and Illert. M. (1981). Integration in spinal neuronal systems. In *Handbook of Physiology*. Sec. 1. Vol. II, Pt. 1, *The Nervous System: Motor Control* (vol. ed., V. B. Brooks) (eds. J. M. Brookhart and V. B. Mountcastle). American Physiological Society, Bethesda, Md., pp. 509–595.

Bawa, P., Binder, M. D., Ruenzel, P., and Henneman, E. (1984). Recruitment order of motoneurons in stretch reflexes is highly correlated with their axonal conduction velocity. *J. Neurophysiol.* 52, 410–420.

Berger, A. J., and Averill, D. B. (1983). Projection of single pulmonary stretch receptors to solitary tract region. *J. Neurophysiol.* 49, 819–830.

Bernstein, N. A. (1926). *General Biomechanics*. Monograph (in Russian). (Cited in Bernstein, 1967.)

Bernstein, N. A. (1967) *The Co-ordination and Regulation of Movements*. Pergamon Press, Oxford.

Bigland-Ritchie, B. R., Dawson, N. J., Johansson, R. S., and Lippold, O. C. J. (1986). Reflex origin for the slowing of motoneurone firing rates in fatigue of human voluntary contractions. *J. Physiol. (Lond.)* 379, 451–459.

Bigland-Ritchie, B. R., Johansson, R., Lippold, O. C. J., Smith, S., and Woods, J. J. (1983). Changes in motoneurone firing rates during sustained maximal voluntary contractions. *J. Physiol. (Lond.)* 340, 335–346.

Binder, M. D., Kroin, J. S., Moore, G. P., and Stuart, D. G. (1977). The response of Golgi tendon organs to single motor unit contractions. *J. Physiol. (Lond.)* 271, 337–349.

Brink, E., Jankowska, E., McCrea, D., and Skoog, B. (1981). Use of sucrose gap for recording postsynaptic population potentials evoked by single interneurons in the spinal cord. *Brain Res.* 223, 165–169.

Brink, E., Jankowska, E., McCrea, D., and Skoog, B. (1983). Inhibitory interactions between interneurones in reflex pathways from group Ia and group Ib afferents in the cat. *J. Physiol. (Lond.)* 343, 361–373.

Burke, R. E. (1981a). Motor units: Anatomy, physiology and functional organization. In *Handbook of Physiology*. Sec. 1, Vol. II, Pt. 1, *The Nervous System: Motor Control.* (vol. ed., V. B. Brooks) (eds. J. M. Brookhart and V. B. Mountcastle). American Physiological Society, Bethesda, Md., pp. 345–422.

Burke, R. E. (1981b). Motor unit recruitment: What are the critical factors? In *Motor*

Unit Types. Recruitment and Plasticity in Health and Disease (ed. J. E. Desmedt). Karger, Basel, pp. 61–84.

Burke, R. E. (1985). Integration of sensory information and motor commands in the spinal cord. In *Motor Control: From Movement Trajectories to Neural Mechanisms. Short Course Syllabus* (ed. P. S. G. Stein). Society for Neuroscience, Bethesda, Md., pp. 44–66.

Burke, R. E., Dum, R. P., Fleshman, J. W., Glenn, L. L., Lev-Tov, A., O'Donovan, M. J., and Pinter, M. J. (1982). An HRP study of the relation between cell size and motor unit type in cat ankle extensor motoneurons. *J. Comp. Neurol.* 209, 17–28.

Burke, R. E., and Edgerton, V. R. (1975). Motor unit properties and selective involvement in movement. In *Exercise and Sport Sciences Reviews* (eds. J. H. Wilmore and J. F. Keogh). Academic Press, New York, pp. 31–81.

Burke, R. E., and Rudomin, P. (1977). Spinal neurons and synapses. In *Handbook of Physiology. The Nervous System. Cellular Biology of Neurons,* Sec. 1. Vol. I. Pt. 2, Chap. 24 (vol. ed., E. R. Kandel) (eds. J. M. Brookhart and V. B. Mountcastle). American Physiological Society, Besthesda, Md., pp. 877–944.

Callister, R. J., Callister, R., and Peterson, E. H. (1989). Histochemical classification of neck and limb muscle fibers in a turtle, *Pseudemys scripta*: a study using microphotometry and cluster analysis techniques. *J. Morphol.* 199, 269–286.

Carpenter, D. O., and Henneman, E. (1966). A relation between the threshold of stretch receptors in skeletal muscle and the diameter of their axons. *J. Neurophysiol.* 29, 353–368.

Clamann, H. P., Gillies, J. D., and Henneman, E. (1974a). Effects of inhibitory inputs on critical firing level and rank order of motoneurons. *J. Neurophysiol.* 37, 1350–1360.

Clamann, H. P., Gillies, J. D., Skinner, R. D., and Henneman, E. (1974b). Quantitative measures of output of a motoneuron pool during monosynaptic reflexes. *J. Neurophysiol.* 37, 1328–1337.

Close, R. I. (1972). Dynamic properties of mammalian skeletal muscles. *Physiol. Rev.* 52, 129–197.

Creed, R. S., Denny-Brown, D., Eccles, J. C., Liddel, E. G. T., and Sherrington, C. S. (1932). *Reflex Activity of the Spinal Cord.* Oxford University Press, London.

Cullheim, S. (1978). Relations between cell body size, axon diameter and axon conduction velocity of cat sciatic alpha-motoneurons stained with horseradish peroxidase. *Neurosci. Lett.* 8, 17–20.

DeLuca, C. J., LeFever, R. S., McCue, M. P., and Xenakis, A. P. (1982). Behaviour of human motor units in different muscles during linearly varying contractions. *J. Physiol. (Lond.)* 329, 113–128.

Denny-Brown, D. (1929). On the nature of postural reflexes. *Proc. R. Soc. Lond. B* 104, 252–301.

Denny-Brown, D. (1949). Interpretation of the electromyogram. *Arch. Neurol. Psychiatry* 61, 99–128.

Denny-Brown, D., and Pennybacker, J. B. (1938). Fibrillation and fasciculation in voluntary muscle. *Brain* 61, 311–333.

Dubose, L., Schelhorn, T. B., and Clamann, H. P. (1987). Changes in contractile speed of cat motor units during activity. *Muscle Nerve* 10, 744–752.

Enoka, R. M., Robinson, G. A., and Kossev, A. R. (1988). A stable, selective electrode for recording single motor-unit potentials in humans. *Exp. Neurol.* 99, 761–764.

Enoka, R. M., and Stuart, D. G. (1984). Henneman's "size principle": Current issues. *Trends Neurosci.* 7, 266–228.

Feldman, J. L., and Grillner, S. (1983). Control of vertebrate respiration and locomotion: A brief account. *Physiologist* 26, 310–316.

Fetz, E. E., Henneman, E., Mendell, L., Stein, R. B., and Stuart, D. G. (1979). Properties of single cells in vertebrate motor systems revealed by spike-triggered averaging. In *Society for Neuroscience, 8th Annual Meeting.* Summaries of Symposia. (BIS Conferene Report 49). BRI Publications, Los Angeles, pp. 11–23.

Forbes, A., and Thatcher, C. (1920). Amplification of action currents with electron tube in recording with string galvanometer. *Am. J. Physiol.* 52, 409.

Fyffe, R. E. W. (1986). The morphological basis of recurrent inhibition in the spinal cord of the cat. *Soc. Neurosci. Abstr.* 12, 250.

Gauthier, G. F., Burke, R. E., Lowey, S., and Hobbs, A. W. (1983). Myosin isozymes in normal and cross-reinnervated cat skeletal muscle fibers. *J. Cell Biol.* 97, 756–771.

Gilliat, R. W. (1981). Dr. Derek Denny-Brown, OBE, MD, DPHIL, FRCP, 1901–1981. *Can. J. Neurol. Sci.* 8, 271–273.

Granit, R. (1956). Reflex rebound by post-tetanic potentiation. Temporal summation-spasticity. *J. Physiol. (Lond.)* 131, 32–51.

Granit, R. (1966). *Charles Scott Sherrington—An Appraisal.* Nelson, London.

Granit, R., Henatsch, H. D., and Steg, G. (1956). Tonic and phasic ventral horn cells differentiated by post-tetanic potentiation in cat extensors. *Acta Physiol. Scand.* 37, 114–126.

Granit, R., Phillips, C. G., Skoglund, S., and Steg, G. (1957). Differentiation of tonic from phasic alpha ventral horn cells by stretch, pinna and crossed extensor reflexes. *J. Neurophsiol.* 20, 470–481.

Grillner, S. (1981). Control of locomotion in bipeds, tetrapods and fish. In *Handbook of Physiology,* Sec. 1. Vol. II. Pt. 2, *The Nervous System: Motor Control* (vol. ed., V. B. Brooks) (eds. J. M. Brookhardt and V. B. Mountcastle). American Physiological Society, Bethesda, Md., pp. 1179–1236.

Grillner, S. (1982). Possible analogies in the control of innate motor acts and the production of sound in speech. In *Speech Motor Control,* Vol. 36, Wenner-Gren Center International Symposium Series (eds. S. Grillner, B. Lindholm, J. Lubker, and A. Persson), Pergamon Press. Oxford, pp. 217–229.

Grillner, S., Stein, P. S. G., Stuart, D. G., Forssberg, H., and Herman, R. M. L. (eds.) (1987). *Neurobiology of Vertebrate Locomotion,* Vol. 45, Wenner-Gren International Symposium Series. Macmillan, London.

Gydikov, A., and Kosarov, D. (1974). Some features of different motor units in human biceps brachii. *Pflugers Arch.* 347, 75–88.

Hamm, T. M., Nemeth, P. M., Solanki, L., Gordon, D. A., Reinking, R. M., and Stuart, D. G. (1988). Association between biochemical and physiological properties in single motor units. *Muscle Nerve* 11, 245–254.

Hamm, T. M., Sasaki, S.-I., Stuart, D. G., Windhorst, U., and Yuan, C.-S. (1987). Distribution of single-axon recurrent inhibitory post-synaptic potentials in a single spinal motor nucleus in the cat. *J. Physiol. (Lond.)* 388, 653-664.

Harris, D. A., and Henneman, E. (1979). Different species of alpha motoneurons in the same pool: Further evidence from effects of inhibition of their firing rates. *J. Neurophysiol.* 42, 927–935.

Harrison, P. J. (1983). The relationship between the distribution of motor unit mechanical properties and the forces due to recruitment and to rate coding for the generation of muscle force. *Brain Res.* 264, 311–315.

Hasan, Z., Enoka, R. M., and Stuart, D. G. (1985). The interface between biomechanics and neurophysiology in the study of movement: Some recent approaches. In *Exercise and Sport Sciences Reviews.* Vol. 13 (ed. R. L. Terjung). Macmillan, New York, pp. 169–234.

Hasan, Z., and Stuart, D. G. (1988). Animal solutions to problems of movement control: The role of proprioceptors. *Ann. Rev. Neurosci.* 11, 199–223.

Hatze, H. A. (1977a). The relative contribution of motor unit recruitment and rate coding to the production of static isometric muscle force. *Biol. Cybern.* 27, 21–25.

Hatze, H. A. (1977b). A myocybernetic control model of skeletal muscle. *Biol. Cybern.* 25, 103–119.

Hatze, H. A. (1979). A teleological explanation of Weber's law and the motor unit size law. *Bull. Math. Biol.* 41, 407–425.

Hatze, H. A., and Buys, J. D. (1977). Energy-optimal controls in the mammalian neuromuscular system. *Biol. Cybern.* 27, 9–20.

Henneman, E. (1957). Relation between size of neurons and their susceptibility to discharge. *Science* 126, 1345–1346.

Henneman, E. (1977). Functional organization of motoneuron pools: The size principle. *Proc. Int. Union Physiol. Sci.* 12, 50.

Henneman, E. (1979). Functional organization of motoneuron pools: the size principle. In *Integration in the Nervous System* (eds. H. Asanuma and V. J. Wilson). Igaku-Shoin, Tokyo. pp. 13–25.

Henneman, E. (1980). Organization of the motoneuron pool: The size principle. In *Medical Physiology,* 14th ed., Vol. 1 (ed. V. B. Mountcastle). Mosby, St. Louis, pp. 718–741.

Henneman, E. (1981). Recruitment of motoneurons: The size principle. In *Motor Unit Types. Recruitment and Plasticity in Health and Disease*, Vol. 9, *Progress in Clinical Neurophysiology* (ed. J. E. Desmedt). Karger. Basel, pp. 26–60.

Henneman, E., Clamann, H. P., Gillies, J. D., and Skinner, R. D. (1974). Rank order of motoneurons within a pool: Law of combination. *J. Neurophysiol.* 37, 1338–1349.

Hennneman, E., and Mendell, L. M. (1981) Functional organization of motoneuron pool and its inputs. In *Handbook of Physiology.* Sec. 1, Vol. II, Pt. 1, *The Nervous System: Motor Control* (vol. ed., V. B. Brooks) (eds. J. M. Brookhart and V. B. Mountcastle). American Physiological Society, Bethesda, Md., pp. 423–507.

Henneman, E., and Olson, C. B. (1965). Relations between structure and function in the design of skeletal muscles. *J. Neurophysiol.* 28, 581–598.

Henneman, E., Shahani, B. T., and Young, R. R. (1976). Voluntary control of human motor units. In *The Motor System: Neurophysiology and Muscle Mechanisms* (ed. M. Shahani). Elsevier, Amsterdam, pp. 73–78.

Herman, R. H., Grillner, S., Stein, P. S. G., and Stuart, D. G. (1976). *Neural Control of Locomotion.* Plenum, New York.

Hermanson, J. W., Lennard, P. R., and Takamoto, R. L. (1986). Morphology and histochemistry of the ambiens muscle of the red-eared turtle (*Pseudemys scripta*). *J. Morphol.* 187, 39–49.

Hirst, G. D. S., Redman, S. J., and Wong, K. (1981). Post-tetanic potentiation and facilitation of synaptic potentials evoked in cat spinal motoneurones. *J. Physiol. (Lond.)* 321, 97–126.

Hoffer, J. A., O'Donovan, M. J., Pratt, C. J., and Loeb, G. E. (1981). Discharge patterns of hindlimb motoneurons during normal cat locomotion. *Science* 213, 466–468.

Houk, J. C., Singer, J. J., and Henneman, E. (1971). Adequate stimulus for tendon organs with observations on mechanics of ankle joint. *J. Neurophysiol.* 34, 1051–1065.

Hunt, C. C. (1951). The reflex activity of mammalian small-nerve fibers. *J. Physiol. (Lond.)* 115, 456–469.

Iles, J. F. (1976). Central terminations of muscle afferents on motoneurones in the cat spinal cord. *J. Physiol. (Lond.)* 262, 91–117.

Jack, J. J. B., Redman, S. J., and Wong, K. (1981). The components of synaptic potentials evoked in cat spinal motoneurones by impulses in single group Ia afferents. *J. Physiol. (Lond.)* 321, 65–96.

Jankowska, E., and Lundberg, A. (1981). Interneurons in the spinal cord. *Trends Neurosci.* 4, 230–233.

Jankowska, E., Roberts, W. J. (1972). An electrophysiological demonstration of the axonal projections of single spinal interneurons in the cat. *J. Physiol. (Lond.)* 222, 597–622.

Kernell, D., and Monster, A. W. (1982). Motoneurone properties and motor fatigue: An intracellular study of gastrocnemius motoneurones of the cat. *Exp. Brain Res.* 46, 197–204.

Kernell, D., and Zwaagstra, B. (1981). Input conductance, axonal conduction velocity and cell size among hindlimb motoneurones of the cat. *Brain Res.* 204, 311–326.

Kirkwood, P. A., and Sears, T. A. (1980). The measurement of synaptic connections in the mammalian central nervous system by means of spike triggered averaging. In *Progress in Clinical Neurophysiology*, Vol. 8, *Spinal and Supraspinal Mechanisms of Voluntary Motor Control and Locomotion* (ed. J. E. Desmedt). Karger, Basel, pp. 44–71.

Kossev, A. R., Robinson, G. A., and Enoka, R. M. (1987). Fatigue-induced changes in the threshold forces of recruitment and derecruitment for low threshold motor units of first dorsal interosseus. *Soc. Neurosci. Abstr.* 13, 873.

Krnjevic, K., and Miledi, R. (1958). Failure of neuromuscular propagation in rats. *J. Physiol. (Lond.)* 140, 440–461.

Kruger, P. (1952). *Tetanus und Tonus der quergestreiften Skelettmuskeln der Wirbeltiere und des Menschen.* Akademische Verlagsgesellschaft, Leipzig.

Kuffler, S. W., and Hunt, C. C. (1949). Small-nerve fibers in mammalian ventral roots. *Proc. Soc. Exp. Biol., N.Y.* 71, 256–257.

Kuffler, S. W., and Hunt, C. C. (1952). The mammalian small-nerve fibers: A system for efferent nervous regulation of muscle spindle discharge. *Res. Publ. Nerv. Ment. Dis.* 30, 24–47.

Lev-Tov, A., Pinter, M. J., and Burke, R. E. (1983). Posttetanic potentiation of group Ia EPSPs: Possible mechanism for differential distribution among medial gastrocnemius motoneurons. *J. Neurophysiol.* 50, 379–398.

Liddell, E. G. T. (1960). *The Discovery of Reflexes.* Oxford University Press, London.

Lindsley, D. B. (1935). Electrical activity of human motor units during voluntary contraction. *Am. J. Physiol.* 114, 90–99.

Loeb, G. E., (1987). Hard lessons in motor control from the mammalian spinal cord. *Trends Neurosci.* 10, 108–113.

Loeb, G. E., and Gans, C. (1986). *Electromyography for Experimentalists*. University of Chicago Press, Chicago.

Luscher, H. -R., Ruenzel, P., Fetz, E., and Henneman, E. (1979). Postsynaptic population potentials recorded from ventral roots perfused with isotonic sucrose: Connections of group Ia and II spindle afferent fibers with large populations of motoneurons. *J. Neurophysiol.* 42, 1146–1164.

Luscher, H. -R., Ruenzel, P., and Henneman, E. (1979). How the size of motoneurones determines their susceptibility to discharge. *Nature* 282, 859–861.

Marey, E. J. (1874). *Animal Mechanism. A Treatise on Terrestrial and Aerial Locomotion*. Appleton-Century-Crofts, New York.

Marey, E. J. (1901). La locomotion animale. In *Traite de Physiologie Biologique*, Masson, Paris, pp. 227–287.

McComas, A. J. (1977). *Neuromuscular Function and Disorders*. Butterworths, Boston.

McDonagh, J. C., Binder, M. D., Reinking, R. M., and Stuart, D. G. (1980). A commentary on muscle unit properties in cat hindlimb muscles. *J. Morphol.* 166, 217–230.

McPhedran, A. M., Wuerker, R. B., and Henneman, E. (1965). Properties of motor units in a homogeneous red muscle (soleus) of the cat. *J. Neurophysiol.* 28, 71–84.

Mendell, L. M., and Henneman, E. (1968). Terminals of single Ia fibers: Distribution within a pool of 300 homonymous motor neurons. *Science* 160, 96–98.

Mendell, L. M., and Henneman, E. (1971). Terminals of single Ia fibers: Location, density and distribution within a pool of 300 homonymous motoneurons. *J. Neurophysiol.* 34, 171–187.

Meyers, D. E. R., and Snow, P. J. (1986). Distribution of activity in the spinal terminations of single hair follicle afferent fibers to somatotopically identified regions of the cat spinal cord. *J. Neurophysiol.* 56, 1022–1038.

Miles, T. S., and Turker, K. S. (1986). Does reflex inhibition of motor units follow the "size principle"? *Exp. Brain Res.* 62, 443–445.

Miller, J. B., and Stockdale, F. E. (1987). What muscle cells know that nerves don't tell them. *Trends Neurosci.* 10, 325–329.

Munson, J. B., Sypert, G. W., Zengel, J. E., Lofton, S. A., and Fleshman, J. W. (1982). Monosynaptic projections of individual spindle group II afferents to type identified medial gastrocnemius motoneurons in the cat. *J. Neurophysiol.* 48, 1164–1174.

Nakao, S., and Sasaki, S. (1980). Excitatory input from interneurons in the abducens nucleus to medial rectus motoneurons mediating conjugate horizontal nystagmus in the cat. *Exp. Brain Res.* 39, 23–32.

Olson, C. B., and Swett, C. P. (1966). A functional and histochemical characterization of motor units in a heterogeneous muscle (flexor digitorum longus) of the cat. *J. Comp. Neurol.* 128, 475–498.

Olson, C. B., and Swett, C. P. (1971). Effect of prior activity on properties of different types of motor units. *J. Neurophysiol.* 34, 1–16.

Rall, W. (1967). Distinguishing theoretical synaptic potentials computed for different somadendritic distributions of synaptic input, *J. Neurophysiol.* 30, 1138–1168.

Rapoport, S., Susswein, A., Uchino, Y., and Wilson, V. J. (1977). Synaptic actions of individual vestibular neurones on cat neck motoneurones. *J. Physiol. (Lond.)* 272, 367–382.

Smith, O. C. (1934). Action potentials from single motor units in voluntary contraction. *Am. J. Physiol.* 108, 629–638.

Spira, M. E., Yarom, Y., and Parnas, I. (1976). Modulation of spike frequency by regions of special axonal geometry and by synaptic inputs. *J. Neurophysiol.* 39, 882–899.

Stalberg, E., and Trontelj, J. (1979). *Single Fibre Electromyography*. Mirvalle Press, Woking, England.

Stein, P. S. G. (ed.) (1985). *Motor Control: From Movement Trajectories to Neural Mechanisms*. Short Course 2 Syllabus. Society for Neuroscience, Washington, D.C.

Stein, R. B., Pearson, K. G., Smith, R. S., and Redford, J. B. (1973). *Control of Posture and Locomotion*, Vol. 7, *Advances in Behavioral Biology*. Plenum Press, New York.

Stuart, D. G. (1985). Summary and challenges for future work. In *Motor Control: From Movement Trajectories to Neural Mechanisms*. Short Course 2 Syllabus (ed. P. S. G. Stein). Society for Neuroscience, Washington, D.C., pp. 95–105.

Stuart, D. G., Binder, M. D., and Enoka, R. M. (1984). Motor unit organization: Application of the quadripartite classification scheme to human muscles. In *Peripheral Neuropathy* (eds. P. J. Dyck, P. K. Thomas, E. H. Lambert, and R. Bunge). W. B. Saunders, Philadelphia, pp. 1067–1090.

Stuart, D. G., and Enoka, R. M. (1983). Motoneurons, motor units, and the size principle. In *The Clinical Neurosciences*. Sec. 5, *Neurobiology* (sec. ed., W. D. Willis) (ed. R. N. Rosenberg). Churchill Livingstone, New York, pp. 471–517.

Stuart, D. G., Enoka, R. M., and Gordon, D. A. (1988). Implications of cat motor-unit studies for the study of human muscle fatigue. *ENA Abstr.* 11, 148.

Sypert, G. W., Fleshman, J. W., and Munson, J. B. (1980). Comparison of monosynaptic actions of medial gastrocnemius group Ia and group II muscle spindle afferents on triceps surae motoneurons. *J. Neurophysiol.* 44, 726–738.

Sypert, G. W., and Munson, J. B. (1981). Basis of segmental motor control: Motoneuron size or motor unit type? *Neurosurgery* 8, 608–621.

Tokizane, T. (1955). Functional differentiation of human skeletal muscle. (In Japanese.) *Kagaku* 25, 229–233.

Tokizane, T., and Shimazu, H. (1964). *Functional Differentiation of Human Skeletal Muscle*. University of Tokyo Press, Tokyo.

Valentini, F. A., and Nelson, P. P. (1985). Mathematical model of muscular fatigue. II. Changes of metabolites level and of force during exercise in relation to a fatigability parameter. *Int. J. Bio-Medical Computing* 17, 197–213.

Van de Graaff, K. M., Frederick, E. C., Williamson, R. G., and Goslow, G. E. (1977). Motor units and fiber types of primary ankle extensors of the skunk. (*Mephitis mephitis*). *J. Neurophysiol.* 40, 1424–1431.

von Euler, C. (1981). The contribution of sensory inputs to the pattern generation of breathing. *Can. J. Physiol. Pharmacol.* 59, 700–706.

Watt, D. G. D., Stauffer, E. K., Taylor, A., Reinking, R. M., and Stuart, D. G. (1976). Analysis of muscle receptor connections by spike-triggered averaging: 1. Spindle primary and tendon organ afferents. *J. Neurophysiol.* 39, 1375–1392.

Wetzel, M. C., and Stuart, D. G. (1976). Ensemble characteristics of cat locomotion and its neural control. *Prog. Neurobiol.* 7, 1–98.

Wuerker, R. B., McPhedran, A. M., and Henneman, E. (1965). Properties of motor units in a heterogeneous pale muscle (m. gastrocnemius) of the cat. *J. Neurophysiol.* 28, 85–99.

Zajac, F. E., and Faden, J. S. (1985). Relationship among recruitment order, axonal conduction velocity, and muscle-unit properties of type-identified motor units in cat plantaris muscle. *J. Neurophysiol.* 53, 1303–1322.

Zengel, J. E., Reid, S. A., Sypert, G. W., and Munson, J. B. (1985). Membrane electrical properties and predictions of motor-unit type of medial gastrocnemius motoneurons in the cat. *J. Neurophysiol.* 53, 1323–1344.

I

PROPERTIES AND FUNCTIONAL ORGANIZATION OF SEGMENTAL MOTOR SYSTEMS

1

The Functional Organization of Muscles, Motor Units, and Tasks

GERALD E. LOEB

THE PROBLEM OF DEFINITION

The mammalian neuromuscular system is generally considered to be organized in a hierarchical manner. Individual muscle fibers are organized into muscle units, each of which is controlled by a single motoneuron, and the ensemble of motoneurons innervating a single muscle is organized into a contiguous nucleus of cell bodies in the spinal cord or brain stem. The force output of the whole muscle may be controlled by both the number of such motor units recruited from this functional pool and the firing rates of the recruited units. Recruitment is deemed to be orderly if the motor units are always recruited in the same order as muscle output increases and derecruited in the inverse order as output decreases, regardless of the nature of the motor task or the source of the command signal.

As detailed elsewhere in this volume, there are strong empirical and theoretical reasons why the recruitment rank of any motoneuron should be correlated with a large number of parameters describing the histological and electrophysiological characteristics of the motoneuron and the histochemical and mechanical properties of the muscle fibers that it innervates. To what extent these correlations derive from causative and/or functional relationships is the subject of considerable debate under the general rubric of the "size principle" (Henneman et al., 1974). However, this chapter deals exclusively with the question of what definitions and conditions must be satisfied before recruitment can be described as orderly, regardless of the mechanisms or advantages of any such regimentation of recruitment order.

Such definitions assume increasing importance as neurophysiologists seek to interpret experimental data on the recruitment of motor units in different muscles and during various tasks. For example, chronic recordings from motor axons projecting to the sartorious muscle in the cat hindlimb suggest that there are three different recruitment groups (Hoffer et al., 1987), even though all of the motoneurons originate in a single, contiguous motor nucleus in the spinal cord (Pratt et al., 1984). These functional subdivisions appear to be related to two separate aspects of the work of the muscle. The sartorius has a distributed insertion; the most anterior part acts to extend the knee, whereas the more medial regions act neutrally or in flexion at the knee (all parts have a similar flexion action at the hip). Motor units composing the medial part form one recruitment group, whereas the mechanically and anatomically homogeneous anterior part contains two other recruitment groups. These latter groups of motor units appear to be related to the two kinematic patterns of work of this part of the muscle during walking: a period of active shortening (concentric work) during the swing phase and a period of active lengthening (eccentric work) during the stance phase. All three groups appear to be recruited together during flexion reflexes elicited by cutaneous nerve stimulation (Loeb et al., 1987a). Recruitment within each group seems to be orderly, but the use of functional as well as purely anatomical criteria to identify these groups may beggar the principle through circular logic.

What, then, is the proper relationship between the functional entity, i.e., the recruitment pool, and the supposedly anatomical entity, i.e., the muscle? We usually presume that an anatomical entity is readily identified by independent criteria, so that it can provide a useful frame of reference for testing hypothesis regarding functional organization. However, the criteria used by anatomists to give a unique name to any particular muscular structure are, in fact, quite subjective and likely to be colored by a knowledge of musculoskeletal function as well as structure.

The cat hindlimb has served as a model system for much research on neuromuscular control. A comparison of various standard anatomical atlases and the terms used in the primary literature suggest that the usage of the word "muscle" is sufficiently consistent so as to be useful, yet sufficiently vague so as to cause substantial confusion. In addition to the previously described complexities in sartorius, consider the following:

The name "biceps femoris" describes a division into two separate heads, anterior and posterior, whereas the insertion actually forms a continuum across the proximal two-thirds of the tibia. The nerve usually has three primary branches (English and Weeks, 1987), and both the anterior and posterior parts of the muscle have intermediate zones with muscle fiber architectures that are similar to each other but distinctly different from those of the remainder of the muscle (Chanaud et al., In press a).

The vastus group of anterior thigh muscles is frequently divided into three muscles (medialis, lateralis, and intermedius). However, the fascial plane between the deep, red intermedius and the two overlying muscles is often incomplete and, in some animals, suggests either that the intermedius is simply a slow compartment of the whole vastus complex or that the two more readily separated superficial muscles, medialis and lateralis, each have a separate deep companion (a fourth name, "vastocrurus," is sometimes used).

The tensor fascia latae is usually treated as one muscle, and appears grossly to be bipinnate, but the two wings have very different muscle fiber architectures and appear to be recruited separately during certain motor behaviors (Pare et al., 1981; Chanaud et al., 1986).

The two heads of the semitendinosus muscle, which are anatomically separate from each other at the levels of the muscle and the muscle-nerves, have abrupt histochemical boundaries dividing each into a predominantly oxidative, deep region and a glycolytic, superficial region with virtually no oxidative fibers (Bodine et al., 1982). Electromyographic (EMG) records from the deep and superficial fascial surfaces of each head during various activities tend to be very different, whereas such records from the corresponding faces of the two heads are modulated almost identically (Chanaud et al., 1986, In press b).

CONSIDERATIONS IN IDENTIFYING MUSCLES

The absence of a formal definition of muscle was acceptable only as long as neurophysiologists confined their attention to muscles like the soleus, which has homogeneous histochemistry, unipinnate fiber architecture, singular origin and insertion, and no distinct nerve branches or internal fascial planes. However, when testing general principles such as orderly recruitment, the ambiguities previously discussed lead to substantial problems. Rather than attempting any formal definition at this time, it seems more useful to describe those factors that must be considered.

Musculoskeletal Architecture (Fig. 1–1)

The arrangement of muscle units and their substituent fibers in any particular muscle is the result of a complex compromise among such diverse factors as the availability of insertion points and their lever arms on the skeleton, the length to be spanned from origin to insertion, the limited range of sarcomere lengths and velocities over which work is efficiently produced, the avoidance of mechanical instabilities, and phylogenetic constraints. Figure 1–1 shows two common architectural patterns that represent effective combinations of these factors, but the factors should be viewed as potentially independent, since many other combinations are known to occur.

By definition, pinnate muscles have their muscle fibers oriented at an angle to the line of the pull of the whole muscle. Although their contractile action is usually described as a parallelogram, the mechanics are actually a complex result of internal hydrostatic pressure and curved fiber paths (Otten, 1988). Their most important mechanical feature is that the fascicles are shorter than the overall muscle path length (origin to insertion), with aponeurotic sheets used to provide attachment points for large numbers of parallel fascicles. This

Musculoskeletal Architecture

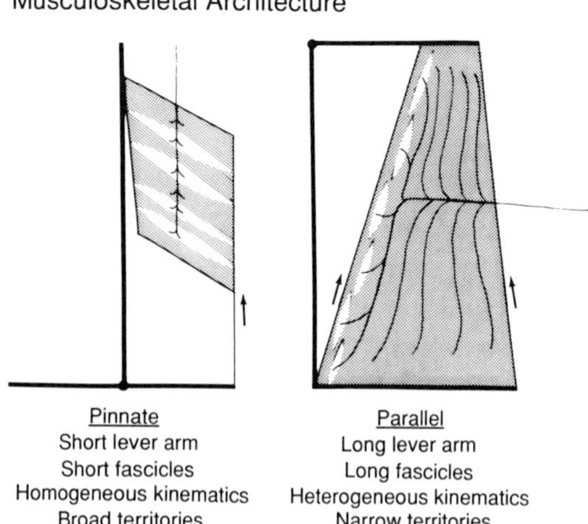

FIG. 1–1.   Two commonly occurring patterns of muscle architecture.

results in a mechanical advantage in the muscle (larger relative motion at the fascicles producing a larger force at the tendon), which is often compensated for by a reverse advantage on the skeleton (short lever arms of attachment magnify small muscle length changes into large limb position changes). The arrangement may be complicated by gradients of fascicle length and orientation, which may be related to differential recruitment, as noted in masseter muscle (Herring et al., 1979).

Parallel-fiber muscles are often more complicated than they first appear. The absence of a mechanical advantage works in their favor when attached to the skeleton with long lever arms or when spanning two or more joints whose motions may sum to produce long muscle length excursions. However, the individual muscle fibers are constrained in their spans by two independent factors, either of which appears to be sufficient to give rise to a series arrangement (Adrian, 1925), as shown in Figure 1–1. The first is a trade-off between the relatively slow conduction velocity of action potentials along muscle fibers and the relatively fast rise time of the mechanical twitch. In the cat, for example, muscle fiber lengths longer than 3–4 cm would not be mechanically stable and appear not to occur, even in muscles with 12-cm fascicle lengths (Loeb et al., 1987b). The second factor is the limited range of sarcomere lengths for which the overlap of actin and myosin filaments permits reasonable tension output. In muscles with very long lever arms, the interdigitated muscle fibers may be able to slide with respect to each other, allowing them to rearrange themselves in order to conserve sarcomere length at different limb positions (Rindos et al., 1984).

Because of their usually broad insertion zones, parallel-fiber muscles may have a substantial gradient of mechanical action from one set of fascicles to another. If muscles cross two or more joints, the relative motions at these joints may cause the net motion in the fascicles during a motor task to change from lengthening to shortening across the width of the muscle. (Consider the parallel muscle in Figure 1–1, where a stretching motion at the upper joint could be turned into a net shortening at the right edge of the muscle by upward rotation of the lower skeletal segment but would remain a net stretch at the left edge of the muscle, where the lower joint has little or no lever arm.) Because muscle fibers and proprioceptors have strongly nonlinear velocity dependencies, the motor control of these regions will pose quite different problems. Regionalized feedback of spindle activity has been reported in such muscles (Botterman et al., 1983; Hamm et al., 1985; see "Intramuscular Compartments" later in this chapter). This, plus the need to synchronize the contraction over the length of a fascicle, may underlie the tendency of units in these muscles to occupy unusually long, narrow territories (Loeb et al., 1987b).

Axial muscles (particularly neck and abdominal) are often divided into a series of compartments that are separated by tendinous inscriptions. These compartments are usually innervated by separate spinal segments as if they were individual muscles (Richmond et al., 1978). This compartmentalized structure may pose substantial coordination problems (Richmond et al., 1985), particularly if the compartments are differentially recruited (Ezure et al., 1983).

Motor Innervation (Fig. 1–2)

The cell bodies of the set of motoneurons innervating a muscle are usually clustered into a single contiguous nucleus. In the spinal cord, the territory occupied by such a nucleus may be very long (up to two segments) and narrow (only one cell wide), with immediately adjacent motoneurons innervating different, even distant, muscles. Among closely related muscles such as the triceps surae, there may be some intermingling of cell bodies (Burke et al., 1977). The position of the cell body along the rostral-caudal axis of the nucleus may be correlated with the location of its muscle unit along the anterior-posterior or medial-lateral axis of the muscle, (see Chapter 2, this volume). This occurs both in muscles with significant mechanical heterogeneity along these axes (e.g., sartorius; Pratt et al., 1984) and in muscles that are more homogeneous (e.g., compartments of the lateral gastrocnemius; reviewed by Kernell, 1986). Thus it is unclear to what extent the highly specific organization of motor nuclei reflects functional as opposed to embryological factors. Compartmentalization of proprioceptive feedback based on physical proximity between the dorsal rootlet entry point of the afferents and the ventral rootlet egress of the motoneurons has been called "location specificity" by Scott and Mendell (1976).

The organization of certain cranial muscles further muddies the issue. The stapedius muscle of the middle ear has a simple bipinnate architecture without anatomical compartmentalization, but its motoneurons are scattered among three subnuclei in the brain stem, each of which is driven by different auditory inputs (Kobler et al., 1987; McCue and Guinan, 1988). The extraocular muscles appear to be supplied by well-defined, coherent motor nuclei, yet each muscle is highly heterogeneous in its muscle fiber architecture (Chiarindini and Davidowitz, 1981). Furthermore, at least some motoneurons apparently branch to

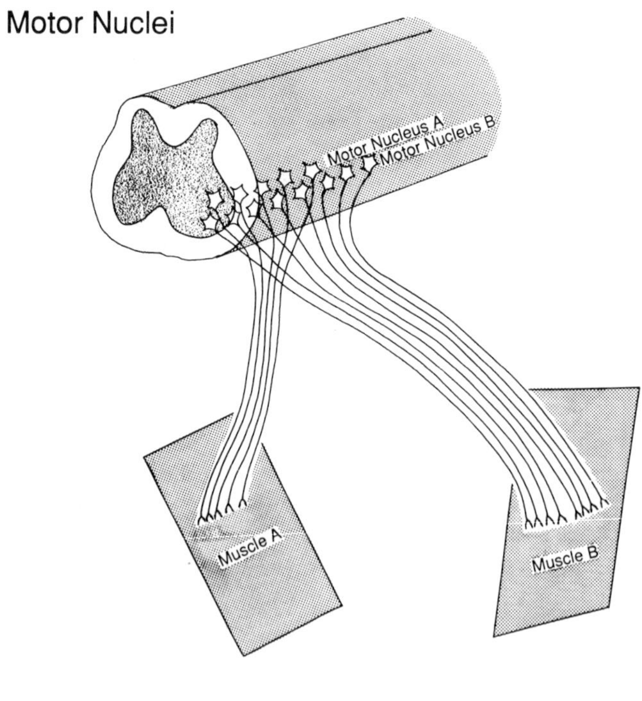

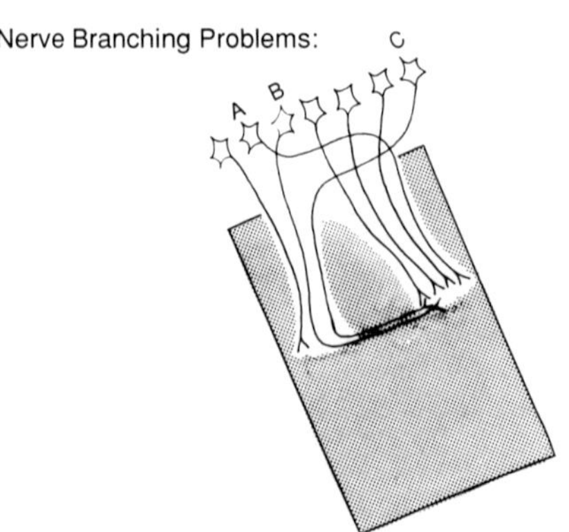

FIG. 1–2. Commonly occurring arrangement of spinal motor nuclei in which long, narrow columns of motoneurons selectively innervate individual muscles. Identification of gradients of innervation related to the rostrocaudal position of individual motoneurons is complicated by peripheral nerve branching patterns, which may be capricious (see text for details).

supply more than one muscle and perhaps even different muscle fiber types (Crandall et al., 1981; Gurahian and Goldberg, 1987).

Finally, it must be noted that the methods for identifying motor nuclei and regionalization of their muscle territories all rely on branching patterns of the peripheral nerves, which may be inconsistent among specimens from the same species (e.g. Loeb et al., 1987b). As shown at the bottom of Figure 1–2, potential problems include "errors" in routing of motor axons before they enter the peripheral nerve (cell A), "errors" in the course of terminal axons within the muscle (cell B), and compensatory "errors" in which a motoneuron in one part of the motor nucleus finds the "correct" region of termination in the muscle but does so via a circuitous route (cell C). Each of these patterns would have a different effect on studies of the structure of motor nuclei and muscle territories that used methods such as electrical stimulation or tracer injection of these nerve branches.

Intramuscular Compartments (Fig. 1–3)

One of the more intensively explored hypotheses regarding segmental motor control concerns the partitioning of homonymous proprioceptive feedback on the basis of intramuscular mechanical compartments (Binder and Stuart, 1980). Scott and Mendell (1976) pointed out that this so-called species specificity must be distinguished from the previously noted location specificity based on correlations between the anatomical gradients along motor nuclei and across muscles. As described earlier under "Musculoskeletal Architecture," gradients of mechanical action or localization of muscle unit territories across the width of muscles may cause regional differences in proprioceptor activity. Servocontrol generally operates best with tight linkages between sensors and actuators, so it is reasonable to expect at least some weighting of the strength of sensory feedback in favor of the closer mechanical linkages, even if the anatomical projections to and from the spinal cord are scrambled in the periphery (Windhorst, 1979).

In principle, the partitioning hypothesis should apply both to muscles with grossly heterogeneous compartments (Fig. 1–3 A, Macro) and to more homogeneous muscles where individual muscle units are known to exert locally powerful effects on mechanically linked spindle and Golgi tendon organs (Fig. 1–3 A, Micro; Cameron et al., 1981). Both should be distinguished from partitioning based on heterogeneous skeletal action (see Fig. 1–3 A, Hetero, and "Musculoskeletal Architecture" earlier in this chapter). In practice, testing has been limited to the macro-partitioning relationships defined by gross nerve branches, and even there, the effects seen are small for spindle feedback (Lucas and Binder, 1984; Lucas et al., 1984; Vanden Noven et al., 1986) and nonexistent for Golgi tendon organs (McCrea, 1986). This form of compartmentalization would seem to be, at most, a minor refinement of the otherwise orderly recruitment of most motor pools as a whole (see also McKeon et al., 1984).

An entirely different form of compartmentalization arises in many muscles that have a nonuniform distribution of muscle fiber types. The deeper regions of these muscles have a disproportionately high percentage of slow-twitch, oxidative muscle fibers (Galvas and Gonyea, 1980; Bodine et al., 1982). In at least some cases, proprioceptors appear to be concentrated in these regions (Richmond and Stuart, 1985). In such muscles, it may be difficult to separate regionalization of motor control based on muscle fiber type, partitioning of sensory feedback, heterogeneity of mechanical action, and gradients along motor nuclei. EMG records purporting to show specialized functions for different

Muscle Compartments

A. Partitioning of Proprioceptive Feedback

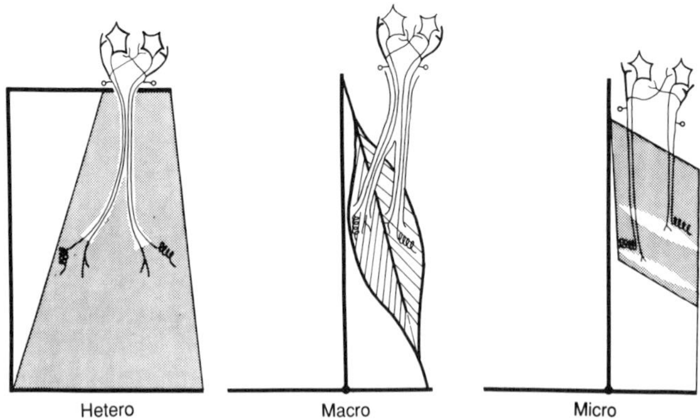

B. Segregation of Muscle Fiber-Types

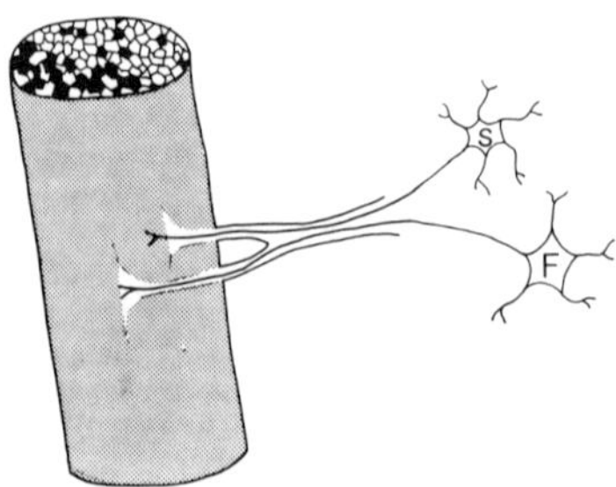

FIG. 1–3. (A) Intramuscular compartments may be based on localized mechanical effects on proprioceptors arising from distributed skeletal action (Hetero), fascial divisions of the muscle mass and nerve branches into gross compartments (Macro), and micromechanical coupling to individual muscle units (Micro). (B) Intramuscular compartments may reflect heterogeneous distributions of motor unit types.

regions of the muscle may actually result from sampling muscle units that are concentrated at a particular recruitment rank in a muscle that, overall, has an orderly and complete pool of recruitable motor units (see Fig. 5.2 in Loeb and Gans, 1986).

Task Groups (Fig. 1–4)

Of all the considerations in defining muscles and motoneuron pools of recruitment, the notion of task groups (Loeb, 1985) is the most problematic. By definition, a task group has no necessary correlate in the anatomy of individual muscles, nerves, or nuclei. A task group is an ensemble of elements (including extra- and intrafusal motoneurons, muscle fibers, and associated proprioceptive afferents) that work together in an orderly manner during the performance of certain kinematic tasks. By virtue of the gross musculoskeletal anatomy of a limb, certain frequently needed trajectories of motion require particular syner-

Task Groups

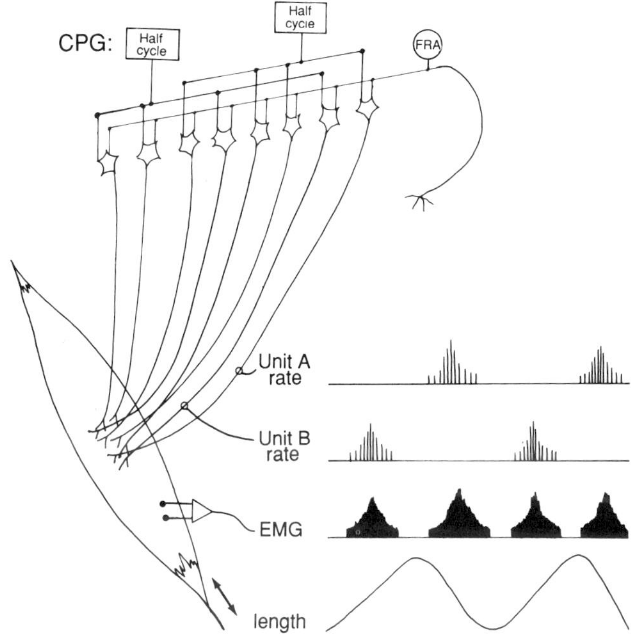

FIG. 1–4. A schematic of the recruitment patterns for motoneurons in the cat anterior sartorius during walking, in which the muscle is recruited twice during each step cycle. One task group of motor units is recruited only during the stance phase, when the muscle is actively lengthening; another task group is recruited only during the swing phase, when the muscle is actively shortening. Stimulation of flexor reflex afferents (FRA) appears to recruit all motor units indiscriminately.

gies of muscular action and result in particular kinematic patterns reflected back to the muscles. Under such circumstances, the required degree of cooperativity argues against strong local servocontrol of individual muscles and in favor of strong, task-specific feedback among the ensemble. However, in some muscles, these same control circuits may be inappropriate for different kinematic tasks. For tasks that occur frequently enough and for which performance must be highly optimized (e.g., locomotion), subsets of these motor elements may be selectively recruited for only those tasks for which their control circuitry (and possibly unit mechanical properties) are appropriate. There also may be tasks that, because of the "uncontrolled" output (e.g., ballistic escape maneuvers), are performed by ensembles of motor units that need not be recruited in their usual order (Kanda et al., 1977; Loeb et al., 1987a).

The task group hypothesis has been applied to the differential recruitment of anterior sartorius motoneurons during the stance and swing phases of walking (described at the beginning of this chapter). It may also be related to changes in recruitment order in human motor units noted during tasks requiring different muscle synergies (first dorsal interosseus muscle during extension versus abduction [Desmedt and Godaux, 1981]; biceps brachii during flexion vs. pronation [Ter Haar Romeny et al., 1984]; Chapter 4, this volume). In the extreme, a proliferation of task groups would be wasteful of muscle mass, redundant in control circuitry, and an impossible impediment in formulating testable hypotheses about neural control. However, if they occur as a coarse-grained strategy of dividing certain motor coordination problems into specialized entities, they offer an attractive escape from the unwieldy problems of developing universal controllers that would need to operate over broad kinematic ranges of highly nonlinear sensor and actuator performance (Loeb, 1985).

A GENERAL APPROACH TO THE MUSCULOSKELETAL APPARATUS

Each of the various factors presented earlier is potentially an independent property of any muscle. As noted under "Musculoskeletal Architecture" (Fig. 1–1), there may be strong associations among particular factors such that certain combinations are seen rarely, if ever. However, it is unwise to assume that any particular muscle is organized similarly to any other muscle on the basis of homologies or other indirect criteria. Muscles that are heterogeneous for any of these factors may be candidates for reclassification into two or more separately controlled entities.

This complexity would seem to place an unduly large experimental burden on the canonical tasks of taxonomy. Interestingly, a similar dilemma has arisen recently in phylogenetic taxonomy, where newly developed assays such as those for DNA homologies are forcing the reclassification of species and genera that had been defined and named on the basis of gross anatomical traits (Lewin, 1987a, 1987b). If the old taxonomy were taken as immutable, the new data would constitute a refutation of the principle of orderly evolution of species. However, that principle is so compelling that it appears better to revise the definition of the items to which the principle applies.

The principle of orderly recruitment is, of course, neither so firmly based nor so widely accepted as that of evolution. However, it does have certain compelling features, including a substantial body of data for which no exceptions are in need of explanation and teleological arguments regarding the optimization of speed and accuracy in motor control and learning. I suggest that the traditional taxonomical tool of the gross anatomist—blunt dissection—is likely to be as subjective and capricious in naming muscles as in naming species. The question of whether to modify our principles or our definitions must be answered by consensus rather than by data alone, but that consensus will need to be informed by many more kinds of data on many more musculoskeletal systems than are now available.

Acknowledgment

The author is grateful to Drs. R. E. Burke and F. J. R. Richmond for critical comments on the manuscript and to Ms. Michele Manley for preparation of the figures.

REFERENCES

Adrian, E. D. (1925). The spread of activity in the tenuissimus muscle of the cat and in other complex muscles. *J. Physiol. (Lond.)* 60, 301–315.

Binder, M. D., and Stuart, D. G. (1980). Motor unit–muscle receptor interactions: Design features of the neuromuscular control system. In *Progress in Clinical Neurophysiology*, Vol. 8., *Spinal and Supraspinal Mechanisms of Voluntary Motor Control and Locomotion* (ed. J. Desmedt). Karger, Basel, pp. 72–98.

Bodine, S. C., Roy, R. R., Meadows, D. A., Zernicke, R. F., Sacks, R. D., Fournier, M., and Edgerton, V. R. (1982). Architectural, histochemical and contractile characteristics of a unique biarticular muscle: The cat semitendinosus. *J. Neurophysiol.* 48, 192–201.

Botterman, B. R., Hamm, T. M., Reinking, R. M., and Stuart, D. G. (1983). Localization of monosynaptic Ia excitatory post-synaptic potentials in the motor nucleus of the cat biceps femoris muscle. *J. Physiol. (Lond.)* 338, 355–377.

Burke, R. E., Strick, P. L., Kanda, K., Kim, C. C., and Walmsley, B. (1977). Anatomy of medial gastrocnemius and soleus motor nuclei in cat spinal cord. *J. Neurophysiol.* 40, 667–680.

Cameron, W., Binder, M., Botterman, B., Reinking, R., and Stuart, D. (1981). "Sensory partitioning" of cat medial gastrocnemius muscle by its muscle spindles and tendon organs. *J. Neurophysiol.* 46, 32–47.

Chanaud, C. M., Pratt, C. A., and Loeb, G. E. (1986). Differential activation within selected cat hindlimb muscles during normal movement. *Neurosci. Abst.* 12, 686.

Chanaud, C. M., Pratt, C. A., and Loeb, G. E. (1986). Differential activation within selected cat hindlimb muscles during normal movement. *Neurosci. Abst.* 12, 686.

Chanaud, C. M., Pratt, C. A., and Loeb, G. E. (In press a). Compartmentalized muscles of the cat hindlimb. III. Heterogeneous architecture of biceps femoris. *Exp. Brain Res.*

Chanaud, C. M., Pratt, C. A., and Loeb, G. E. (In press b). Compartmentalized muscles of the cat hindlimb. VI. The roles of histochemical and mechanical heterogeneity in differential recruitment. *Exp. Brain Res.*

Crandall, W. F., Goldberg, S. J., Wilson, J. S., and McClung, J. R. (1981). Muscle units divided among retractor bulbi muscle slips and between the lateral rectus and retractor bulbi muscles in cat. *Exp. Neurol.* 71, 251–260.

Desmedt, J. E., and Godaux, E. (1981). Spinal motoneuron recruitment in man: Rank deordering with direction but not with speed of voluntary movement. *Science* 214, 933–936.

English, A. W., and Weeks, O. I. (1987). An anatomical and functional analysis of cat biceps femoris and semitendinosus muscles. *J. Morphol.* 191, 161–175.

Ezure, K., Fukushima, K., Schor, R. H., and Wilson, V. J. (1983). Compartmentalization of the cervicocollic reflex in cat splenius muscle. *Exp. Brain Res.* 51, 397–404.

Galvas, P. E., and Gonyea, W. (1980). Motor end plate and nerve distribution of a histochemically compartmentalized pennate muscle in the cat. *Am. J. Anat.* 159, 147–156.

Gurahian, S. M., and Goldberg, S. J. (1987). Fatigue of lateral rectus and retractor bulbi motor units in cat. *Brain Res.* 415, 281–292.

Hamm, T. M., Koehler, W., Stuart, S. G., and Vanden Noven, S. (1985). Partitioning of monosynaptic Ia excitatory postsynaptic potentials in the motor nucleus of the cat semimembranosus muscle. *J. Physiol.* (Lond.) 369, 379–398.

Henneman, E., Clamann, H. P., Gillies, J. D., and Skinner, R. D. (1974). Rank order of motoneurons within a pool: Law of combination. *J. Neurophysiol.* 37, 1338–1349.

Herring, S. W., Grimm, A. F., and Brimm, B. R. (1979). Functional heterogeneity in a multipinnate muscle. *Am. J. Anat.* 154, 563–576.

Hoffer, J. A., Loeb, G. E., Sugano, N., Marks, W. B., O'Donovan, M. J., and Pratt, C. A. (1987). Cat hindlimb motoneurons during locomotion. III. Functional segregation in sartorius. *J. Neurophysiol.* 57, 554–562.

Kanda, K., Burke, R. E., and Walmsley, B. (1977). Differential control of fast and slow twitch motor units in the decerebrate cat. *Exp. Brain Res.* 29, 57–74.

Kernell, D. (1986). Organization and properties of spinal motoneurons and motor units. *Prog. Brain Res.* 64, 21–30.

Kobler, J. B., Vacher, S. R., and Guinan, J. J., Jr. (1987). The recruitment order of stapedius motoneurons in the acoustic reflex varies with sound laterality. *Brain Res.* 425, 372–375.

Lewin, R. (1987a). Africa: Cradle of modern humans. *Science* 237, 1292–1295.

Lewin, R. (1987b). When does homology mean something else? *Science* 237, 1570.

Loeb, G. E. (1985). Motoneuron task groups—coping with kinematic heterogeneity. *J. Exp. Biol.* 115, 137–146.

Loeb, G. E., and Gans. C. (1986). *Electromyography for Experimentalists*. University of Chicago Press, Chicago.

Loeb, G. E., Marks, W. B., and Hoffer, J. A. (1987a). Cat hindlimb motoneurons during locomotion. IV. Participation in cutaneous reflexes. *J. Neurophysiol.* 57, 563–573.

Loeb, G. E., Pratt, C. A., Chanaud, C. M., and Richmond, F. J. R. (1987b). Distribution and innervation of short, interdigitated muscle fibers in parallel-fibered muscles of the cat hindlimb. *J. Morphol.* 191, 1–15.

Lucas, S. M., and Binder, M. D. (1984). Topographic factors in distribution of homonymous group Ia afferent input to cat medial gastrocnemius motoneurons. *J. Neurophysiol.* 51, 50–63.

Lucas, S. M., Cope, T. C., and Binder, M. D. (1984). Analysis of individual Ia-afferent EPSPs in a homonymous motoneuron pool with respect to muscle topography. *J. Neurophysiol.* 51, 64–74.

McCrea, D. A. (1986). Spinal cord circuitry and motor reflexes. *Exerc. Sport Sci. Rev.* 14, 105–142.

McCue, M. P., and Guinan, J. J. Jr. (1988). Anatomical and functional segregation in the stapedius motoneuron pool of the cat. *J. Neurophysiol.* 60, 1160–1180.

McKeon, B., Gandevia, S., and Burke, D. (1984). Absence of somatotopic projection of muscle afferents onto motoneurons of same muscle. *J. Neurophysiol.* 51(2), 185–194.

Otten, B. (1988). Concepts and models of functional architecture in skeletal muscle. *Exerc. Sport Sci. Rev.* 16, 89–138.

Pare, E. B., Stern, J. T., and Schwartz, J. M. (1981). Functional differentation within the tensor fasciae latae. *J. Bone Joint Surg.* 63, 1457–1471.

Pratt, C. A., Yee, W. J., Chanaud, C. M., and Loeb, G. E. (1984). Organization of the cat sartorius motoneuron pool. *Neurosci. Abst.* 10, 629.

Richmond, F. J. R., MacGillis, D. D. R., and Scott, D. A. (1985). Muscle-fiber compartmentalization in cat splenius muscles. *J. Neurophysiol.* 53, 868–885.

Richmond, F. J. R., Scott, D. A., and Abrahams, V. C. (1978). Distribution of motoneurons to the neck muscles, biventer cervicis, splenius and complexus in the cat. *J. Comp. Neurol.* 181, 451–463.

Richmond, F. J. R., and Stuart, D. G. (1985). Distribution of sensory receptors in the flexor carpi radialis muscle of the cat. *J. Morphol.* 183, 1–13.

Rindos, A. J., Loeb, G. E., Richmond, F. J., and Morris, O. (1984). Architectural features of short, series muscle fibers in cat sartorius and tenuissimus muscles. *Neurosci. Abst.* 10, 629.

Scott, J. G., and Mendell, L. M. (1976). Individual EPSPs produced by single triceps surae Ia afferent fibers in homonymous and heteronymous motoneurons. *J. Neurophysiol.* 39, 679–692.

Ter Haar Romeny, B. M., Denier, J. J., Van der Gon, C. C., and Gielen, A. M. (1984). Relation between location of a motor unit in the human biceps brachii and its critical firing levels for different tasks. *Exp. Neurol.* 85, 631–650.

Vanden Noven, S., Hamm, T. M., and Stuart, D. G. (1986). Partitioning of mono-synaptic Ia excitatory postsynaptic potentials in the motor nucleus of the cat lateral gastrocnemius muscle. *J. Neurophysiol.* 55, 569–586.

Windhorst, U. (1979). A possible partitioning of segmental muscle stretch reflex into incompletely de-coupled parallel loops. *Biol. Cybern.* 34, 205–213.

2

Spinal Motoneurons and Their Muscle Fibers: Mechanisms and Long-Term Consequences of Common Activation Patterns

DANIEL KERNELL

This chapter provides a brief but fairly general survey of a number of findings from our own present and (if still relevant) past experimental work on motoneurons and motor units of the cat's hindlimb. It then gives special attention to the way in which the known usage of motoneurons and motoneuron pools is promoted by their physiological properties and anatomical organization. Questions about the following topics will be the main concern:

1. Recruitment gradation.
2. Rate gradation.
3. The combination of recruitment and rate modulation.
4. Long-term consequences of motoneuronal activity patterns.

RECRUITMENT GRADATION

Recruitment Strategies

In the majority of voluntary or reflex contractions that have been studied, the most easily activated alpha motoneurons tend to be those with the thinnest axons. In accordance with the "size principle" of Henneman (Henneman et al.,

1965; Henneman, 1980; Henneman and Mendell, 1981; Bawa et al., 1984), a progressive increase in force is, statistically speaking, commonly produced by the activation of progressively more thickly axoned cells (see Chapter 5, this volume). One of the reasons for the functional importance of this ascending size order of recruitment lies in the fact that axonal size commonly correlates with essential contractile properties of the motor units (Burke, 1981; Henneman and Mendell, 1981): The thinnest axons tend to innervate units that are relatively slow, weak, and fatigue resistant. Conversely, the thickest motor axons, which are more difficult to recruit, tend to have units that are fast and strong. Thus, the ascending size order of recruitment represents a case of what one might also more generally term a "property-related recruitment strategy." Even though some properties of motoneurons and muscle units vary independently of axonal conduction velocity (e.g., differences between fast-twitch units with regard to their fatigue resistance, motoneuronal input resistance, and motoneuronal excitability: Burke et al., 1973; Dum and Kennedy, 1980; Fleshman et al., 1981; Kernell and Monster, 1981), axonal and other aspects of neuronal size are, without doubt, essential factors in the quantitative and statistical analysis of the organization and behavior of motoneuron-muscle unit populations (see Chapters 9 and 10, this volume). The size principle may be seen as a valuable summarizing concept (a "conceptual tool"), pointing to the important fact that so many of the properties of motoneurons and muscle units are mutually interrelated and covarying with aspects of neuronal size (see Henneman, 1980; Henneman and Mendell, 1981). There remain, however, many intriguing questions (Enoka and Stuart, 1984), including the problem of what the possible *causal* links are between motoneuronal size and the various functional properties implicated in the size principle (see Lüscher et al., 1979).

There is much evidence indicating that, besides the property-related recruitment order, there is also a "task-related recruitment strategy" (Loeb, 1984; Chapter 1, this volume). Thus, even among units that exert their force in the same direction, different motor tasks often seem to show a preference for different individual units within the same muscle (Desmedt and Godeaux, 1981; Ter Haar Romeny et al., 1984; Hoffer et al., 1987; Chapter 4, this volume). The two main types of recruitment strategy that I have mentioned should *not* be seen as mutually exclusive alternatives; they are probably both active in parallel (Loeb, 1984). According to the property-related strategy, the small-axoned, slow units are most easily mobilized in the majority of motor acts. The task-related strategy might then determine precisely which of the various slow, small-axoned units would be preferentially activated in a given task. In this context, it is of interest to mention that when we studied recruitment in a lumbrical mucle of the cat (Kernell and Sjöholm, 1975), we used two synaptic inputs that differed with respect to their preference for individual units. Statistically speaking, however, both sources of synaptic activation produced the same standard type of property-related recruitment order (ascending size order according to electromyography [EMG], stimulation of the motor cortex vs. a skin reflex).

Following these introductory comments on recruitment strategies, we will consider some of the mechanisms involved.

Motoneuronal Membrane Properties and Size-Related Recruitment Strategies

The ease with which an individual motoneuron in a pool may become activated during a given motor act must depend on the combination of at least two groups of factors: (1) the extent to which the cell is favored by that particular set of active synapses and (2) the ease with which the cell is fired by excitatory synaptic current (see also Chapters 9 and 10, this volume). As the ascending size order of recruitment occurs so often and in combination with so many different types of synaptic organization (Henneman and Mendell, 1981), the second factor becomes particularly interesting: Do small-axoned, slow motoneurons have membrane properties that make them more easily excited than larger and faster cells?

Many years ago, I found that motoneurons with slow axonal conduction velocity also had high input resistance and a low current threshold for the activation of repetitive impulse firing (Kernell, 1966a). The differences in current threshold were probably caused, to an important extent, by the differences in input resistance: If the various cells had to become depolarized to about the same extent in order to start firing, then less current would obviously be needed to discharge those with a high input resistance than for those with a lower one (cf. Ohm's law). Originally, these differences were thought to have a fairly simple explanation (Kernell, 1966a): They could have been produced by differences in soma-dendrite size. As demonstrated by Cullheim (1978), as well as in our own laboratory (Kernell and Zwaagstra, 1981), motoneurons with thin axons do indeed also tend to have a relatively small soma. Furthermore, motoneurons with a small soma tend, on average, to possess relatively thin proximal dendrites (Kernell, 1966a; Zwaagstra and Kernell, 1981; Ulfhake and Kellerth, 1981, 1983). If other conditions remain constant, a small membrane area presents a greater electrical resistance than a larger area. Continued experimental analysis demonstrated, however, that size was not the only factor involved.

When we first investigated the relationship between electrical properties and anatomy in the same neurons, we estimated cell size simply on the basis of measurements of the dimensions of the intracellularly labeled soma and proximal dendrites (Kernell and Zwaagstra, 1981). We then found that the ratio between input conductance and soma area was significantly higher for large-axoned than for small-axoned cells (Table 2–1). This remained true ($p < 0.05$) even if cells with an input resistance of ≥ 4 MΩ were excluded from the calculations (see comments by Gustafsson and Pinter, 1984a). If all the cells had had the same shape and had differed only in linear scaling, the conductance/area ratio would instead have been *lower* for large cells than for smaller ones (for detailed arguments, see Kernell and Zwaagstra, 1981). The observed difference in the conductance/size ratio did not seem to be explained by any difference with respect to the relative supply of dendrites, because the ratio between Σ (dendritic stem diameter$^{1.5}$) and soma area was the same for both groups of cells (see $\Sigma d^{1.5}/A_s$ in Table 2–1). Hence, we concluded that the high input conductance of the fast, large-axoned motoneurons was caused, to an

Table 2–1 Relation between input conductance and size in spinal motoneurons of different axonal conduction velocity

Parameter	Cells with slow axons	Cells with fast axons	P
Axonal cond. vel. (m/s)	<90	≥90	
AHP duration (ms)	158 ± 48	90 ± 24	<0.001
Soma diameter (μm)	39.5 ± 5.1	54.7 ± 6.9	<0.001
G_{in}/A_s (mS cm^{-2})	6.6 ± 3.1	12.8 ± 5.1	<0.001
$\Sigma d^{1.5}/A_s$ (cm$^{-0.5}$)	1.9 ± 0.6	1.9 ± 0.4	ns
n	17	20	

Source: From results of Kernell and Zwaagstra (1981).

Note: Experimental results indicating that the differences in input conductance between small and large (or slow and fast) motoneurons cannot be accounted for by differences in size. For comparisons to recruitment experiments, the cells have been grouped according to their axonal conduction velocity (with a dividing line arbitrarily chosen at 90 m/s). Results are from lumbosacral spinal motoneurons of the cat. After the completion of intracellular physiological measurements, the cells were labeled with procion dye or horseradish peroxidase. Dimensions of the cell body and proximal dendrites were measured from reconstructions based on serial sections of labeled cells. Means ± S.D. Statistical significance of the differences was evaluated by the t-test (P = probability; ns = not significant).

Abbreviations: cond. vel. = conduction velocity; AHP = afterhyperpolarization; G_{in} = neuronal input conductance (reciprocal of input resistance); A_s = soma area (taken to be four times the cross-sectional area); d = stem dendrite diameter.

important extent, by low specific membrane resistivity. In essence, such a view received support from the results of a number of other laboratories (Burke et al., 1982; Gustafsson and Pinter, 1984a; Ulfhake and Kellerth, 1984; Chapter 9, this volume; see also Barrett and Crill, 1974). Our conclusion was, however, based on an assumption that was reasonable but not yet directly proven: that for dendrites of the same membrane properties, the respective input conductances would vary in proportion to the stem diameters raised to a power of 1.5, as would be the case for corresponding equivalent cylinders (Rall, 1959, 1977). This assumption may be tested by calculations performed on completely reconstructed dendritic trees (Rall, 1959). In a recent series of experiments, we performed such calculations for a population of 52 dendrites from four motoneurons of the cat's triceps surae (Kernell and Zwaagstra, 1989b). In double-logarithmic plots, there was a very good correlation between the calculated input conductance and the dendritic stem diameter ($r = \sim +0.90$). Irrespective of the assumed value for membrane resistivity, the average slope was 1.5, i.e., dendritic input conductance was indeed proportional to the 1.5th power of the stem diameter. This was true in spite of the fact that, from some other points of view, the properties of the reconstructed dendrites differed from those of Rall's (1959, 1977) equivalent-cylinder model of a dendritic tree.

Our complete reconstructions were made in four motoneurons that were chosen to represent most of the range of size-related properties in the triceps surae pool (range of input resistance for the four cells: 0.7–4.0 MΩ). Even though our sample was small, we obtained a statistically significant correlation ($p < 0.01$) between the measured neuronal input resistance and the calculated value for membrane resistivity (computed on the basis of the measured input resistance and the anatomical measurements; Rall, 1959). Thus, these more direct measurements confirmed that high motoneuronal input resistance is caused not only by small size but also, to an appreciable extent, by high specific membrane resistivity.

The existence of systematic differences in specific membrane resistivity between large- and small-axoned motoneurons has important consequences for the potential reflex excitability of these various cells. Even if a given class of activated excitatory synapses were randomly distributed among the cells of a motoneuron pool, the differences in specific membrane resistivity would cause a greater depolarization to be produced in small-axoned than in large-axoned cells (Kernell and Zwaagstra, 1981). Hence, even in the absence of any specificity in the distribution of synapses within a motoneuron pool, the ascending size order of recruitment would tend to appear. We feel that these results help to explain why the ascending size order of recruitment is so commonly encountered in motor physiology (see Chapters 4, 10, and 16, this volume).

Differences in membrane resistivity are also likely to be largely responsible for the fact that, for the cat's triceps surae, motoneurons of fast-twitch, fatigue-resistant (FR) units are electrically more excitable than those of the fast-twitch, fatigue-sensitive (FF) ones (Fleshman et al., 1981; Kernell and Monster, 1981). These two classes of motoneurons do not differ significantly in axon or soma size (Burke et al., 1973, 1982; Ulfhake and Kellerth, 1982), but the input resistance is higher for FR than for FF units (Fleshman et al., 1981; see similar findings for flexor motoneurons—Dum and Kennedy, 1980).

Besides being dependent on membrane resistivity, electrical excitability is also influenced by subthreshold rectification processes, as well as by variation in voltage threshold and/or resting membrane potential. Although some studies indicate that there may indeed be systematic differences in the amount of threshold depolarization required for motoneurons of different functional types (Fleshman et al., 1981; Gustafsson and Pinter, 1984b), such differences might commonly be less marked than those referring to membrane resistivity (cf. Pinter et al., 1983).

Motoneuronal Soma Position and Property-Related Recruitment Strategies

Our conclusion that differences in membrane properties are important for recruitment behavior does not, of course, mean that this is the only factor involved. Differences in synaptic distribution, as well as in synaptic activation efficiency (cf. Lüscher et al., 1979; Chapters 17 and 18, this chapter), are also likely to be of great importance. There is ample evidence indicating that various sets of synapses exist that may tend to sharpen or neutralize, or even partly reverse, the apparently intrinsic tendency for an ascending size order of recruitment (e.g., Burke, 1968; Burke et al., 1970; Garnett and Stephens, 1981). Furthermore, within a given pool, different task-group strategies of recruitment may show a preference for different combinations of individual motoneurons (e.g., Desmedt and Godeaux, 1981; Ter Haar Romeny et al., 1984; Hoffer et al., 1987). Such variations must depend on differences in synaptic organization.

Central synapses are often (but not always) organized on topographical principles (e.g., Lüscher et al., 1980). Hence, we have been interested in finding out to what extent the spatial organization of motoneurons and motoneuron pools might be relevant for recruitment strategies. For instance, we wondered whether motoneurons that belonged to different categories with respect to their property- or task-related recruitment tend to lie in different portions of the motoneuron pool. We have investigated such questions for the motoneurons innervating the peroneus longus muscle (PerL) of the cat's hindlimb. This muscle is suitable for such studies concerning central aspects of motoneuronal organization, because peripherally all the PerL muscle units are mechanically equivalent with respect to force direction: They are all connected to the foot via the same long, slender tendon.

In an initial anatomical study, the PerL motoneurons were retrogradely labeled with horseradish peroxidase, and soma sizes were measured. We found no marked relationship between the size of a cell body and its rostrocaudal position within the pool (Kernell et al., 1985; see Burke et al., 1977; Clamann and Kukulka, 1977). We then proceeded to study the intraspinal position of peroneal motoneurons in relation to the contractile properties of their muscle units (Kernell et al., 1985). The relative rostrocaudal site of the studied motoneurons was deduced from the exit level of their ventral root filaments. A summary of results is shown in Figure 2–1. The distribution was significantly different from random: There was a weak tendency for slowness and fatigue resistance to be somewhat better represented caudally than rostrally, and, unexpectedly, the units with *intermediate* fatigue resistance appeared to be most common rostrally. This difference in location between intermediate and other units was statistically significant for the six most evidently intermediate cases with a fatigue index of 35–65%, all of which had a rostral location (two-tailed Fisher test, $p = 0.035$). These six units came from four different animals; hence, the results could not be explained as being due to a simple sampling accident. If true for other muscles as well, such an uneven spatial distribution of F(int) units might perhaps help to explain why the percentage of such units

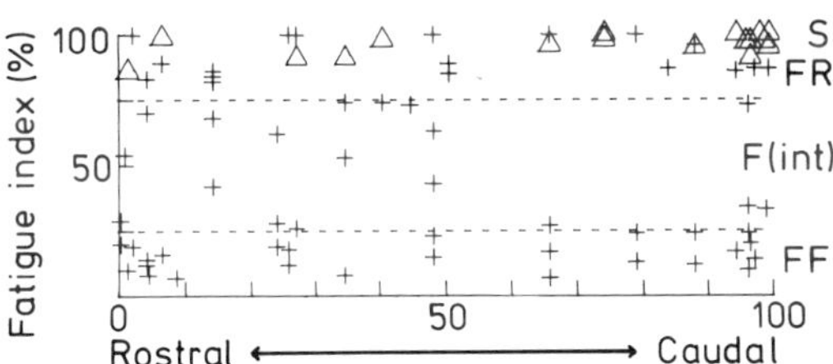

FIG. 2–1. Graph illustrating the intrapool distribution of motoneurons innervating different functional types of muscle unit. Data from the Per L of the cat. Fatigue resistance (fatigue index, percent) are plotted versus the relative rostrocaudal site of exit from the spinal cord of the respective ventral root filament (abscissa) for slow-twitch (triangles) and fast-twitch (crosses) units. Fatigue index and slow versus fast classification according to Burke et al. (1973; "sag" criterion for slow versus fast). Horizontal interrupted lines drawn through fatigue index values of 25 and 75%, respectively. Rostrocaudal site given in terms of a "rostrocaudal index," calculated as described by Kernell et al. (1985). (Data from results of Kernell et al., 1985; illustration from Kernell, 1986, reproduced with permission.)

varies so much among different published materials (see the discussion of Reinking et al., 1975).

Although the lengthwise distribution of motoneuronal types was not random, it was not distinct enough to serve as a topographical basis for a type-specific innervation: Fast and slow units were intermingled in all parts of the pool (Fig. 2–1). The nonrandomness of this intermixture might, however, suggest that rostral and caudal PerL units were subjected to different types of daily use (see the later discussion).

Motoneuronal Soma Position and Task-Related Activation Strategies

For many muscles, there is an evident correlation between the rostrocaudal position of a motoneuron within its spinal pool and the intramuscular site of its nerve endings (e.g., Swett et al., 1970). We used the technique of glycogen depletion to investigate this relationship in the cat's PerL (Donselaar et al., 1985). We found that rostral portions of the PerL motoneuron pool distributed their endings predominantly to anterior muscle portions, and vice versa. This meant that we could use localized EMG recordings from anterior and posterior muscle portions to study, in an indirect way, the distribution of activity between the rostral and caudal portions of the intraspinal motoneuron pool. In recent experiments, we used this approach to investigate whether different synaptic inputs to the motoneurons of a given muscle tend to distribute their excitation to different rostrocaudal portions of the pool (Kandou and Kernell, 1989).

The measurements were performed in cats anesthetized with pentobarbitone. We caused long-lasting contractions to occur by means of repetitive stimulation of either (1) the contralateral motor cortex or (2) the superficial peroneal nerve, evoking a classical flexion reflex. EMG was simultaneously recorded from anterior and posterior muscle portions. The contractions were relatively weak, and we could quantify the EMG with respect to the mean spike size as well as with regard to the total number of spikes per unit time. The main results are summarized in Figure 2–2. In this graph, ratios are shown between EMG measurements that were obtained from anterior and posterior muscle electrodes. Most of these anteroposterior ratios tended to be below unity, i.e., both synaptic inputs had some preference for motoneurons innervating posterior muscle portions. This posterior preference was, however, significantly more marked for contractions evoked via stimulation of the motor cortex than for those elicited via the flexion reflex. Considering the somatotopic relationships between PerL motoneurons and their muscle fibers (see preceding paragraph), these results strongly suggested that the two synaptic inputs differed from each other with respect to their rostrocaudal distribution within the spinal cord. Thus, at least for the peroneus longus muscle of the cat, topographical factors do indeed seem to be of importance for task-related aspects of motoneuronal activation (cf. also Ter Haar Romeny et al., 1984).

The Spatial Distribution of Motoneuronal Dendrites:
A Factor of Importance for Recruitment Strategies?

Until now, the discussion of topography has been restricted to the organization of neuronal cell bodies. However, at least 97% of the receptive surface area

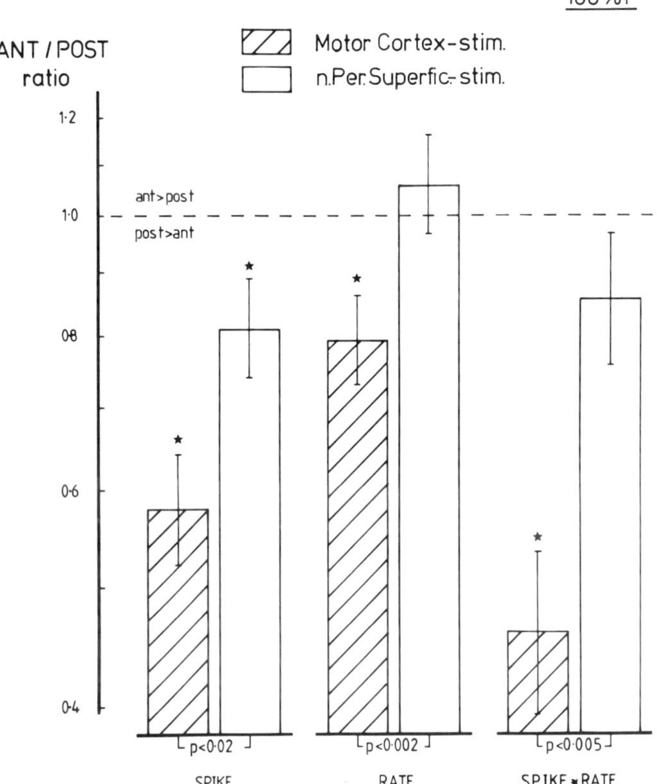

FIG. 2–2. Illustration demonstrating that different means of activating a motoneuron pool may lead to different distributions of intramuscular activity. Measurements of EMG activity were performed in the cat Per L when it was activated by repetitive electrical stimulation of the contralateral motor cortex (hatched columns) or by the skin portion of the superficial peroneal nerve (open columns). EMGs were simultaneously recorded from anterior and posterior muscle portions. The multiunit discharges were weak enough for counting and measuring the amplitude of individual spikes. The graph shows means ± S.E.M. ($n = 13$) for anteroposterior ratios of three types of EMG quantification: *left*, measurement of mean peak-to-peak spike amplitude (SPIKE), as normalized in relation to the maximum compound spike; *middle*, measurement of total number of spikes per 500-ms sampling period (RATE); *right*, the product of SPIKE and RATE. Calculations of means and S.E.M. performed on logarithms for the respective anteroposterior ratios; scale of plot logarithmic. Asterisks indicate that the respective anteroposterior ratio was significantly different from 1.0 (*t*-test, $P < 0.05$). Significance of difference between values of neighboring columns indicated in the graph (two-way ANOVA test). Within the range of force levels tested, the relative force level was not important for the illustrated differences between contractions evoked by cortical and peroneal nerve stimulation. (From results of Kandou and Kernell, 1989.)

of a motoneuron is composed of its dendrites. Thus, it should also be considered whether the dendrites of small and large (or slow and fast) motoneurons, for instance, may show systematic differences in their topography.

Several years ago, we found that motoneurons with large cell bodies also tended, on average, to have dendrites with relatively large stem diameters (Kernell, 1966a; Zwaagstra and Kernell, 1981; see also Ulfhake and Kellerth, 1981,

1983). If large dendritic trees were simply upscaled versions of the smaller ones, then the relative proportion of surface area beyond a given absolute distance would be greater for the thick- than for the thin-stemmed dendrites. With this in mind, we used intracellularly labeled motoneurons of triceps surae for the spatial analysis of dendritic trees (Kernell and Zwaagstra, 1989a). Our results confirmed the existence of a good correlation between total dendritic surface area and dendritic stem diameter (see Ulfhake and Kellerth, 1981, 1983; Cullheim et al., 1987). Thus, the stem diameter was indeed a good predictor of the total size of a dendritic tree. On the other hand, there was a remarkable absence of any significant correlation between dendritic stem diameter and the percentage of total surface area beyond a given distance from the cell body (e.g., 500, 750, or 1000 μm). We used the term "remoteness" for this type of measure, indicating the extent to which the dendritic surface area is located far from the soma. We found that dendrites of the same total size and stem diameter often differed markedly in remoteness, i.e., similarly sized dendrites displayed fundamental differences in their spatial layout. As a coarse analogy, one might think of different kinds of ordinary trees: A poplar and an oak may, for instance, turn out to have the same total surface area, but the poplar will then presumably reach farther from the ground.

We found two major clusters of dendritic properties: (1) a *size-related cluster* within which parameters were correlated with dendritic stem diameter but not with dendritic remoteness and (2) a *remoteness-related cluster* within which properties were correlated with dendritic remoteness but not with dendritic stem diameter. The size-related cluster included the total membrane area, the total cumulative length, the total number of branch points, and (consequently) the total number of terminal endings (see Ulfhake and Kellerth, 1981, 1983; Cullheim et al., 1987). The remoteness-related cluster included the mean somatofugal distance to the branchpoints and to terminations, the maximum distance from soma to termination and, somewhat less distinctly, the mean length of terminal branches.

The relative independence between measures of remoteness and size was also observed for comparisons among the dendrites of single individual motoneurons. There were, however, marked differences in mean remoteness between the sets of dendrites belonging to different cells: For our four completely reconstructed motoneurons, the mean percentage of total area beyond 750 μm ranged from 6.2 to 30.9%. Our results suggested that the relationship between remoteness and motoneuronal size or speed might be relatively weak. In our material, the two cells with the highest degree of remoteness actually represented the two extremes with respect to input resistance, duration of afterhyperpolarization and axonal conduction velocity. Such observations, albeit preliminary, made us doubt whether motoneuronal differences in dendritic remoteness would turn out to be organized in such a way as to promote size- or other property-related recruitment strategies. An alternative possibility, which should be experimentally evaluated, is that differences between motoneurons with respect to their mean dendritic remoteness are associated with the task group organization of the respective cells.

RATE GRADATION

Tension–Rate Relation of Muscle Units

In skeletal muscle fibers, isometric force increases with activation rate according to a markedly sigmoid curve (Cooper and Eccles, 1930). The steep intermediate region of this "tension–frequency curve" is positioned at lower rates for motor units and muscles with a slow twitch than for those with a faster twitch (Cooper and Eccles, 1930; Kernell et al., 1975, 1983b). These isometric aspects of muscle "speed" are probably related mainly to the kinetics of sarcoplasmic calcium movements (see Kugelberg and Thornell, 1983). How are the properties of motoneurons matched to their tasks in the rate modulation of muscle tension?

Frequency–Current Relation of Motoneurons

As motoneurons become activated during a maintained contraction, they typically discharge at fairly regular intervals. Such maintained repetitive discharges are evoked by persistent activating currents produced by the summation of many asynchronous postsynaptic events (see Granit et al., 1966). The discharge-generating action of these postsynaptic currents may be well imitated by currents that are injected through the tip of an intracellular microelectrode (Granit et al., 1963a, 1963b, 1966; Kernell, 1965b, 1965a, 1965c, 1969). Experiments using this technique have demonstrated several different ways in which the repetitive properties of motoneurons are well matched to the response properties of their muscle fibers. The main points are enlisted and briefly commented upon in the following paragraphs.

1. *Minimum discharge rate.* In discussing rate gradation, it is important to realize that motoneurons have not only a maximum possible rate of discharge but also a minimum one below which no regular firing is maintained (Kernell, 1965c). As motoneurons are gradually recruited during a weak contraction of slowly increasing strength, each cell starts firing regularly at its own characteristic minimum rate, which tends to be similar for cells with a similar recruitment threshold. As the contractile force is enhanced, the firing rate also typically tends to increase for already discharging units (e.g., Kernell and Sjöholm, 1975). The minimum firing rate of a motoneuron typically corresponds to the lower end of the steep region of the tension–frequency relation of its motor unit (Kernell, 1965c, 1966b, 1979, 1983; Kernell and Sjöholm, 1975). Due to this "rate match" between motoneurons and mucle fibers, an increase in the discharge rate of an already recruited motoneuron will automatically lead to a significant increase in motor unit force.

The minimum rate of regular motoneuronal firing is mainly determined by the time course of the afterhyperpolarization (AHP): At the minimum frequency, the impulse intervals are similar to the total duration of this afterpotential (Kernell, 1965c). The rate match between motoneuron and muscle is largely achieved by a match between the time courses of the motoneuronal AHP and the motor unit twitch: Both phenomena are typically of about the same duration (cf. Fig. 3 of Kernell, 1983). Interestingly, not only the twitch (see section Tension–Rate Relation of Muscle Units) but also the AHP reflects a calcium-dependent function; the AHP duration of spinal motoneurons may depend predominantly on the deactivation kinetics of a calcium-dependent potassium permeability (Krnjević et al., 1978; Barrett et al., 1980; see, however, Gustafsson and Pinter, 1985).

2. *Maximum discharge rate.* The maximum possible impulse frequency that a motoneuron may maintain (e.g., during at least 0.5–1 sec) is not determined by its AHP but must depend on the spike-generating properties of its membrane (proneness for inactivation of voltage-dependent sodium channels?). Earlier studies showed that motoneurons may indeed commonly be made to discharge at rates high enough to produce a tetanic tension close to the maximum one of their muscle fibers (Kernell, 1965c, 1966b). This maximum rate is also higher for AHP-fast than for AHP-slow motoneurons (maximum rate of the "secondary range"; Kernell, 1965c).

3. *Shape of the frequency–current curve.* At the very highest submaximal forces of a muscle, the tension–frequency relation becomes less steep. This decrease in the tension–frequency slope is partly compensated for by the fact that, at such high rates of discharge, the frequency–current (f–I) slope of motoneurons tends to become steeper (secondary range; Kernell, 1965b, 1965c).

4. *Initial adaptation.* The "gain" (f–I slope) of a motoneuron is much higher just after the abrupt onset of a step of stimulating current than later on. Thus, motoneurons are more sensitive to *changes* in excitation than to the steady-state excitation level. One of the consequences of this dynamic sensitivity is that, for all stimulation intensities except juxtathreshold ones, a motoneuron that is activated by a step of direct current tends to start off with a few high-rate intervals before it settles down to more regular firing. This "initial adaptation" (Granit et al., 1963a; Kernell, 1965a) probably depends, to an important extent, on the nonlinear "summation" of successive AHP-related conductance changes (Kernell, 1968, 1972; Kernell and Sjöholm, 1973; Baldissera and Gustafsson, 1974; Barrett et al., 1980). The initial burst enables the motoneurons to achieve a high rate of rise of force at the sudden onset of a contraction. These dynamic aspects of motoneuronal sensitivity and neuron–muscle matching have been explored in detail in a series of experiments by Baldissera et al. (1987 and earlier).

5. *Late adaptation.* Following the initial adaptation, there is a more gradual decline in the firing rate during the course of constant stimulation. This "late adaptation" is not associated with any evident gain changes (Granit et al., 1963b; Kernell, 1965a), and the drop in firing rate is particularly marked during the first 0.5–1 min of a maintained stimulation period (maximally 4 min studied; Kernell and Monster, 1982a). In the same neuron, the extent of late adaptation is greater at high starting rates than at lower ones. This relationship with the discharge rate is what one would expect if the late adaptation were dependent upon the cumulative aftereffects of many consecutive spikes. The frequency dependence of late adaptation is also important for motoneuron–muscle matching. As a result of differences in the minimum rate, slow-twitch gastrocnemius motoneurons would start discharging at a lower rate than fast-

twitch ones if all cells were activated by the same weak suprathreshold current intensity. Consequently, under these circumstances, the slow-twitch neurons also showed a much less marked late adaptation than the fast-twitch ones (Kernell and Monster, 1982b). Due to their modest amount of late adaptation, the slow-twitch motoneurons are particularly well suited for the maintenance of long-lasting, steady postural contractions.

During the initial minute of a maximum voluntary contraction, there is a progressive fall in the motoneuronal discharge rate similar to that of the late adaptation during constant-current stimulation. Although much of the frequency change during a maximum voluntary contraction may be caused by reflex mechanisms (Woods et al., 1987), the late adaptation is likely to be important in this context as well.

Interestingly, there seem to be no differences between FF and FR motoneurons with respect to their late adaptation. Motoneurons that differ mainly with respect to the fatigue sensitivity of their muscle fibers also differ in electrical excitability (current threshold for activation; Fleshman et al., 1981; Kernell and Monster, 1981), but apparently not in their other discharge properties. Although the motoneurons of FF units are presumably used mainly for relatively brief activity periods (Hennig and Lømo, 1985), even cells of this class have been made to fire repetitively for several minutes (Kernell and Monster, 1982b).

COMBINED EFFECTS OF RECRUITMENT AND RATE MODULATION

Since the pioneering studies of Adrian and Bronk (1929), it has been known that rate and recruitment gradation may be used in parallel during voluntary or reflex contractions. This is also what one would expect if the motoneuron population were driven by sets of axons that delivered their respective synapses to most or all of the individual members of the pool (see the data for Ia axons in Mendell and Henneman, 1971). For a long time, however, the literature was unclear with respect to the relative importance of these two strategies of force gradation. When discussing this point, it is relevant to note that, at least for several different muscles, there is good evidence that (1) the maximum possible force can be mobilized voluntarily or reflexly (e.g., Merton, 1954; Milner-Brown et al., 1973; Woods et al., 1987) and (2) motoneurons firing at their minimum rate of maintained discharge will typically elicit a mean force of only about 10–25% of the maximum (i.e., the mean force produced by a series of nonsumming twitches; calculations and measurements at optimum muscle length: Kernell, 1966b, 1979, 1983; Kernell and Sjöholm, 1975; see also Milner-Brown et al., 1973). Hence, if motoneurons always kept firing at their minimum rate, about 75–90% of the total muscle force will remain unattainable. In this sense, rate modulation is actually responsible for the greater part of the whole range of possible force modulation (for the detailed analysis of a particular case, see Milner-Brown et al., 1973). The precise balance between the two strategies at different relative force levels may, however, vary considerably among muscles.

Thus, in biceps brachii, recruitment of new motoneurons continues up to a force as high as 80% of the maximum voluntary contraction, while in the adductor pollicis, most of the pool is apparently recruited already at a force of 30–50% of maximum (Kukulka and Clamann, 1981).

The extent to which rate and recruitment gradation will actually be used together over a range of lower force levels depends on how closely clustered the various recruitment thresholds are. If all these thresholds, expressed in terms of the summed excitatory input to the whole pool (cf. Kernell, 1976), were very close together, then little rate increase would take place in parallel with the recruitment of successive motoneurons (see Figs. 2–4 of Kernell, 1976). Hence, in such a muscle, a relatively large proportion of the initial force increase would be the result of recruitment gradation.

Interestingly, the balance between recruitment and rate gradation would not be changed by recurrent inhibition unless that inhibition had a particular distribution among the members of the pool (Kernell, 1976).

LONG-TERM CONSEQUENCES OF MOTONEURONAL ACTIVITY PATTERNS

Up to now, two main types of motoneuron–muscle unit match have been discussed: (1) a *recruitment match*, whereby the recruitment order of motoneurons is matched, in a functionally relevant manner, to the contractile properties of their muscle units (i.e., weak before strong, slow before fast, FR before FF: Burke, 1981; Henneman and Mendell, 1981), and (2) a *rate match*, whereby the rates of the neuronal frequency–current curve are matched to the rates of the tension–frequency curve of the muscle unit. The recruitment match seems, to an important extent, to reflect a match between the motoneuronal membrane resistivity (and, hence, electrical excitability) and the muscle unit speed, endurance, and maximum force. The rate match reflects a match between the time courses of the motoneuronal AHP and the muscle unit twitch ("twitch speed"). It should be noted that muscle unit *speed* is a factor in both kinds of match.

How might these various kinds of motoneuron–muscle unit match be explained? To what extent might the match be the long-term consequence of differential muscle unit "training," as caused by the activity patterns of various classes of motoneuron? With this general question in mind, we have embarked on an ongoing series of experiments concerning the effects of long-term stimulation on muscle properties. Preceding studies had clearly shown that a fast muscle could be made slower if it were treated continuously at a slow pulse rate (e.g., 10 Hz) for several weeks (Salmons and Vrbová, 1969; for other references, see reviews: Salmons and Henriksson, 1981; Pette and Vrbová, 1985; Chapter 14, this volume). However, the importance of different stimulation parameters in obtaining specific types of physiological effect remained unclear. Does, for instance, the rate match between motoneurons and their muscle units result from *rate-specific* effects of activity on contractile speed?

Our chronic stimulation experiments were performed on cats whose experimental hindlimb had been made insensitive by the use of a dorsal rhizotomy (no pain, no reflex discharges). In itself, this preparatory operation (combined with an ipsilateral hemispinalization) had surprisingly small effects on the investigated muscle properties (Eerbeek et al., 1984; Donselaar et al., 1987). Our chronic stimulation patterns were given in different amounts and at different pulse rates for various groups of cats, and the total duration of treatment was 4 or 8 weeks. The daily amounts varied between 0.5% and ≥50% of the total time, and the pulse rates were between 5 and 100 Hz. At the end of a period of chronic stimulation, the isometric contractile properties and the EMG behavior were investigated for one of the chronically activated muscles (PerL) and for its contralateral control. Thereafter, the muscles were removed and prepared for subsequent morphometric and histochemical analysis. The results led to the following main conclusions (Eerbeek et al., 1984; Donselaar et al., 1987; Kernell et al., 1987a, 1987b).

1. *Isometric speed.* Physiologically, our studies concerned measurements of twitch time course, as well as of the tension–frequency relation. Histochemically, we looked at muscle composition with respect to myosin ATPase. Our results confirmed that very large daily amounts of chronic stimulation (≥50% of the time) turns a mixed hindlimb muscle into a markedly slow one with a homogeneous histochemical composition (see Salmons and Henriksson, 1981; Pette and Vrbová, 1985). Contrary to our own initial expectations, which were inspired by preceding publications concerning other kinds of preparations (see Salmons and Vrbová, 1969; Lømo et al., 1980), the effects of chronic stimulation on muscle speed were *not* dependent on the pulse rate used during the chronic treatment (see Fig. 2–3). Even bursts at rates of 100 Hz had an appreciable slowing effect on muscle contraction, and 100-Hz activation did not counteract any of the slowing effects produced by 10-Hz stimulation. Physiologically, weak slowing effects were seen already for a stimulation pattern covering only 0.5% of the daily time.

2. *Maximum tetanic force.* We confirmed that very large amounts of daily

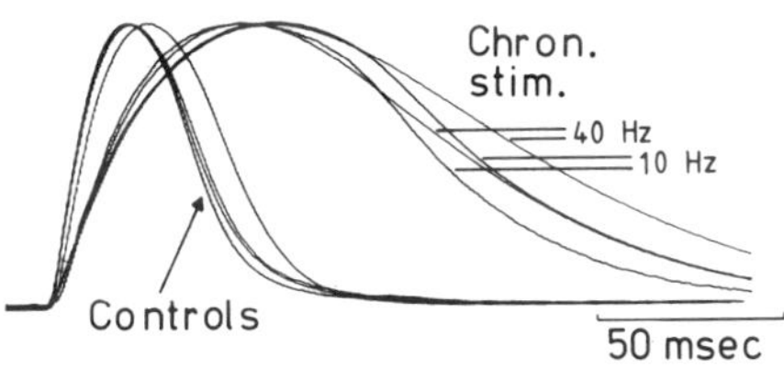

FIG. 2–3. Records illustrating the relative unimportance of the stimulus rate for long-term effects of activation on the twitch speed of the cat fast muscle (Per L). The twitches were from eight different muscles of four different animals. Records labeled "Chron. stim." were from left-side muscles subjected to large daily amounts of long-term activation at pulse rates of 40 Hz (two cases) and 10 Hz (two cases), respectively. In each animal, the chronic activation covered 50% of the daily time during 8 weeks. Records labeled "Controls" were from the right-side muscles of the same animals. All records are averages of 10 sweeps each. In order to facilitate comparisons of time courses, the twitches are displayed at a common time scale, but with normalized amplitudes. (From Eerbeek et al., 1984, reproduced with permission.)

activation tended to make a muscle considerably weaker and that part of this weakening was caused by a decrease in fiber diameter (see Salmons and Henriksson, 1981; Pette and Vrbová, 1985). Furthermore, we found that the weakening and the shrinkage in fiber diameter were both dependent on the pulse rates used during chronic activation. For the maintenance of fiber size and maximum force, high pulse rates, producing strong contractions, tended to be more beneficial than slower rates. In mixture patterns of treatment, the weakening effects of 10-Hz activation could even be neutralized by the addition of brief 100-Hz bursts.

3. *Fatigue resistance and EMG behavior*. We confirmed that large daily amounts of chronic stimulation produced a marked increase in contractile fatigue resistance (see Salmons and Henriksson, 1981; Pette and Vrbová, 1985). Furthermore, we added the new observation that chronic stimulation is also effective in counteracting the "EMG depression" that is commonly associated with contractile fatigue (i.e., the gradual decrease in amplitude of the successive compound muscle action potentials that are evoked by nerve stimulation during a fatigue test). Further analysis showed, however, that there was no strong link between the EMG depression and the contractile fatigue (see Chapter 13, this volume): EMG depression could also be markedly affected by daily amounts of stimulation (0.5%) that were too small to produce any pronounced change in contractile fatigue (Kernell et al., 1987b).

4. *Combined effects*. The contractile properties of a normal mixed cat muscle are typically dominated by those of relatively fatigue-sensitive units, i.e., FF and F(int) (Burke, 1981). In the PerL the FF and F(int) units together are responsible for 77% of the maximum force (Kernell et al., 1983a). In general, chronic stimulation tends to affect the FF–F(int)-dominated muscle such that all of its properties are shifted toward those of the units which are normally most heavily used: the S units. The stimulated muscle becomes slower, weaker, and more fatigue resistant. This shift occurs such that moderate amounts of daily activity cause a mild slowing and a marked increase in fatigue resistance, i.e., a shift from an FF muscle to an FR muscle. An increase from moderate (~5%) to large (≥50%) amounts of daily activation causes little further enhancement in standard measures of fatigue resistance but produces a marked decrease in speed and force, i.e., a shift from an FR muscle to an S muscle. As far as is known, the amounts of stimulation time required for these changes are compatible with the daily activity patterns of normal motoneurons. For instance, FR muscles were produced by daily amounts of activity of ~5%, which is similar to the amount of spontaneous daily firing observed for presumed FR motoneurons in the rat (Hennig and Lømo, 1985; no data are yet available for the cat). Our findings are consistent with the idea that the normal match between the properties of motoneurons and muscle units is markedly dependent on differential muscle-training effects caused by motoneuronal activity patterns. However, it should be stressed that our findings do not necessarily mean that activity is the *only* factor of relevance for the differentiation of muscle unit properties. During the ontological development of muscle, nonneuronal factors are known to be of great importance for differentiation (e.g.,

Miller and Stockdale, 1987). Such factors might, for instance, be responsible for setting the "adaptive range" within which the adult muscle properties may become further adjusted by means of long-term effects of usage.

In the adult, usage-dependent changes would be needed for the continuous adjustment of muscle unit properties to alterations in motor behavior. Usage-dependent changes might also be responsible for much of the remarkable recovery of motoneuron–muscle unit matching after reinnervation (cf. Gordon and Stein, 1982).

Our results from experiments with chronic stimulation have shown that the speed, maximum force, and fatigue resistance of a muscle are differentially sensitive to different types of stimulation parameters. Hence, these various contractile properties could, to some extent, be independently influenced by activity. Most kinds of stimulation effect varied with the daily *amount* of activation. In addition, the stimulation effects of maximum contractile force were markedly dependent on *pulse rate,* and the effects on contractile speed were relatively much more dependent on the total daily duration of contiguous activity periods ("block duration," Kernell et al., 1987a). Pulse rate was unimportant and block duration was of only limited significance in influencing fatigue resistance. These observations suggest that there may be many different intracellular links between long-term muscle (or nerve) activation and the biochemical events that were ultimately responsible for the respecification of muscle properties; the respecification could not all be exclusively dependent on, for instance, changes in intracellular calcium concentration.

Effects of Long-Term Activation on Motoneurons

Little is still known about the long-term effects of usage changes on motoneurons. Functional properties of motoneurons may be altered by spinalization (e.g., Czéh et al., 1978; Munson et al., 1986), as well as by muscle activation (Czéh et al., 1978). In general, however, the properties of motoneurons seem to be less usage dependent than those of their muscle fibers. In our experimental situation (dorsal roots cut), the chronic nerve stimulation would cause muscles to contract and evoke antidromic discharges of their motoneurons, but there would be few direct effects on the intraspinal synaptic activity (presumably mainly some activation of recurrent inhibition). This type of chronic stimulation had little or no effect on the size or oxidative enzyme activity of the respective motoneuronal cell bodies (succinate dehydrogenase histochemistry; Donselaar et al., 1986). Furthermore, in preliminary experiments, we found no evidence for any marked effects on the duration of AHP (Kernell and Eerbeek, unpublished observations). Among 22 motoneurons of peroneal nerves that had been subjected to heavy chronic stimulation (daily amount, 50%; duration, 4 weeks), the mean AHP duration was 72 $\pm$ 21 ms (S.D.), and half the number of cells still had an AHP with a duration as brief as 60 ms or less, which is similar to that of the fastest class of normal motoneurons (AHP measured from the onset of the spike; see Eccles et al., 1958). It should be noted, however, that in normal motor training the associated activation of intraspinal synapses might conceivably have much stronger effects on motoneuron properties than those evoked by the motoneuronal action potentials themselves (see Kernell and Peterson, 1970).

REFERENCES

Adrian, E. D., and Bronk, D. W. (1929). The discharge of impulses in motor nerve fibres. Part II. The frequency of discharge in reflex and voluntary contractions. *J. Physiol. (Lond.)* 67, 119–151.

Baldissera, F., Campadelli, P., and Piccinelli, L. (1987). The dynamic response of cat gastrocnemius motor units investigated by ramp current injection into their motoneurones. *J. Physiol. (Lond.)* 387, 317–330.

Baldissera, F., and Gustafsson, B. (1974). Firing behaviour of a neurone model based on the afterhyperpolarization conductance time course and algebraical summation. Adaptation and steady state firing. *Acta Physiol. Scand.* 92, 27–47.

Barrett, E. F., Barrett, J. N., and Crill, W. E. (1980). Voltage-sensitive outward currents in cat motoneurones. *J. Physiol. (Lond.)* 304, 251–276.

Barrett, J. N., and Crill, W. E. (1974). Specific membrane properties of cat motoneurones. *J. Physiol. (Lond.)* 239, 301–324.

Bawa, P., Binder, M. D., Ruenzel, P., and Henneman, E. (1984). Recruitment order of motoneurons in stretch reflexes is highly correlated with their axonal conduction velocity. *J. Neurophysiol.* 52, 410–420.

Burke, R. E. (1968). Group Ia synaptic input to fast and slow twitch motor units of cat triceps surae. *J. Physiol. (Lond.)* 196, 605–630.

Burke, R. E. (1981). Motor units: Anatomy, physiology and functional organization. In *Handbook of Physiology—The Nervous System II*, Part 1 (ed. V. B. Brooks). American Physiological Society, Bethesda, Md., pp. 345–422.

Burke, R. E., Dum, R. P., Fleshman, J. W., Glenn, L. L., Lev-Tov, A., O'Donovan, M. J., and Pinter, M. J. (1982). An HRP study of the relation between cell size and motor unit type in cat ankle extensor motoneurons. *J. Comp. Neurol.* 209, 17–28.

Burke, R. E., Jankowska, E., and Ten Bruggencate, G. (1970). A comparison of peripheral and rubrospinal synaptic input to slow and fast twitch motor units of triceps surae. *J. Physiol. (Lond.)* 207, 709–732.

Burke, R. E., Levine, D. N., Tsairis, P., and Zajac, F. E. (1973). Physiological types and histochemical profiles in motor units of the cat gastrocnemius. *J. Physiol. (Lond.)* 234, 723–748.

Burke, R. E., Strick, P. L., Kanda, K., Kim, C. C., and Walmsley, B. (1977). Anatomy of medial gastrocnemius and soleus motor nuclei in cat spinal cord. *J. Neurophysiol.* 40, 667–680.

Clamann, H. P., and Kukulka, C. G. (1977). The relation between size of motoneurons and their position in the cat spinal cord. *J. Morphol.* 153, 461–466.

Cooper, S., and Eccles, J. C. (1930). The isometric responses of mammalian muscles. *J. Physiol. (Lond.)* 69, 377–385.

Cullheim, S. (1978). Relations between cell body size, axon diameter and axon conduction velocity of cat sciatic alpha-motoneurons stained with horseradish peroxidase. *Neurosci. Lett.* 8, 17–20.

Cullheim, S., Fleshman, J. W., Glenn, L. L., and Burke, R. E. (1987). Membrane area and dendritic structure in type-identified triceps surae alpha motoneurons. *J. Comp. Neurol.* 255, 68–81.

Czéh, G., Gallego, R., Kudo, N., and Kuno, M. (1978). Evidence for the maintenance of motoneurone properties by muscle activity. *J. Physiol. (Lond.)* 281, 239–252.

Desmedt, J. E., and Godaux, E. (1981). Spinal motoneuron recruitment in man: Rank deordering with direction but not with speed of voluntary movement. *Science* 214, 933–936.

Donselaar, Y., Eerbeek, O., Kernell, D., and Verhey, B. A. (1987). Fibre sizes and histochemical staining characteristics in normal and chronically stimulated fast muscle of cat. *J. Physiol. (Lond.)* 382, 237–254.

Donselaar, Y., Kernell, D., and Eerbeek, O. (1986). Soma size and oxidative enzyme activity in normal and chronically stimulated motoneurones of the cat's spinal cord. *Brain Res.* 385, 22–29.

Donselaar, Y., Kernell, D., Eerbeek, O., and Verhey, B. A. (1985). Somatotopic relations between spinal motoneurones and muscle fibres of the cat's musculus peroneus longus. *Brain Res.* 335, 81–88.

Dum, R. P., and Kennedy, T. T. (1980). Physiological and histochemical characteristics of motor units in cat tibialis anterior and extensor digitorum longus muscles. *J. Neurophysiol.* 43, 1615–1630.

Eccles, J. C., Eccles, R. M., and Lundberg, A. (1958). The action potentials of the alpha motoneurones supplying fast and slow muscles. *J. Physiol. (Lond.)* 142, 275–291.

Eerbeek, O., Kernell, D., and Verhey, B. A. (1984). Effects of fast and slow patterns of tonic long-term stimulation on contractile properties of fast muscle in the cat. *J. Physiol. (Lond.)* 352, 73–90.

Enoka, R. M., and Stuart, D. G. (1984). Henneman's "size principle": Current issues. *Trends Neurosci.* 7, 226–228.

Fleshman, J. W., Munson, J. B., Sypert, G. W., and Friedman, W. A. (1981). Rheobase, input resistance and motor-unit type in medial gastrocnemius motoneurons in the cat. *J. Neurophysiol.* 46, 1326–1338.

Garnett, R., and Stephens, J. A. (1981). Changes in the recruitment threshold of motor units produced by cutanous stimulation in man. *J. Physiol. (Lond.)* 311, 463–473.

Gordon, T., and Stein, R. B. (1982). Reorganization of motor-unit properties in reinnervated muscles of the cat. *J. Neurophysiol.* 48, 1175–1190.

Granit, R., Kernell, D., and Lamarre, Y. (1966). Algebraical summation in synaptic activation of motoneurones firing within the "primary range" to injected currents. *J. Physiol. (Lond.)* 187, 379–399.

Granit, R., Kernell, D., and Shortess, G. K. (1963a). Quantitative aspects of repetitive firing of mammalian motoneurones, caused by injected currents. *J. Physiol. (Lond.)* 168, 911–931.

Granit, R., Kernell, D., and Shortess, G. K. (1963b). The behaviour of mammalian motoneurones during long-lasting orthodromic, antidromic and trans-membrane stimulation. *J. Physiol. (Lond.)* 169, 743–754.

Gustafsson, B., and Pinter, M. J. (1984a). Relations among passive electrical properties of lumbar alpha-motoneurones of the cat. *J. Physiol. (Lond.)* 356, 401–431.

Gustafsson, B., and Pinter, M. J. (1984b). An investigation of threshold properties among cat spinal alpha-motoneurones. *J. Physiol. (Lond.)* 357, 453–483.

Gustafsson, B., and Pinter, M. J. (1985). Factors determining the variation of the afterhyperpolarization duration in cat lumbar alpha-motoneurones. *Brain Res.* 326, 392–395.

Henneman, E. (1980). Organization of the motoneuron pool. The size principle. In *Medical Physiology*, Vol. I (ed. V. B. Mountcastle). C. V. Mosby, St. Louis, pp. 718–741.

Henneman, E., and Mendell, L. M. (1981). Functional organization of motoneuron pool and its inputs. In *Handbook of Physiology—The Nervous System*, II, Part 1 (ed. V. B. Brooks). American Physiological Society, Bethesda, Md., pp. 423–507.

Henneman, E., Somjen, G., and Carpenter, D. O. (1965). Functional significance of cell size in spinal motoneurons. *J. Neurophysiol.* 28, 560–580.

Hennig, R., and Lømo, T. (1985). Firing patterns of motor units in normal rats. *Nature* 314, 164–166.

Hoffer, J. A., Loeb, G. E., Sugano, N., Marks, W. B., O'Donovan, M. J., and Pratt, C. A. (1987). Cat hindlimb motoneurons during locomotion. III. Functional segregation in sartorius. *J. Neurophysiol.* 57, 544–562.

Kandou, T. W. A., and Kernell, D. (1989). Distribution of activity within the cat's peroneus longus muscle when activated in different ways via the central nervous system. *Brain Res.*, in press.

Kernell, D. (1965a). The adaptation and the relation between discharge frequency and current strength of cat lumbosacral motoneurones stimulated by long-lasting injected currents. *Acta Physiol. Scand.* 65, 65–73.

Kernell, D. (1965b). High-frequency repetitive firing of cat lumbosacral motoneurones stimulated by long-lasting injected currents. *Acta Physiol. Scand.* 65, 74–86.

Kernell, D. (1965c). The limits of firing frequency in cat lumbosacral motoneurones possessing different time course of afterhyperpolarization. *Acta Physiol. Scand.* 65, 87–100.

Kernell, D. (1966a). Input resistance, electrical excitability, and size of ventral horn cells in cat spinal cord. *Science* 152, 1637–1640.

Kernell, D. (1966b). The repetitive discharge of motoneurones. In *Muscular Afferents and Motor Control,* (ed. R. Granit). Almqvist and Wiksell, Stockholm, pp. 351–362.

Kernell, D. (1968). The repetitive impulse discharge of a simple neurone model compared to that of spinal motoneurones. *Brain Res.* 11, 685–687.

Kernell, D. (1969). Synaptic conductance changes and the repetitive impulse discharge of spinal motoneurones. *Brain Res.* 15, 291–294.

Kernell, D. (1972). The early phase of adaptation in repetitive impulse discharges of cat spinal motoneurones. *Brain Res.* 41, 184–186.

Kernell, D. (1976). Recruitment, rate modulation and the tonic stretch reflex. *Prog. Brain Res.* 44, 257–265.

Kernell, D. (1979). Rhythmic properties of motoneurones innervating muscle fibres of different speed in m. gastrocnemius medialis of the cat. *Brain Res.* 160, 159–162.

Kernell, D. (1983). Functional properties of spinal motoneurons and gradation of muscle force. In *Motor Control Mechanisms in Health and Disease* (ed. J. E. Desmedt). Raven Press, New York, pp. 213–226.

Kernell, D. (1986). Organization and properties of spinal motoneurones and motor units. *Prog. Brain Res.* 64, 21–30.

Kernell, D., Donselaar, Y., and Eerbeek, O. (1987b). Effects of physiological amounts of high- and low-rate chronic stimulation on fast-twitch muscle of the cat hindlimb. II. Endurance-related properties. *J. Neurophysiol.* 58, 614–627.

Kernell, D., Ducati, A., and Sjöholm, H. (1975). Properties of motor units in the first deep lumbrical muscle of the cat's foot. *Brain Res.* 98, 37–55.

Kernell, D., Eerbeek, O., and Verhey, B. A. (1983a). Motor unit categorization on basis of contractile properties: An experimental analysis of the composition of the cat's m. peroneus longus. *Exp. Brain Res.* 50, 211–219.

Kernell, D., Eerbeek, O., and Verhey, B. A. (1983b). Relation between isometric force and stimulus rate in cat's hindlimb motor units of different twitch contraction time. *Exp. Brain Res.* 50, 220–227.

Kernell, D., Eerbeek, O., Verhey, B. A., and Donselaar, Y. (1987a). Effects of physiological amounts of high- and low-rate chronic stimulation on fast-twitch muscle of the cat hindlimb. 1. Speed- and force-related properties. *J. Neurophysiol.* 58, 598–613.

Kernell, D., and Monster, A. W. (1981). Threshold current for repetitive impulse firing in motoneurones innervating muscle fibres of different fatigue sensitivity in the cat. *Brain Res.* 229, 193–196.

Kernell, D., and Monster, A. W. (1982a). Time course and properties of late adaptation in spinal motoneurones in the cat. *Exp. Brain Res.* 46, 191–196.

Kernell, D., and Monster, A. W. (1982b). Motoneurone properties and motor fatigue. An intracellular study of gastrocnemius motoneurones of the cat. *Exp. Brain Res.* 46, 197–204.

Kernell, D., and Peterson, R. P. (1970). The effect of spike activity versus synaptic activation on the metabolism of ribonucleic acid in a molluscan giant neurone. *J. Neurochem.* 17, 1087–1094.

Kernell, D., and Sjöholm, H. (1973). Repetitive impulse firing: Comparisons between neurone models based on "voltage clamp equations" and spinal motoneurones. *Acta Physiol. Scand.* 87, 40–56.

Kernell, D., and Sjöholm, H. (1975). Recruitment and firing rate modulation of motor unit tension in a small muscle of the cat's foot. *Brain Res.* 98, 57–72.

Kernell, D., Verhey, B. A., and Eerbeek, O. (1985). Neuronal and muscle unit properties at different rostro-caudal levels of cat's motoneurone pool. *Brain Res.* 335, 71–79.

Kernell, D., and Zwaagstra, B. (1981). Input conductance, axonal conduction velocity and cell size among hindlimb motoneurones of the cat. *Brain Res.* 204, 311–326.

Kernell, D., and Zwaagstra, B. (1989a). Size and remoteness: Two relatively independent parameters of dendrites, as studied for spinal motoneurones of the cat. *J. Physiol. (Lond.)*, in press.

Kernell, D., and Zwaagstra, B. (1989b). Dendrites of cat's spinal motoneurones: Relationship between stem diameter and predicted input conductance. *J. Physiol. (Lond.)*, in press.

Krnjević, K., Puil, E., and Werman, R. (1978). EGTA and motoneuronal afterpotentials. *J. Physiol. (Lond.)* 275, 199–223.

Kugelberg, E., and Thornell, L. -E. (1983). Conduction time, histochemical type, and terminal cisternae volume of rat motor units. *Muscle Nerve* 6, 149–153.

Kukulka, C. G., and Clamann, H. P. (1981). Comparison of the recruitment and discharge properties of motor units in human brachial biceps and adductor pollicis during isometric contractions. *Brain Res.* 219, 45–55.

Loeb, G. E. (1984). The control and responses of mammalian muscle spindles during normally executed motor tasks. *Exercise Sport Sci. Rev.* 12, 157–204.

Lømo, T., Westgaard, R. H., and Engebretsen, L. (1980). Different stimulation patterns affect contractile properties of denervated rat soleus muscles. In *Plasticity of Muscle* (ed. D. Pette). De Gruyter, Berlin, pp. 297–309.

Lüscher, H. -R., Ruenzel, P., and Henneman, E. (1979). How the size of motoneurones determines their susceptibility to discharge. *Nature* 282, 859–861.

Lüscher, H. -R., Ruenzel, P., and Henneman, E. (1980). Topographic distribution of terminals of IA and group II fibers in spinal cord, as revealed by postsynaptic population potentials. *J. Neurophysiol.* 43, 968–985.

Mendell, L. M., and Henneman, E. (1971). Terminals of single Ia fibers: Location, density and distribution within a pool of 300 homonymous motoneurons. *J. Neurophysiol.* 34, 171–187.

Merton, P. A. (1954). Voluntary strength and fatigue. *J. Physiol. (Lond.)* 123, 553–564.

Miller, J. B., and Stockdale, F. E. (1987). What muscle cells know that nerves don't tell them. *Trends Neurosci.* 10, 325–329.

Milner-Brown, H. S., Stein, R. B., and Yemm, R. (1973). Changes in firing rate of human motor units during linearly changing voluntary contractions. *J. Physiol. (Lond.)* 230, 371–390.

Munson, J. B., Foehring, R. C., Lofton, S. A., Zengel, J. E., and Sypert, G. W. (1986). Plasticity of medial gastrocnemius motor units following cordotomy in the cat. *J. Neurophysiol.* 55, 619–634.

Pette, D., and Vrbová, G. (1985). Neural control of phenotypic expression in mammalian muscle fibres. *Muscle Nerve* 8, 676–689.

Pinter, M. J., Curtis, R. L., and Hosko, M. J. (1983). Voltage threshold and excitability among variously sized cat hindlimb motoneurons. *J. Neurophysiol.* 50, 644–657.

Rall, W. (1959). Branching dendritic trees and motoneuron membrane resistivity. *Exp. Neurol.* 1,491–527.

Rall, W. (1977). Core conductor theory and cable properties of neurons. In *Handbook of Physiology,* Sect. 1, Vol. I, Part 1 (ed., E. R. Kandel). American Physiological Society, Bethesda, Md., pp. 39–97.

Reinking, R. M., Stephens, J. A., and Stuart, D. G. (1975). The motor units of cat medial gastrocnemius: Problem of their categorisation on the basis of mechanical properties. *Exp. Brain Res.* 23, 301–313.

Salmons, S., and Henriksson, J. (1981). The adaptive response of skeletal muscle to increased use. *Muscle Nerve* 4, 94–105.

Salmons, S., and Vrbová, G. (1969). The influence of activity on some contractile characteristics of mammalian fast and slow muscles. *J. Physiol. (Lond.)* 201, 535–549.

Swett, J. E., Eldred, E., and Buchwald, J. S. (1970). Somatotopic cord-to-muscle relations in efferent innervation of cat gastrocnemius. *Am. J. Physiol.* 219, 762–766.

Ter Haar Romeny, B. M., Denier van der Gon, J. J., and Gielen, C. C. A. M. (1984). Relation between location of a motor unit in the human biceps brachii and its critical firing levels to different tasks. *Exp. Neurol.* 85, 631–650.

Ulfhake, B., and Kellerth, J. -O. (1981). A quantitative light microscopic study of the dendrites of cat spinal alpha-motoneurons after intracellular staining with horseradish peroxidase. *J. Comp. Neurol.* 202, 571–583.

Ulfhake, B., and Kellerth, J. -O. (1982). Does alpha-motoneuron size correlate with motor unit type in cat triceps surae? *Brain Res.* 251, 201–209.

Ulfhake, B., and Kellerth, J. -O. (1983). A quantitative morphological study of HRP-labelled cat alpha-motoneurones supplying different hindlimb muscles. *Brain Res.* 264, 1–19.

Ulfhake, B., and Kellerth, J. -O. (1984). Electrophysiological and morphological measurements in cat gastrocnemius and soleus alpha-motoneurones. *Brain Res.* 307, 167–179.

Woods, J. J., Furbush, F., and Bigland-Ritchie, B. (1987). Evidence for a fatigue-induced reflex inhibition of motoneuron firing rates. *J. Neurophysiol.* 58, 125–137.

Zwaagstra, B., and Kernell, D. (1981). Sizes of soma and stem dendrites in intracellularly labelled alpha-motoneurones of the cat. *Brain Res.* 204, 295–309.

3

Properties and Control
of the Neck Musculature

V. C. ABRAHAMS, P. K. ROSE,
AND F. J. R. RICHMOND

The primary motor function of the neck musculature is to move the head. The motor system that controls head movement assumes particular significance because of the important role of head position in the operation of the special senses. The eyes, the ears, and the olfactory apparatus are all carried on the head. In addition, the face of fur-bearing mammals carries two sets of specialized cutaneous receptors. First are the vibrissae, which have at their base a complex of receptors (Andres, 1966). Second is the rhinarium, the glabrous skin around the nostrils. This skin contains a dense accumulation of cutaneous receptors organized in a fashion similar to that of primate digital skin (Abrahams et al., 1987). Thus, under many circumstances, the operation of the motor control system of the head must be integrated with the operation of a number of sensory systems. The most thoroughly studied of these systems is that of gaze control, in which movements of the head and eye are combined in order that the visual system can foveate an object in space. In most considerations of the gaze control system, the organization of head motor control has been considered secondarily to oculomotor control (Harris, 1980; Roucoux et al., 1980). In consequence, little attention has been paid to the head motor system and its intrinsic physiology until quite recently. As the complexities of the head motor system have become apparent, the term sometimes used by oculomotor physiologists, the "head motor plant," appears less and less appropriate. Nor is it always appropriate to consider head movement solely within the context of gaze control. For example, in cats there is a range of head movements in activities such as grooming, feeding, fighting, exploration, and aversion when head motor control cannot be subordinated to the requirements of a gaze control system. In this chapter, we concentrate on the details of the head motor plant.

It is paradoxical that the first systematic studies related to the head motor system were stimulated by curiousity about its sensory rather than its motor apparatus. The demonstration of tonic neck reflexes in the decerebrate cat (Magnus, 1926) led to a search for the receptors underlying the reflex. Early experiments showed that the reflex originated with unspecified receptors lying in close proximity to neck joints (McCouch et al., 1951). McCouch et al. were cautious in identifying the receptors and suggested that they might originate from either the joint capsule or connective and muscle tissues closely adherent to the vertebral column. Their findings were frequently interpreted to mean that the receptors of the neck lay within the vertebral joints themselves. However, later anatomical studies provided evidence that the receptor population in neck muscles might also play a role. In particular, neck muscles have been found to contain a remarkable abundance of muscle spindles in all species so far studied, including the human (Voss, 1958; Cooper and Daniel, 1963), the cat (Richmond and Abrahams, 1975a; Richmond and Bakker, 1982), and the rat (Thompson, 1970).

ELEMENTS OF THE NECK MUSCLE SENSORY SYSTEM

Receptor Wealth and Specialization in Neck Muscles

Neck muscles are now known to have not only an abundance but also an unusually complex system of muscle proprioceptors (Richmond and Abrahams, 1975b; Richmond and Bakker, 1982). In the cat, neck muscles that play a role in head movement have muscle spindle and Golgi tendon organ densities unmatched elsewhere in muscles of equivalent size (Richmond and Bakker, 1982). For example, the densities of muscle spindles in cat intervertebral muscles range from 100 to 500 spindles per gram of muscle tissue. In comparison, cat limb muscles have densities ranging from 5 to 20 spindles per gram (Richmond et al., 1988). Receptor densities similar to those of the large dorsal neck muscles have been observed in fine muscles of the digits, but because the digital muscles are small, their total receptor content is low (Chin et al., 1962). Neck muscle receptors also have a range of morphological specializations not commonly seen in other skeletal muscles. The typical textbook diagram of a cat muscle spindle shows an isolated receptor with a grouping of intrafusal fibers consisting of two bag and five to seven chain fibers. Spindles with this morphology are common in cat hindlimb muscles, but such isolated spindles constitute a minority in the neck. More commonly in neck muscles, spindles occur in aggregates of 2–12 receptors arranged in chain-like arrays and often linked by structural elements (Richmond and Abrahams, 1975b; Bakker and Richmond, 1982; Richmond and Bakker, 1982). Some spindle units in these complexes appear to have a specialized internal organization. For example, 25–40% of spindle units in many dorsal and deep neck muscles lack a bag_1 fiber in their intrafusal fiber complement (Bakker and Richmond, 1981). The bag_1 fiber is the intrafusal fiber that is specifically implicated in the transduction of the large dynamic response typical of the spindle primary ending. Spindles lacking a bag$_1$ fiber should have a much weakened dynamic response (Bakker and Richmond, 1981), and the existence of such spindle properties in neck muscles has been reported (Richmond and Abrahams, 1979; Price and Dutia, 1987). Both the aggregation of spindles and the range of transductive specialization seen within individual spindles of the aggregate suggest that the system of proprioceptors in neck muscles may provide a richness and breadth of sensory information greater than that provided by skeletal muscle receptors elsewhere in the body.

Receptor Wealth and Reflex Strength

What roles might be served by this complex spindle system? Other chapters in this volume draw attention to the motoneuron as a significant target for spindle afferent fibers. The presence of large numbers of neck muscle spindles raises the expectation that neck motoneurons have a strong monosynaptic excitatory connection and thus that neck muscles should exhibit a powerful monosynaptic stretch reflex. Yet, as early as 1897, Sherrington observed that stimulating the C2 dorsal root or branches of the root in the decerebrate cat did not cause a demonstrable stretch reflex in dorsal neck extensor muscles. Quite the opposite: The stimulation caused the high-held head to drop (an observation inconsistent with the presence of strong excitatory reflexes, either monosynaptic or multisynaptic).

Since that time, many studies have showed an apparent weakness of the monosynaptic reflex of neck motoneurons. Abrahams et al. (1975) showed that the excitation of neck motoneurons by electrical stimulation of neck muscle nerves rarely led to short-latency motoneuron excitation. Monosynaptic excitatory postsynaptic potentials (EPSPs) have been consistently recorded intracellularly in neck motoneurons, but the composite EPSPs are much smaller than might be expected given the large number of muscle spindles in each dorsal neck muscle. For example, stimulation of the medial gastrocnemius muscle nerve leads to an average monosynaptic EPSP of 4.6 mV in medial gastrocnemius motoneurons (Eccles et al., 1957). Stimulation of the segmental nerves innervating the large dorsal neck muscles, each supplying approximately the same number of muscle spindle afferents as the medial gastrocnemius muscle nerve, evokes composite EPSPs averaging only 400 μV in dorsal neck motoneurons (range, 350–3100 μV: Rapoport, 1979; Brink et al., 1981). The relatively small size of composite EPSPs recorded in dorsal neck motoneurons may be a consequence of the highly selective projection of single neck muscle spindle afferents to neck motoneurons. Recent experiments using spike-triggered averaging techniques have shown that only a small fraction of motoneurons supplying a single neck muscle receive functional contacts from individual neck muscle afferents (Keirstead and Rose, 1988a). This arrangement is in contrast to the more widespread projection of individual hindlimb muscle spindle afferents, in which each afferent contacts up to 100% of the motoneurons in a single motoneuron nucleus (Henneman and Mendell, 1981; Chapters 16–18, this volume).

In general, the anatomical features of primary afferent fibers leaving neck muscles resemble those seen elsewhere in the spinal cord (Abrahams et al., 1984; Bakker et al., 1984, 1985). The fibers track both rostrally and caudally, with caudally directed projections less extensive than rostrally directed ones (Bakker and Abrahams, 1988). Numbers of collaterals are dropped off, some of which project immediately to the central cervical nucleus. Fine afferents appear to project to laminae I and V. Individual neck muscle spindle afferents, injected intra-axonally with horseradish peroxidase, have a rich projection to the intermediate layers of the spinal cord, particularly in and around the central cervical nucleus. There is also a major projection to the ventral horn, including the region of the motoneuron nuclei (Keirstead and Rose, 1988b). Each collateral may provide as many as 300 boutons to the region occupied by neck motoneuron dendrites. Although individual primary afferent collaterals are widely spaced (on average, 3.3 mm apart), each collateral gives rise to an arborization in the ventral horn that extends, on average, for 1400 μ in the rostrocaudal plane. Thus there is no obvious anatomical reason to explain the low projection frequency of individual neck muscle afferents to motoneurons and, correspondingly, the weakness of the monosynaptic reflex. The anatomical evidence indicates that the potential for powerful monosynaptic activation is present but that activation is not readily observed in the experimental paradigms so far used. Despite the apparent weakness of the monosynaptic connection, neck muscle receptors do appear to participate in a complex cervical spinal reflex, the cervico-collic reflex (Peterson et al., 1981; Ezure et al., 1983).

ELEMENTS OF THE NECK MUSCLE MOTOR SYSTEM

Compartmentalization: Motoneuronal Recruitment as a Cooperative Effort

As well as describing the frequency and types of neck receptors, early studies of the cat neck musculature (Richmond and Abrahams, 1975a) showed that the large dorsal neck muscles, biventer cervicis, splenius, and complexus are complex architecturally. Each muscle is intersected by tendinous inscriptions that to a greater or lesser degree divide each muscle into compartments. In biventer cervicis, compartments are separate subvolumes of fibers that use the inscriptions as sites of origin and insertion. Thus the muscle as a whole is composed of several "mini-muscles" linked in series (Armstrong et al., 1988; Richmond and Armstrong, 1988). In other muscles, such as splenius, tendinous inscriptions cross only one part of the muscle, but an in-series arrangement of fibers can still be seen in the remaining noninscripted regions. The in-series compartments of fibers are further distinguished from each other because they are supplied by separate muscle nerve bundles that originate from different segmental levels of the cervical spinal cord. As shown in Figure 3–1, the biventer cervicis is innervated from four cervical segments, but its motor axons are grouped into five separate nerve bundles. Glycogen depletion experiments have shown that each nerve bundle serves a specific compartment of motor units that are usually confined to one of the muscle compartments delimited by the tendinous inscriptions (Armstrong et al., 1988).

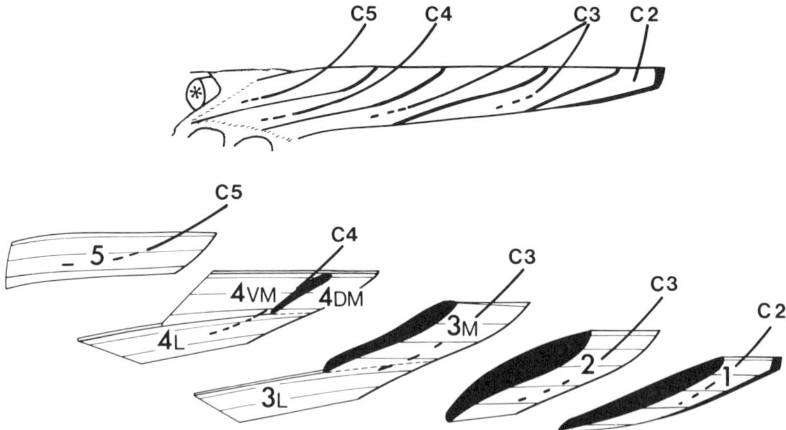

FIG. 3–1. Diagram illustrating the compartmentalization and innervation of the dorsal neck muscle, biventer cervicis. *Top*: The relationships between the innervation of the muscle and individual compartments. *Bottom*: exploded view of the muscle to show the organization of the compartments. Note that the compartment innervated by the caudal branch of the C3 nerve is divided into a medial (3M) and a lateral (3L) subcompartment. The compartment innervated by the C4 nerve is also complex, with a ventromedial (4VM), dorsomedial (4DM), and a lateral compartment (4L).

Thus, for these large dorsal neck muscles to act as a unit, activity in the serially ordered compartments must be synchronized. Activity in one compartment alone will only serve to stretch the fibers in neighboring compartments and thus produce little or no tension at the muscle ends.

Neck Muscle Motoneurons

The motoneurons of neck muscle have only recently come under intensive study. In general, their spinal location in the cat resembles that of motoneurons in the lumbosacral cord, with the majority clustered in lamina IX of the ventral horn (Richmond et al., 1978; Abrahams and Keane, 1984). The motoneurons located in one spinal segment mainly give rise to axons that leave the spinal cord in the corresponding segmental ventral root (Richmond et al., 1978). Nevertheless, there are numerous aspects of cat neck motoneuron distribution and morphology that are distinctive. First, a significant proportion of neck motoneurons lie outside of the classical motoneuron pools in lamina IX. The earliest experiments based on the retrograde transport of horseradish peroxidase (HRP) used the chromogen 3,3′-diaminobenzidine (DAB) (Richmond et al., 1978) and showed that neck motoneurons were present on the medial wall of the ventral horn as far dorsal as the commissural nucleus fund the centrodorsal nucleus, and were also present close to the central canal. Later HRP transport studies, using the more sensitive chromogen 3,3′, 5,5′-tetramethylbenzidine (TMB) (Abrahams and Keane, 1984), showed an even more extensive distribution of neck motoneurons. Some were found in the white matter adjacent to the medial part of the ventral horn, some in the intermediate gray, and a few in the contralateral intermediate gray (Fig. 3–2), findings recently confirmed by Callister

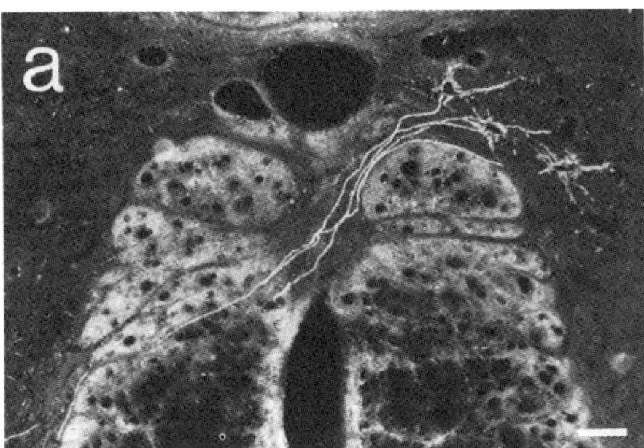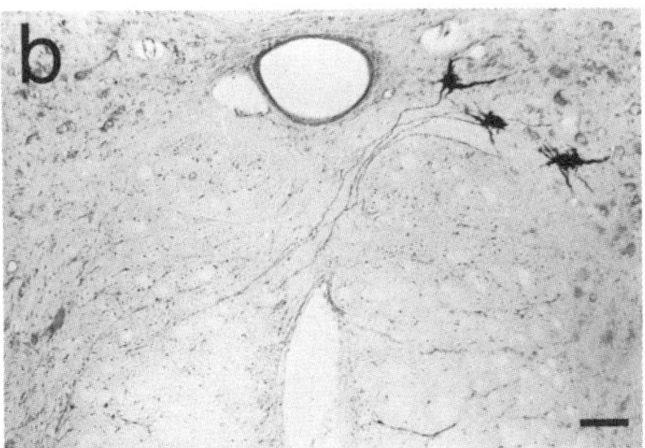

FIG. 3–2. Demonstration of contralateral neck motoneurons in the upper cervical cord of the cat. The cells were stained by retrograde transport after exposure of contralateral nerves supplying the biventer cervicis and complexus muscles to HRP. Note that the reaction product has filled both cell bodies and axons. (a) Dark-field illumination; (b) bright-field illumination. (Reproduced with permission from Abrahams and Keane, *J. Comp. Neurol.*, 1984, 223, 448–456.)

et al. (1987). The neck motoneuron pool deep in the ventral horn had the usual bimodal size distribution, but the motoneurons lying outside the main motor nucleus were uniformly small (Richmond et al., 1978; Abrahams and Keane, 1984). Studies carried out on other spinal segments (Eccles et al., 1960; Bryan et al., 1972; Cullheim, 1978; Cullheim and Ulfhake, 1979; Westbury, 1982), have shown that fusimotor neurons are smaller than alpha motoneurons, and so it is a reasonable assumption that the small neck motoneurons lying outside the main motoneuron pool are fusimotor neurons.

The morphology of neck motoneurons located in the classical motoneuron nuclei has been investigated extensively, using the technique of intracellular staining with HRP (Rose, 1981; Keirstead and Rose, 1983; Vanner and Rose, 1984; Rose et al., 1985). As Figure 3–3 shows, the dendritic trees of these motoneurons are large and complex. However, despite their complexity, the distribution of the dendrites is not random. Dendritic trees of motoneurons innervating the same muscle are usually arranged in the same pattern. For example, motoneurons innervating the neck muscle, biventer cervicis, always have four major dendritic projections. One is directed rostrally, another caudally, one dorsomedially, and one dorsolaterally. Motoneurons supplying other muscles usually have a different dendritic structure. For example, splenius motoneurons, in addition to the four major dendritic projections characteristic of biventer cervicis motoneurons, have a rich projection of dendrites ventral and ventrolateral to their somata. Some exceptions do exist, and it has not been possible to find any major differences between the distribution of dendrites of biventer cervicis and complexus motoneurons, motoneurons that occupy the same region of the ventral horn (Richmond et al., 1978; Rose, 1981; Abrahams and Keane, 1984).

Trapezius muscle motoneurons exist as three morphologically distinct populations, each with its own unique dendritic distribution. These distribution patterns are not associated with the innervation of the three heads of the trapezius muscle—clavotrapezius, acromiotrapezius, and spinotrapezius. Instead, the anatomical differences depend on the position of the motoneurons within

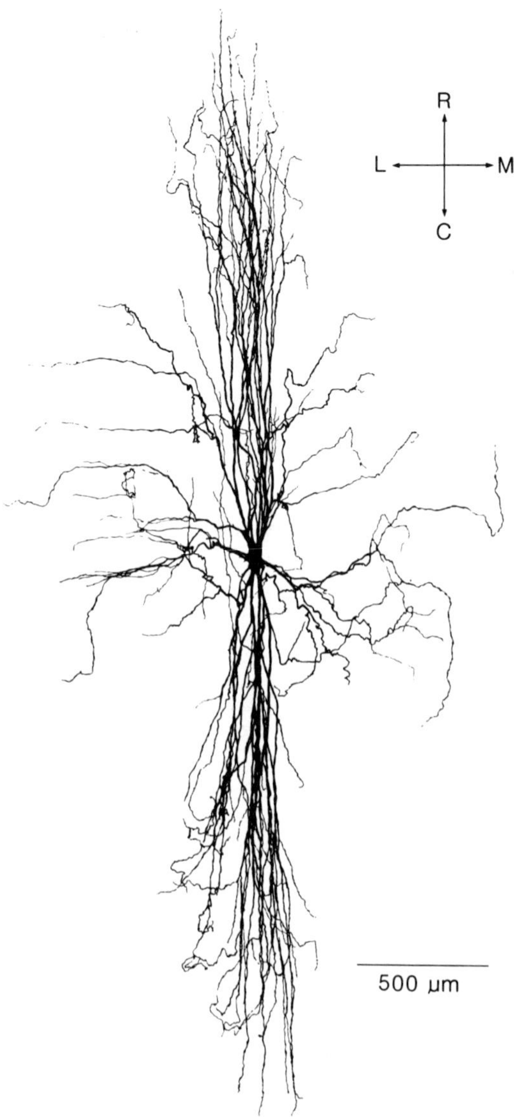

FIG. 3–3. Reconstruction of the dendritic tree of a clavotrapezius motoneuron located at the border of C2 and C3. Horizontal view. R, rostral; C, caudal; M, medial; L, lateral. (Modified from Vanner and Rose, 1984.)

the elongated trapezius motoneuron nucleus. Rostrally located motoneurons have a different dendritic pattern than motoneurons located in the medial portions of the nucleus, and motoneurons in the caudal parts of the nucleus have a different dendritic pattern again.

It has also been found that individual primary dendritic branches of biventer cervicis motoneurons have one of two branching patterns (Rose, 1982). Approximately half of the primary dendrites have branches that are confined to a small region of the territory occupied by the complete dendritic tree. Thus, these dendrites may have branches either dorsolateral to the cell body or rostral to the cell body, but not in both zones. The remaining dendrites have branches that occupy a wider territory, and at least one primary dendrite of each motoneuron has branches distributed throughout most of the region occupied by the complete dendritic tree. The proportion of each type of dendrite is remarkably consistent from motoneuron to motoneuron. Thus, the branching pattern of individual dendrites, as well as the dendritic tree as a whole, appear to be predictable.

It is not yet clear why neck motoneurons have such ordered dendritic patterns. Ramon y Cajal (1909) was the first to suggest that different regions of the dendritic tree of spinal motoneurons might be contacted by different afferent systems. Although this view is still popular (Sprague and Ha, 1964; Scheibel and Scheibel, 1970; Szekely, 1976), the evidence for such an arrangement in neck motoneurons is indirect. It is known that the termination zones of axons of many descending systems that contact neck motoneurons, e.g., vestibulospinal and reticulospinal axons (Wilson and Peterson, 1981), are small and do not project to all the territory occupied by the dendrites of a single neck motoneuron (Nyberg-Hansen, 1966; Petras, 1967). Many of these observations, however, are based on older anterograde degeneration techniques that may give an incorrect answer, since they fail to reveal the total extent of the termination zones of descending axons (see, for example, Martin et al., 1979, Holstege and Kuypers, 1982; Shinoda et al., 1986).

Electron microscopic studies have shown that the somata and proximal dendrites of biventer cervicis and complexus motoneurons are in contact with axon terminals whose morphology is different from that of axon terminals located on distal dendrites (Rose and Neuber, 1987). Over half of the axon terminals found on the soma and proximal dendrites (less than 240 μm from the soma) contain tightly packed vesicles that are either spherical or pleomorphic in shape. In contrast, these boutons are rare on distal dendrites (more than 540 μm from the soma). This would suggest that there is some order in the distribution of afferents on the dendritic tree of neck motoneurons.

NECK MUSCLES IN HEAD MOVEMENT IN THE CONSCIOUS CAT

Consequences of In-Series Organization

The in-series organization of compartments and motor units in neck muscles is not just an anatomical curiosity; it is an important feature that has functional implications for the control of neck motoneurons. Unless the recruitment of motoneurons in individual muscles is coordinated so that contractions occur in an ordered fashion in the serially linked compartments, tension cannot be developed efficiently between the muscle ends. Electromyographic (EMG) studies in chronically implanted animals show that when dorsal neck muscles contract, very similar patterns of EMG activity can be recorded concurrently in each of their serial compartments (Fig. 3–4) (Abrahams and Richmond,

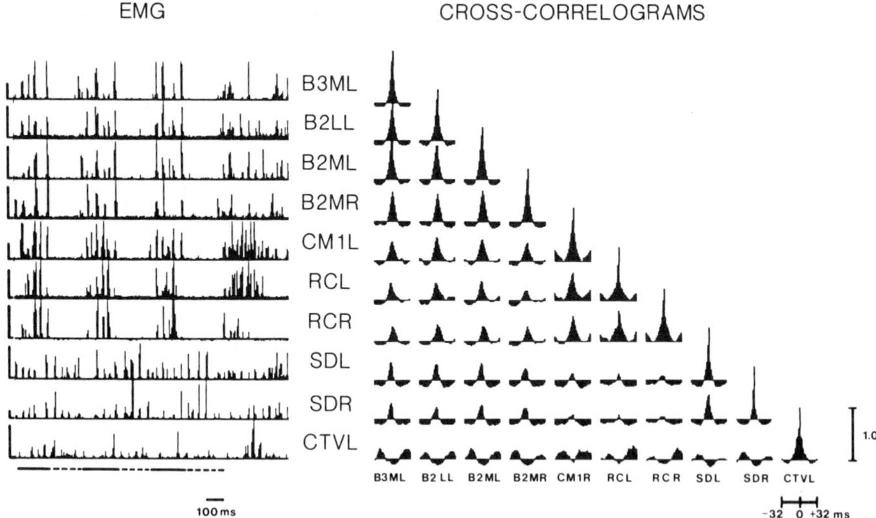

FIG. 3–4. EMG activity and associated cross-correlograms. The EMG records were made during grooming behavior in which the cat licked its paws. Bars at the bottom of the left-hand record indicate head extension. These movements are associated with rhythmic EMG bursts. The matrix of the cross-correlograms shown on the right gives a measure of the synchronization of activity in the muscle pairs indicated. The plot at the right-hand end of each line is the autocorrelation function. Narrow, strongly positive peaks indicate strong synchronization. Negative correlation (below the baseline) indicates alternation of EMG spike bursts. CTVL, left centrotransversarius; SDL, spinalis dorsi, left; SDR, spinalis dorsi, right; RCL, rectus capitis posterior major, left; RCR, rectus capitis posterior major, right; CMIL, complexus, compartment 1, left; B3ML, biventer cervicis, compartment 3 medial, left; B2LL, biventer cervicis, compartment 2 lateral, left; B2ML, biventer cervicis, compartment 2 medial, left; B2MR, biventer cervicis, compartment 2 medial, right. (Reproduced with permission from Vestibulospinal control of posture and locomotion, *Progress in Brain Research*, Pompeiano and Allum, eds., Elsevier, 1988.)

1988). The motor commands responsible for neck muscle contraction thus appear to distribute their effects synchronously to several segmental levels, so that motoneurons supplying different compartments can be recruited in a very similar way. This patterning of EMG activity presumably reflects the capacity of the motor system to match the force development in different linked regions of the muscle in order to balance the tension development in different muscle parts.

Different Levels of Synchronization of Motoneuron Recruitment in Neck Muscles

The coordinated recruitment of motoneurons supplying different in-series compartments represents only one level of synchronization that occurs in the motoneuron nuclei of neck muscles. A second level of motor unit synchronization occurs on a millisecond-by-millisecond basis during some types of head movement and results in the nonrandom firing of motoneurons in a range of concurrently active neck muscles (Loeb et al., 1987). This specialized pattern of synchronization, shown in Figure 3–4, has two features that must be considered when trying to understand the central mechanisms responsible for motoneuron recruitment. First, sets of motor units in a single muscle appear to fire rhythmically in bursts that occur at a single frequency close to 30 Hz. This pattern is distinctly different from that observed in limb muscles, where motoneurons fire asynchronously at frequencies that vary widely (Severin et al, 1967; Hoffer et al., 1981, 1987; DeLuca et al., 1982). Second, the same rhythmical pattern of bursting is simultaneously recorded in most other active muscles. The neural origin of this fine-grained pattern of synchronization is not yet understood. It is perhaps significant that this pattern can be lost if recruitment levels increase markedly or if the nature of the movement is changed. It is less readily observed in muscles with higher proportions of fast fibers such as the clavotrapezius and splenius, although synchronization can be detected in the splenius during certain types of head movements. Synchronization is most apparent in neck muscles acting to produce vertical movements of the head, and this synchronization disappears when similar movements are made with the head turned far to the left or the right. Interestingly, the ventral intervertebral muscles, which are often considered functionally as antagonists to the dorsal musculature, have an episodic pattern of bursting that is out of phase with that of dorsal muscles when the dorsal and ventral muscles are called upon to contract simultaneously. "Short-term synchronization" with features similar to those of the patterns described here has been reported in studies of recruitment in the respiratory motor system (Davies et al., 1985). In the respiratory system, short-term synchrony is thought to derive, at least in part, from the synchronized firing of premotor neurons that relay respiratory commands from higher centers. In the neck, this explanation becomes less plausible because the short-term synchronization extends across so many muscles and occurs during complex movements when the overall phasing of recruitment for different muscles is not at all the same, despite a strong pattern of fine-grained synchrony. The possibility must be explored that propriospinal circuitry may be arranged to ensure the synchronized recruitment of motoneurons throughout many motoneuron nuclei.

The questions of motor control that are posed by the neck musculature are many. The interrelationships between oculomotor and head motor control are still imperfectly understood, as are the interrelationships between head motor control and the other sensory inputs. The complex functional interrelationships within individual compartments of the same muscles, and between the many different muscles that are directly involved in any head movement, whether reflex or voluntary action, are still poorly understood. Suffice it to say that the head motor plant is a very complex plant indeed.

REFERENCES

Abrahams, V. C., Hodgins, M., and Downey, D. (1987). Morphology, distribution, and density of sensory receptors in the glabrous skin of the cat rhinarium. *J. Morphol.* 191, 109–114.

Abrahams, V. C., and Keane, J. (1984). Contralateral, midline, and commissural motoneurons of neck muscles: A retrograde HRP study in the cat. *J. Comp. Neurol.* 223, 448–456.

Abrahams, V. C., and Richmond, F. J. R. (1988). Specialization of sensorimotor organisation in the neck muscle system in Vestibulospinal control of posture and locomotion. *Prog. Brain Res.* 76, 125–135.

Abrahams, V. C., Richmond, F. J. R., and Keane, J. (1984). Projections from C2 and C3 nerves supplying muscles and skin of the cat neck: A study using transganglionic transport of horseradish peroxidase. *J. Comp. Neurol.* 230, 142–154.

Abrahams, V. C., Richmond, F. J. R., and Rose, P. K. (1975). Absence of monosynaptic reflex in dorsal neck muscles of the cat. *Brain Res.* 92, 130–131.

Andres, K. H. (1966). Über die feinstruktur der rezeptoren an sinushaaren. *Z. Zellforschung. Mikrosk. Anat.* 75, 339–365.

Armstrong, J. B., Rose, P. K., Vanner, S., Bakker, G. J., and Richmond, F. J. R. (1988). Compartmentalization of motor units in the cat neck muscle, biventer cervicis. *J. Neurophysiol.* 60, 30–45.

Bakker, D. A., and Abrahams, V. C. (1988). Central projections from nuchal afferent systems. In *Control of Head Movement* (ed. B. Peterson and F. J. R. Richmond). Oxford University Press, pp. 63–75.

Bakker, G. J., and Richmond, F. J. R. (1981). Two types of muscle spindles in cat neck muscles: A histochemical study of intrafusal fiber composition. *J. Neurophysiol.* 45, 973–986.

Bakker, D. A., and Richmond, F. J. R. (1982). Muscle spindle complexes in muscles around upper cervical vertebrae in the cat. *J. Neurophysiol.* 48, 62–74.

Bakker, D. A., Richmond, F. J. R., and Abrahams, V. C. (1984). Central projections from cat suboccipital muscles: A study using transganglionic transport of horseradish peroxidase. *J. Comp. Neurol.* 228, 409–421.

Bakker, D. A., Richmond, F. J. R., Abrahams, V. C., and Courville, J. (1985). Patterns of primary afferent termination in the external cuneate nucleus from cervical axial muscles in the cat. *J. Comp. Neurol.* 241, 467–479.

Brink, E. E., Jinnai, D., and Wilson, V. J. (1981). Pattern of segmental monosynaptic input to cat dorsal neck motoneurons. *J. Neurophysiol.* 46, 496–505.

Bryan, R. N., Trevino, D. L., and Willis, W. D. (1972). Evidence for a common location of alpha and gamma motoneurons. *Brain Res.* 38, 193–96.

Callister, R. J., Brichta, A. M., and Peterson, B. W. (1987). Quantitative analysis of the cervical musculature in rats: Histochemical composition and motor pool organization. II. Deep dorsal muscles. *J. Comp. Neurol.* 255, 369–385.

Chin, N. K., Cope, M., and Pang, M. (1962). Number and distribution of spindle capsules in seven hindlimb muscles of the cat. In *Symposium on Muscle Receptors* (ed. D. Barker). Hong Kong University Press, Hong Kong, pp. 241–248.

Cooper, S., and Daniel, P. M. (1963). Muscle spindles in man, their morphology in the lumbricals and the deep muscles of the neck. *Brain* 86, 563–594.

Cullheim, S. (1978). Relations between cell body size, axon diameter and axon conduction velocity of cat sciatic alpha-motoneurons stained with horseradish peroxidase. *Neurosci. Lett.* 8, 17–26.

Cullheim, S., and Ulfhake, B. (1979). Observations on the morphology of intracellularly stained gamma-motoneurons in relation to their axon conduction velocity. *Neurosci. Lett.* 13, 47–50.

Davies, J. G. M., Kirkwood, P. A., and Sears, T. A. (1985). The distribution of monosynaptic connections from inspiratory bulbospinal neurons to inspiratory motoneurons in the cat. *J. Physiol.* 368, 63–87.

Deluca, C. J., Lefever, R. S., McCue, M. P., and Xenapis, A. P. (1982). Behavior of human motor units in different muscles during linearly varying contractions. *J. Physiol.* 329, 113–128.

Eccles, J. D., Eccles, R. M., Iggo, A., and Lundberg, A. (1960). Electrophysiological studies on gamma motoneurons. *Acta Physiol. Scand.* 50, 32–40.

Eccles, J. C., Eccles, R. M., and Lundberg, A. (1957). The covergence of monosynaptic excitatory afferents on to many different species of alpha motoneurons. *J. Physiol.* 137, 22–50.

Ezure, K., Fukushima, K., Schor, R. H., and Wilson, V. J. (1983). Compartmentalization of the cervicocollic reflex in cat splenius muscle. *Exp. Brain Res.* 51, 397–404.

Harris, L. (1980). The superior colliculus and movements of the head and eyes in cats. *J. Physiol.* 300, 367–391.

Henneman, E., and Mendell, L. M. (1981). Functional organization of motoneuron pool and its inputs. In *Handbook of Physiology*, Vol. I Sect. I., *The Nervous System* (ed. V. E. Brooks). American Physiological Society, Bethesda, Md., pp. 423–507.

Hoffer, J. A., O'Donovan, M. J., Pratt, C. A., and Loeb, G. E. (1981). Discharge patterns in hind limb motoneurons during normal cat locomotion. *Science* 213, 466–468.

Hoffer, J. A., Sugano, N., Loeb, G. E., Marks, W. B., O'Donovan, M. J., and Pratt, C. A. (1987). Cat hindlimb motoneurons during locomotion: II. Normal activity patterns. *J. Neurophysiol.* 57, 530–553.

Holstege, G., and Kuypers, H. G. J. M. (1982). The anatomy of brainstem pathways to the spinal cord of the cat. A labeled amino acid tracing study. *Prog. Brain Res.* 57, 145–157.

Keirstead, S. A., and Rose, P. K. (1983) Dendritic distribution of splenius motoneurons in the cat: Comparison of motoneurons innervating different regions of the muscle. *J Comp. Neurol.* 219, 273–284.

Keirstead, S. A., and Rose, P. K. (1988a). Monosynaptic projections of single muscle spindle afferents to neck motoneurons in the cat. *J. Neurosci.* 8, 3945–3950.

Keirstead, S. A., and Rose, P. K. (1988b). Structure of the intraspinal projections of single, identified muscle spindle afferents from neck muscle of the cat. *J. Neurosci.* 8, 3413–3426.

Loeb, G. E., Yee, W. J., Pratt, C. A., Chanaud, C. M., and Richmond, F. J. R. (1987). Cross-correlation of EMG reveals widespread synchronization of motor units during some slow movements in intact cats. *J. Neurosci. Methods* 21, 239–249.

Magnus, R. (1926). Physiology of posture. *Lancet* 211, 531–536.

Martin, G. F., Humberston, A. O., Jr., Laxson, L. C., Panneton, W. M., and Tschismadia, I. (1979). Spinal projections from the mesencephalic and pontine reticular formation in the North American opossum: A study using axonal transport techniques. *J. Comp. Neurol.* 187, 373–400.

McCouch, G. P., Deering, I. D., and Ling, T. H. (1951). Location of receptor for tonic neck reflexes. *J. Neurophysiol.* 14, 191–195.

Nyberg-Hansen, R. (1966). Functional organization of descending supraspinal fiber systems to the spinal cord. Anatomical observations and physiological correlations. *Ergeb. Anat. Entwicklungsgesch.* 39, 6–42.

Peterson, B. W., Bilotto, G., Fuller, J. H., Goldberg, J., and Leeman, B. (1981). Interaction of vestibular and neck reflexes in the control of gaze. In *Progress in Oculomotor Research* (ed. A. F. Fuchs and W. Becker). Elsevier/North Holland, New York, pp. 335–342.

Petras, J. M. (1967). Cortical, tectal and tegmental fiber connections in the spinal cord of the cat. *Brain Res.* 6, 275–324.

Price, R. F., and Dutia, M. B. (1987). Properties of cat neck muscle spindles and their excitation by succinylcholine. *Exp. Brain Res.* 68, 619–630.

Ramon y Cajal, S. (1909). *Histologie de système nerveux de l'homme et des vertebrés,* Vol. 2. Maloin, Paris, pp. 712–717.

Rapoport, S. R. (1979). Reflex connections of motoneurons of muscles involved in head movement in the cat. *J. Physiol.* 289, 311–327.

Richmond, F. J. R., and Abrahams, V. C. (1975a). Morphology and enzyme histochemistry of dorsal muscles of the cat neck. *J. Neurophysiol.* 38, 1312–1321.

Richmond, F. J. R., and Abrahams, V. C. (1975b). Morphology and distribution of muscle spindles in dorsal muscles of the cat neck. *J. Neurophysiol.* 38, 1322–1339.

Richmond, F. J. R., and Abrahams, V. C. (1979). Physiological properties of muscle spindles in dorsal neck muscles of the cat. *J. Neurophysiol.* 42, 604–617.

Richmond, F. J. R., and Armstrong, J. B. (1988). Fiber architecture and histochemistry in the cat neck muscle, biventer cervicis. *J. Neurophysiol.* 60, 46–59.

Richmond, F. J. R., and Bakker, D. A. (1982). Anatomical organisation and sensory receptor content of soft tissues surrounding upper cervical vertebrae in the cat. *J. Neurophysiol.* 48, 49–61.

Richmond, F. J. R., Bakker, D. A., and Stacey, M. J. (1988). The sensorium: Receptors of neck muscles and joints. In *Control of Head Movement* (ed. B. Peterson and F. J. R. Richmond). Oxford University Press, New York, pp. 49–62.

Richmond, F. J. R., Scott, D. A., and Abrahams, V. C. (1978). Distribution of motoneurons to the neck muscles, biventer cervicis, splenius and complexus in the cat. *J. Comp. Neurol.* 181, 451–464.

Rose, P. K. (1981). Distribution of dendrites from biventer cervicis and complexus motoneurons stained intracellularly with horseradish peroxidase in the adult cat. *J. Comp. Neurol.* 197, 395–409.

Rose, P. K. (1982). Branching structure of motoneuron stem dendrites: A study of neck muscle motoneurons intracellularly stained with horseradish peroxidase in the cat. *J. Neurosci.* 2, 1596–1607.

Rose, P. K., Keirstead, S. A., and Vanner, S. J. (1985). A quantitative analysis of the geometry of cat motoneurons innervating neck and shoulder muscles. *J. Comp. Neurol.* 239, 89–107.

Rose, P. K., and Neuber, M. (1987). Differences in the morphology and frequency of axon terminals on proximal and distal dendrites of neck motoneurons in the cat. *Soc. Neurosci. Abst.* 13, 1695.

Roucoux, A. D., Guitton, D., and Crommelinck, A. (1980). Stimulation of the superior colliculus in the alert cat. II. Eye and head movements evoked when the head is unrestrained. *Exp. Brain Res.* 39, 75–85.

Scheibel, M. E., and Scheibel, A. B. (1970). Of pattern and place in dendrites. *Int. Rev. Neurobiol.* 13, 1–26.

Severin, F. V., Shik, M. L., and Orlovskii, G. N. (1967). Work of the muscles and single motor neurons during controlled locomotion. *Biophysics* 12, 762–772.

Sherrington, C. S. (1897). Decerebrate rigidity and reflex coordination of movements. *J. Physiol.* 22, 319–332.

Shinoda, Y., Ohgaki, T., and Futami, T. (1986). The morphology of single lateral vestibulospinal tract axons in the lower cervical spinal cord of the cat. *J. Comp. Neurol.* 249, 226–241.

Sprague, J. M., and Ha, H. (1964). The terminal fields of dorsal root fibres in the lumbrosacral spinal cord of the cat, and the dendritic organization of the motor nuclei. *Prog. Brain Res.* 11, 120–154.

Szekely, G. (1976). The morphology of motoneurons and dorsal root fibers in the frog's spinal cord. *Brain Res.* 103, 275–290.

Thompson, J. (1970). Parallel spindle systems in the small muscles of the rat tail. *J. Physiol.* 211, 781–789.

Vanner, S. J., and Rose, P. K. (1984). Dendritic distribution of motoneurons innervating the three heads of the trapezius muscle in the cat. *J. Comp. Neurol.* 226, 96–110.

Voss, H. (1958). Zahl und anordnung der muskelspindeln in den unteren Zungenbein- muskeln dem M. sternocleidomastoideus und den mauch- und tiefennackmu- skeln. *Anat. Anz.* 105, 265–275.

Westbury, D. R. (1982). A comparison of the structures of alpha and gamma spinal motoneurons of the cat. *J. Physiol.* 325, 79–91.

Wilson, V. J., and Peterson, B. W. (1981). Vestibulospinal and reticulospinal systems. In *Handbook of Physiology*, Vol. II, Sect. I, *The Nervous System* (ed. V. B. Brooks). American Physiological Society, Bethesda, Md., pp. 667–701.

II

THE ORDERLY RECRUITMENT OF MOTOR UNITS

4

Motor Unit Recruitment in Humans

BLAIR CALANCIE AND PARVEEN BAWA

Contraction of skeletal muscle represents the ultimate expression of the motor division of the mammalian central nervous system (CNS). The resulting muscle output may be directed to articulations of the bones and produce joint rotation or gliding (such as knee extension), or it may act on soft tissues in which muscle fibers originate and/or are inserted (such as lip movements during speech). A primary task of the CNS in its regulation of motor output, then, is to achieve adequate control of the movement parameters produced by muscle contraction.

The group of alpha motoneurons innervating an entire muscle is called the motoneuron "pool" for that muscle. Each motoneuron of the pool innervates a number of muscle fibers of the corresponding muscle to form the motor unit. One way to increase the force output from a muscle is to increase the number of active motor units within the motoneuron pool, a mechanism termed "recruitment." Once a motor unit is recruited, further increases in its force output can be achieved by causing the discharge rate to rise, a mechanism termed "rate coding." The relative importance of recruitment and rate coding for the control of muscle parameters, including force, seems to vary with the muscle examined (Milner-Brown et al., 1973b; Harrison, 1983).

After the initial observations by Denny-Brown (1929) on the recruitment order of slow versus fast muscles, the first systematic studies on patterns of motor unit recruitment in animals were done by Henneman and co-workers (Henneman, 1957; Henneman et al., 1965, 1974). It was demonstrated that in decerebrate or chloralose-anesthetized cats, a net excitatory input to a motoneuron pool led to the recruitment of motor units in order of increasing conduction velocity (Clamann et al., 1974; Henneman and Mendell, 1981; Bawa et al., 1984). Since axonal conduction velocity and diameter are directly related (Hursh, 1939; Burke et al., 1982), it follows that smaller motoneurons within a pool show higher susceptibility to discharge than larger motoneurons. This relationship has become known as Henneman's "size principle" of motoneuron recruitment (Henneman et al., 1965).

The functional significance of this size principle is of real importance for how the CNS controls force production. It is now well known that muscle units innervated by small motoneurons tend to produce small twitch and tetanic forces but are highly resistant to fatigue (Henneman and Olson, 1965; Burke, 1967, 1981). Conversely, large motoneurons tend to produce high twitch and tetanic tensions but are easily fatigued. The orderly recruitment of small before large motoneurons would then allow for smooth increments of force at any level of contraction (Henneman and Olson, 1965; Harrison, 1983). Moreover, movements or behaviors requiring only small forces could be continued for long periods with little or no fatigue.

Various presynaptic and postsynaptic mechanisms underlying this strong correlation between motor unit size and recruitment order have been suggested (Burke, 1981; Sypert and Munson, 1981; Luscher et al., 1983; Gustafsson and Pinter, 1985; Henneman, 1985; Heckman and Binder, 1988; Chapters 9, 10, and 17, this volume). These studies have concentrated on electrophysiological and morphological properties of motoneurons and their inputs, and as such have relied almost exclusively on animal models.

The animal studies cited previously have typically used invasive surgical techniques designed to allow testing of a variety of excitatory and inhibitory inputs to different motoneuron pools. Obviously, such invasive procedures are not possible with human subjects, but the latter provide their own important advantage over animals; that is, the range of behaviors available to study patterns of recruitment is far more extensive and subtle in humans. The validity of the size principle in human subjects has been tested through an examination of motor unit recruitment and derecruitment patterns produced by various inputs to motoneuron pools. These inputs include (1) voluntary contractions, (2) reflex contractions, and (3) recruitment following stimulation of the motor cortex. In the following discussion, results both in support of and contrary to the size principle for motoneuron recruitment in humans will be reviewed for each of these inputs to the motoneuron pool.

VOLUNTARY CONTRACTIONS

Slow Ramp Contractions

Adrian and Bronk (1929) were the first to report on the discharge pattern of single motor units in human subjects, using concentric needle electrodes. Later studies showed that during slowly increasing voluntary contractions, the electromyographic (EMG) potentials increased in amplitude with progressively stronger contractions (Denny-Brown and Pennybacker, 1938; Kugelberg and Skoglund, 1946; Buchthal et al., 1954). This recruitment pattern was believed to be a statistical artifact of the recording method. That is, the small EMG potentials first seen during the initial portion of a slowly increasing contraction were considered to be due to the activity of muscle fibers distant to the recording electrode. Recruitment of larger potentials following increases in contraction strength was thought to reflect activity in nearby fibers (Kugelberg and Skoglund, 1946; Buchthal et al., 1954). The fact that this recruitment pattern was not a function of the spatial relationship between recording electrode and active muscle fibers, but rather was entirely consistent with Henneman's size principle, was pointed out by Olson et al. (1968).

The first demonstration of orderly recruitment of motor units in humans can be credited to Stein and co-workers (Milner-Brown et al., 1973a). These authors used the spike-triggered averaging (STA) technique (Mendell and Henneman, 1971; Stein et al., 1972) to extract the average-twitch waveform produced by the contraction of identified single motor units of the first dorsal interosseous (FDI) muscle from the force fluctuations of the whole muscle. This information allowed these authors to compare directly the twitch amplitudes and contraction times of single motor units with the voluntary force, or recruitment force "threshold," at which the unit began to discharge. The measurement of threshold was done during a slowly increasing isometric contraction from rest. A positive and significant linear correlation was found between the twitch tension of a motor unit and its recruitment threshold. Furthermore, the number of units with small twitch tensions greatly exceeded the number with larger twitch tensions (Milner-Brown et al., 1973a), as had previously been shown in the cat (Henneman and Olson, 1965). These findings led Milner-Brown et al. (1973a) to conclude that slow isometric contractions in the human FDI muscle led to orderly recruitment of motor units, in accordance with the size principle.

Figure 4–1 shows an example of orderly recruitment for motor units from the flexor carpi radialis muscle of four subjects, two male (panel A) and two female (panel B). Motor unit twitch amplitude was obtained using the STA

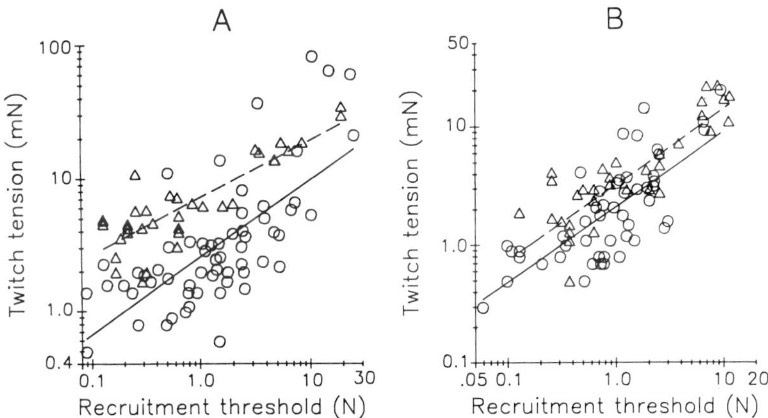

Fig. 4–1. Log-log plot of twitch tension (mN) versus recruitment threshold (N) for single motor units of the flexor carpi radialis muscle in four subjects. A first-order linear regression was calculated and plotted for the least-squares differences between points. A significant correlation between twitch tension and recruitment threshold was found for all subjects. (A) Results from two male subjects ($r = 0.67$, ○; 0.76, △). (B) Results from two female subjects ($r = 0.74$, ○; 0.84, △).

technique. A given value was plotted against the unit's recruitment threshold as measured during the initial rising phase of a slow isometric contraction. For each subject, a significant positive correlation was observed between these parameters, indicating that small motoneurons are the first to be recruited at the onset of contraction, while larger cells are recruited only at higher levels of voluntary effort.

Indicators of motor unit size besides twitch amplitude include the motor axon or muscle fiber conduction velocity (Freund et al., 1975; Andreasson and Arendt-Nielson, 1987; Dengler et al., 1988); and the amplitude of the evoked EMG waveform measured with intramuscular electrodes (Goldberg and Derfler, 1977; Sussman et al., 1977; Eriksson et al., 1984). Using these different criteria, orderly recruitment of motor units during slow contractions has been reported in a wide variety of muscles, including the temporalis (Yemm, 1977), masseter (Goldberg and Derfler, 1977; Yem, 1977; Desmedt and Godaux, 1979), digastric (Sussman et al., 1977), extensor digitorum communis (Monster and Chan, 1977; Thomas et al., 1978), abductor pollicus brevis (Schmidt and Thomas, 1981; Thomas et al., 1987), first dorsal interosseous (Milner-Brown et al., 1973a; Freund et al., 1975; Stephens and Usherwood, 1977; Schmidt and Thomas, 1981; DeLuca et al., 1982; Thomas et al., 1986), adductor pollicis (Hainaut et al., 1981), abductor digiti minimi (Tanji and Kato, 1973), deltoid (DeLuca et al., 1982), flexor carpi radialis (Calancie and Bawa, 1985b), extensor indicis (Freund et al., 1975; Henneman et al., 1976), tibialis anterior (Desmedt and Godaux, 1977b), and vastus lateralis (Cremer et al., 1983) muscles.

Thus, there seems to be general agreement that motor unit recruitment during slow voluntary contractions takes place in accordance with the size principle. Exceptions to this conclusion have been few, and usually involve cases where the muscle being studied is not acting as a prime mover but is working as a synergist in a particular movement. For example, Desmedt and Godaux (1981) found that 8% of the 142 pairs of motor units recorded from the FDI muscle consistently reversed their recruitment order in contractions producing flexion compared to abduction of the index finger. The correlation coefficient between motor unit twitch tension and recruitment threshold was significantly higher for abduction (where FDI acts as the prime mover) than for flexion (where FDI acts as a synergist) of the index finger (Desmedt and Godaux, 1981). This "deordering" of motor unit recruitment during flexion was explained in terms of differences in the distribution of central connections onto the FDI motoneuron pool when acting as a prime mover (for which input was evenly distributed) as opposed to a synergist (for which input was selectively distributed).

Results similar to those of Desmedt and Godaux (1981) for the FDI muscle were obtained by Thomas et al. (1986), who extended these studies to include the abductor pollicis brevis (APB) muscle (Thomas et al., 1987). These authors found that the rank orders of recruitment for motor units during contractions in different directions of the FDI and APB muscles were correlated for both muscles but were not identical, indicating some direction-dependent reversals of recruitment order between different motor units.

As a last example, "disorderly" recruitment between motor unit pairs was observed in the extensor digitorum muscle by Thomas et al. (1978). In these cases, some motor unit pairs whose action potentials were "visible" at the same recording site acted on separate digits, resulting in distorted threshold readings. Thus, the disorderly recruitment observed was probably a result of mechanical artifact, rather than an exception to the size principle (Thomas et al., 1978).

There is evidence from animal experiments that some portions of a muscle, and the motor units within those portions, may be involved in motor tasks quite distinct from the tasks to which other units of the muscle contribute (Loeb, 1985; Chapter 1, this volume). An example of such organization in human subjects has been shown in the biceps brachii, which contributes to both flexion and supination of the forearm. Recordings from the long head of the biceps revealed populations of motor units that discharged exclusively for specific tasks, while other units discharged during several tasks (Ter Haar Romeny et al., 1982). Furthermore, the locations of these populations were confined to specific portions of the muscle (Ter Haar Romeny et al., 1984). These findings support the concept of "task-specific" motor unit subpopulations within multifunctional muscles, raising the possibility that the size principle may govern the order of motor unit recruitment within subpopulations of a pool, but that it may not apply universally across the entire motoneuron pool.

One should, however, remember that multifunctional muscles contribute not only to two or three directions of force (for example, flexion and abduction of the index finger for the FDI) but to a continuum of movement directions. The use of "task groups," then, necessitates a continuum of patterns of central connectivities onto the same motoneuron pool (Desmedt, 1980) or requires a large number of task groups for one muscle. At present, the organization and distribution of excitatory connections from the motor cortex onto alpha motoneurons are not well understood, although these problems are being actively investigated (Fetz and Cheney, 1980; Cheney et al., 1985; Lemon and Mantel, 1987; Chapter 20, this volume). Thus, at present, it is difficult to know how much consideration should be given to task groups as an explanation for disorderly recruitment.

An alternative explanation for these observed recruitment reversals between motor unit pairs is the change in the mechanical output of the muscle unit when measured in different directions of contraction. That is, the reported twitch tensions extracted by STA are seldom, if ever, corrected for the lever length and the direction of the force vector of each motor unit. Consider three motor units, A, B, and C, in a muscle whose fibers are primarily aligned in different directions, as shown in Figure 4–2. Also consider that for all movements, the recruitment order from resting is, first, A, then B, then C, and the maximal twitch tensions of these units, when measured along their main axes of contraction, are 0.5, 0.75, and 1.0 g, respectively. When the muscle acts as a prime mover, the twitch tensions extracted from the three units are 0.47, 0.75, and 0.94 g, respectively. The recruitment threshold and twitch tensions show a good correlation during isometric contraction in this direction. However, when the muscle acts as a synergist at an angle of 50 degrees, the observed twitch tensions are 0.43, 0.48, and 0.34 g, respectively. In this case, it would appear that the "smallest" motor unit, C, has the highest threshold.

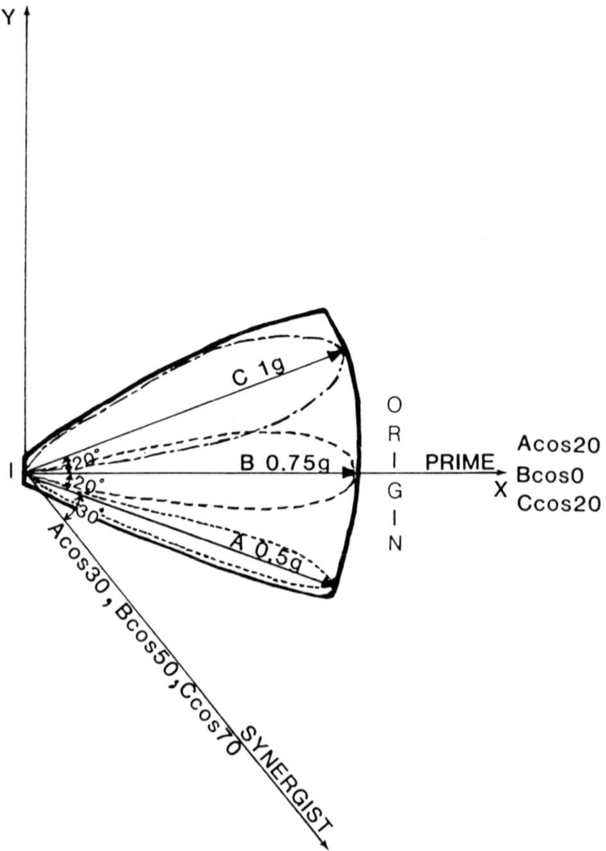

Fig. 4–2. Schematic representation of the influence of muscle geometry on force output. The thick continuous line marks the boundary of a muscle in the X–Y plane. The insertion of the muscle is shown at I, and the muscle fibers originate in a broad band. The boundaries of three muscle units, A, B, and C, are shown by dotted lines; they exert their optimal forces along −20, 0, and 20 degrees, respectively. The muscle acts as a prime mover if it exerts force along 0 degrees and as a synergist when it exerts force at −50 degrees. All contractions are considered in one plane.

Even though the order of recruitment of these units within the motoneuron pool is the same in each case, the correlation of recruitment threshold and twitch tension is very different. Thomas et al. (1986, 1987) observed that for FDI and APB motor units, the twitch tensions, when measured in the prime direction of contraction, exceeded those for each muscle acting as a synergist in another direction of contraction. However, the absolute number of reversals was relatively small. This raises the question of whether or not these few reversals are of any real significance in influencing the strategies employed by the CNS for motoneuron recruitment, or instead can be attributed to low levels of "noise" within the system.

Fast Ballistic Contractions

Recruitment according to the size principle is intuitively appealing in describing the control of slowly increasing contractions starting from rest. That is, force increments have been shown to be approximately linear with increasing effort (Milner-Brown et al., 1973a), and the effects of fatigue are minimized by ensuring that the fatigable units do not begin contributing to force production until well after the contraction is initiated.

By the same reasoning, it is tempting to speculate that contractions that reach their peak force quickly might be best accomplished by the exclusive recruitment of fast-twitch, fatigable units. The rapid contraction time would allow faster movement times, and the duration of the contraction would be short enough to prevent any significant fatigue effect. Indeed, this type of recruitment pattern for *whole muscle* has been reported during the rapid paw shake of a cat hindlimb in response to cutaneous stimulation of the pad (Smith et al., 1980). In this case, the slowly contracting soleus muscle remains virtually silent during the rapidly alternating limb movements (cycle time approximately 88 ms) that form the paw shake. It is believed that participation of the soleus would slow down the maximum rate of this alternating behavior and interfere with its usefulness.

The previous example (Smith et al., 1980) does not address the question of selective recruitment of motor unit types *within* a pool during rapid movements. There have been reports that under certain conditions it is possible for human subjects to "learn" how to influence the recruitment order of motor units with different thresholds (Basmajian, 1963). Typically, these conditions occur during the production of rapid contractions, and when the subject has both visual and audible feedback of the unit's discharge.

This position was gradually adopted by Grimby, Hannerz, and co-workers in a series of papers beginning in the late 1960s. These authors began by describing occasional reversals of recruitment order during slow contractions in human subjects (Ashworth et al., 1967), a point that Henneman and co-workers also reported in animal experiments (Henneman et al., 1965). Subsequent reports led to descriptions of motor unit "rotations," where the first unit to discharge during a rapid contraction then fell silent, while the second unit that discharged in the initial phase of the contraction continued to discharge during a plateau in the contraction strength (Grimby and Hannerz, 1968). Even more extreme was the outcome of a later study, where for rapid voluntary contractions it was concluded that "normal man can select in advance the recruitment order of motor units most appropriate for the work intended" (Hannerz and Grimby, 1973, p. 275). In other words, the recruitment order of motoneurons was not fixed due to an even distribution of excitatory input from all sources (Henneman and Mendell, 1981; Henneman, 1985), but was instead under constant central influence, and in some cases could be modified by volitional control.

Desmedt and Godaux carried out a rigorous series of studies to address the question of disorderly recruitment during rapid contractions, and for the most part were unable to repeat the findings of Grimby and Hannerz. These authors found that the relative order of recruitment of motor unit pairs from the tibialis anterior during slow ramp contractions was the same as that for fast ballistic contractions (Desmedt and Godaux, 1977a). There were occasional recruitment reversals (about 11% of trials), but these almost always involved units with similar recruitment thresholds as measured during slow ramp contractions (Desmedt and Godaux, 1977b). Similar results were reported for motor units in the vastus lateralis during rapid alternating knee flexion and extension (Cremer et al., 1983).

Nonisometric or Dynamic Contractions

In daily use, most muscles contribute to a mixture of isometric, lengthening, and shortening contractions. However, the great majority of studies of motor unit recruitment patterns in humans have been restricted to the examination of isometric contractions. There is some evidence to suggest that less constrained movements, which may include multiple degrees of freedom, take place with more frequent "reversals" in the orderly recruitment of motoneurons than are seen during isometric contractions.

For example, Thomas et al. (1987) examined recruitment order during isometric contractions of the FDI and APB muscles during isometric contractions and showed orderly motor unit recruitment (Thomas et al., 1986, 1987). Following this, they had subjects open and close a pair of scissors and looked at the recruitment order between pairs of units in either muscle. These authors concluded that, for the most part, orderly recruitment was preserved during these movements for both motoneuron pools (Thomas et al., 1987). However, there were still many cases in which recruitment reversals were seen, both for unit pairs of similar voluntary threshold and for units with widely dissimilar thresholds. To illustrate, 100% orderly recruitment was demonstrated in only 36% and 22% of the unit pairs from FDI and APB muscles, respectively; other unit pairs showed at least some reversals during these shortening contractions. No doubt the distribution of axonal conduction velocities contributed to at least some of these reversals, whereby as much as 5–10 ms latency difference at the muscle may occur for two motoneurons that discharged simultaneously in the spinal cord (Desmedt and Godaux, 1981; Thomas et al., 1987). However, Thomas et al. (1987) could not rule out the possibility that the increased complexity of the motor task may have contributed to the relatively high incidence of reversals seen in that study.

A conclusion that the recruitment pattern of motor units during shortening contractions can be *very* different from that seen during isometric contractions was reached by Kato et al. (1985). They found that motor units in the tibialis anterior muscle had characteristic muscle *lengths* (or angles of ankle rotation) at which they were recruited. The recruitment order of units was not fixed among units with similar length "ranges," but did tend to be orderly between units with widely dissimilar length ranges. This conclusion is similar to that for the recruitment order during slow isometric contractions of motor units with similar force thresholds: When they do occur, reversals involve units with similar thresholds but do not occur between units with widely separated thresholds.

The recruitment order of motor units from the parasternal intercostal muscles was examined in a group of subjects producing voluntary hyperventilation (Watson and Whitelaw, 1987). It was found that units with low thresholds often exhibited reversals after several cycles of breathing. This disorderly recruitment reverted to normal approximately 10 min after hyperventilation ended. At no time, however, was there evidence of reversals between units of widely dissimilar thresholds; that is, there were no "major shifts between slow and fast motor units" (Watson and Whitelaw, 1987).

Thus, at this point, there is little evidence to suggest that motor unit recruitment order during nonisometric contractions differs markedly from that during isometric contractions. Although the absolute number of reversals observed is higher in nonisometric contractions, these examples typically involve units with similar thresholds. Since normal movements are likely to involve movements in more than one direction, it may be that the reversals that have been reported (Thomas et al., 1987; Watson and Whitelaw, 1987) are attributable to at least some of the factors discussed earlier under "Slow Ramp Contractions."

REFLEX CONTRACTIONS

Muscle Afferents

The majority of the previously mentioned studies from various laboratories support the concept of a stereotyped recruitment pattern of motor units for voluntary contractions in humans. A variety of reflex inputs to motoneuron pools have also been used to examine recruitment, and again a stereotypical recruitment pattern of small-to-large motoneurons has typically been observed, at least for some types of reflex input.

The tonic vibration reflex (TVR) was elicited from motoneurons of the masseter and soleus muscles in normal subjects. The recruitment order observed was consistent with that of voluntary contractions, in support of the size principle (Desmedt and Godaux, 1975, 1978). The same authors examined the pattern of reflex *inhibition* of soleus motoneurons first recruited during the H-reflex and then derecruited by vibration of the Achilles tendon. They demonstrated orderly derecruitment consistent with the size principle (Desmedt and Godaux, 1978).

An afferent input that is arguably more "physiological" than vibration is that produced by the tendon tap. Buller et al. (1980) showed that taps to the belly of the first or second dorsal interosseous muscle caused an increased probability of short-latency discharge of tonically active motor units. Furthermore, these units that were most responsive to the afferent input were also the first to be recruited during a slow voluntary isometric contraction. These authors also saw a small increase in response probability at a long latency following the tendon tap and suggested that this latter response represented the contribution of the "functional stretch reflex" (Melville Jones and Watt, 1971).

The previously mentioned study by Buller et al. (1980) did not fully explore the reflex response patterns of motor units, since these authors examined only the tonically firing units and did not examine the recruitment order during the late component of this reflex. We studied the reflex discharge pattern of motor units from the flexor carpi radialis for a variety of background contraction strengths and for different magnitudes of ramp wrist extensions produced by a torque motor (Calancie and Bawa, 1985a, 1985b). Figure 4–3 summarizes these findings. The top panel (A) shows the averaged EMG from wrist flexors following ramp wrist extension. As with other upper limb muscles, there are two distinct periods of reflex responses: short latency (SL, or "M1"; onset 25 ms poststimulus and long latency (LL, or "M2–3"; onset, 50–60 ms poststimulus). The short-latency reflex has been interpreted as corresponding to the

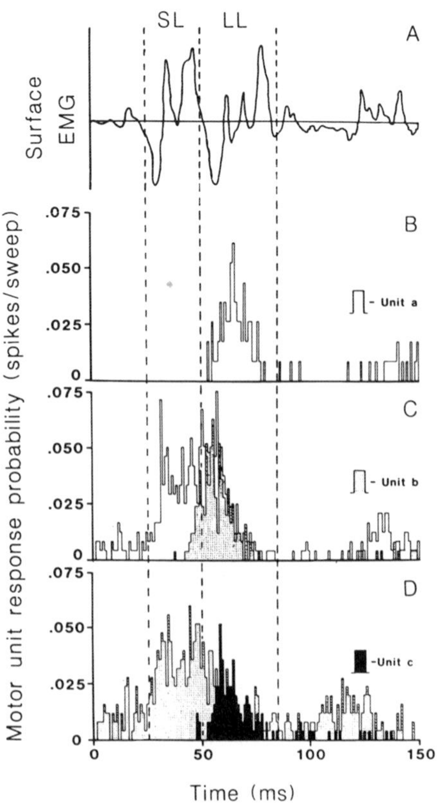

Fig. 4–3. (A) Average unrectified surface EMG from wrist flexor muscles in response to a sudden wrist extension via a torque motor. Two distinct periods of reflex activity are seen: SL, 25–50 ms; LL, 50–90 ms. Below are poststimulus time histograms showing the discharge pattern of three single motor units from the flexor carpi radialis recorded simultaneously in response to different background contractions (preloads) and wrist perturbation magnitudes (loads). The thresholds for recruitment during voluntary contraction were 114, 189, and 810 g for units **a**, **b**, and **c**, respectively. (B) The combination of no preload and a moderate load caused recruitment of only unit **a**. (C) Following a stronger preload (but the same load), unit a now discharges during the SL period, and unit **b** is recruited to discharge during the LL period. (D) Both preload and load have been further increased to cause recruitment of unit c during the LL portion of the stretch reflex.

familiar spinal monosynaptic reflex. The origin of the long-latency reflex remains controversial. It may involve polysynaptic pathways, including a transcortical reflex arc (Phillips, 1969; Marsden et al., 1976) or may include contributions from cutaneous (Darton et al., 1985) or other afferents (Cody et al., 1987).

Motor unit recordings from the flexor carpi radialis following rapid wrist extension revealed that when a unit just began to discharge during the stretch reflex, it did so almost totally during the long-latency period. This is shown in the poststimulus time histograms of unit discharge in panels B, C, and D of Figure 4–3 for units **a**, **b**, and **c**, respectively. With increases in either the background contraction (preload) or magnitude of the wrist perturbation (load), the response probability of a unit increased and the latency to discharge decreased. Making the unit tonic by increasing the preload resulted in a reflex response confined mostly to the short-latency period. Furthermore, additional units began to discharge under these conditions, always starting during the long-latency period. The recruitment order observed during the stretch reflex was identical to that seen during voluntary isometric contractions. That is, the three units illustrated had recruitment thresholds during a slow voluntary ramp contraction of 114, 189, and 810 g, respectiveley. Finally, under any combination of loading conditions, the reflex response probability of the lower-threshold unit virtually always exceeded that of the higher-threshold unit. From these observations, we concluded that motor unit recruitment during both the long- and short-latency components of the stretch reflex was in accordance with the size principle (Calancie and Bawa, 1985b).

Cutaneous Afferents

While the evidence in support of orderly motor unit recruitment following activation of muscle afferents is good, this conclusion does not appear to describe fully the recruitment pattern following inputs to the motoneuron pool arising from *cutaneous* receptors. Garnett and Stephens (1980, 1981) examined the effects of index finger digital nerve stimulation on the discharge properties and recruitment thresholds of motor units from the FDI muscle. Following a period of stimulation of the digital nerves, the voluntary recruitment threshold for low-threshold units increased, while high-threshold units showed a reduction in threshold for voluntary discharge (Garnett and Stephens, 1981). These authors concluded that the distribution of input to the motoneuron pools for cutaneous afferents may be different from that seen for muscle afferents, and may be preferentially organized with respect to motor unit type (Garnett and Stephens, 1980).

It could be argued that such cutaneous stimulation as employed by Garnett and Stephens (1980, 1981) is unphysiological, making the results difficult to interpret (Meinck et al., 1983). However, findings similar in essence to those reported by Garnett and Stephens were published by Kanda and Desmedt (1983). These authors recorded motor unit pairs from the FDI muscle during precision grip and found that 20% of the units studied showed reductions in threshold to voluntary contraction following cutaneous stimulation caused by rubbing the volar tips of the thumb and index finger against each other. All of the units that showed threshold changes were high-threshold ones, such that recruitment reversals were often seen. The great majority of low-threshold units were unaffected by the stimulation. Kanda and Desmedt (1983) concluded that cutaneous stimulation facilitates the recruitment of high-threshold units while apparently delaying the recruitment of low-threshold motor units.

In a study on the influence of a different category of cutaneous receptors, the effect of noxious stimulation of the lower lip on the tonic discharge of motor units recorded from the masseter muscle was examined (Miles and Turker 1986; Miles et al., 1987). These authors reported that motoneurons that were discharging at a constant rate of 10 pulses per second (pps) were equally inhibited by the stimulation. They concluded that it is the firing rate, rather than the motoneuron size, that determines the cell's susceptibility to inhibition, a conclusion that clearly contradicts the size principle of recruitment. However, an alternative explanation for these findings is that they do indeed support the original observation by Henneman et al. (1965) on orderly derecruitment of motoneurons for inhibitory inputs to a pool. With a constant excitatory input to a motoneuron pool, small motoneurons are at a higher level of excitation (and thus have a higher discharge rate) than large ones. An inhibitory input silences those motoneurons whose threshold for tonic discharge has just been exceeded, which tend to be the larger motoneurons. In the paradigm of Miles and co-workers, each motoneuron's inhibitability was tested by first raising its excitation to approximately the same level (i.e., causing it to discharge at 10 pps). Under such conditions, each motoneuron was equally inhibited by the noxious stimulus to the lip, suggesting a functionally equivalent distribution of inhibitory input to all motoneurons of the pool (see Chapter 10, this volume), leading to derecruitment in accordance with the size principle (Henneman and Mendell, 1981).

TRANSCUTANEOUS CORTICAL STIMULATION

Until the beginning of the 1980s, it was possible to activate motor units in only two ways: either through voluntary contractions or by accessing a reflex pathway with appropriate afferent stimulation. A third method has now emerged that results in reliable, consistent, noninvasive stimulation of motor areas of the cerebral cortex, using either electrical (Merton and Morton, 1980; Marsden et al., 1983; Rossini et al., 1985; Amassian et al., 1987) or magnetic (Barker et al., 1985; Hess et al., 1986; Barker et al., 1987; Hess et al., 1987) stimulation. This method avoids the difficulties in obtaining identical voluntary contractions for examining central motor output. Electrodes or a coil are positioned on or immediately above the scalp overlying the precentral motor region. Adequate stimulation results in short-latency contraction of muscle groups on the contralateral side of the body. Electrical stimulation is stronger and hence more effective in eliciting limb muscle contractions than current versions of magnetic stimulation. Considering the novelty of the technique and the ethical considerations associated with its use, very little work has appeared on motor unit recruitment using this method of activation.

In a recent study, Calancie et al. (1987) examined the discharge of motor units from wrist flexor and extensor muscles in response to different strengths of electrical cortical stimulation. In the majority of cases, only one motor unit was discharging rhythmically and repetitively (i.e., tonic discharge) at the time of application of cortical stimulation, and no attempts were made to examine the discharge properties of two or more motor units firing simultaneously. The question of orderly motoneuron recruitment was not of primary interest in this study, and the authors stated that they could not determine whether or not orderly recruitment occurred, due to an inability to establish reliably the relative thresholds to cortical stimulation of motor unit *pairs*.

However, there were some cases in which the discharge pattern and threshold of a unit, when tonic, were compared to the properties of the same unit made nontonic by a reduction in the background contraction. In these instances, the one unit that had been tonic was the first to be recruited at the threshold for cortical stimulation when nontonic. This is shown in Figure 4–4. The tonic unit discharged in response to a weak (30% of maximum output, corresponding to ~250 V and 200 mA) stimulus strength in approximately 50% of the trials (left side). When nontonic following a partial relaxation of the background contraction, an identical stimulus (30%) failed to elicit any unit discharge (not shown). It was only when the stimulus strength was increased to 40% that

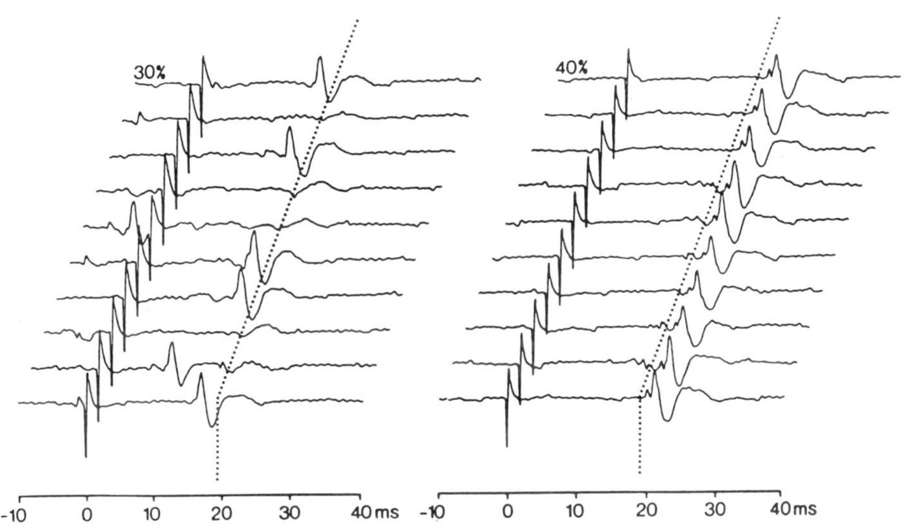

Fig. 4–4. Individual traces of the discharge of a motor unit from the flexor carpi radialis in response to transcranial cortical stimulation. Stimulation is at time 0 and can be seen in each trace as the stimulus artifact. The dotted line crosses each trace at 19 ms. The left panel illustrates a unit that was discharging tonically at the time of stimulus and, in some cases, responded to the stimulus at a latency of ~17 ms. Reducing the preload to cause this unit to fall silent and then increasing the strength of the cortical stimulus resulted in the same unit being the first to discharge (right), indicating the same recruitment order for voluntary contraction as for transcranial cortical stimulation.

recruitment was seen (right side), and then the same unit as before was recruited. This pattern was consistently observed, indicating that the motor pathways accessed by the cortical stimulus lead to a recruitment order consistent with that seen during voluntary contractions. That is, motor unit recruitment in wrist flexors and extensors following transcranial cortical stimulation occurs in accordance with the size principle. A similar conclusion for motor units of the abductor digiti quinti and tibialis anterior muscles can be made based on observations reported in a recent paper by Zidar et al. (1987).

DISCUSSION AND CONCLUSIONS

Some of the situations described earlier, in which it appears that the size principle does not adequately describe the recruitment pattern of human motor units, may reflect limitations of the measuring techniques themselves. For example, in animal experiments, forces are measured directly at the tendon, whereas in human subjects, only torques about a joint are measurable. The twitch tensions computed from torque values are difficult to establish. Passive viscoelastic properties of the joint and the soft tissue also affect the measured torques.

In addition, the twitch mechanical parameters (twitch tension and contraction time) obtained with the STA technique are differentially affected for different muscle units because of partial fusion of force (Calancie and Bawa, 1986). That is, the minimum rhythmic firing rates of motor unit discharge used for STA affect the apparent contraction times and twitch amplitudes of low-threshold (presumably slow-twitch) motor units more than those of higher-threshold (fast-twitch) motor units. This effect enhances the apparent correlation between twitch tension and recruitment threshold for a population of motor units with widely dissimilar mechanical parameters (Calancie and Bawa, 1986).

Another difficulty can arise due to cross-talk between different muscles or muscle sections. It is generally assumed that a microelectrode inserted in a particular muscle is detecting activity only from that muscle, and that the neighboring muscles are electrically insulated from each other. However, this may not always be the case. For example, if one elicits a stretch reflex in the triceps surae muscle group of a decerebrate cat and then cuts the muscle nerve to the medial gastrocnemius (MG), it is still possible to record distinct motor unit potentials with a microelectrode inserted in the MG on the far side of the soleus. Clearly, this is soleus-lateral gastrocnemius (LGS) activity being recorded from within an inactive MG muscle due to volume conduction (Binder and Bawa, unpublished observations). Such a situation has been demonstrated when testing motor unit recruitment during contractions in different directions (e.g., Thomas et al., 1978).

Further difficulties can be seen in determining the absolute threshold to motor unit recruitment during a slowly increasing isometric contraction. Typically, the estimate of recruitment thresholds is made at the beginning of a contraction. However, once a unit has been discharging for several minutes, it is not unusual for its apparent threshold to either increase or decrease, as shown in Figure 4–5. Oscilloscope tracings are shown for three motor units discharging simultaneously, whose thresholds were in the order of increasing action potential size. The four panels represent four different times following the initiation of the contraction. The largest unit was recruited initially at a threshold force of ~ 1N (panel B), and its discharge was maintained at its minimum rhythmic firing rate. Panel C shows the force and EMG 5 min after the onset of the contraction; it can be seen that although the largest unit continued to discharge, the total force declined and the smaller units had ceased to discharge. Following momentary relaxation (at which time all units stopped firing) with subsequent contraction, panel D shows that all three motor units were again discharging and that the order of recruitment was the same as that seen in panels A and B. However, the threshold force had declined substantially for all three units, with the largest unit being most affected. Thus, measurement of the recruitment threshold of these units following repetitive discharge may sometimes give values quite different from those seen at the onset of contraction preceded by a period of rest, and may lead to erroneous cases of recruitment reversals.

Such observations of gradual changes in the threshold for tonic discharge of motor units are common, and one can only speculate on the underlying mechanisms governing these changes. Segmental mechanisms, namely, Ib inhibition, presynaptic inhibition, Renshaw cell inhibition, and thyxotropic properties of the passive tissues, may contribute to these observations.

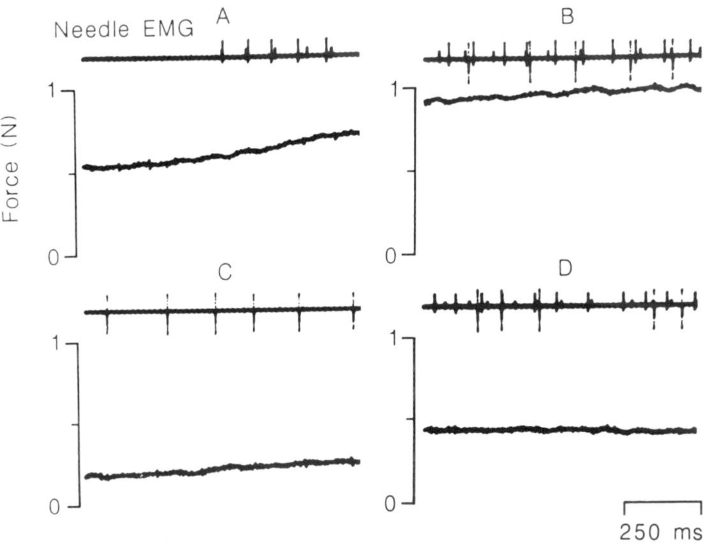

Fig. 4–5. Motor unit discharge (top) and force of wrist flexion (bottom) at four different times following the beginning of a voluntary isometric contraction. The thresholds for the two smaller unit potentials are almost identical at about 0.6 N (A), and the threshold for the largest unit potential (B) is approximately 1.0 N. The subject found that the force required to maintain tonic discharge of this large unit declined over time, while the two smaller units stopped discharging completely (C). Following a brief relaxation with subsequent contraction (D), the recruitment order was identical to that first observed, but the absolute force thresholds at which the units were recruited had declined considerably.

Thus, at present, the stereotyped recruitment order of small-before-large motor units is strongly supported for muscle contraction and the production of force in humans. Deviations from this pattern during voluntary contractions, although demonstrated on occasion, are not easily reproduced. Unequivocal paradigms, in which an experimenter can repeatedly demonstrate reversals in recruitment order between different motor units, have yet to be formulated. Thus, we feel that the size principle continues to provide an adequate basis for the investigation of mechanisms underlying the control of movement in humans and animals.

Acknowledgments

The continuing support from the Natural Sciences and Engineering Research Council (NSERC) for P. Bawa is gratefully acknowledged. B. Calancie, now with The Miami Project and the Department of Neurological Surgery, University of Miami, was a Post-doctoral Fellow of the Alberta Heritage Foundation for Medical Research at the time of writing.

REFERENCES

Adrian, E. D., and Bronk, D. W. (1929). The discharge of impulses in motor nerve fibers. Part II. The frequency of discharge in reflex and voluntary contractions. *J. Physiol. (Lond.)* 67, 119–151.

Amassian, V. E., Stewart, M., Quirk, G. J., and Rosenthal, J. L. (1987). Physiological basis of motor effects of a transient stimulus to cerebral cortex. *Neurosurgery* 20, 74–93.

Andreassen, S., and Arendt-Nielsen, L. (1987). Muscle fibre conduction velocity in motor units of the human anterior tibial muscle: A new size principle parameter. *J. Physiol. (Lond.),* 391, 561–571.

Ashworth, B., Grimby, L., and Kugelberg, E. (1967). Comparison of voluntary and reflex activation of motor units. *J. Neurol. Neurosurg Psychiatry,* 30, 91–98.

Barker, A. T., Freeston, I. L., Jalinous, R., and Jarratt, J. A. (1987). Magnetic stimulation of the human brain and peripheral nervous system: An introduction and the results of an initial clinical evaluation. *Neurosurgery* 20, 100–109.

Barker, A. T., Jalinous, R., and Freeston, I. L. (1985). Non-invasive magnetic stimulation of human motor cortex. *Lancet* 1, 1106–1107.

Basmajian, J. V. (1963). Control and training of individual motor units. *Science* 141, 440–441.

Bawa, P., Binder, M. D., Ruenzel, P., and Henneman, E. (1984). Recruitment order of motoneurons in stretch reflexes is highly correlated with their axonal conduction velocity. *J. Neurophysiol.* 52, 410–420.

Buchthal, F., Pinelli, P., and Rosenfalck, P. (1954). Action potential parameters in normal human muscle and their physiological determinants. *Acta Physiol. Scand.* 32, 219–229.

Buller, N. P., Garnett, R., and Stephens, J. A. (1980). The reflex responses of single motor units in human hand muscles following muscle afferent stimulation. *J. Physiol. (Lond.)* 303, 337–349.

Burke, R. E. (1967). Motor unit types of cat triceps surae muscle. *J. Physiol. (Lond.)* 193, 141–160.

Burke, R. E. (1981). Motor units: Anatomy, physiology, and functional organization.

In *Handbook of Physiology. The Nervous System* (ed. V. B. Brooks), Vol. 2, Sect. 1, American Physiological Society, Bethesda, Md., pp. 345–442.

Burke, R. E., Dum, R. P., Fleshman, J. W., Glenn, L. L., Lev-Tov, A., O'Donovan, M. J., and Pinter, M. J. (1982). An HRP study of the relation between cell size and motor unit type in cat ankle extensor motoneurons. *J. Comp. Neurol.* 209, 17–28.

Calancie, B., and Bawa, P. (1985a). Firing patterns of human flexor carpi radialis motor units during the stretch reflex. *J. Neurophysiol.* 53, 1179–1193.

Calancie, B., and Bawa, P. (1985b). Voluntary and reflexive recruitment of flexor carpi radialis motor units in humans. *J. Neurophysiol.* 53, 1194–1200.

Calancie, B., and Bawa, P. (1986). Limitations of the spike-triggered averaging technique. *Muscle Nerve* 9, 78–83.

Calancie, B., Nordin, M., Wallin, U., and Hagbarth, K.-E. (1987). Motor-unit responses in human wrist flexor and extensor muscles to transcranial cortical stimuli. *J. Neurophysiol.* 58, 1168–1185.

Cheney, P. D., Fetz, E. E., and Palmer, S. S. (1985). Patterns of facilitation and suppression of antagonist forelimb muscles from motor cortex sites in the awake monkey. *J. Neurophysiol.* 53, 805–820.

Clamann, H. P., Gillies, J. D., Skinner, R. D., and Henneman, E. (1974). Quantitative measures of output of a motoneuron pool during monosynaptic reflexes. *J. Neurophysiol.* 37, 1328–1337.

Clamann, H. P., Ngai, A. C., Kukulka, C. G., and Goldberg, S. J. (1983). Motor pool organization in monosynaptic reflexes: Responses in three different muscles. *J. Neurophysiol.* 50, 725–742.

Cody, F. W. J., Goodwin, C. N., and Richardson, H. C. (1987). Effects of ischaemia upon reflex electromyographic responses evoked by stretch and vibration in human wrist flexor muscles. *J. Physiol. (Lond.)* 391, 589–609.

Cremer, S. A., Gregor, R. J., and Edgerton, V. R. (1983). Voluntarily induced differential alteration in force threshold of single motor units of the human vastus lateralis. *EMG Clin. Neurophysiol.* 23, 627–641.

Darton, K., Lippold, O. C. J., Shahani, M., and Shahani, U. (1985). Long-latency spinal reflexes in humans. *J. Neurophysiol.* 53, 1604–1618.

DeLuca, C. J., LeFever, R. S., McCue, M. P., and Xenakis, A. P. (1982). Behaviour of human motor units in different muscles during linearly varying contractions. *J. Physiol. (Lond.)* 329, 113–128.

Dengler, R., Stein, R. B., and Thomas, C. K. (1988). Axonal conduction velocity and force of single human motor units. *Muscle Nerve.* 11:136–145.

Denny-Brown, D. (1929). Nature of postural reflexes. *Proc. R. Soc. Lond.* Series B 104, 252–301.

Denny-Brown, D., and Pennybacker, J. B. (1938). Fibrillation and fasciculation in voluntary muscle. *Brain* 61, 311–334.

Desmedt, J. E. (1980). Patterns of motor commands during various types of voluntary movement in man. *TINS* 3, 265–268.

Desmedt, J. E., and Godaux, E. (1975). Vibration-induced discharge patterns of single motor units in the masseter muscle in man. *J. Physiol. (Lond.)* 253, 429–442.

Desmedt, J. E., and Godaux, E. (1977a). Fast motor units are not preferentially activated in rapid voluntary contractions in man. *Nature* 267, 717–719.

Desmedt, J. E., and Godaux, E. (1977b) Ballistic contractions in man: Characteristic recruitment pattern of single motor units of the tibialis anterior muscle. *J. Physiol. (Lond.)* 264, 373–393.

Desmedt, J. E., and Godaux, E. (1978). Mechanism of the vibration paradox: Excitatory and inhibitory effects of tendon vibration on single soleus motor units in man. *J. Physiol. (Lond.)* 285, 197–207.

Desmedt, J. E., and Godaux, E. (1979). Recruitment patterns of single motor units in the human masseter muscle during brisk jaw clenching. *Arch. Oral Biol.* 24, 171–178.

Desmedt, J. E., and Godaux, E. (1981). Spinal motoneuron recruitment in man: Deordering with direction, but not with speed of voluntary movement. *Science* 214, 933–936.

Eriksson, P.-O., Stalberg, E., and Antoni, L. (1984). Flexibility in motor-unit firing pattern in the human temporal and masseter muscles related to type of activation and location. *Arch. Oral Biol.* 29, 707–712.

Fetz, E. E., and Cheney, P. D. (1980). Postspike facilitation of forelimb muscle activity by primate corticomotoneuronal cells. *J. Neurophysiol.* 44, 751–772.

Freund, H. J., Budingen, H. J., and Dietz, V. (1975). Activity of single motor units from human forearm muscles during voluntary isometric contractions. *J. Neurophysiol.* 38, 933–946.

Garnett, R., and Stephens, J. A. (1980). The reflex responses of single motor units in human first dorsal interosseous muscle following cutaneous afferent stimulation. *J. Physiol. (Lond.)* 303, 351–364.

Garnett, R., and Stephens, J. A. (1981). Changes in the recruitment threshold of motor units produced by cutaneous stimulation in man. *J. Physiol. (Lond.)* 311, 463–473.

Goldberg, L. J., and Derfler, B. (1977). Recruitment order, spike amplitude and twitch tension of single motor units in human masseter muscle. *J. Neurophysiol.* 40, 879–890.

Grimby, L., and Hannerz, J. (1968). Recruitment order of motor units in voluntary contraction: Changes induced by proprioceptive afferent activity. *J. Neurol. Neurosurg. Psychiatry* 31, 565–564.

Gustafsson, B., and Pinter, M. J. (1985). On factors determining orderly recruitment of motor units: A role for intrinsic membrane properties. *TINS* 8, 431–433.

Hainaut, K., Duchateau, J., and Desmedt, J. E. (1981). Differential effects on slow and fast motor units of different programs of brief daily muscle training in man. In *Progress in Clinical Neurophysiology* (ed. J. E. Desmedt), Vol. 9. Basel, Karger, pp. 241–249.

Hannerz, J., and Grimby, L. (1973). Recruitment order of motor units in man: Significance of pre-existing state of facilitation. *J. Neurol. Neurosurg. Psychiatry* 36, 275–281.

Harrison, P. J. (1983). The relationship between the distribution of motor unit mechanical properties and the forces due to recruitment and to rate coding for the generation of muscle force. *Brain Res.* 264, 311–315.

Heckman, C. J., and Binder, M. D. (1988). Analysis of effective synaptic currents generated by homonymous Ia afferent fibers in motoneurons of the cat. *J. Neurophysiol.* 60:1946–1966.

Henneman, E. (1957). Relation between size of neurons and their susceptibility to discharge. *Science* 126, 1345–1347.

Henneman, E. (1985). The size-principle: A deterministic output emerges from a set of probabilistic connections. *J. Exp. Biol.* 115, 105–112.

Henneman, E., Clamann, H. P., Gillies, J. D., and Skinner, R. D. (1974). Rank-order of motoneurons within a pool: Law of combination. *J. Neurophysiol.* 37, 1338–1349.

Henneman, E., and Mendell, L. M. (1981) Functional organization of motoneuron pool and its inputs. In *Handbook of Physiology, The Nervous System*, Vol. II (ed. V. B. Brooks). American Physiological Society, Bethesda, Md., pp. 423–507.

Henneman, E., and Olson, C. B. (1965). Relations between structure and function in the design of skeletal muscles. *J. Neurophysiol.* 28, 581–598.

Henneman, E., Shahani, B. T., and Young, R. R. (1976). Voluntary control of human motor units. In *The Motor System: Neurophysiology and Muscle Mechanisms* (ed. M. Shahani). Elsevier, Amsterdam, pp. 73–78.

Henneman, E., Somjen, G., and Carpenter, D. O. (1965). Functional significance of cell size in spinal motoneurons. *J. Neurophysiol.* 28, 560–580.

Hess, C. W., Mills, K. R., and Murray, N. M. F. (1986). Magnetic stimulation of the human brain: Facilitation of motor responses by voluntary contraction of ipsilateral and contralateral muscles with additional observations on an amputee. *Neurosci. Lett.* 71, 235–240.

Hess, C. W., Mills, K. R., and Murray, N. M. F. (1987). Responses in small hand muscles from magnetic stimulation of the human brain. *J. Physiol. (Lond.)* 388, 397–419.

Hursh, J. B. (1939). Conduction velocity and diameter of nerve fibers. *Am. J. Physiol.* 127, 131–139.

Kanda, D., and Desmedt, J. E. (1983). Cutaneous facilitation of large motor units and motor control of human fingers in precision grip. In *Advances in Neurology. Motor Control Mechanisms in Health and Disease* (ed. J. E. Desmedt). Raven Press, New York, pp. 253–261.

Kato, M., Murakami, S., and Yasuda, K. (1985). Behavior of single motor units of human tibialis anterior muscle during voluntary shortening contraction under constant load torque. *Exp. Neurol.* 90, 238–253.

Kugelberg, E., and Skoglund, C. R. (1946). Natural and artificial activation of motor units—a comparison. *J. Neurophysiol.* 9, 399–412.

Lemon, R. N., and Mantel, G. W. H. (1987). Direct facilitation by corticospinal neurons of single motor units in the hand muscles of the conscious monkey. *Soc. Neurosci. Abstr.* 13, 243.

Loeb, G. E. (1985). Motoneuron task groups: Coping with kinematic heterogeneity. J. Exp. Biol. 115, 137–146.

Luscher, H.-R., Ruenzel, P., and Henneman, E. (1983). Composite EPSPs in motoneurons of different sizes before and during PTP: Implications for transmission failure and its relief in Ia projections. *J. Neurophysiol.* 49, 269–289.

Marsden, C. D., Merton, P. A., and Morton, H. B. (1976). Stretch reflex and servo action in a variety of human muscles. *J. Physiol. (Lond.)* 259, 531–560.

Marsden, C. D., Merton, P. A., and Morton, H. B. (1983). Direct electrical stimulation of corticospinal pathways through the intact scalp in human subjects. In *Advances in Neurology. Motor Control Mechanisms in Health and Disease*, Vol. 39 (ed. J. E. Desmedt). Raven Press, New York, pp. 387–392.

Meinck, H. M., Benecke, R., Kuster, S., and Conrad, B. (1983). Cutaneomuscular (flexor) reflex organization in normal man and in patients with motor disorders. In *Advances in Neurology. Motor Control Mechanisms in Health and Disease*, Vol. 39 (ed. J. E. Desmedt). Raven Press, New York, pp. 787–796.

Melville Jones, G., and Watt, D. G. D. (1971). Observations on the control of stepping and hopping movements in man. *J. Physiol. (Lond.)* 219, 709–729.

Mendell, L. M., and Henneman, E. (1971). Terminals of single Ia fibers: Location, density and distribution within a pool of 300 homonymous motoneurons. *J. Neurophysiol.* 34, 171–187.

Merton, P. A., and Morton, H. B. (1980). Stimulation of the cerebral cortex in the intact human subject. *Nature* 285, 227.

Miles, T. S., and Turker, K. S. (1986). Does reflex inhibition of motor units follow the "size principle"? *Exp. Brain Res.* 62, 443–445.

Miles, T. S., Turker, K. S., and Nordstrom, M. A. (1987). Reflex responses of motor units in human muscle to electrical stimulation of the lip. *Exp. Brain Res.* 65, 331–336.

Milner-Brown, H. S., Stein, R. B., and Yemm, R. (1973a). The orderly recruitment of human motor units during voluntary isometric contractions. *J. Physiol. (Lond.).* 230, 359–370.

Milner-Brown, H. S., Stein, R. B., and Yemm, R. (1973b). Changes in firing rate of human motor units during linearly changing voluntary contractions. *J. Physiol. (Lond.)* 230, 371–390.

Monster, A. W., and Chan, H. (1977). Isometric force production by motor units of extensor digitorum communis muscle in man. *J. Neurophysiol.* 40, 1432–1443.

Olson, C. B., Carpenter, D. O., and Henneman, E. (1968). Orderly recruitment of muscle action potentials: Motor unit threshold and EMG amplitude. *Arch. Neurol.* 19, 591–597.

Phillips, C. G. (1969). Motor apparatus of the baboon's hand. *Proc. R. Soc. Lond. (Biol.)* 173, 141–174.

Rossini, P. M., Marciani, M. G., Caramia, M., Roma, V., and Zarola, F. (1985). Nervous propagation along "central" motor pathways in intact man: Characteristics of motor responses to "bifocal" and "unifocal" spine and scalp noninvasive stimulation. *EEG Clin. Neurophysiol.* 61, 272–286.

Schmidt, E. M., and Thomas, J. S. (1981). Motor unit recruitment order: Modification under volitional control. In *Progress in Clinical Neurophysiology,* Vol. 9 (ed. J. E. Desmedt). Basel, Karger, pp. 145–148.

Smith, J. L., Betts, B., Edgerton, V. R., and Zernicke, R. F. (1980). Rapid ankle extensions during paw shakes: Selective recruitment of fast ankle extensors. *J. Neurophysiol.* 43, 612–620.

Stein, R. B., French, A. S., Mannard, A., and Yemm, R. (1972). New methods for analyzing motor function in man and animals. *Brain Res.* 40, 187–192.

Stephens, J. A., and Usherwood, T. P. (1977). The mechanical properties of human motor units with special reference to their fatigability and recruitment threshold. *Brain Res.* 125, 91–97.

Sussman, H. M., MacNeilage, P. F., and Powers, R. K. (1977). Recruitment and discharge patterns of single motor units during speech production. *J. Speech Hear. Res.* 20, 613–630.

Sypert, G. W., and Munson, J. B. (1981). Basis of segmental motor control: Motoneuron size or motor unit type? *Neurosurgery* 8, 608–621.

Tanji, J., and Kato, M. (1973). Firing rate of individual motor units in voluntary contraction of abductor digiti minimi in man. *Exp. Neurol.* 40, 771–783.

Ter Haar Romeny, B. M., Denier van der Gon, J. J., and Gielen, C. C. A. M. (1982). Changes in recruitment order of motor units in the human biceps muscle. *Exp. Neurol.* 78, 360–368.

Ter Haar Romeny, B. M., Denier van der Gon, J. J., and Gielen, C. C. A. M. (1984). Relation between location of a motor unit in the human biceps brachii and its critical firing levels for different tasks. *Exp. Neurol.* 85, 631–650.

Thomas, C. K., Ross, B. H., and Calancie, B. (1987). Human motor-unit recruitment during isometric contractions and repeated dynamic movements. *J. Neurophysiol.* 57, 311–324.

Thomas, C. K., Ross, B. H., and Stein, R. B. (1986). Motor-unit recruitment in human first dorsal interosseous muscle for static contractions in three directions. *J. Neurophysiol.* 55, 1017–1029.

Thomas, J. S., Schmidt, E. M., and Hambrecht, F. T. (1978). Facility of motor unit control during tasks defined directly in terms of unit behaviors. *Exp. Neurol.* 59, 384–395.

Watson, T. W. J., and Whitelaw, W. A. (1987). Voluntary hyperventilation changes recruitment order of parasternal intercostal motor units. *J. Appl. Physiol.* 62, 187–193.

Yemm, R. (1977). The orderly recruitment of motor units of the masseter and temporal muscles during voluntary isometric contraction in man. *J. Physiol. (Lond.)* 265, 163–174.

Zidar, J., Trontelj, J. V., and Mihelin, M. (1987). Percutaneous stimulation of human corticospinal tract: A single-fiber EMG study of individual motor unit responses. *Brain Res.* 422, 196–199.

5

Coupling of Recruitment Order to the Force Produced by Motor Units: The "Size Principle Hypothesis" Revisited

FELIX E. ZAJAC

Beginning with Denny-Brown's observations some 60 years ago (Denny-Brown, 1929), and continuing during the last 30 years under the impetus provided by Henneman (e.g., Henneman, 1957), the relationship between the orderly recruitment of motor units and their size has often been referred to as the "size principle" (for reviews, see Burke, 1981b; Henneman, 1981; Henneman and Mendell, 1981; Stuart and Enoka, 1983; Enoka and Stuart, 1984; Burke, 1986). Specifically, there are data suggesting an orderly recruitment according to the size of the motoneurons (actually, according to measures of the diameter of their motor axons; see the later discussion) and other data suggesting an ordering according to the size of the innervated muscle units (actually, according to the measures of a unit's force-generating capability; see the later discussion). Thus, the size principle has come to mean (e.g., Henneman, 1977):

> The recruitment of motoneurons belonging to a motor pool (i.e., the α-motoneurons innervating a single muscle) is ordered according to both the size of the motoneurons and the size of their innervated muscle units.

If true, the size principle of motor unit recruitment would have enormous implications not only for neural control of movement vis à vis the orderly recruitment of motor units (see Chapter 4, this volume) but also on the functional coupling between the organization of the motoneurons constituting a motor pool and the organization of their innervated muscle units (see Chapter 2, this book).

However, motor axon diameter (as indicated by axonal conduction velocity) and muscle unit size (as indicated by maximum isometric strength, P_0) are now believed to be unrelated among the fast-contracting motor unit sub-population, at least in large hindlimb muscles of the cat; furthermore, the fast-contracting motor unit subset is now known to comprise up to 75% of the motor pool of these muscles (for reviews and a historical perspective, see Wuerker et al., 1965; Burke et al., 1973; Stephens and Stuart, 1975; Burke et al., 1976b; Gerlach et al., 1976; Proske and Waite, 1976; Dum and Kennedy, 1980; Burke, 1981b; Fleshman et al., 1981; Dum et al., 1982; Stuart and Enoka, 1983). These findings are seemingly paradoxical to the de facto definition of the size principle (Burke, 1981b). How can some studies of the whole motor pool of these same muscles, which have putatively included the high-threshold, fast-contracting units in their sample, show that recruitment of motoneurons is highly correlated with measures of motor axon diameter, whereas other studies show that recruitment of muscle units is highly correlated with measures of muscle unit size?

A brief review of these issues, and of recent work that has focused on resolving this paradox, follows. A formal definition of the size principle, applicable to the recruitment of either the slow- or fast-contracting motor unit subsets, and to the whole motor unit population as well, is then proposed. The proposed definition of the size principle is:

> Motor units of a motor pool are recruited in strict accordance with the force-generating properties of their muscle units (i.e., muscle unit size).

Analysis of the data collected to resolve the paradox suggests that only slow-contracting motor units of a motor pool are recruited in strict accordance with *both* motor axon size and muscle unit size. Finally, in reexamining the techniques commonly used to study and analyze motor unit recruitment, I offer precautions to be taken in the design of recruitment studies and the interpretation of recruitment data, and suggest studies that would hopefully identify measures of motoneuron size compatible with the more general de facto definition of the size principle for recruitment of motor units.

CORRELATION OF RECRUITMENT ORDER WITH MOTONEURON SIZE

To test for a correlation of recruitment order with motoneuron size, investigators must first choose the variable to be used as an indicator of motoneuron size. With one exception, measures of axon diameter have been used, including the axon's conduction velocity (CV) and the extracellular spike discharge amplitude recorded from the ventral root or the peripheral nerve in which the axon resides (see the later discussion). More direct indices of motoneuron size (such as soma diameter, soma input conductance, soma or dendritic membrane area) have not been used. The reason is, of course, that the motoneuron under study would have to be penetrated to determine these cellular properties, and probably during the recruitment study as well. In fact, the recruitment study may even require the simultaneous penetration of another cell. Not only would such a study be a formidable task, but the results would be inconclusive since a motoneuron's threshold to recruitment might be severely affected by the penetration (Clamann and Goldberg, 1975).

Studies have indeed found that the recruitment order of motor units is correlated with motor axon size. Henneman and his colleagues (Henneman, 1957; Henneman et al., 1965b, 1965c; Somjen et al., 1965; Clamann et al., 1974a; Henneman et al., 1974; Clamann and Henneman, 1976; Binder et al., 1983; Bawa et al., 1984) found a correlation, and at times a very high one, between size and the recruitment order of hindlimb motoneurons in decerebrate cats during either reflex or supraspinal excitation of motoneuronal pools. Clamann et al. (1983) also found a correlation between recruitment and the size of the cat hindlimb motoneurons, but this time afferent volleys from dorsal root stimulation were used to excite the motor pool. In humans, the recruitment order of units in hand muscles has been found to be correlated with axonal CV during voluntary isometric contraction (Freund et al., 1975), and in foot muscles during locomotion as well (Grimby, 1986).

Based on the correlations found in these studies, and assuming that motor axon diameter is a good indicator of motoneuron size (Cullheim, 1978; Kernell and Zwaagstra, 1981; see Chapter 2, this volume), it was postulated that the relative size of a motoneuron determines to a large extent its recruitment threshold (see Chapters 9 and 10, this volume).

CORRELATION OF RECRUITMENT ORDER WITH MUSCLE UNIT SIZE

Other studies have investigated the relationship, and indeed have found a correlation, between muscle unit size and the orderly recruitment of motor units (Chapter 4, this volume). With only a few exceptions, variables associated with the twitch of the muscle unit have been used as measures of muscle unit size, including twitch amplitude (P_{tw}), contraction speed (sometimes estimated from spike-triggered averaging (Milner-Brown et al., 1973a), and the motor unit action potential amplitude recorded from the synchronized firing of the unit's muscle fibers. However, the twitch is not stable; it is short-term, time-history dependent (e.g., it can be in a potentiated state after a tetanus; Burke et al., 1973, 1976a). In addition, spike-triggered averaging may underestimate the twitch if the background firing rate of the unit is high. Finally, the motor unit action potential amplitude depends on the location of the fibers in the muscle relative to the electrode.

A more stable and intuitively satisfying index of muscle unit size is the maximum isometric force that a unit can develop (P_0). The reason for the appeal is that P_0 is short-term stable; i.e., P_0 adapts slowly compared to the twitch to use or disuse of the muscle unit as long as the unit is not in a fatigued state. (Presumably P_0 depends only on the maximum number of cross-bridges per sarcomere; Huxley, 1974). It should also be mentioned that even if P_{tw} were stable, the recruitment order's correlation with P_{tw} might differ from its correlation with P_0 because units have different twitch-to-tetanus (P_{tw}/P_0) ratios (Burke et al., 1973). However, P_0 has hardly been used as an index of muscle unit size in recruitment studies because, once again, the technical obstacles are often insurmountable. To measure a muscle-unit's P_0, the tension response of the muscle to a high-frequency pulse train delivered in isolation to the unit is required, either before or after its threshold to recruitment has been recorded. In only a few cases in animals has success been achieved, and the data show that a correlation between P_0 and recruitment order does indeed exist (Mizote, 1982; Zajac and Faden, 1985; see the later discussion).

Using the more common indices of the twitch as measures of muscle-unit size, studies have shown that the orderly recruitment of motor units is correlated with the "twitch size" of their muscle units. Henneman and colleagues (Olson et al., 1968) found the order to be correlated with twitch muscle unit size in decerebrate cats during spinal reflexes and supraspinal excitation. Barmack (1977) also found a correlation in rabbit extraocular muscles during vestibular-induced reflexes. Complementing these studies on recruitment order during reflex and stimulus-induced contractions, other studies show that correlations exist during voluntarily induced contractions. These studies include voluntary control of monkey forearm and masseter muscles (Humphrey et al., 1977; Clark et al., 1978) and human hand and jaw muscles (Milner-Brown et al., 1973b; Tanji and Kato, 1973; Desmedt and Godaux, 1977; Stephens and Usherwood, 1977).

Based on the correlations found in these other studies, it has also been proposed that the size of the innervated muscle units is coupled to the orderly recruitment of motoneurons. Naturally, then, investigators have come to believe that recruitment order of motoneurons is coupled with *both* their size and the size of their innervated muscle units. This belief has been reinforced by studies showing that motoneurons with fast-conducting motor axons *tend* to belong to motor units that generate large forces (Wuerker et al., 1965; Burke, 1967; Burke et al., 1973).

THE SIZE PRINCIPLE HYPOTHESIS: A PARADOX

For the recruitment of motor units belonging to the whole motor pool to be *strictly* ordered according to both motoneuron and muscle unit size, a very high to perfect correlation ought to exist between axonal CV and tetanic tension P_0 among the whole set of motor units, assuming that axonal CV and P_0 are good indices of motoneuron and muscle unit size, respectively. Though strong correlations had been found in small cat lumbrical muscles (Appelberg and Emonet-Denand, 1967; Emonet-Denand et al., 1971) and in the homogeneous cat soleus muscle (Gerlach et al., 1976), axonal CV and P_0 were found to be, at best, weakly correlated among the entire set of motor units of large mixed muscles of the cat (Burke, 1967; Mosher et al., 1972; Gerlach et al., 1976; Proske and Waite, 1976; Goslow et al., 1977b; Stephens and Usherwood, 1977). It appears that the low correlation found among the whole motor unit pool manifests itself because a correlation is absent among the numerous fast-contracting motor unit subset, even though a very high correlation exists among the slow-contracting subset (Wuerker et al., 1965; Burke et al., 1973; Stephens and Stuart, 1975; Burke et al., 1976b; Gerlach et al., 1976; Proske and Waite, 1976; Dum and Kennedy, 1980; Fleshman et al., 1981; Dum et al., 1982).

It thus became evident that the orderly recruitment of units within the fast-contracting motor unit subset could *not* be in strict accordance with *both* motor axon size (i.e., axonal CV) and muscle unit size (i.e., P_0), though such a strict ordering to both could occur within the slow-contracting motor unit subset. The questions that then naturally arose were:

1. With which of the two sizes, if either one, is the orderly recruitment of fast-contracting units in strict accordance?

2. If recruitment is in strict accordance with one index, how do we account for the correlations found between recruitment order and the other index in those investigations where presumably fast-contracting as well as slow-contracting motor units are included in the studied sample?

3. Is there one hypothesis that can unify the strict ordering of recruitment of motor units so as to be applicable to the slow-contracting motor unit subset, the fast-contracting subset, and the whole motor unit population of a motor pool?

RECRUITMENT ORDER AMONG FAST-CONTRACTING MOTOR UNITS

To resolve the paradox, the recruitment order of the fast-contracting motor units must be studied, for it is within this subpopulation that motor axon size (i.e., axonal CV) is uncorrelated with muscle unit size (i.e., P_0)—at least in many mixed muscles of the cat hindlimb; see the previous discussion). However, there is only one substantive published report in which the recruitment order of fast-contracting and other type-identified motor units was studied and their axonal CV and muscle unit properties were measured (Zajac and Faden, 1985). Since the resolution of the paradox has important implications for the functional coupling between motoneuronal organization and muscle unit organization, why is there only report? The reason is that many technical obstacles potentially hinder the completion of such a conceptually simple experiment (Zajac and Faden, 1985). Some of these obstacles are:

1. Fast-contracting motor units must be studied. These units correspond to the motor units with high thresholds to recruitment. Techniques to recruit these units and simultaneously record their unitary discharges are few (Clamann et al., 1974b; Zajac and Faden, 1985).

2. The functional threshold to recruitment of each unit studied must be found. Either the unit's absolute rank in the recruitment order must be established (e.g., Clamann et al., 1974b) or at least two high-threshold (fast-contracting) motor units must be recorded from simultaneously (Zajac and Faden, 1985).

3. *Both* motor axon size (i.e., axonal CV) and muscle unit size (i.e., P_0) of each motor unit studied must be ranked relative to each other one if pairs of units are studied, or else the absolute sizes must be ascertained if functional thresholds to recruitment of units are measured singly.

4. Recordings must be stable and techniques nontraumatic as the recruitment order of units is established and their motoneuron and muscle unit properties are ascertained.

5. Half of the data, even if only fast-contracting units are studied, will probably be meaningless in resolving the paradox. The reason is that axonal CV and P_0, assuming that they are used as size indices, are uncorrelated (see the earlier discussion). Therefore, only half of all pairs of units selected at random will have the characteristic needed to discern whether recruitment is better ordered according to axonal CV or P_0. The required characteristic is, of course, that the weaker unit of the pair is the one with the faster axonal CV, for only then will the unit with the lower functional threshold to recruitment be either the weaker or the slower unit, but not both.

Overcoming these obstacles, Zajac and Faden (1985) established the recruitment order in 20 pairs of fast-contracting cat plantaris (PL) motor units during homonymous reflexes (Table 5–1). In all 20 pairs, the weaker unit had the lower functional threshold to recruitment. However, the lower-threshold unit had the slower-conducting motoneuron in only 9 pairs; in 10 pairs, the faster-contracting unit had the lower threshold; in 1 pair, the axonal CVs of the two units were indistinguishable.

These data support the notion that the recruitment order of fast-contracting motor-units is in strict accordance with muscle unit size P_0 (Stephens and Stuart, 1975; Zajac and Faden, 1979; Fleshman et al., 1981; Sypert and Munson, 1981; Stuart and Enoka, 1983). These data do *not* support the notion that recruitment order of fast-contracting motor units is in strict accordance with motor axon size (i.e., axonal CV). In fact, for the subpopulation of fast-contracting units, the data support the notion that recruitment order is random with respect to axonal CV. Consistent with the randomness found between recruitment order and axonal CV, they found in a separate study (Phase I of Zajac and Faden, 1985) that the weaker unit had the slower axonal CV with $p = 0.52$. This separate study defined the relationship between axonal CV and P_0 by performing a pairwise analysis on an unbiased population of PL motor units.

RELATIONSHIP OF RECRUITMENT ORDER TO MOTOR AXON SIZE AND MUSCLE UNIT SIZE IN SLOW AND MIXED MOTOR UNIT POPULATIONS

In all 22 pairs of slow- and mixed-contracting unit pairs studied (Table 5–1), Zajac and Faden (1985) again found the weaker unit to have the lower functional threshold to recruitment. In contrast to fast-contracting unit pairs, however, in which only half of the low-threshold units of the pair had the slower axonal CV, 21 of the 22 low-threshold units in slow- and mixed-contracting unit pairs had the slower-conducting axons. The finding that the low-threshold unit to recruitment had the slower axonal CV in 21 of the 22 pairs can be accounted for by probability, as was the case with fast-contracting unit-pairs; i.e., the weaker unit has the slower axonal CV, with $p = 0.95$, and $p = 0.97$

Table 5–1 Relationship of recruitment threshold to axonal CV and P_0 for pairs of cat plantaris motor units

Type of units in pair	Number of pairs	Number of pairs with lower-threshold unit having:			
		Slower CV	Faster CV	Smaller P_0	Larger P_0
Fast, fast (types F, F)	20[a]	9	10	20	0
Slow, slow (types S, S)	9	8	1	9	0
Slow, fast (types S, F)	13	13	0	13	0

Source: Adapted from Zajac and Faden (1985).

[a]For one pair, CVs were identical.

in slow- and mixed-contracting unit pairs, respectively. Thus, these data on slow- and mixed-contracting unit pairs are also compatible with the hypothesis that recruitment order is in strict accordance with muscle unit size P_0.

RELATIONSHIP OF RECRUITMENT ORDER TO MOTOR UNIT TYPE AND FATIGABILITY

Henneman and colleagues were one of the earlier groups to develop criteria for classifying slow- and fast-contracting motor units (Wuerker et al., 1965). A widely used classification scheme of somewhat more recent vintage has been the one developed by Burke et al. (1973) (see also Chapter 11, this volume), where the type S group corresponds to the slow-contracting, very highly resistant-to-fatigue units; the type FR group to the fast-contracting, highly resistant-to-fatigue units; and the type FF group to the fast-contracting, fatigue-susceptible units. (For clarity, the type FI group, which is the group of fast-contracting units with intermediate resistance to fatigue, is included here with the type FF group.) This classification scheme requires, among other tests, that the amount of "fatigue" be measured at the end of two minutes of stimulation (called the "fatigue index").

Contraction strength (P_0) has been found to be correlated with motor unit type and fatigability (Burke et al., 1973; Goslow et al., 1977a; Dum and Kennedy, 1980; McDonagh et al., 1980; Fleshman et al., 1981; Dum et al., 1982). Furthermore, a pairwise analysis of medial gastrocnemius (MG) and PL unit pairs has substantiated the relationship between unit type and strength (Zajac and Faden, 1985); i.e., there is a very high probability ($p > 0.95$) of finding the type FR unit in a type FR-FF pair and of finding the type S unit in either an S-FR or an S-FF pair to have the lower contraction strength (P_0). Since investigators have suggested that recruitment is ordered according to P_0, it is no surprise that an ordering according to motor unit type has been suggested as well (Burke and Edgerton, 1975; Stephens and Usherwood, 1977; Walmsley et al., 1978; Burke, 1981a; Fleshman et al., 1981; Henneman and Mendell, 1981; Stuart and Enoka, 1983).

These suggestions have been substantiated by Zajac and Faden (1985), who found a strict ordering by type in the 21 pairs of mixed-type units studied (i.e., S > FR > FF; Table 5–2). Also, in all 19 pairs whose units had different fatigue indices, the unit least susceptible to fatigue had the lower functional threshold to recruitment.

RECRUITMENT ORDER IS IN STRICT ACCORDANCE TO MOTOR UNIT CONTRACTION STRENGTH P_0: A HYPOTHESIS

It is desirable to state a formal definition of the size principle hypothesis that is applicable to the whole motor pool of motor units, not just to the slow-contracting motor unit subset. The direct evidence on the recruitment order of units of a large mixed muscle thus supports a strict ordering of recruitment according to either contraction strength P_0, unit type, or fatigability (Zajac and Faden, 1985). The least restrictive of these three hypotheses is that the order is according to unit type, since there are, by definition, many more units than there are types in a motor pool. Since fatigue, and indices of fatigue, are conceptually vague and more difficult to define and reach a consensus (see Chapter 13, this volume), it appears that a constructive formal definition of the size principle hypothesis should be:

> The recruitment order of motor units of a muscle is ranked in strict accordance to the isometric contraction strengths of the motor units.

In another study comparing the recruitment order of three pairs of motor units to the size of both their motor axons (i.e., axonal CV) and their muscle units (i.e., P_0), Mizote (1982) also found that the order is in strict accordance with the P_0. However, the lower threshold unit to recruitment in two of the three pairs also had the slower axonal CV (in the other pair, the CVs were the same). Thus, Mizote's data support the hypothesis proposed here, but since the number of pairs studied by them is few, their study does not help to resolve the paradox.

Table 5–2 Relationship between recruitment threshold and unit type for pairs of cat plantaris motor units

Type of low-threshold unit in pair	Type of high-threshold unit in pair	Number of occurrences for this type of pair	Number of exceptions for this type of pair
S	FR	8	0
S	FF	5	0
FR	FF	8	0

Source: Adapted from Zajac and Faden (1985).

HOW EXPERIMENTAL DESIGN CAN OBSCURE THE LACK OF CORRELATION BETWEEN MOTOR AXON SIZE AND RECRUITMENT ORDER AMONG THE NUMEROUS FAST-CONTRACTING MOTOR UNITS

The formal definition of the size principle hypothesis just presented implies that if a correlation exists between recruitment order and some other variable (e.g., a measure of motor axon size), it is because a correlation exists between this variable and contraction strength (P_0). However, as stated before, a low to nonexistent correlation exists between P_0 and axonal CV in the fast-contracting motor unit subpopulation in many cat hindlimb muscles, including the MG and PL, even though the fast-contracting subset (i.e., F = FR + FF) in each of these mixed calf muscles can comprise up to 75% of the whole population (Burke et al., 1973; Burke, 1981b). How, then, do I account for the correlations found between recruitment and motor axon size in past recruitment studies of cat calf muscles (e.g., PL and MG)?

I believe the answer to this question is that the experimental design of recruitment studies is generally flawed, obscuring the lack of correlation between motor axon size and recruitment order in the numerous fast-contracting motor unit subset. The following analysis shows how such an "obstruction" can occur in the cat PL and MG motor pools. The reason the PL and MG muscles are chosen for illustration is that the many studies showing a correlation between recruitment order and motor axon size have focused on the cat triceps surae and PL muscles (Clamann et al., 1974a, 1974b; Clamann and Henneman, 1976; Binder et al., 1983; Bawa et al., 1984). In addition, the physiological and anatomical properties of the motor units of these muscles have been extensively studied (see Burke, 1981), ensuring high confidence in the probability estimates needed in the following analysis.

Suppose that a recruitment study of PL unit pairs is performed and two units are selected at random from the whole motor pool. The probability of selecting either an S or an F unit is $p = 0.39$ and $P = 0.61$, respectively; i.e., the distribution of PL motor unit types is assumed to be 39 and 61% (Zajac and Faden, 1985). Thus, the probability of finding either a type S-S, S-F, F-F pair is:

S-S pair:	$p = (0.39)\,(0.39)$	$= 0.15$
S-F pair:	$p = 2\,(0.39)\,(0.61)$	$= 0.48$
F-F pair:	$p = (0.61)\,(0.61)$	$= 0.37$

Notice that the likelihood of finding a fast-contracting pair is only $p = 0.37$ when units are randomly selected from the whole motor pool, even though fast-contracting units constitute 61% of the motor pool.

The probability of finding the weaker unit of a pair of PL units to be also the unit with the slower axonal CV depends on the types of units in the pair; the following probability estimates have been found (Zajac and Faden, 1985):

S-S pair:	$p = 0.95$
S-F pair:	$p = 0.97$
F-F pair:	$p = 0.52$

Notice, as stated in a previous section, that the probability of finding the weaker unit to be also the slower unit is very high among slow-contracting and mixed unit pairs. Among fast-contracting unit pairs, however, only by chance will the weaker unit of the pair have the slower-conducting motor axon.

Let us assume that motor units belonging to a whole motor pool are recruited in strict accordance to P_0, compatible with the formal definition of the size principle stated earlier. Then, in a recruitment study of PL unit pairs, one should expect to find the unit of the pair with the lower functional threshold to recruitment to have the slower axonal CV with the following probability:

$$p = (0.15)(0.95) + (0.48)(0.97) + (0.37)(0.52)$$
$$= 0.80$$

This prediction agrees well with the high correlation found between the recruitment order of PL motoneurons and their axonal CVs during potentiated, homonymous reflexes, a situation where high- and low-threshold motoneurons are recruited, and thus where the whole motor pool is indeed sampled (Clamann and Henneman, 1976). Notice that the reason the overall probability ($p = 0.80$) is much higher than chance is that type S-S and type S-F pairs are expected to be studied reasonably frequently ($p = 0.15 + 0.48 = 0.63$), and the weaker unit of these pairs has a very high probability of being also the slower-conducting unit ($p > 0.95$).

If the population of units studied during recruitment happens to be restricted to type S and type FR units, as occurs during unpotentiated PL reflexes (Zajac and Faden, 1985) and as expected during unpotentiated MG reflexes as well (Burke, 1981b), such an analysis of PL unit pairs shows that the slower unit is expected to have the lower threshold to recruitment, with $p = 0.91$ (Zajac and Faden, 1985). A similar analysis on a restricted population of MG unit pairs shows that the slower unit is expected to have the lower threshold to recruitment, with $p = 0.81$, again given the hypothesis that units are recruited in strict accordance with P_0 (Zajac and Faden, 1985). This prediction also agrees with the reported incidence of $p = 0.86$ that the smaller motor axon has the lower recruitment threshold during unpotentiated reflexes of cat calf muscles (Henneman et al., 1965b). These predictions are, however, low when compared with the data of Bawa et al. (1984), who found the slower-conducting motor axon in 36 of 37 MG pairs to have the lower threshold to recruitment. The motor units in their study were, however, not type identified. If their sample had been biased towards the type S-FR pairs, the number of pairs in which the slower-conducting axon is expected to be recruited first would be 35 of 37, using these probability estimation techniques and assuming that motor units are recruited strictly according to P_0.

Again, it should be mentioned that if one studies only pairs of units among the fast-contracting motor unit subset, which comprises 61% and 75% of the population of PL and MG units, respectively, one should expect to find only by chance ($p = 0.52$ and $p = 0.50$, respectively) the motoneuron with the lower functional threshold to recruitment to be the one having the slower-conducting axon, given the hypothesis proposed here. And indeed, this has been found for the PL type F population of motor units (see the earlier discussion).

To summarize, one should expect to find the lower-threshold unit to recruitment of a pair of units to be not only the weaker but also the one with the slower-conducting motor axon, assuming that motor units are indeed recruited in strict accordance with contraction strength P_0 and randomly selected from the whole motor pool during the experiment. However, if one analyzes the recruitment order among only the fast-contracting units, which constitute the majority of the motor unit population (at least in many cat hindlimb muscles), one should expect only by chance to find the lower-threshold unit of a pair to be also the one with the slower-conducting motor axon.

CONCLUDING REMARKS

When recruitment of motoneurons is compared with measurements of both the size of their motor axons (i.e., axonal CV) and their innervated muscle units (i.e., P_0), the recruitment order of the whole motoneuronal pool is found to be in strict accordance with the force-generating properties of the innervated muscle units. One also finds that the order is in strict accordance with the type and the fatigability of the muscle units. For only the slow-contracting motor unit subset of the motor pool do the data support the hypothesis that recruitment is ordered according to the size of the motoneurons' motor axons. The recruitment order among the fast-contracting motor unit subset appears to depend hardly, if at all, on motor axon size.

How are the conclusions from other studies on mixed muscles that suggest an ordering of motoneuron recruitment according to the size of their motor axons reconciled, especially when the recruitment of high-threshold (and putatively fast-contracting) units has been included in their samples of studied motor units? I submit that these recruitment studies are designed so as to mask unintentionally the incompatibility of recruitment order according to motor axon size among fast-contracting motor units. An examination of the experimental paradigm commonly used to study recruitment (see the previous section) suggests that fast-contracting motor unit pairs are probably encountered uncommonly, and even when they are, the incompatibility should arise only half the time. The single, unequivocal way to unmask the incompatibility is to restrict the recruitment study and analysis to the fast-contracting motor unit subpopulation (e.g., Zajac and Faden, 1985).

Of course, the force-generating properties of the innervated motor units do not cause the recruitment of the parent motoneurons. It is both the intrinsic properties of motoneurons and the distribution and properties of synapses onto motoneurons that affect a motoneuron's recruitment threshold (see Chapter 10, this volume). The de facto definition of the size principle implies that motoneuron size determines a motoneuron's functional threshold to recruitment. I propose that recruitment of only the slow-contracting motor unit subset is in (almost) strict accordance with motor axon size. Assuming that motor axon size is indicative of motoneuron size (see Chapter 2, this volume), I submit that motoneuron size as measured this way, is a major determinant of a motoneuron's threshold to recruitment among slow-contracting motor units but not among fast-contracting units.

Could it be that measures of motoneuron size other than motor axon size might better predict recruitment order, especially among the numerous fast-contracting motor unit subset? Indeed, input conductance of motoneurons innervating cat hindlimb muscles has been found to be related to motor unit type (Dum and Kennedy, 1980, Fleshman et al., 1981) and, together with motoneuronal rheobase (and/or other motoneuronal properties), can almost perfectly discriminate motor unit type (Zengel et al., 1985). Furthermore, these relations among motoneuronal properties and motor unit type reappear after reinnervation (Foehring et al., 1986) and cross-reinnervation of a mixed muscle by a mixed nerve (Foehring et al., 1987). Specific membrane resistivity may also be unit type dependent (Kernell and Zwaagstra, 1981; Burke et al., 1982). Besides these physiological parameters, measures of anatomical cell size also suggest a linkage between cell size and motor unit type (Burke et al., 1982, Ulfhake and Kellerth, 1982), though the number of motor units studied is small.

Since recruitment order is linked to motor unit type, and since these intrinsic anatomical and physiological measures are correlated with unit type, these measures are candidate determinants of recruitment. However, hypothesizing that recruitment is strictly coupled with contraction strength P_0 is a much more restrictive hypothesis than a match between recruitment order and unit type. I thus believe that the following would be a fruitful approach to the delineation of the intrinsic properties responsible for a motoneuron's functional threshold to recruitment; the approach is to search among the fast-contracting motor unit subset for motoneuronal properties that singly or together give a nearly perfect correlation with P_0, and then determine if these same properties can predict P_0 in slow-contracting units as well (see Zengel et al., 1985). The reason for suggesting a search first among the fast-contracting motor unit subset is that the challenge may well lie within this subset, since no correlation between motor axon size and recruitment order exists among fast-contracting motor units.

It is a great tribute to Elwood Henneman that it has become necessary to define more precisely the size principle for recruitment of motor units. His work and that of his colleagues stimulated many studies outside his laboratory on the recruitment of motor units, on the relationship between recruitment and motor unit properties, and even on the properties of motor units themselves. One reason the size principle has appealed to so many is that it has had a significant impact on major issues of motor control and the coupling of motoneuronal organization (cellular organization within the CNS) to muscle fiber organization (cellular organization peripheral to the CNS). My belief that the size principle hypothesis needs to be defined more precisely implies that we have learned a great deal about motor units and their recruitment order and attests to the stature of the size principle for recruitment of motor units.

Acknowledgments

I thank Dr. Joel Faden, my collaborator in the work to which much reference is made, and Kristin Bennett for assistance in typing. Supported by NIH grant NS 17662 and the Veterans Administration.

REFERENCES

Appelberg, B., and Emonet-Denand, F. (1967). Motor units of the first superficial lumbrical muscle of the cat. *J. Neurophysiol.* 30, 154–160.

Barmack, N. H. (1977). Recruitment and suprathreshold frequency modulation of single extraocular muscle fibers in the rabbit. *J. Neurophysiol.* 40, 779–790.

Bawa, P., Binder, M. D., Ruenzel, P., and Henneman, E. (1984). Recruitment order of motoneurons in stretch reflexes is highly correlated with their axonal conduction velocity. *J. Neurophysiol.* 52, 410–420.

Binder, M. D., Bawa, P., Ruenzel, P., and Henneman, E. (1983). Does orderly recruitment of motoneurons depend on the existence of different types of motor units? *Neurosci. Lett.* 36, 55–58.

Burke, R. E. (1967). Motor unit types of cat triceps surae muscle. *J. Physiol. (Lond.)* 193, 141–160.

Burke, R. E. (1981a). Motor unit recruitment: What are the critical factors? In *Progress in Clinical Neurophysiology*, Vol. 9: *Motor Unit Types, Recruitment and Plasticity in Health and Disease*, (ed. J. E. Desmedt). Karger, Basel, pp. 61–84.

Burke, R. E. (1981b). Motor units: Anatomy, physiology and functional organization. In *Handbook of Physiology. The Nervous System*, Vol. II, Sect. 1, Pt. 1 (ed. V. B. Brooks). American Physiological Society, Bethesda, Md., pp. 345–422.

Burke, R. E. (1986). The control of muscle force: Motor unit recruitment and firing patterns. In *Human Muscle Power* (ed. N. J. Jones, N. McCartney, and A. J. McComas). Human Kinetics Publishers, Champaign, Ill., pp. 97–109.

Burke, R. E., Dum, R. P. Fleshman, J. W., Glenn, L. L., Lev-Tov, A., O'Donovan, M. J., and Pinter, M. J. (1982). An HRP study of the relation between cell size and motor unit type in cat ankle extensor motoneurons. *J. Comp. Neurol.* 209, 17–28.

Burke, R. E., and Edgerton, V. R. (1975). Motor unit properties and selective involvement in movement. *Exer. Sport Sci. Rev.* 3, 31–81.

Burke, R. E., Levine, D. N., Tsairis, P., and Zajac, F. E. III (1973). Physiological type and histochemical profiles in motor units of the cat gastrocnemius. *J. Physiol. (Lond.)* 234, 723–748.

Burke, R. E., Rudomin, P., and Zajac, F. E. III (1976a). The effect of activation history on tension production by individual muscle units. *Brain Res.* 109, 515–529.

Burke, R. E., Rymer, W. Z., and Walsh, J. V. (1976b). Relative strength of synaptic inputs from short-latency pathways to motor units of defined type in cat medial gastrocnemius. *J. Neurophysiol.* 39, 447–458.

Clamann, H. P., Gillies, J. D., and Henneman, E. (1974a). Effects of inhibitory inputs on critical firing level and rank order of motoneurons. *J. Neurophysiol.* 37, 1350–1360.

Clamann, H. P., Gillies, J. D., Skinner, R. D., and Henneman, E. (1974b). Quantitative measures of output of a motoneuron pool during monosynaptic reflexes. *J. Neurophysiol.* 37, 1328–1337.

Clamann, H. P., and Goldberg, S. J. (1975). Uncertainty of recruitment order when tested with intracellular techniques. *Neurosci. Abstr.* 1, 261.

Clamann, H. P., and Henneman, E. (1976). Electrical measurement of axon diameter and its use in relating motoneuron size to critical firing level. *J. Neurophysiol.* 39, 844–851.

Clamann, H. P., Nagai, A. C., Kukulka, C. G., and Goldberg, S. J. (1983). Motor pool organization in monosynaptic reflexes: Responses in three different muscles. *J. Neurophysiol.* 50, 725–742.

Clark, R. W., Luschei, E. S., and Hoffman, D. S. (1978). Recruitment order, contractile characteristics, and firing patterns of motor units in temporalis muscle of monkeys. *Exp. Neurol.* 61, 31–52.

Cullheim, S. (1978). Relations between cell body size, axon diameter and axon conduction velocity of cat sciatic α-motoneurons stained with horseradish peroxidase. *Neurosci. Lett.* 8, 17–20.

Denny-Brown, D. (1929). On the nature of postural reflexes. *Proc. R. Soc. Lond. Series B,* 104, 252–301.

Desmedt, J. E., and Godaux, E. (1977). Fast motor units are not preferentially activated in rapid voluntary contractions in man. *Nature (Lond.)* 267, 717–719.

Dum, R. P., Burke, R. E., O'Donovan, M. J., Toop, J., and Hodgson, J. A. (1982). Motor-unit organization in flexor digitorum longus muscle of the cat. *J. Neurophysiol.* 43, 1108–1125.

Dum, R. P., and Kennedy, T. T. (1980). Physiological and histochemical characteristics of motor units in cat tibialis anterior and extensor digitorum longus muscles. *J. Neurophysiol.* 43, 1615–1630.

Emonet-Denand, F., Laporte, Y., and Proske, U. (1971). Contraction of muscle fibers in two adjacent muscles innervated by branches of the same motor axon. *J. Neurophysiol.* 34, 132–138.

Enoka, R. M., and Stuart, D. G. (1984). Henneman's "size principle": Current issues. *Trends Neurosci.* 7, 226–227.

Fleshman, J. W., Munson, J. B., Sypert, G. W., and Friedman, W. A. (1981). Rheobase, input resistance, and motor unit type in medial gastrocnemius motoneurons in the cat. *J. Neurophysiol.* 46, 1326–1338.

Foehring, R. C., Sypert, G. W., and Munson, J. B. (1986). Properties of self-reinnervated motor units of medial gastrocnemius of cat. 1. Long-term reinnervation. *J. Neurophysiol.* 5, 931–946.

Foehring, R. C., Sypert, G. W., and Munson, J. B. (1987). Motor-unit properties following cross-reinnervation of cat lateral gastrocnemius and soleus muscles with medial gastrocnemius nerve. II. Influence of muscle on motoneurons. *J. Neurophysiol.* 57, 1227–1245.

Freund, H., Budingen, H. J., and Dietz, V. (1975). Activity of single motor units from human forearm muscles during voluntary isometric contractions. *J. Neurophysiol.* 38, 933–946.

Gerlach, R. L., Stauffer, E. K., Goslow, G. E., Jr., and Stuart, D. G. (1976). Relation between nerve axon size and muscle unit size and speed in motor units of cat hindlimb muscles. *Electromyogr. Clin. Neurophysiol.* 16, 177–190.

Goldberg, L. J., and Derfler, B. (1977). Relationships among recruitment order, spike amplitude, and twitch tension of single motor units in human masseter muscle. *J. Neurophysiol.* 40, 879–890.

Goslow, G. E., Cameron, W. E., and Stuart, D. G. (1977a). The fast twitch motor units of cat ankle flexors. 1. Tripartite classification on basis of fatigability. *Brain Res.* 134, 35–46.

Goslow, G. E., Cameron, W. E., and Stuart, D. G. (1977b). The fast twitch motor units of cat ankle flexors. 2. Speed–force relations and recruitment order. *Brain Res.* 134, 47–58.

Grimby, L. (1986). Single motor unit discharge during voluntary contraction and locomotion. In *Human Muscle Power* (ed. N. J. Jones, N. McCartney, and A. J. McComas). Human Kinetics Publishers, Champaign, Ill. pp. 111–130.

Henneman, E. (1957). Relation between size of neurons and their susceptibility to discharge. *Science* 126, 1345–1346.

Henneman, E. (1977). Functional organization of motoneuron pools: The size principle. *Proc. Int. Union Physiol. Sci.* 12, 50.

Henneman, E. (1981) Recruitment of Motoneurons: The size principle. In *Progress in Clinical Neurophysiology*, Vol. 9: *Motor Unit Types, Recruitment and Plasticity in Health and Disease* (ed. J. E. Desmedt). Karger, Basel, pp. 26–60.

Henneman, E., Clamann, H. P., Gillies, J. D., and Skinner, R. D. (1974). Rank order of motoneurons within a pool: law of combination. *J. Neurophysiol.* 37, 1338–1349.

Henneman, E., and Mendell, L. M. (1981). Functional organization of motoneuron pool and its inputs. In *Handbook of Physiology. The Nervous System*, Vol. II, Sect. 1, Pt. 2 (ed. V. B. Brooks). American Physiological Society, Bethesda, Md., pp. 423–507.

Henneman, E., Somjen, G., and Carpenter, D. O. (1965a). Relations between structure and function in the design of skeletal muscles. *J. Neurophysiol.* 28, 581–598.

Henneman, E., Somjen, G., and Carpenter, D. O. (1965b). Functional significance of cell size in spinal motoneurons. *J. Neurophysiol.* 28, 560–580.

Henneman, E., Somjen, G., and Carpenter, D. O. (1965c). Excitability and inhibitability of motoneurons of different sizes. *J. Neurophysiol.* 28, 599–620.

Humphrey, D. R., Rominski, J., and Bundacz, A. M. (1977). Patterns of motor unit recruitment in a single forearm muscle of monkey in relation to the dynamics of voluntary contraction. *Soc. Neurosci. Abstr.* 3, 272.

Huxley, A. F. (1974). Review lecture: Muscular contraction *J. Physiol. (Lond.)* 243, 1–43.

Kernell, D., and Zwaagstra, B. (1981). Input conductance, axonal conduction velocity and cell size among hindlimb motoneurones of the cat. *Brain Res.* 204, 311–326.

McDonagh, J. C., Binder, M. D., Reinking, R. M., and Stuart, D. G. (1980). Tripartite declassification of motor units of cat tibialis posterior. *J. Neurophysiol.* 44, 696–712.

McPhedran, A. M., Wuerker, R., and Henneman, E. (1965). Properties of motor units in a homogeneous red muscle (soleus) of the cat. *J. Neurophysiol.* 28, 71–84.

Milner-Brown, H. S., Stein, R. B., and Yemm, R. (1973a). The contractile properties of human motor units during voluntary isometric contractions. *J. Physiol. (Lond.)* 228, 285–306.

Milner-Brown, H. S., Stein, R. B., and Yemm, R. (1973b) The orderly recruitment of human motor units during voluntary isometric contractions. *J. Physiol. (Lond.)* 230, 359–370.

Mizote, M. (1982). The effect of digital nerve stimulation on recruitment order of motor units in the first deep lumbrical muscle of the cat. *Brain Res.* 248, 245–255.

Mosher, C. G., Gerlach, R. L., and Stuart, D. G. (1972). Soleus and anterior tibial motor units of the cat. *Brain Res.* 44, 1–11.

Olson, C. B., Carpenter, D. O., and Henneman, E. (1968). Orderly recruitment of muscle action potentials. *Arch. Neurol.* 19, 591–597.

Proske, U., and Waite, P. M. E. (1976). The relation between tension and axonal conduction velocity for motor units in the medial gastrocnemius muscle of the cat. *Exp. Brain Res.* 26, 325–326.

Reinking, R. M., Stephens, J. A., and Stuart, D. G. (1975). The motor units of cat medial gastrocnemius: Problem of their categorization on the basis of mechanical properties. *Exp. Brain Res.* 23, 301–313.

Somjen, S., Carpenter, D. O., and Henneman, E. (1965). Responses of motoneurons of different sizes to graded stimulation of supraspinal centers of the brain. *J. Neurophysiol.* 28, 958–965.

Stein, R. B., French, A. S., Mannard, A., and Yemm, R. (1972). New methods for analyzing motor function in man and animals. *Brain Res.* 40, 187–192.

Stephens, J. A., and Stuart, D. G. (1975). The motor units of cat medial gastrocnemius: Speed–size relations and their significance for the recruitment order of motor units. *Brain Res.* 91, 177–195.

Stephens, J. A., and Usherwood, T. P. (1977). The mechanical properties of human motor units with special reference to their fatigability and recruitment threshold. *Brain Res.* 125, 91–97.

Stuart, D. G., and Enoka, R. M. (1983). Motoneurons, motor units and the size principle. In *The Clinical Neurosciences. Neurobiology* (ed. R. N. Rosenburg). Churchill Livingstone, New York, pp. 471–517.

Sypert, G. W., and Munson, J. B. (1981). Basis of segmental motor control: Motoneuron size or motor unit type? *Neurosurgery* 8, 608–621.

Tanji, J., and Kato, M. (1973). Recruitment of motor units in voluntary contractions of a finger muscle in man. *Exp. Neurol.* 40, 759–770.

Ulfhake, B., and Kellerth, J.-O. (1982). Does α-motoneuron size correlate with motor unit type in cat triceps surae? *Brain Res.* 251, 201–209.

Walmsley, B., Hodgson, J. A., and Burke, R. E. (1978). Forces produced by medial gastrocnemius and soleus muscles during locomotion in freely moving cats. *J. Neurophysiol.* 41, 1203–1216.

Wuerker, R. B., McPhedran, A., and Henneman, E. (1965). Properties of motor units in a heterogeneous pale muscle (m. gastrocnemius) of the cat. *J. Neurophysiol.* 28, 85–99.

Yemm, R. (1977). The orderly recruitment of motor units of the masseter and temporal muscles during voluntary isometric contraction in man. *J. Physiol. (Lond.)* 265, 163–174.

Zajac, F. E., and Faden, J. S. (1979). Tetanic tension appears to be a perfect predictor for recruitment of plantaris (PL) motor units in the cat. *Soc. Neurosci. Abstr.* 5, 392.

Zajac, F. E., and Faden, J. S. (1985). Relationship among recruitment order, axonal conduction velocity, and muscle-unit properties of type-identified motor units in cat plantaris muscle. *J. Neurophysiol.* 53, 1303–1322.

Zengel, J. E., Reid, S. A., Sypert, G. W., and Munson, J. B. (1985). Membrane electrical properties and prediction of motor-unit type of medial gastrocnemius motoneurons in the cat. *J. Neurophysiol.* 53, 1323–1344.

6

Orderly Recruitment of Phrenic Motoneurons

ALBERT J. BERGER

Quiet breathing is a stereotyped, rhythmic act mediated principally by contraction of the main skeletal muscle of respiration, the diaphragm. The diaphragm is innervated by the phrenic nerves, whose motoneuronal cell bodies are located in the cervical spinal cord. Inspiratory-phase activity of these motoneurons leads to progressive contraction of the diaphragm. This contraction produces a smooth, downward displacement of the abdominal contents, which results in a more negative intrapleural pressure and ultimately produces expansion of the lungs and alveoli. A great advantage of using this motor system to study motor unit recruitment is that natural inspiratory-phase phrenic motoneuronal activity is present in reduced, tractable experimental preparations such as the anesthetized or decerebrate cat. This activity can be altered simply by changing the descending respiratory drive from the brain stem, such as by chemical means (hypercapnia or hypoxia) or mechanical means by tapping the epipharynx to produce an aspiration or sniff reflex that results in rapid, brief diaphragmatic contractions (Korpás and Tomori, 1979). Further, phrenic inspiratory activity is of supraspinal origin, and populations of premotor cells residing in the medulla oblongata, as well as the monosynaptic connections from these cells to the phrenic motoneurons, have been identified (Fedorko et al., 1983; Lipski et al., 1983; Merrill and Fedorko, 1984; Davies et al., 1985; Monteau et al., 1985).

The advantages of studying this system to understand the control of motor unit activity were recognized early. In 1928, in one of the first studies in which the activity of single mammalian motoneurons was recorded, Adrian and Bronk investigated the inspiratory-phase discharge properties of phrenic motoneurons, making some very important observations on the range of discharge frequency and on the unimportance of proprioceptive inputs to phrenic motor activity.

Unfortunately, no clear evidence was reported for progressive recruitment of motoneurons during inspiration. The authors concluded that discharge frequency increases account for the graded increases in diaphragmatic contraction.

Seven years before this seminal study, based upon indirect measurements involving whole phrenic nerve recordings, Gasser and Newcomer (1921) had come to an alternative conclusion: "the gradual even contraction of the diaphragm is occasioned by the calling into activity of more and more nerve fibers as inspiration deepens." This statement provided the fundamental view that recruitment of phrenic motoneurons is also important in explaining the natural behavior of the system. Thus, even at this early stage in the understanding of motor unit regulation in this motor system, the roles of both rate modulation and recruitment had been identified.

This chapter describes the recruitment process in the phrenic motor pool and provides an explanation of some possible mechanisms responsible for this phenomenon. Much of the work described here is based on attempts to investigate the applicability to the phrenic motor pool of the size principle originally presented by Henneman (1957). Many of the experiments used to investigate this problem in the phrenic motor pool are similar to those first used by Henneman and his collaborators to study neuronal recruitment in lumbosacral motor pools. Unless otherwise stated, all studies discussed were performed in decerebrate or anesthetized cats.

ANATOMICAL ORGANIZATION OF THE PHRENIC MOTOR POOL

The following discussion summarizes the important anatomical features of the cat phrenic motor pool. Phrenic motoneurons are located in the ventral portion of the ventral horn (Rexed's lamina IX) from the caudal end of C4 to the caudal end of C6. The phrenic motor column, containing the motoneuronal somas, is organized into a longitudinally oriented cylinder with a diameter of approximately 200 to 300 μm (Webber et al., 1979; Cameron et al., 1983; Berger et al., 1984). On either side of the cord, there are approximately 500 to 700 phrenic motoneurons (Duron et al., 1978; Webber et al., 1979; Berger et al., 1984). The distribution of motoneuronal somal sizes is approximately unimodal (Webber et al., 1979), as is the distribution of phrenic motor axon diameters (Duron et al., 1978). This result suggests a paucity of γ-motoneurons in this pool, which is in direct contrast to what is known of lumbosacral motoneuron pools (Burke et al., 1977). In parallel with this conclusion, there are few muscle spindles in the diaphragm; in one study, only seven and nine spindles were found in two diaphragms, respectively (Duron et al., 1978). There is a somatotopic relationship between the rostrocaudal location of a motoneuronal cell body and the portion of the diaphragm that it innervates (Duron et al., 1979). Specifically, rostral motoneurons innervate more ventral portions of the muscle, whereas caudal motoneurons innervate more dorsal regions. Cell bodies of phrenic motoneurons aggregate in clusters along the rostrocaudal axis that defines the phrenic motor column, in contrast to medial gastrocnemius motoneurons, which, when examined in the same cats, exhibited none of this clustering (Berger et al., 1984). The functional relevance of the clustering is not understood.

Another interesting anatomical feature is the presence of marked bundling of phrenic motoneuronal dendrites; again, the functional relevance of this feature is not known (Dekker et al., 1973; Cameron et al., 1983; Lipski et al., 1985). However, it has been speculated that this bundling could provide a means of motoneuronal synchronization, possibly through chemical or electrical interactions between dendrites, or that it may be a structural feature that provides for efficient sharing of common synaptic inputs. Although triceps surae α-motoneuronal dendrites exhibit radial symmetry about their cell bodies (Cullheim et al., 1987b), this is not the case for phrenic motoneurons (Cameron et al., 1983; Lipski et al., 1985). Dendrites from these latter cells project preferentially to various regions in both the gray and white matter of the cervical cord. The main region of dendritic projection is within the cylinder that defines the phrenic motor column itself.

RECRUITMENT

Figure 6–1 illustrates the spontaneous discharge pattern of diaphragmatic motor units recorded from the costal region of the diaphragm during quiet breathing. Some motor units begin to fire at the beginning of inspiration, whereas others are recruited as inspiration progresses. Still others (not illustrated) do not fire at all during quiet breathing, but may do so under specific reflex conditions when additional diaphragmatic effort is required (Jodkowski et al., 1987). This task-specific recruitment is analogous to that existing in the hindlimb, where some motor units are active during standing, others are recruited during walking, and still others are recruited during jumping (Burke, 1981a; Sypert and Munson, 1981). The distribution of firing onset times with respect to the onset of whole phrenic nerve activity during inspiration is approximately bimodal (Hillaire et al., 1972; Donnelly et al., 1985; Dick et al., 1987). Cells that begin their activity approximately at the onset of phrenic nerve activity are termed "early phrenic motoneurons." Cells that begin to fire after 10–20% of the inspiratory phase has been completed are termed "late phrenic motoneurons." Motor unit behavior is stereotyped from inspiration to inspiration. That is, the time at which a unit is recruited is approximately constant; in addition, the spike discharge pattern is approximately the same from cycle to cycle (Fig. 6–1).

After a motor unit is recruited, its discharge frequency increases as inspiration progresses. Thus, both recruitment and frequency modulation are responsible for the progressive increase of negative intrapleural pressure that characterizes inspiration and that ultimately results in an increase in lung volume (Fig. 6–1). The integrated phrenic motoneuronal and diaphragmatic motor unit activities exhibit a crescendo as inspiration progresses. Following the peak of inspiratory activity, most electrical activity ceases abruptly and the diaphragm remains quiescent until the start of the next inspiration.

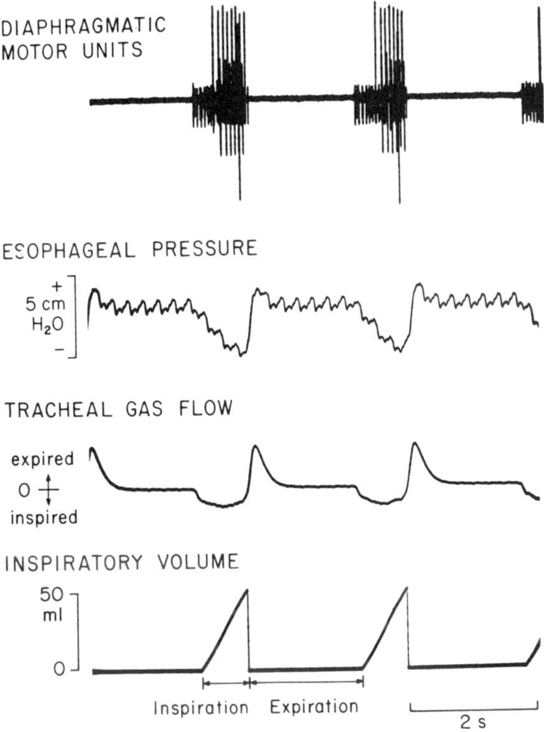

Fig. 6–1. Discharge pattern of diaphragmatic motor units and its relationship to intrathoracic pressure and lung volume changes during quiet breathing. Note the presence of both early- and late-onset motor units. Esophageal pressure changes in the same direction and by approximately the same magnitude during each breathing cycle, as does intrapleural pressure. Small-amplitude, high-frequency waves in the esophageal pressure trace are due to heart movements. Tracheal gas flow measured by a pneumotachograph connected to the tracheal cannula. Tidal volume derived by integrating the inspiratory-phase gas flow.

A major purpose of our research is to explain why some phrenic motoneurons fire earlier than others during inspiration. In essence, the question is: What is the mechanism for the recruitment order of these motoneurons? Basically, there have been two views on this subject. One holds that the recruitment can be explained using Henneman's size principle, i.e., that properties of motoneurons themselves, correlated with cell size, are responsible for the order of recruitment. The other holds that differences in synaptic inputs are responsible for recruitment order. As explained later, a combination of the two views probably best describes the factors determining the order of phrenic motoneuronal recruitment during inspiration.

SIZE PRINCIPLE

Certain observations support the use of the size principle to account for the orderly recruitment of phrenic motoneurons. Extracellular recording of two or more phrenic motor axons using a single recording electrode has shown that axons beginning their inspiratory discharge first had significantly smaller spike amplitudes than those whose discharge began later (Hilaire et al., 1972; Iscoe et al., 1976). There were exceptions to this finding, which is expected, because of technical limitations arising from multiunit extracellular recording from a single nerve fascicle. Further, multiunit recordings have shown that later-recruited diaphragmatic motor units have shorter contraction times and greater tetanic tensions than earlier-recruited motor units (Büdingen and Yasargil, 1972). Using intracellular injection of horseradish peroxidase (HRP), early- and late-recruited phrenic motoneurons were shown to be morphologically distinct. This finding was based upon differences in somal size, the regions to which the dendrites projected, and dendritic complexity (Cameron et al., 1985; see also Webber and Pleschka, 1976). A recent report on type-identified triceps surae α-motoneurons (Cullheim et al., 1987a) has shown that slow-twitch (type S) motoneurons have less complex dendritic trees and a significantly smaller mean total membrane surface area than fast-twitch (type F) motoneurons.

Recently, we employed an experimental approach devised by Henneman and his colleagues (Bawa et al., 1984) to compare the size (i.e., axonal conduction velocities) and recruitment order of pairs of diaphragmatic motor units (Dick et al., 1987). We recorded activity from pairs of diaphragmatic motor units and used two-point, delayed spike-triggered averaging (STA) of whole phrenic nerve activity to determine, with high accuracy, the axonal conduction velocity of each of the motor units (Dick et al., 1987). This method has the advantage that recruitment times and axonal conduction velocities are measured simultaneously for the motor units of a pair. Thus, pairwise comparisons of both axonal conduction velocity and recruitment order minimized experimental uncertainty. Results showed that inspiratory-phase recruitment time for a single motor unit is significantly correlated with axonal conduction velocity (correlation coefficient $r = 0.72$, $p < 0.0001$). This is shown in Figure 6–2A, where recruitment time is normalized to take into account the variability of inspiratory duration over the course of any one experiment and between experiments. Therefore, motor units that started to discharge early in inspiration had slower conduction velocities than those that started to discharge later. Figure 6–2B compares the axonal conduction velocities of simultaneously recorded diaphragmatic motor units pairs. For 93% (155/166) of motor unit pairs for which the difference in axonal conduction velocity was >1 m/s, we observed that the slower-conducting motor unit was recruited before the faster-conducting unit. The results presented in Figure 6–2 were independent of whether or not the dorsal roots were intact. These results support the applicability of Henneman's size principle to those portions of the phrenic motor pool that are active during quiet breathing. It is likely (see the later discussion) that in this circumstance only some of the diaphragmatic motor units are active.

In the hindlimb, a high correlation exists between order of recruitment and axonal conduction velocity for S motor units, but no such correlation was found for F motor units (Zajac and Faden, 1985). It has also been observed in cats walking at slow to moderate speeds, during which the S units and the smaller F units (the so-called FR, or fast-twitch, fatigue-resistant units) are active, that

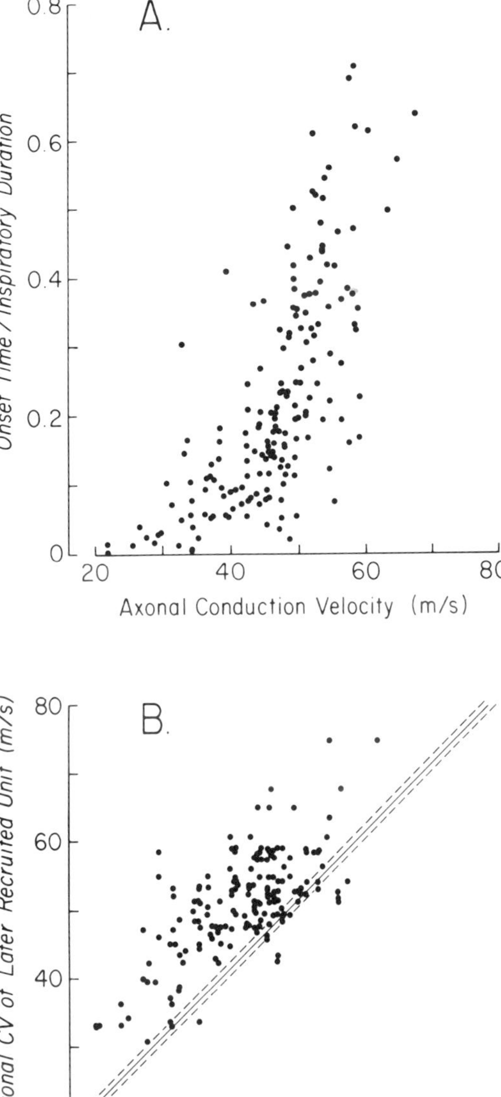

Fig. 6–2. Relationships between diaphragmatic motor unit recruitment and motor unit axonal conduction velocity. (A) Relative firing onset time during inspiration plotted against axonal conduction velocity for single motor units. Motor units recruited later in inspiration have greater axonal conduction velocity. (B) Pairwise comparison of axonal conduction velocity of later recruited versus earlier recruited diaphragmatic motor units that were simultaneously recorded. For each pair, the abscissa is the conduction velocity of the earlier recruited motor unit; the ordinate is the conduction velocity of the later recruited unit. Points above the line of identity (solid line) are for pairs of motor units where the earlier recruited motor unit has a conduction velocity lower than that of the later recruited unit. Dashed lines are confidence limits in conduction velocity measurements (± 1 m/s). Points outside these lines represent motor units whose conduction velocities were significantly different. (Modified from Dick et al., 1987.)

a good correlation exists between recruitment and axonal conduction velocity for these types of motor units (Hoffer et al., 1987). During running and jumping, the larger F motor units, including FI (fast-twitch intermediate) and FF (fast-twitch fatigable), are active (Burke, 1981b). These results in the hindlimb, which indicate that recruitment order is highly correlated with axonal conduction velocity for S units but not for the larger F units, has relevance for the phrenic motor pool when assessing which types of motor units are active during quiet breathing, where, as described earlier, there is a very good correlation between recruitment order and axonal conduction velocity.

Recently, we have determined the electrical properties of antidromically identified phrenic motoneurons whose membrane potentials were recorded intracellularly (Jodkowski et al., 1987). These electrical properties, including input resistance (R_n) and rheobase (I_{rh}), were measured during hypocapnic apnea. In this condition, the cells are neither spiking nor receiving phasic synaptic inputs. Figure 6–3A shows the relationship between I_{rh} and R_n for the overall population of 38 phrenic motoneurons in this study. In addition to the existence of an inverse relationship between these variables (see also Zengel et al., 1985), it is of interest that the distribution of data points is not uniform. Few phrenic motoneurons have an R_n near 1.3 MΩ. Therefore, we classified phrenic motoneurons into two groups based on R_n. One class of neurons was termed "type L" for low R_n (<1.3 MΩ), and a second class of neurons was termed "type H" for high R_n (>1.3 MΩ). Type L cells had a significantly higher I_{rh} (mean, 13.7 nA) than type H cells (mean, 5.3 nA). Following the determination of electrical properties, we elevated inspired CO_2 to initiate respiratory rhythmogenesis. During this procedure, we were able to maintain stable intracellular recordings for a subset ($n = 14$) of the cells, and for each of these, we determined the maximal inspiratory-phase synaptic depolarization, as well as whether the cell had an inspiratory-phase spike discharge. Figure 6–3B summarizes the results of this experiment. Type L cells had low synaptic depolarization and were not recruited to fire. In contrast, type H cells had significantly greater synaptic depolarization, and four of six were recruited to fire. Clearly of interest would be whether these two different groups of motoneurons were from motor units with different contractile properties.

Previously, Zengel et al. (1985), in studying medial gastrocnemius motor units, observed that a combination of I_{rh} and R_n was an excellent predictor of motor unit type determined on the basis of contractile properties. They found that an I_{rh}/R_n ratio of 7 separated the type S ($I_{rh}/R_n < 7$) from the type F ($I_{rh}/R_n > 7$) motor units. The dashed line in Figure 6–3A passes through the origin and has a slope (I_{rh}/R_n) equal to 7. Clearly, this line divides the phrenic motoneuronal population into two groups that were determined previously by using $R_n = 1.3$ MΩ alone. Further, if we extrapolate the results of Zengel et al. (1985) in the hindlimb to the phrenic motor pool, we would predict that most, if not all, type L phrenic motoneurons are type F motor units and that type H phrenic motoneurons are primarily type S motor units. Thus, in quiet breathing, the active diaphragmatic motor units are mostly type S. This conclusion is based on circumstantial evidence and awaits direct testing.

The low density of data points in the vicinity of the $I_{rh}/R_n = 7$ line (Fig.

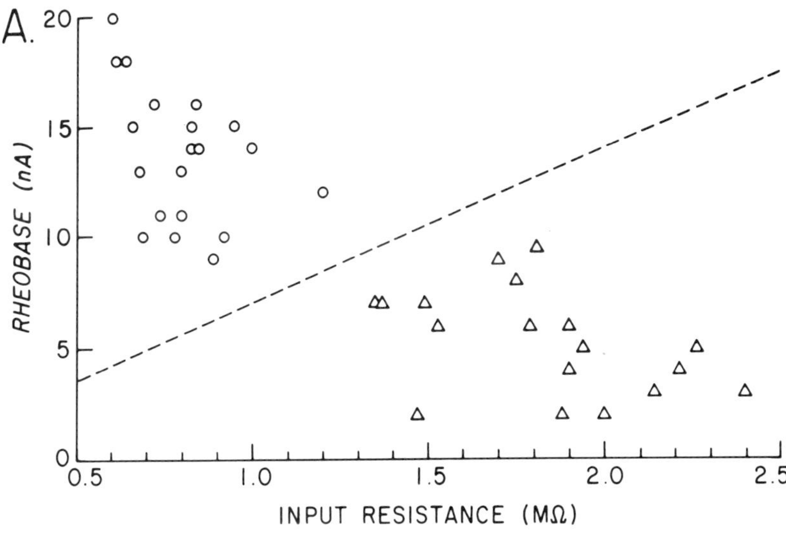

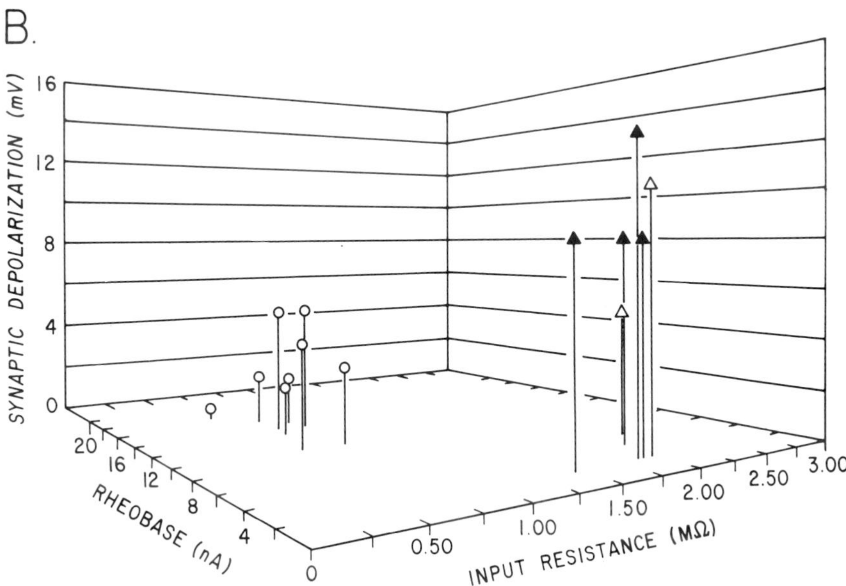

Fig. 6–3. Relationship of rheobase, input resistance, inspiratory-phase synaptic drive, and recruitment for phrenic motoneurons. (A) Relationship between rheobase and input resistance for 38 phrenic motoneurons determined during hypocapnic apnea. Different symbols represent different subpopulations of phrenic motoneurons (*circles*: low input resistance cells; *triangles*: high input resistance cells). Dashed line (*y* = 7*x*) derived from data of Zengel et al. (1985). (B) Amplitude of inspiratory-phase synaptic depolarization induced by elevating end-tidal CO_2 versus rheobase and input resistance for 14 phrenic motoneurons. *Circles*: low input resistance cells; *triangles*: high input resistance cells. *Open symbols*: cells not recruited to fire; *filled triangles*: cells recruited to fire during inspiration. (Modified from Jodkowski et al., 1987.)

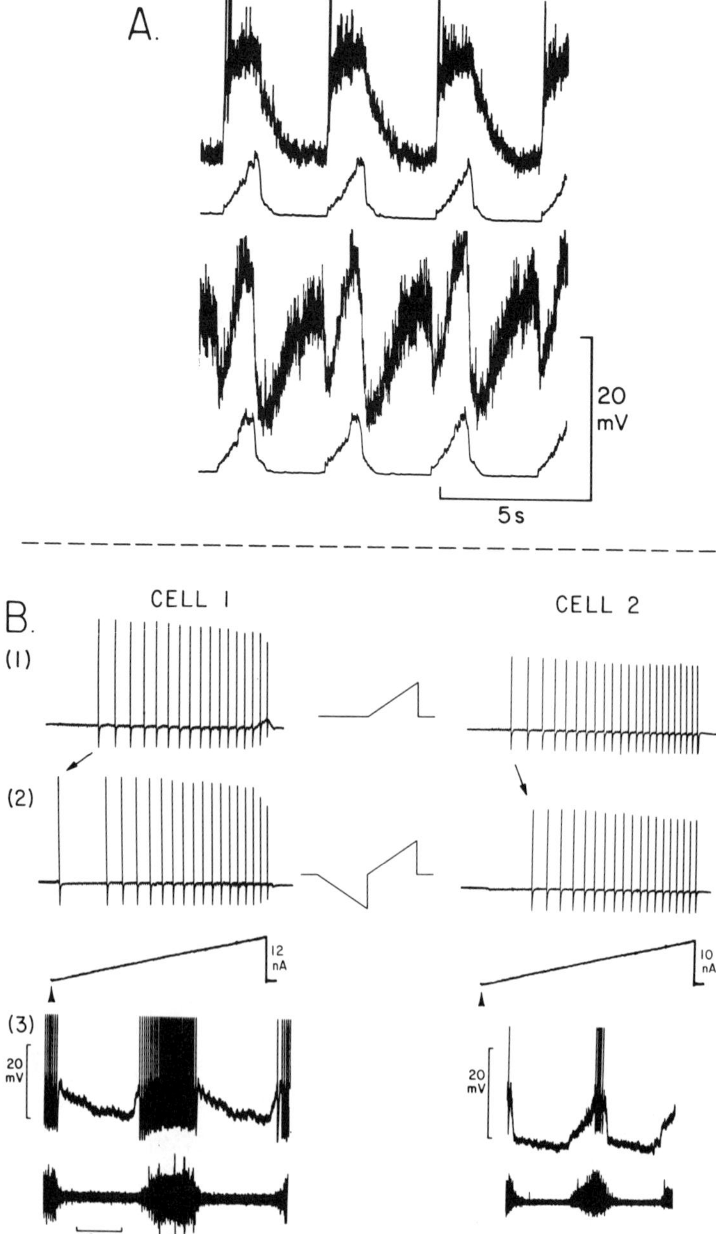

Fig. 6–4. Possible effect of expiratory-phase inhibition of phrenic motoneurons on their inspiratory-phase recruitment. (A) Effect of hyperpolarizing current injection on the membrane potential trajectory of an early-firing phrenic motoneuron. *Upper record (two traces)*: control record; note the slow wave of increasing hyperpolarization throughout expiration and the rapid initial depolarization and firing at the start of inspiration. *Lower record*: from the same cell, but while passing 10 nA hyperpolarizing current. Note the reversal of the expiratory-phase hyperpolarizing wave to a depolarizing wave, thereby demonstrating active expiratory-phase inhibition. *Upper trace, each record*: membrane potential (only partial spikes can be seen); *lower trace*: integrated

6–3A) suggests that type FR motor units may be lower in frequency in this motor system compared with the medial gastrocnemius system, where a more even distribution of points has been observed (Zengel et al., 1985). Data of Fournier and Sieck (1988), which are based on a relatively small population of motor units, indicate that only 4% of diaphragmatic motor units are of type FR. In contrast, in the medial gastrocnemius, 20–30% of motor units are of this type (Burke, 1981a; Fleshman et al., 1981).

SYNAPTIC INPUTS

Preferential connectivity between different types of bulbospinal inspiratory premotor neurons and phrenic motoneurons has been proposed as a mechanism for ordering motor unit recruitment (Monteau et al., 1985). In this case, early-recruited inspiratory bulbospinal neurons are more likely to provide stronger synaptic input to early than to late-recruited phrenic motoneurons. Similarly, late-recruited inspiratory bulbospinal neurons may have increased connectivity with late-recruited versus early-recruited motoneurons. Such preferential connectivity has been demonstrated from one population of medullary inspiratory bulbospinal neurons, the dorsal respiratory group neurons, using intracellular STA of phrenic motoneurons (Monteau et al., 1985). This mechanism cannot be the only one responsible for the orderly recruitment of phrenic motoneurons, because monosynaptic excitatory connections from this population of bulbospinal neurons provide only a small fraction of the total inspiratory-phase depolarization required by a phrenic motoneuron to reach spike threshold (Davies et al., 1985; Jodkowski et al., 1987). Further, when the presence of preferential connectivity has been tested by other, albeit less direct, methods, it has not been found (Davies et al., 1985; Donnelly et al., 1985; Dick et al., 1987). It is therefore uncertain whether there are preferential inspiratory synaptic inputs to phrenic motoneurons.

Another possible synaptic mechanism that may influence spike discharge has as its basis the presence of expiratory-phase inhibition of phrenic motoneurons and the effect of this inhibition upon the subsequent inspiratory-phase spike discharge. In 1979, it was demonstrated directly that during expiration

---

whole phrenic nerve activity. Calibrations same for both records. (Reprinted from Berger, 1979). (B) Effect of ramp current injections on early-firing (left column, cell 1) and late-firing (right column, cell 2) phrenic motoneurons. (1): Effect of 1-sec positive-current ramp injection on firing pattern (ac-coupled records here and in (2); schematic form of the ramp is shown between the two records). (2): Effect of identical 1-sec positive-current ramp, as in (1), but preceded by a negative-current ramp of the same duration and absolute peak amplitude. *Upper traces*: spike records; *lower traces*: positive-current ramp trajectories for both (1) and (2). Each of the arrowheads points to the onset of the positive ramp. Note the shift in the latency of the first spike, indicated at the arrow in each record, with application of the negative-current ramp. (3): Rhythmic, respiratory-related membrane potential changes and inspiratory-phase firing for the same cells as in (1) and (2), but after elevation of end-tidal CO_2. *Upper traces*: membrane potential (dc-coupled records), spikes truncated; *lower traces*: whole phrenic nerve activity. Time calibration is the same for the left- and right-hand records in (3). (Reprinted from Jodkowski et al., 1988).

both early- and late-onset phrenic motoneurons are actively inhibited (Berger, 1979). This inhibition is particularly strong in early onset motoneurons, as shown in Figure 6–4A, where, for such a cell, continuous hyperpolarizating current injection clearly reversed the expiratory-phase hyperpolarization to one that becomes a ramp depolarization. Further, the inspiratory-phase membrane depolarization trajectory was also markedly influenced by this hyperpolarizing current injection; the cell no longer showed a rapid depolarization leading to spike discharge at the start of inspiration. This result led to the hypothesis that expiratory-phase inhibitory synaptic input can influence the subsequent inspiratory-phase recruitment (Berger, 1979).

Recently, we tested this hypothesis by injecting negative- and positive-current ramps into otherwise quiescent phrenic motoneurons during hypocapnic apnea to simulate synaptic inputs (Jodkowski et al., 1988). We compared the time to the first spike from the start of the depolarizing current ramp under two conditions: (1) where only a depolarizing ramp of current was given and (2) where it was immediately preceded by a hyperpolarizing current ramp of the same duration and absolute peak amplitude as the subsequent depolarizing ramp. The hyperpolarizing and depolarizing current ramps were intended to simulate the pattern of expiratory-phase inhibition and inspiratory-phase excitation of phrenic motoneurons, respectively. In different cells, we found that compared to depolarizing current ramps alone, the onset of discharges could be advanced or retarded during the depolarizing current ramp if that ramp were preceded by a hyperpolarizing ramp. Figure 6–4B shows the results of ramp current injections in two phrenic motoneurons. Figure 6–4B, (1) and (2) [left-hand records—cell 1], spike onset is advanced to the very beginning of the depolarizing ramp following release of the hyperpolarizing current. This early spike onset compares with a spike onset that is delayed almost 250 ms from the start of the depolarizing ramp alone. In contrast, for the motoneuron shown in Figures 6–4B(1) and 6–4B(2) [right-hand records—cell 2], the hyperpolarizing ramp led to a 70-ms retardation of spike onset. In these same motoneurons, the functional importance of these effects to spike recruitment was suggested when we were able to raise the end-tidal CO_2 level, initiating respiratory rhythm and motoneuronal discharge. Figure 6–4B(3) (left-hand records) shows that cell 1, with spike onset advancement, turned out to be an early-onset phrenic motoneuron, whereas cell 2 [Fig. 6–4B(3) (right-hand record)], with spike onset retardation, was a late-onset phrenic motoneuron. Thus, these results demonstrate that synaptic input can influence spike recruitment in phrenic motoneurons and that expiratory-phase inhibition may be an important factor in determining subsequent inspiratory-phase spike onset.

The ionic mechanisms responsible for these effects have yet to be determined but clearly are worthy of further study. It is possible that the rebound excitation and advancement of spike onset may be due to the inward current responsible for anomalous rectification or a low-threshold calcium conductance, both of which have been observed in vitro (Llinás and Yarom, 1981; Spain et al., 1987). Spike onset retardation may be due to activation of the so-called A-current, which is a transient outward current (Rogawski, 1985). Thus, differences in the balance of currents activated by expiratory-phase inhibition of phrenic motoneurons may in part determine their recruitment order.

In summary, our studies have demonstrated that the orderly recruitment of phrenic motoneurons during inspiration is determined primarily by intrinsic properties of these motoneurons in accord with Henneman's size principle. Further, I_{rh} and R_n values were found to predict whether a phrenic motoneuron was recruited to fire during inspiration. Finally, presynaptic factors, such as expiratory-phase inhibition and the extent to which this inhibition may activate inward and outward currents, were suggested as affecting the onset of spike discharge during the subsequent inspiratory burst.

Acknowledgments

This work was supported by National Institutes of Health Javits Neuroscience Investigator Award NS 14857. Special thanks also go to Dr. T. E. Dick for his review of the manuscript and to Hanna Atkins for editing and preparing the illustrations.

REFERENCES

Adrian, E. D., and Bronk, D. W. (1928). The discharge of impulses in motor nerve fibres. Part I. Impulses in single fibres of the phrenic nerve. *J. Physiol. (Lond.)* 66, 81–101.

Bawa, P., Binder, M. D., Ruenzel, P., and Henneman, E. (1984). Recruitment order of motoneurons in stretch reflexes is highly correlated with their axonal conduction velocity. *J. Neurophysiol.* 52, 410–420.

Berger, A. J. (1979). Phrenic motoneurons in the cat: Subpopulations and nature of respiratory drive potentials. *J. Neurophysiol.* 42, 76–90.

Berger, A. J., Cameron, W. E., Averill, D. B., Kramis, R. C., and Binder, M. D. (1984). Spatial distributions of phrenic and medial gastrocnemius motoneurons in the cat spinal cord. *Exp. Neurol.* 86, 559–575.

Büdingen, H. J., and Yasargil, G. M. (1972). Die funktionelle Organisation der motorischen Einheiten des Zwerchfells. *Pflügers Arch.* 332, 218–231.

Burke, R. E. (1981a). Motor units: Anatomy, physiology, and functional organization. In *Handbook of Physiology*, Vol. II, Part 1, Sect. 1, *The Nervous System* (ed. V. B. Brooks), American Physiological Society, pp. 345–422.

Burke, R. E. (1981b). Motor unit recruitment: What are the critical factors? In *Motor Unit Types, Recruitment and Plasticity in Health and Disease. Progress in Clinical Neurophysiology*, Vol. 9 (ed. J. E. Desmedt), Karger, Basel, pp. 61–84.

Burke, R. E., Strick, P. L., Kanda, K., Kim, C. C., and Walmsley, B. (1977). Anatomy of medial gastrocnemius and soleus motor nuclei in cat spinal cord. *J. Neurophysiol.* 40, 667–680.

Cameron, W. E., Averill, D. B., and Berger, A. J. (1983). Morphology of cat phrenic motoneurons as revealed by intracellular injection of horseradish peroxidase. *J. Comp. Neurol.* 219, 70–80.

Cameron, W. E., Averill, D. B., and Berger, A. J. (1985). Evidence for differential inputs to phrenic motoneurons based on dendritic morphology. In *Neurogenesis of Central Respiratory Rhythm*, (ed. A. L. Bianchi and M. Denavit-Saubié). MTP Press, Lancaster, U.K., pp. 230–233.

Cullheim, S., Fleshman, J. W., Glenn, L. L., and Burke, R. E. (1987a). Membrane area and dendritic structure in type-identified triceps surae alpha motoneurons. *J. Comp. Neurol.* 255, 68–81.

Cullheim, S., Fleshman, J. W., Glenn, L. L., and Burke, R. E. (1987b). Three-dimensional architecture of dendritic trees in type-identified α-motoneurons. *J. Comp. Neurol.* 255, 82–96.

Davies, J. G. McF., Kirkwood, P. A., and Sears, T. A. (1985). The distribution of monosynaptic connexions from inspiratory bulbospinal neurones to inspiratory motoneurons in the cat. *J. Physiol. (Lond.)* 368, 63–87.

Dekker, J. J., Lawrence, D. G., and Kuypers, H. G. J. M. (1973). The location of longitudinally running dendrites in the ventral horn of the cat spinal cord. *Brain Res.* 51, 319–325.

Dick, T. E., Kong, F.-J., and Berger, A. J. (1987). Correlation of recruitment order with axonal conduction velocity for supraspinally driven diaphragmatic motor units. *J. Neurophysiol.* 57, 245–259.

Donnelly, D. F., Cohen, M. I., Sica, A. L., and Zhang, H. (1985). Responses of early and late onset phrenic motoneurons to lung inflation. *Respir. Physiol.* 61, 69–83.

Duron, B., Jung-Caillol, M. C., and Marlot, D. (1978). Myelinated nerve fiber supply and muscle spindles in the respiratory muscles of cat: Quantitative study. *Anat. Embryol.* 152, 171–192.

Duron, B., Marlot, D., Larnicol, N., Jung-Caillol, M. C., and Macron, J. M. (1979). Somatotopy in the phrenic motor nucleus of the cat as revealed by retrograde transport of horseradish peroxidase. *Neurosci. Lett.* 14, 159–163.

Fedorko, L., Merrill, E. G., and Lipski, J. (1983). Two descending medullary inspiratory pathways to phrenic motoneurones. *Neurosci. Lett.* 43, 285–291.

Fleshman, J. W., Munson, J. B., Sypert, G. W., and Friedman, W. A. (1981). Rheobase, input resistance, and motor-unit type in medial gastrocnemius motoneurons in the cat. *J. Neurophysiol.* 46, 1326–1338.

Fournier, M. and Sieck, G. C. (1988). Mechanical properties of muscle units in the cat diaphragm. *J. Neurophysiol.* 59, 1055–1066.

Gasser, H. S., and Newcomer, H. S. (1921). Physiological action currents in the phrenic nerve. An application of the thermionic vacuum tube to nerve physiology. *Am. J. Physiol.* 57, 1–26.

Henneman, E. (1957). Relations between size of neurons and their susceptibility to discharge. *Science* 126, 1345–1347.

Hilaire, G., Monteau, R., and Dussardier, M. (1972). Modalités du recrutement des motoneurones phréniques. *J. Physiol. (Paris)* 64, 457–478.

Hoffer, J. A., Loeb, G. E., Marks, W. B., O'Donovan, M. J., Pratt, C. A., and Sugano, N. (1987). Cat hindlimb motoneurons during locomotion. I. Destination, axonal conduction velocity, and recruitment threshold. *J. Neurophysiol.* 57, 510–529.

Iscoe, S., Dankoff, J., Migicovsky, R., and Polosa, C. (1976). Recruitment and discharge frequency of phrenic motoneurons during inspiration. *Respir. Physiol.* 26, 113–128.

Jodkowski, J. S., Viana, F., Dick, T. E., and Berger, A. J. (1987). Electrical properties of phrenic motoneurons in the cat: Correlation with inspiratory drive. *J. Neurophysiol.* 58, 105–124.

Jodkowski, J. S., Viana, F., Dick, T. E., and Berger, A. J. (1988). Repetitive firing properties of phrenic motoneurons in the cat. *J. Neurophysiol.* 60, 687–702.

Korpás, J., and Tomori, Z. (1979). The sniff-like aspiration reflex. In *Progress in*

Respiration Research, Vol. 12: *Cough and Other Respiratory Reflexes,* (ed. H. Herzog). Karger, Basel, pp. 224–250.

Lipski, J., Fyffe, R. E. W., and Jodkowski, J. (1985). Recurrent inhibition of cat phrenic motoneurons. *J. Neurosci.* 5, 1545–1555.

Lipski, J., Kubin, L., and Jodkowski, J. (1983). Synaptic action of R_β neurons on phrenic motoneurons studied with spike-triggered averaging. *Brain Res.* 288, 105–118.

Llinás, R., and Yarom, Y. (1981). Electrophysiology of mammalian inferior olivary neurones *in vitro.* Different types of voltage-dependent ionic conductances. *J. Physiol. (Lond.)* 315, 549–567.

Merrill, E. G., and Fedorko, L. (1984). Monosynaptic inhibition of phrenic motoneurons: A long descending projection from Bötzinger neurons. *J. Neurosci.* 4, 2350–2353.

Monteau, R., Khatib, M., and Hilaire, G. (1985). Central determination of recruitment order: Intracellular study of phrenic motoneurons. *Neurosci. Lett.* 56, 341–346.

Rowgawski, M. A. (1985) The A-current: How ubiquitous a feature of excitable cells is it? *Trends Neurosci.* 8, 214–219.

Spain, W. J., Schwindt, P. C., and Crill, W. E. (1987). Anomalous rectification in neurons from cat sensorimotor cortex in vitro. *J. Neurophysiol.* 57, 1555–1576.

Sypert, G. W., and Munson, J. B. (1981). Basis of segmental motor control: Motoneuron size or motor unit type? *Neurosurgery* 8, 608–621.

Webber, C. L., Jr., and Pleschka, K. (1976). Structural and functional characteristics of individual phrenic motoneurons. *Pflügers Arch.* 365, 113–121.

Webber, C. L., Jr., Wurster, R. D., and Chung, J. M. (1979). Cat phrenic nucleus architecture as revealed by horseradish peroxidase mapping. *Exp. Brain Res.* 35, 395–406.

Zajac, F. E., and Faden, J. S. (1985). Relationship among recruitment order, axonal conduction velocity, and muscle-unit properties of type-identified motor units in cat plantaris muscle. *J. Neurophysiol.* 53, 1303–1322.

Zengel, J. E., Reid, S. A., Sypert, G. W., and Munson, J. B. (1985). Membrane electrical properties and prediction of motor-unit type of medial gastrocnemius motoneurons in the cat. *J. Neurophysiol.* 53, 1323–1344.

III
PROPERTIES OF MOTONEURONS

Perspectives on Neuron Modeling

WILFRID RALL

Many different neuronal models have been created for different purposes. In my research, I have usually tried to include in the model the most essential features of what we know about anatomy and physiology, and use it to predict the results of certain experiments. The art comes in deciding how much detail can be judged nonessential for each particular purpose; such detail can then be smoothed (idealized) to help focus attention on the variables chosen for study. Once such an idealized model is formulated mathematically, computational experiments with this model can be used to make explicit predictions for different sets of model parameters. These predictions should be tested against the results of suitably controlled laboratory experiments. With luck, qualitative agreement may provide the encouragement to pursue improved values for the model parameters, and these may provide even quantitative agreement with the experiment. Alternatively, one may be lucky in a different way; by discovering a basic flaw in the model, one may be led to create a different model with better prospects for success. In the process of exploring the properties of successful models, one can gain insights that provide a deeper understanding of the model system, and these insights may contribute both to the design of better experiments and to a better understanding of the biological system.

Much of this chapter is concerned with models of individual motoneurons, some with idealized dendritic branching, others with arbitrary branching, and some with soma shunt conductance; there is also consideration of the degrees of freedom in a large, multicompartmental model of such individual neurons. However, the unifying theme of the present volume also suggests a brief review of some earlier efforts at modeling populations of motoneurons.

FRACTIONAL POOL DISCHARGE: MONOSYNAPTIC INPUT–OUTPUT RELATION

My earliest news of Elwood Henneman came in 1954 on the day I presented my first seminar at the National Institutes of Health (NIH). Based on my Ph.D. research, this seminar included experimental results and a model for monosynaptic input–output relations in a motoneuron pool. One of the points emphasized was the need to scale the output magnitude (synchronous output volley recorded from the ventral root) relative to an elusive maximum (i.e., a complete synchronous discharge from all of the motoneurons in the pool); such scaling provides an estimate of fractional pool discharge. In the discussion following the seminar, someone mentioned that Henneman had also been concerned with estimating fractional pool discharge. It seems that both he and I had come to pursue this interest quite independently. We both explored various experimental approaches to measurement of complete pool discharge, and both recognized that posttetanic potentiation of this monosynaptic reflex (Lloyd, 1949; Eccles and Rall, 1950) provides a valuable means of demonstrating that the usual unpotentiated output represents incomplete pool discharge (Rall, 1951, 1954, 1955a, 1955b; Henneman, 1954; see also Jefferson and Benson, 1953).

My interest in this problem arose during an apprenticeship with Professors J. C. Eccles and A. K. McIntyre in Dunedin, New Zealand (1949–53). It followed from the pioneering study of the monosynaptic input–output relation that Lloyd had begun with the segmental reflex (Lloyd, 1943, 1945). On the basis of experiments by Lloyd and McIntyre in New York, and our experiments in Dunedin (Brock et al. 1951), I knew that it was important to restrict the input to a muscle nerve (triceps surae). Compared with dorsal root stimulation, this had two important advantages: (1) this restricted the input–output study to a pair of synergic motoneuron pools, in contrast to the nonfunctional combination of motoneuron pools provided by the segmental reflex (which includes antagonist and incomplete pools), and (2) the longer afferent conduction distance (from the hindlimb) helped to separate the effective portion from the ineffective portion of the input volley, because direct synapses to the motoneuron pool are made only by the group Ia afferent axons (which have the largest diameters, lowest electrical thresholds, and highest conduction velocities). Axons of group Ib and group II are also active in a maximal afferent volley, but they make no contribution to the effective input of the monosynaptic reflex because they make no direct synapses to the motoneuron pool; these ineffective axons have smaller diameters, higher electrical thresholds, and lower conduction velocities, such that their contamination of the experimental input record is greatest for large afferent volleys produced by large electrical stimuli. However, because groups Ia and Ib overlap in their threshold distributions, it was essential to determine the relation between the effective input and the experimental input record (Rall, 1955b). These points deserve emphasis because they were not recognized in another input-output study (Rosenblueth et al., 1949); consequently, those authors misinterpreted the plateau of their input–output relation as indicative of output saturation (i.e., complete discharge of their segmental pool); this error greatly complicated their effort to produce a theoretical model that could match their input–output curves.

Convincing evidence that the output plateau does not represent saturation (complete pool discharge) was provided by experiments that achieved four levels of reflex excitability in a single preparation (Rall, 1955b). These four levels were obtained by means of two depths of anesthesia, each used with and without brief tetanic conditioning. The four resulting input–output curves (see the left side of Fig. 7–1) all show an output plateau for experimental inputs greater than 70% of the maximum recorded afferent volley. It is important to understand that each output plateau corresponds to a different fraction of total pool discharge (approximately 37, 60, 72, and 84%). In other words, none of these curves showed output saturation; each plateau resulted from the ineffectiveness of the higher-threshold afferent axons (belonging to groups Ib and II), which contributed most of the upper 40% of the experimental input record. For small inputs, the effective component of the input volley (carried only by group Ia axons) grew linearly with the experimental input record (see the linear part of the dashed curve at the left in Fig. 7–1). Then, over the mid-range (from 20 to 70% of maximal experimental input), the normalized effective input curve bent and reached a maximum where the experimental input record was only 70% of its maximum. The shape of this dashed curve was verified by experiments with graded monosynaptic facilitation and with graded subthreshold synaptic potentials (of the motoneuron pool) recorded in the ventral root. Once

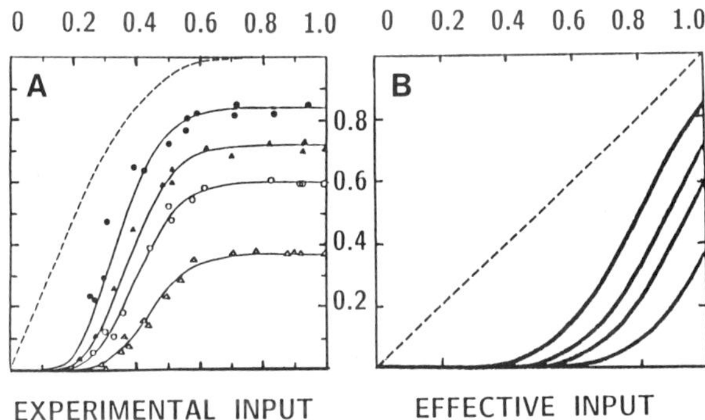

Fig. 7–1. Output as fractional pool discharge versus two different measures of input. Each input–output curve shows an output plateau in (A); transformed curves show no plateau in (B). The four solid curves in (A) were fitted to data of output versus the experimental input record (diphasic amplitude measured from intact dorsal root). The dashed line represents a normalized curve of "effective input" plotted against the experimental input record; this was based on observations of graded monosynaptic facilitation and on ventral root synaptic potentials; the linear relation for small inputs corresponds to recruitment of low-threshold group Ia fibers in the afferent muscle nerve. The ineffectiveness of increasing the experimental input volley from 60% to 100% of its maximum can be understood as resulting from the fact that the higher-threshold afferent fibers are ineffective because they belong to groups II and Ib and do not make synapses on these motoneurons. The five curves in (B) are transformed from the five curves in (A); each experimental input value (abscissa in A) was replaced (in B) by its effective input value, as defined by the ordinates on the dashed line in (A). This figure combines Figures 2 and 6 of Rall (1955b). Straight-line fitting of the transformed data was shown in Figure 4 of Rall (1955a).

this dashed curve was understood, it was not surprising that the transformed input–output curves (at the right in Fig. 7–1) did not exhibit a plateau, because here the outputs were plotted as functions of the effective input. This transformation was the key to success in fitting the data with a relatively simple theoretical model (Rall, 1955a, 1955b).

In this model, it was assumed that the distribution of activated synaptic knobs could be treated as random over the motoneuron population. Suppose that each neuron has the same number, N, of potential synaptic sites (e.g., $N = 5000$) and that each site has the same probability, γ, of being occupied by a synapse belonging to the monosynaptic pathway (e.g., $\gamma = 0.02$); then the average number of relevant synapses per motoneuron is γN (e.g., $\gamma N = 100$). The effective input, β, ranges from 0 to 1, and for any particular value of β, we assume that $\beta\gamma$ defines the probability that a synaptic site receives an activated synapse (belonging to this pathway); thus, the average number of such activated synapses per motoneuron is $n = \beta\gamma N$ (e.g., n equals 100, 75, and 50 for β values of 1, 0.75, and 0.5, respectively). Because these probabilities were assumed to be independent, the result is a binomial (nearly Poisson) distribution of the motoneuron population with respect to the number, n, of activated synapses that each receives; the variance of this distribution is very close to n (e.g., $\mathrm{var}(n) \approx 100$ when $\beta = 1$).

A motoneuron was assumed to fire an impulse when the number of its simultaneously activated synapses, n, exceeded some threshold number, h. The value of h was assumed to have a variability that could result both from inherent variability of motoneuron excitability and from background synaptic activity in other synapses. Because this variability in h was assumed to be independent of the variability in n, it was reasonable to approximate the combined variability of the motoneurons, with respect to their n-h values, as a normal distribution with a variance, $\mathrm{var}(n\text{-}h) = \mathrm{var}(n) + \mathrm{var}(h)$. In this case, good results were obtained for a normal distribution with a standard deviation very close to $\sigma = \gamma N/5$, (e.g., $\sigma = 20$).

The normal distributions in Figure 7–2 are shown with $\sigma = 20$, but to simplify the diagram, these distributions are shown as though all of the combined variability were in the value of n (the number of synapses activated on an individual motoneuron). This permitted the threshold to be shown as though it were fixed at its average value, $\bar{h}$. The diagrams at the left illustrate how this normal distribution becomes shifted (relative to $\bar{h}$) for different values of effective input ($\beta = 0.5, 0.75,$ and 1.0). In each case, the shaded area of the distribution corresponds to the output, ω, as fractional pool discharge ($\omega = 0.05, 0.40,$ and 0.84, respectively). The resulting input–output curve is shown at the right in Figure 7–2.

This model has basically two theoretical parameters; both are scaled to the number, γN, the average number of (direct group Ia) synapses per motoneuron (e.g., $\gamma N = 100$). One of these two parameters is the standard deviation, $\sigma/\gamma N$, of the motoneuron population with respect to the difference variable, n-h (i.e., the difference between the number, n, of synapses activated on a particular motoneuron and the threshold number, h, required to fire that neuron). The other basic parameter is the average threshold value, $\bar{h}/\gamma N$. It was satis-

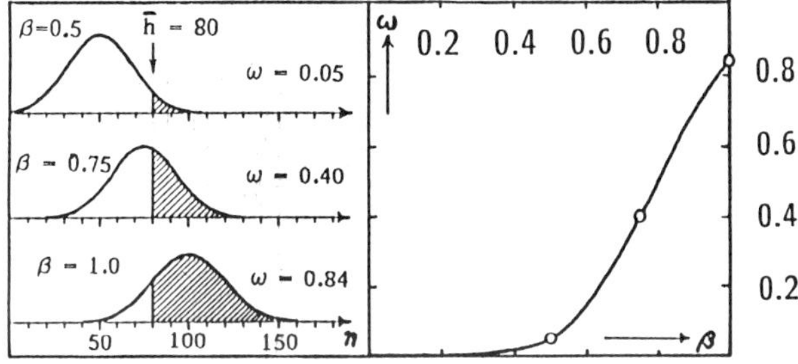

Fig. 7–2. Schematic illustration of a mathematical model that gives output (ω) as fractional pool discharge versus effective input (β). At the left, the three input values, β = 0.5, 0.75, and 1.0, result in three normal distributions of the motoneuron population with respect to the number (n) of synapses activated on a motoneuron; these normal distributions are centered about mean values of 50, 75, and 100, with a standard deviation of 20; the mean threshold value is shown as 80, for the number of activated synapses needed to fire a motoneuron spike. The fractional pool discharge is shown as the shaded area under each normal distribution curve; this is the fraction of the motoneuron population for which the number of activated synapses exceeds threshold. These fractions are shown as ω = 0.84 for β = 1, ω = 0.40 for β = 0.75, and ω = 0.05 for β = 0.5 at the left, and by the open circles on the input–output curve at the right. (Figure 1 in Rall, 1955a.)

fying to find that one of these parameters had the same value for all four of the input–output curves shown in Figure 7–1; i.e., $\sigma/\gamma N = 1/5$. Because of this, each input–output curve could be obtained by resetting the value of the other parameter, $\bar{h}/\gamma N$; four values, very close to 0.80, 0.88, 0.95, and 1.07, yielded the four input–output curves of Figure 7–1.

The agreement found between theory and experiment thus implied that the shift to a deeper level of anesthesia (in the experiment) was matched by an increase in the value of a single model parameter (the average threshold, $\bar{h}$, in the motoneuron population) without a significant change in the variance or standard deviation of the population with respect to n-h. In addition, the effect of brief tetanic conditioning was matched by a decrease in the effective value of that same model parameter (or by an increase in the effective value of n). It may be noted that complications, such as possible departures from a normal distribution, and the possible role of higher densities of activated synapses in local zones of the soma surface were addressed in the original paper (Rall, 1955a) and found to result in similar input–output curves.

Because this model also predicted how the factor of output potentiation should depend on the level of fractional pool discharge (Fig. 5 of Rall, 1955a), it was pointed out that this could be developed into a method of estimating fractional pool discharge. Further, an extension of the model to include distinctions between homonymous and heteronymous synapses was shown to yield agreement with "cross-facilitation" of one motor pool by input from heteronymous afferents, in contrast to little or no monosynaptic "cross-discharge" in the absence of homonymous input (Figs. 6 and 7 of Rall, 1955a). A related modeling effort (Rall and Hunt, 1956) was able to account for experimental observations of the firing indices of individual motoneurons, in relation to motoneuron pool discharge, during repeated trials, for several different levels of reflex excitability.

Looking back about 33 years, it seems fair to say that these early efforts did succeed in providing explicit models that corresponded reasonably well with the general concept of spatial summation in motoneuron pools, originally introduced by Denny-Brown and Sherrington (1928) and discussed by Lloyd (1945) in terms of an "excited zone," a "discharge zone," and a "subliminal fringe." The discharge zone corresponds to the shaded area in Figure 7–2, while the subliminal fringe is composed of motoneurons in a band just to the left of the vertical threshold line; the excited zone probably includes the entire population for effective inputs greater than 50% of maximum.

One result of this study was to show that the shape of the input–output curve does not require spatial summation to be the very local process envisaged by Lorente de Nó (1938) and by Lloyd (1945). Moreover, another theoretical model, for passive electrotonic spread over a spherical soma, led to the conclusion that the membrane depolarization becomes essentially uniform over the closed soma surface by the time the synaptic potential reaches its maximum amplitude (Rall, 1953, 1955a, 1959); this result weighed against the validity of very local spatial summation on the motoneuron soma surface. It is interesting that the concept of local synaptic interactions has recently returned in a different context, namely, for synapses on excitable dendritic spines at distal dendritic locations (Rall and Segev, 1987, 1988).

In concluding this section on motoneuron populations, it is important to point out several limitations of these early models. No distinction was then made between motoneurons of different size or functional type; these important distinctions have been explored by Henneman and by other contributors to this volume. The assumption of random synaptic distributions was a convenience that was justified by ignorance of actual synaptic distributions. In addition, no distinction was made between different sequences of afferent fiber recruitment, and no consideration was given to distinguishing between synapses at different (proximal to distal) dendritic locations in the motoneuron population. The task of incorporating such considerations into a more comprehensive model of a motoneuron pool provides an interesting challenge for future modeling.

FAMILY OF DENDRITIC BRANCHING MODELS

There is no one model for dendritic neurons. A variety of models has been used to solve different problems. Some models involve only cylinders; others involve tapered core conductors or dendritic trees with unequal branch lengths. A different but important approach divides the neuron into sets of connected compartments that can be assigned different surface areas, different membrane properties, and different synaptic inputs (Rall, 1964; Perkel and Mulloney, 1978). Because compartmental models are not restricted to uniform membranes or to constraints on branch diameters and lengths, they can be used to investigate the effects of various deviations from more idealized models.

DENDRITIC TREE INPUT CONDUCTANCE: EQUIVALENT CYLINDER OR NOT?

One particularly useful model is the idealized dendritic tree whose branching is constrained to permit transformation of the tree to an equivalent cylinder. The three essential constraints are as follows: (1) every branch is represented as a cylinder with the same uniform membrane properties; (2) at every branch point, the diameters of the daughter branches may be unequal, but the sum of their $d^{3/2}$ values must equal the $d^{3/2}$ value of the parent branch; and (3) individual branch lengths are not constrained, provided that all terminal branches terminate with the same boundary condition at the same electrotonic distance from the origin of the dendritic tree.

Because many dendritic trees have electrotonic lengths, L in the range from 0.5 to 1.5, it is appropriate to seek some general insights about the relations between dendritic input conductance, G_D, dendritic surface area, A_D, and dendritic membrane conductivity, G_{md}, for several different examples of dendritic trees with such L values. These examples, summarized in Table 7–1, include equivalent cylinders of three different lengths and two types of deviation from equivalence to a cylinder. In terms of ratios of input conductance and surface area, it can be seen that there is relatively little difference between most of these cases. This leads to the insight that results for the simplest cases provide good estimates for the more complicated cases. Such estimates are all we need for some purposes; in addition, they provide good initial values for further computation when higher precision is required.

Expressions for calculating the input conductance of a uniform cylinder of finite electrotonic length, $L = \ell/\lambda$, depend on the boundary conditions (Rall, 1959). When the distal end of the cylinder is sealed, the input conductance at the proximal end is less than the reference value, G_∞, by a factor that equals $\tanh(L)$. Here it may be useful to note that the hyperbolic tangent and its inverse are conveniently available on several inexpensive pocket calculators. When L is very small, the value of the hyperbolic tangent essentially equals L, while at the other extreme, large L values (from 4 to ∞) give the asymptotic value of $\tanh(L) = 1$. For intermediate L values of 0.5, 1.0, and 1.5, $\tanh(L)$ has the values shown in the first numerical column of Table 7–1 (the column headed by "G_D/G_∞"). Note that the difference between the first two values is 0.30, while the next difference is 0.143, leaving less than 0.10 for an increase in L from 1.5 to infinity. This illustrates both the nonlinearity of the hyperbolic tangent function and the biophysical fact that the input conductance increases little with further increases in dendritic electrotonic length.

The dendritic surface area, A_D, increases linearly with L, as shown by the next column of Table 7–1, which expresses the surface areas of these three cylinders relative to that for $L = 1$. Because the input conductance increases less than linearly with L, the ratio, G_D/A_D, does not remain constant; it decreases with increasing L, as shown in the next column of the table. This ratio has the physical dimensions of conductance per unit area (S/cm^2). In the limit, as L is made very small, the numerical part of this ratio approaches 1.0; this can be given the following physical interpretation: The steady-state depolari-

Table 7–1   Dendritic input conductance, surface area, G_D/A_D and L_{def}

Dendritic Tree	$G_D/G_\infty{}^a$	$A_D/(\pi\lambda_o d_o)^b$	$G_D/A_D{}^c$	$L_{def}{}^d$
Equiv. cylinder				
$L = 0.5$	0.462	0.50	0.924 G_{md}	0.50
$L = 1.0$	0.762	1.0	0.762 G_{md}	1.00
$L = 1.5$	0.905	1.5	0.603 G_{md}	1.50
Cyl. + taper^e				
L: 0–0.5–1.12	0.60	0.70	0.86 G_{md}	0.69
L: 0–0.6–1.22	0.66	0.80	0.83 G_{md}	0.79
Eight thin cylinders connected in parallel, with staggered lengths^f				
L: 0.4, …, 1.1	0.616	0.75	0.82 G_{md}	0.72
L: 0.5, …, 1.2	0.672	0.85	0.79 G_{md}	0.81
7×0.5; 1×2.0	0.525	0.69	0.76 G_{md}	0.58

^{a}This ratio equals tanh(L) for a uniform cylinder with a sealed end at L. Note that G_∞ is the limiting value of G_D for a semi-infinite extension of the cylinder (trunk cylinder of dendritic tree).

^{b}This ratio equals 1.0 for $L = 1$, because $\pi\lambda d$ equals the area of the cylindrical surface of length λ and diameter d; the subscript, o, designates the original cylinder.

^{c}The numerical portion of this entry is the quotient of the two numbers at the left; it is the factor, F_{dga}, defined by Equation (7–1); also, G_{md} equals $G_\infty/(\pi\lambda d)$ and represents the membrane conductivity (S/cm^2), being the reciprocal of membrane resistivity (ohm cm^2).

^{d}This effective L value for a dendritic tree is defined by Equation (7–3). These numbers are inverse hyperbolic tangents of the values for G_D/G_∞ shown in the first column of numbers.

^{e}Diameter held constant from $x = 0$ to $x = 0.5\lambda_o$ in the first case, and to $x = 0.6\lambda_o$ in the second case; then it was tapered by means of stepwise diameter reductions (for $\Delta x = 0.1\lambda_o$) to relative diameters of 0.8, 0.6, 0.4, and then 0.2 for the terminal segment. Note that the reduced-diameter segments have λ values that are smaller than the original λ_o; consequently, the terminal L value is 1.12 in the first case and 1.22 in the second case. For these two cases, G_D was calculated by the iterative procedure described in Rall (1959) for stepwise changes in diameter.

^{f}Eight thin cylinders of equal diameter, but unequal length, connected in parallel. The first case has a set of L values ranging from 0.4 to 1.1 in steps of 0.1; the second case differs only by replacing $L = 0.4$ with $L = 1.2$; the third case has seven cylinders with $L = 0.5$, plus one cylinder with $L = 2$. For all cases, the thin diameter was set equal to one-fourth of the large original diameter, d_o, because then the sum of the 3/2 power of the eight thin diameters equaled the 3/2 power of d_o. This choice also yielded matching cylindrical surface areas if all eight thin cylinders had the same electrotonic length, L, as the large cylinder; then the thin cylinders were half as long as the large cylinder, but their combined circumference was twice that of the large cylinder, making their surface areas equal. Such matching of areas was expected, because the large cylinder was electrotonically equivalent to the eight thin cylinders of equal L. Relative to such matching, the departure from equivalence to the large cylinder was achieved by setting the thin cylinders to unequal lengths.

zation of very short dendritic trees approaches isopotentiality, and with complete isopotentiality, the ratio G_D/A_D exactly equals the dendritic membrane conductance per unit area, G_{md} (assumed to be uniform). The values tabulated in this column are less than 1.0, showing the effect of dendritic nonisopotentiality during a steady-state input conductance measurement. For L values between 0.5 and 1.0, the correction factor lies between 0.76 and 0.925; furthermore, this range holds for all of the more complicated cases included in the lower part of this table. In fact, a middle value $G_D/A_D = 0.84\ G_{md}$, differs by less than 10% from most of the examples in this table.

    Thus, we have a robust result: The ratio of dendritic input conductance to dendritic surface area is smaller than dendritic membrane conductivity by a factor, F_{dga}, that can be expressed as

$$F_{dga} = \frac{G_D}{A_D G_{md}} = \frac{\tanh(L)}{L} \tag{7-1}$$

where the expression containing G_D provides a general definition of this factor, while the expression containing $\tanh(L)$ provides the exact result for dendritic trees that are equivalent to cylinders (the subscript, *dga*, is meant to indicate dendritic conductance and area). From the results already discussed, along with Table 7–1, we can express the approximation (within 10%) as

$$F_{dga} \approx 0.84 \qquad \text{for } (0.5 < L_{def} < 1.0) \tag{7–2}$$

which applies to a variety of dendritic trees that deviate from equivalence to a cylinder, provided that the effective dendritic electrotonic length, L_{def}, lies in the range between 0.5 and 1.0; however, it is now necessary to provide a definition of L_{def} for dendritic trees with unequal branch lengths or with taper. Because we already have an explicit interactive method (Rall, 1959) for calculating G_D/G_∞ for any dendritic tree with specified branching or (stepwise) taper, the most useful definition of L_{def} is the following:

$$L_{def} = \tanh^{-1}\left(\frac{G_D}{G_\infty}\right) \tag{7–3}$$

where the subscript, *def*, is meant to indicate effective dendritic; in addition, $\tanh^{-1}$ designates the inverse hyperbolic tangent. This definition means that L_{def} is the L value for a cylinder that has the same G_∞ as the trunk of the dendritic tree, and the same G_D as the tree. The last column of Table 7–1 lists the values of L_{def} for all these cases.

Now, returning to Equation (7–1), the real reason for focusing on this factor is that it provides a key to estimating the unknown dendritic membrane conductivity. If we have good values for the dendritic surface area and the dendritic input conductance, and if we have reasons to suppose that the effective L is between 0.5 and 1.0, we can use the approximate result (Eqs. 7–1 and 7–2) to provide an estimate of the dendritic membrane conductivity (assumed to be uniform) with an error that will probably be less than 10%. It should be pointed out, however, that because this holds for one dendritic tree, its usefulness is limited by the fact that we rarely measure the input conductance of one dendritic tree alone. Usually there are several dendritic trees connected to a soma, and we must consider the input conductance of these dendritic trees to be in parallel not only with each other but also with the soma membrane and with a soma shunt conductance if microelectrode penetration of the soma membrane is present; see the discussion in the next section.

DENDRITIC NEURON MODEL WITH SOMA SHUNT CONDUCTANCE

The neuron soma is often depicted as a sphere, but the precision of the spherical shape is irrelevant, because we assume the soma membrane potential to be uniform (isopotential). What is important about the soma is its surface area, its parallel membrane conductance and capacitance per unit area, and the shunt conductance that results when its membrane is penetrated by a microelectrode. Although recognized in cases of obvious injury, this shunt conductance was often dismissed as negligible when recording conditions seemed stable. It had been thought that a good resting potential would provide evidence of negligible leakage conductance. However (as pointed out to me by Julian Jack and Stephen Redman), that argument is no longer valid: One should expect the puncture to cause entry of calcium (Ca) ions, which would then open the Ca-dependent channels for K^+ ions, and for Cl^- ions (Krnjevic et al., 1978; Owen et al., 1984); these channels would tend to restore the resting potential and would add to the total shunt conductance. While most of these complications may be avoided when a patch electrode (with a giga-ohm seal) is used for whole cell recording, this technique seems applicable only to certain favorable situations and needs careful controls.

The effect on theoretical transients of introducing a different soma conductance value was treated by Iansek and Redman (1973); shunt conductance at one end of a cylinder of finite length was treated by Rall (1969). The publications of Durand (1984) and Kawato (1984), as well as unpublished results of mine, have dealt with the effects of large soma shunt conductances on the transient properties of a soma-dendritic model; also, some of the steady-state aspects were discussed by Rall (1977, p. 91).

Here we focus on how the soma shunt conductance complicates the task of estimating neuronal membrane resistivity. The input conductance, G_N, of the neuron is the sum of the soma conductance and the combined input conductance of n dendritic trees:

$$G_N = G_s + \sum_j^n G_{D_j} \tag{7-4}$$

The soma conductance can be expressed

$$G_s = G_{\text{shunt}} + G_{ms}A_s = \beta G_{md}A_s \tag{7-5}$$

where the expression at the far right constitutes a definition of β, a parameter that can be thought of as the soma shunting factor. For large shunt conductances, β can be as large as 1000; for a zero shunt conductance, $\beta = 1$, if the membrane conductivity is the same for somatic and dendritic membrane.

The combined conductance of the n dendritic trees can be expressed as

$$\sum_j^n G_{D_j} = G_{md} \sum_j^n (F_{dga_j}A_{D_j}) \approx G_{md}F_{dga}A_{CD} \tag{7-6}$$

where the approximation, at the right, implies that all the trees have essentially the same value of the factor, F_{dga} (defined by Eq. 7–1) and A_{CD} represents the combined surface area of all of the dendritic trees; if there are two groups of dendrites with different effective electrotonic lengths (implying different values of F_{dga}), these groups should be summed separately. By combining Equations (7–4) to (7–6), we can also obtain the expressions

$$G_N = G_{md}(\beta A_s + F_{dga}A_{CD}) = G_{md}A_s(\beta + \rho\beta) \tag{7-7}$$

where

$$\rho = \frac{\sum G_{D_j}}{G_s} = \frac{F_{dga}A_{CD}}{\beta A_s} \qquad (7\text{--}8)$$

is the parameter representing the dendritic to soma conductance ratio. It may be noted that, as somatic shunting is increased (i.e., both G_s and β are increased), the value of ρ must decrease. In fact, it is the product, $\rho\beta$, that remains constant, because this depends only on the surface areas and the factor, F_{dga}, as shown by the expression

$$\rho\beta = \frac{F_{dga}A_{CD}}{A_s} \qquad (7\text{--}9)$$

The fact that $\rho\beta$ remains constant (at the value of ρ for $\beta = 1$) provides a valuable point of reference while dealing with uncertainties about the value of the soma shunting factor, β. For example, consider a particular neuron for which $\rho\beta = 16$, based on the measurement of surface area (plus an estimate of F_{dga}; see Eqs. 7–1 and 7–9). Before microelectrode penetration, the intact neuron would have $\beta = 1$ and $\rho = 16$; however, with microelectrode penetration, a somatic shunting factor, $\beta = 10$, for example, would cause the value of ρ to be reduced to $\rho = 1.6$; also, the value of G_N would be increased by a factor of about 1.5; more exactly, this factor is $(10 + 16)/(1 + 16) = 1.53$, based on a change in the factor $\beta + \rho\beta$ in Equation (7–7). Still larger somatic shunting, such as $\beta = 160$, would imply that $\rho = 0.1$, and the value of G_N would be increased by a factor of about 10; more exactly, this factor is $(160 + 16)/(1 + 16) = 10.35$ relative to its unshunted control value.

A general expression for the ratio of an actual input conductance, G_N, relative to its reference value, G_{N1}, (for $\beta = 1$), can be written as follows:

$$\frac{G_N}{G_{N1}} = \frac{(\beta + \rho\beta)}{(1 + \rho\beta)} = \frac{R_{N1}}{R_N} \qquad (7\text{--}10)$$

The inverse ratio for input resistance has been included for those who prefer to think of input resistance ratios rather than input conductance ratios. For any dendritic neuron whose value of $\rho\beta$ is known, Equation (7–10) provides a compact result that defines the effect of different somatic shunting factors, β, on the measured input conductance.

ESTIMATING MEMBRANE CONDUCTIVITY FROM EXPERIMENTAL DATA

By rearranging Equation (7–7), we have an expression for calculating the dendritic membrane conductivity,

$$G_{md} = \frac{G_N}{\beta A_s + F_{dga}A_{CD}} \qquad (7\text{--}11)$$

where all symbols have been defined with Equations (7–1) to (7–7).

For zero soma shunting and $G_{ms} = G_{md}$, we have $\beta = 1$, and Equation (7–11) provides an estimate of G_{md} from measurements of the neuronal input conductance and the membrane surface area of the soma and combined dendrites, provided that one has a good value for F_{dga}, such as the 0.84 value that was pointed out earlier, as good within 10% for all dendritic trees whose effective L values lie between 0.5 and 1; see Equation (7–2) and Table (7–1).

However, we are usually faced with two unknowns, β and G_{md}, and we do not know the value of L. There are many pairs of values of these two unknowns that can satisfy Equation (7–7) or (7–11) for the same values of input conductance and membrane surface area, and we must find a way of solving for the best pair.

Any particular choice of G_{md}, together with detailed measurement of dendritic branching (and a value for the intracellular specific resistance, R_i), allows us to calculate the input conductance, G_D, and the effective electrotonic length, L_{def}, for each dendritic tree. However, to test the consistency of such L values with an experiment, one needs to consider the additional data provided by experimental voltage transients.

An ideally simple solution to this problem occurs when all of the trees correspond to equivalent cylinders of the same electrotonic length. By using a voltage clamp at the soma, complication by the soma shunt is completed in the first few microseconds after clamp onset; the two longest time constants can be used to estimate the common L value of these dendritic trees (Eq. 33 of Rall, 1969); also, this L value, together with either of these time constants, implies a τ_m value for these dendrites (Eq. 32 of Rall, 1969). If we assume that $C_m = 1$ μF/cm^2, we then have an estimate of $G_{md} = C_{md}/\tau_{md}$. Also, this G_{md} value can be cross-checked by calculating the dendritic L value that it implies (using the anatomy and a value for R_i) to see if it agrees with the L value implied by the time constants under voltage clamp. This G_{md} value can also be used, together with the steady-state G_N measurement, to obtain an estimate of the soma shunting factor, β (from Eq. 7–7 or 7–11). Once β is estimated, it can be checked against the two longest τ values that are theoretically predicted under the current clamp with somatic shunting; these τ values have been discussed by Durand (1984) and Kawato (1984). These τ values were also defined by Equation (43) of Rall (1969), provided that the leakage parameter, $h = G_L/G_\infty$, used there, is replaced by the ratio of G_s to combined dendritic G_∞; that ratio can be designated $1/\rho_\infty$, or, more explicitly, $[\rho \coth(L)]^{-1}$.

However, when the dendritic trees have different L values, and when the trees are not equivalent to cylinders, the theoretical transient solutions become more complicated. There are additional component terms in the sum of exponential decays; these additional terms involve additional time constants that can be understood to result from the several unequal L values. By considering many examples of current clamp transients, we found that where the several L values differ by less than 20%, the coefficients of the additional decay terms have very small magnitudes; these coefficients are so small that these decay terms are not detected when peeling the overall exponential decay (especially in the presence of experimental noise); also, the value of L_{peel} (defined as the estimate of L obtained when the equivalent cylinder formula, for both ends sealed, is used with the τ_0/τ_1 ratio obtained by peeling the transient) was found to be close to that expected for the weighted average (or effective) L value (Segev and Rall, 1983; Holmes and Rall, 1987). However, when L values (associated with significant $d^{3/2}$ values) differ by more than 20%, the coefficients of some additional decay terms can become significant in magnitude; then (depending on the noise level) one may peel τ values implying larger L_{peel} values that correspond approximately to the sum of two of the component L values. An explanation of this (see Rall, 1969, pp. 1496–1497) has been verified by the computation of many additional examples (Segev and Rall, 1983; Holmes and Rall, 1987), but further discussion of this topic seems beyond the scope of this chapter.

An alternative to fitting the different τ values expected for current clamping and voltage clamping is to compute such transients for appropriately chosen models and then attempt to adjust the model parameters to provide a fit to the experimentally recorded transients; this approach has been explored by Clements and Redman (1988) and by Fleshman, et al. (1988). Several of us have discussed the pros and cons of various methods of using the transient experimental data to provide good estimates of corresponding model parameters, but this evaluation is not yet complete. We are still evaluating the non-uniqueness of such solutions and the complications in the transients that arise with different kinds of deviations from the idealized equivalent cylinder (Holmes and Rall, 1987).

DEGREES OF FREEDOM IN MULTICOMPARTMENTAL MODELS

Now that many laboratories have experience in using horseradish peroxidase (HRP) to visualize and measure the details of extensive dendritic branching, and many of these laboratories also have access to large computers, investigators have begun to extend the early results obtained with small compartmental models (Rall, 1964) to simulations in which the branched neuron morphology is represented by 1000 or more compartments (e.g., Bunow et al., 1985; Segev et al., 1985; Clements and Redman, 1988; Fleshman et al., 1988). Simulations of various electrophysiological properties and responses can now be computed with such compartmental models. These models offer several important advantages: (1) There is no need to make simplifying assumptions about the branching pattern; one can specify as much of the observed detail as one chooses. (2) There is no need to assume uniform membrane properties; one can specify different properties for each compartment in terms of the ion channel densities of several channel types. (3) One can also specify how synaptic inputs are distributed to the various compartments. These advantages also bring disadvantages, not only in increased programming effort and computer time, but also because of the large number of degrees of freedom present in the model before suitable constraints are specified. These degrees of freedom and constraints will be discussed later. But first, we note that in order to specify nonuniform membrane properties realistically, we need data that are not presently available; similarly, for synaptic input distributions, most of the data needed are not available. However, by making explicit assumptions to specify several possible distributions of membrane properties and synaptic inputs, we can gain insight by computing and comparing the consequences of different sets of specifications (e.g., Rall, 1964, 1967).

We distinguish two rather different kinds of applications for multicompartmental-neuron models. One, called the "forward problem," is to compute the responses for a particular model with particular values specified for every parameter of the model. The other, called the "inverse problem," is to estimate the unknown values of key parameters by requiring the model to match one or more sets of experimental data. It is noteworthy that a more general inverse problem, namely, to deduce the model itself from the data, is impossible without the imposition of constraints; one may be able to demonstrate that one type of model fits data better than some specified alternative model type, but one can never know that all possible alternative model types have been considered. In practice, we impose constraints (either explicitly or implicitly), which reduce the universe of possible models to a few alternatives. For the restricted inverse problem, where consideration is restricted to only one type of model (such as a specified class of compartmental models), the problem of estimating the unknown values of the parameters is usually impossible until one imposes constraints that reduce the number of unknowns (degrees of freedom). Such considerations are relevant to the question: How can a compartmental model be matched to the neuron it is meant to simulate?

Example of a Model with 1011 Compartments

Suppose that the dendrites are represented by 1000 compartments and that we add 11 more, 1 for the soma and 10 for the axon hillock, initial segment, and first few nodes of the axon. Until we specify a variety of constraints, the model composed of these 1011 compartments can represent more than 10,000 degrees of freedom. With the help of Table 7–2, we can identify these degrees of freedom and discuss the steps by which their number can be reduced.

Membrane Surface Area

Each compartment has a membrane surface area that must be specified. Thus we show 1011 degrees of freedom in column A of row 1 in Table 7–2. If this were just a formal model, we could decide to make all compartments the same size; imposing that constraint would reduce those 1011 degrees of freedom to 1. However, if we aim to match this model to the HRP anatomy of a particular neuron, we can say that the area of each compartment is specified by the measurements, leaving zero degrees of freedom, as shown in column C of row 1. But can we know the correct values for the membrane surface area without evaluating the shrinkage of the tissue?

Table 7–2 Degrees of freedom for model with 1011 compartments
with constraints

	Constraints	A Least	B Moderate	C Severe
1	Membrane surface area	1,011	1	0
2	Shrinkage correction	3	1	0–1
3	Branching type	300	3–20	0
4	Membrane capacitance	1,011	1	0–1
5	Membrane conductance	3,066	15	1
6	Somatic shunt	1	1	0–1
7	Intracel. resistivity	5	1	0–1
8	Synaptic input	6,006	6–30	0
9	Sum of above	11,403	29–70	1–5

Shrinkage

It is known that some shrinkage results from the preparation of tissues for
histological study. Although some workers have neglected this when tabulating
their measurements, others have made corrections for as much as 10–20%
shrinkage in linear dimensions. Such shrinkage can have significant consequences for the values estimated for various parameters, such as membrane
resistivity and the length constants for different branch segments. The unknown
shrinkage provides at least one degree of freedom, shown in column B of row
2. When there is evidence of differential shrinkage, the areas of various compartments could be subject to different correction factors; this is indicated
by showing three degrees of freedom in column A of row 2. In those cases
where careful control observations provide a good estimate of the shrinkage,
or where we are not trying to match experimental morphology, we have zero
degrees of freedom, shown in column C of row 2.

Branching Type

So far, we have said little about compartmental connectivity (the branching
type). The possible number of branching patterns is immense. For example,
suppose that we restrict our consideration to a branching family characterized
by 100 terminal branches, each of which might be different in its diameter, its
length, and the dimensionless electrotonic distance, L, of its terminal from the
soma. This would imply at least the 300 degrees of freedom shown in column
A of row 3. This number could be increased further by considering differences
in the types and orders of proximal branching. On the other hand, if the branching is completely specified by matching HRP morphology, these degrees of
freedom are reduced to zero, as shown in column C of row 3. For column B,
we really wish to distinguish only a few significantly different types of branching, as indicated by the following questions. (1) Does the branching satisfy
constraints corresponding to an equivalent cylinder? If so, do all of the dendritic trees have the same value of L? If so, we would have one degree of
freedom, corresponding to the unknown value of L. (2) Are there 2 (or more)
sets of dendritic trees of different length or type (e.g., apical and basal den-

drites of a pyramidal cell, or perhaps 10 different trees of a motoneuron)? If so, what is their relative electrotonic length and their relative surface area; also, do they correspond to equivalent cylinders, or to tapers, or to several cylinders of unequal length? Such classification would involve from 3 to 20 degrees of freedom, as indicated in column B or row 3.

Membrane Capacitance

If we wish to simulate voltage transients in the neuron, we must specify the membrane capacitance of each compartment; that could imply the 1011 degrees of freedom shown in column A of row 4. However, it is usual to assume that the membrane capacitance per unit area is the same over all of the neuron; imposing this constraint reduces these degrees of freedom to one, as shown in column B of row 4. Many modelers assume (at least initially) that C_m should be set to 1.0 μF/cm^2 (Cole, 1968) in all compartments; when this constraint is imposed, we are left with zero degrees of freedom. However, if one has excellent experimental data, one should let the value of C_m be among the parameters to be estimated from fitting the transients; hence we show zero to one degree of freedom in column C of row 4.

Membrane Conductance

For steady states as well as transients, we must specify the membrane conductance of each compartment; this would imply 1011 degrees of freedom, except that in many of these compartments, membrane conductance is composed of various densities of different ionic channel types. If we suppose, for example, that there are three types of channels whose density should be considered, we would have 3033 degrees of freedom; also, the 11 compartments assigned to the soma, initial segment, and axon might need several kinetic parameters to define their nonlinear properties (perhaps 33 parameters); this would imply the 3066 degrees of freedom shown in column A of row 5. However, for intermediate models, we might be inclined to specify one set of three densities for the soma, another for all proximal dendritic compartments, still another for all distal dendritic compartments, and perhaps two more sets for the axon hillock and the initial segment; that would account for the 15 degrees of freedom shown in column B of row 5. If this model were also to be used to study the effects of different synaptic input patterns, we would need additional degrees of freedom for these synaptic conductances, as shown in row 8. On the other hand, if we were willing to make the simplifying assumption of a uniform, passive membrane everywhere, this would reduce the degrees of freedom to one, as shown in column C of row 5.

Somatic Shunt

It is well known that penetration of the membrane by a micropipette can cause disastrous damage to a neuron. Even when a neuron survives penetration and seems stable, it is likely that some electric leakage continues to be present; see further comments in the earlier section on "Dendritic Neuron Model with Soma Shunt Conductance." It should now be regarded as essential to include a somatic shunt conductance in the model when fitting experimental data obtained with penetration by a conventional microelectrode; this adds one degree of freedom to the model. Because some experiments do not require intracellular recording, and some forward computations can neglect the shunt, we show zero to one degrees of freedom in row 6.

Intracellular Resistivity

In these compartmental models, the coupling resistance between any two compartments is supposed to correspond to the intracellular resistance along the core conductor between the midpoints of the two membrane regions. The magnitude of this resistance depends on geometry and the intracellular resistivity, R_i. The value of this resistivity for mammalian neurons has not been measured. Although the values measured for marine invertebrates range from 30 to 70 Ωcm, it is important to remember that intracellular cations are about one-third as concentrated in mammals as in marine invertebrates; this suggests a larger resistivity, say from 90 to 210 Ωcm, for mammalian neurons. Uncertainty about this value is responsible for the single degree of freedom shown in column B of row 7. If one also considers that cytoplasmic organelles can increase the effective intracellular resistivity in different regions (especially in constricted regions, such as dendritic spine stems, or the constrictions associated with varicose processes), one might get the five degrees of freedom shown in column A of row 7. However, in the future, when we have careful measurements of this resistivity for various regions of the neuron, or if we impose a particular resistivity value as an arbitrary constraint, we will be left with zero degrees of freedom; hence, we show zero to one degrees of freedom in column C of row 7.

Synaptic Input

In general, any of 1001 compartments could receive synaptic input at any given time. For both synaptic excitation and inhibition, we need three parameters to define the reversal potential, the peak conductance, and one or more parameters (such as α) that define the conductance time course; this explains the 6006 degrees of freedom shown in column A of row 8. This represents only the degrees of freedom in spatial pattern, and could be multiplied manyfold by combining these with several possible temporal patterns. However, in many cases, we may be interested in only a few synaptic input patterns corresponding perhaps to only two to five locations with different input combinations; this could imply 12 to 30 degrees of freedom, as shown in column B of row 8. On the other hand, in the simplest experiments, we apply no synaptic input, and we show zero degrees of freedom in column C of row 8.

Sum of Degrees of Freedom in Each Column

In row 9 of Table 7–2, we have collected the total degrees of freedom implied by the preceding numbers in each of the three columns. As already noted, a completely unconstrained model with 1011 compartments would have many times the 11,403 degrees of freedom that were enumerated in producing column A. The point of this exercise is to show that the moderate and reasonable constraints imposed on the model in producing column B only reduce the degrees of freedom to the range from 29 to 70. This leaves far too many unknowns for the task of attempting to match theory to experiment. Thus, it is important to be aware of the severe constraints that were needed to reduce the degrees of freedom to the range from one to five, shown in column C.

Perhaps the message is that the apparent flexibility of the large multicompartment model must be reduced by the imposition of severe constraints before there is any hope of matching its parameters to an experiment. When it is so constrained, it becomes equivalent, in many respects, to one of the simple models discussed earlier in this chapter. Awareness of this can help us gain a better perspective on what is involved in estimating the values of key parameters from experimental data. It is very important to remember that when there are too many degrees of freedom, it may be easy to find parameter sets that fit the data, but such solutions are not unique and may be far from optimal. To avoid such pitfalls, it is better to reduce the degrees of freedom severely at first, and to make use of anatomical information as well as both steady-state and transient electrophysiological data; then the problem becomes similar to that discussed earlier in the paragraphs following Equation (7–11).

CONCLUDING PERSPECTIVE

This chapter is not meant to provide a comprehensive perspective on all of my modeling efforts. For example, the field potentials produced by antidromic activation of the olfactory bulb and the recognition of dendrodendritic synaptic interactions (Rall and Shepherd, 1968; Rall, 1970; cf. Klee and Rall, 1977) were not discussed. Also omitted are the excitatory postsynaptic potential (EPSP) shape index loci (Rall et al., 1967) for different dendritic locations of synaptic input, the theoretical basis for various equalizing time constants related to cylinder length (Rall, 1969) and to several orders of dendritic branching (Rinzel and Rall, 1974), as well as effects on impulse propagation resulting from both gradual and abrupt changes in core conductor geometry (Goldstein and Rall, 1974), effects of voltage clamping the soma of a dendritic neuron (Rall and Segev, 1985), and the functional implications of excitable dendritic spines (Miller et al., 1985; Shepherd et al., 1985; Rall and Segev, 1987, 1988; Segev and Rall, 1988).

The three different subject areas (presented in this chapter) do have an important point in common. It has to do with the relation between the theoretical model and experimental reality. The model is designed to match the biology in its most essential features, but significant experimental difficulties must also be taken into account (such as the effect of somatic shunting or the effect of an ineffective input component). We seek qualitative and approximately quantitative agreement, because good qualitative matching is more important than high precision or mathematical overkill. The input–output study by Rosenblueth et al. (1949) had the benefit of two unusually talented mathematicians, but this collaborative study foundered because of a basic misunderstanding of the data; the authors assumed that their output was saturating, because they did not fully appreciate the overlap between effective and ineffective components of the input, and they overlooked the biological reality offered by different levels of reflex excitability. The dendritic tree examples (in Table 7–1) are all idealized to different degrees, but they all imply a similar value for the factor, F_{dga} (see Eqs. 7–1 and 7–2). This approximate result is robust, and efforts at higher precision may be wasted as long as one is confronted by the uncertainties due to unknown somatic shunting. Similarly, the discussion of the 1011-compartment model highlights how the number of degrees of freedom must be reduced, either by using good data or by imposing arbitrary constraints; this example also shows that (as we get sufficiently comprehensive data) we should try to resolve the often overlooked uncertainties about shrinkage and the values of C_m and R_i. The sophistication of a model needs to be matched to the sophistication of the data; then one has reason to hope for an evolution of better experiments and better models.

Acknowledgment

I am pleased to acknowledge helpful comments by William Holmes and Steven Baer on earlier drafts of this chapter, as well as recent discussions of some of these issues with a number of colleagues, including Julian Jack, Stephen Redman, Idan Segev, John Rinzel, William Holmes, and Robert Burke.

REFERENCES

Brock, L. G., Eccles, J. C., and Rall, W. (1951). Experimental investigations on the afferent fibres in muscle nerves. *Proc. R. Soc. (Biol.)*, 138, 453–475.

Bunow, B., Segev, I., and Fleshman, J. W. (1985). Modeling the electrical behavior of anatomically complex neurons using a network analysis program: Excitable membrane. *Biol. Cybern.* 53, 41–56.

Clements, J. D., and Redman, S. J. (1989). Cable properties of cat spinal motoneurones measured by combining voltage clamp, current clamp and intracellular staining. *J. Physiol. (Lond.)*, 409, 63–87.

Cole, K. S. (1968). *Membranes, Ions and Impulses.* University of California Press, Berkeley.

Denny-Brown, D. E., and Sherrington, C. S. (1928). Subliminal fringe in spinal flexion. *J. Physiol. (Lond.)* 66, 175–180.

Durand, D. (1984). The somatic shunt cable model for neurons. *Biophys. J.* 46, 645–653.

Eccles, J. C., and Rall, W. (1950) Post-tetanic potentiation of responses of motoneurones. *Nature* 166, 465.

Fleshman, J. W., Segev, I., and Burke, R. E. (1988). Electrotonic architecture of type-identified α-motoneurons in the cat spinal cord. *J. Neurophysiol.* 60, 60–85.

Goldstein, S., and Rall, W. (1974). Changes of action potential shape and velocity for changing core conductor geometry. *Biophys. J.* 14, 731–757.

Henneman, E. (1954). Maximal discharge of a motoneuron pool during potentiation. *Fed. Proc.* 13, 69.

Holmes, W. R., and Rall, W. (1987). Estimating the electrotonic structure of neurons which cannot be approximated as equivalent cylinders. *Soc. Neurosci. Abst.* 13, (422.7).

Iansek, R., and Redman, S. J. (1973). An analysis of the cable properties of spinal motoneurones using a brief intracellular current pulse. *J. Physiol. (Lond.)* 234, 613–636.

Jefferson, A., and Benson, A. (1953). Some effects of post-tetanic potentiation of monosynaptic responses of spinal cord of cat. *J. Neurophysiol.* 16, 381–396.

Kawato, M. (1984). Cable properties of a neuron model with non-uniform membrane resistivity. *J. Theoret. Biol.* 111, 149–169.

Klee, M., and Rall, W. (1977). Computed potentials of cortically arranged populations of neurons. *J. Neurophysiol.* 40, 647–666.

Krnjevic, K., Puil, E., and Werman, W. (1978). EGTA and motoneurone after-potentials. *J. Physiol. (Lond.)* 275, 199–233.

Lloyd, D. P. C. (1943). Reflex action in relation to pattern and peripheral source of afferent stimulation. *J. Neurophysiol.* 6, 111–120.

Lloyd, D. P. C. (1945). On the relation between discharge zone and subliminal fringe in a motoneuron pool supplied by a homogenous presynaptic pathway. *Yale J. Biol. Med.* 18, 117–121.

Lloyd, D. P. C. (1949). Post-tetanic potentiation of response in monosynaptic reflex pathways of the spinal cord. *J. Gen. Physiol.,* 33, 147–170.

Lorente de Nó, R. (1938). Synaptic stimulation as a local process. *J. Neurophysiol.* 1, 194–207.

Miller, J. P., Rall, W., and Rinzel, J. (1985). Synaptic amplification by active membrane in dendritic spines. *Brain Res.* 325, 325–330.

Owen, D. G., Segal, M., and Barker, J. L. (1984). A Ca-dependent Cl-conductance in cultured mouse spinal neurones. *Nature* 311, 567–570.

Perkel, D. H., and Mulloney, B. (1978). Electrotonic properties of neurons: Steady-state compartmental model. *J. Neurophysiol.* 41, 621–639.

Rall, W. (1951). Input–output relation of a monosynaptic reflex. *Proc. Univ. Otago Med. Sch.* 29, 17–18.

Rall, W. (1953). Electrotonic theory for a spherical neurone. *Proc. Univ. Otago Med. Sch.* 31, 14–15.

Rall, W. (1954). Monosynaptic reflex input–output analysis. *J. Physiol. (Lond.)* 125, 30–31.

Rall, W. (1955a). A statistical theory of monosynaptic input–output relations. *J. Cell. Comp. Physiol.* 46, 373–412.

Rall, W. (1955b). Experimental monosynaptic input–out relations in the mammalian spinal cord. *J. Cell. Comp. Physiol.* 46, 413–438.

Rall, W. (1959). Branching dendritic trees and motoneuron membrane resistivity. *Expt. Neurol.* 2, 503–532.

Rall, W. (1964). Theoretical significance of dendritic trees for neuronal input–output relations. In *Neural Theory and Modeling* (ed. R. Reiss). Stanford University Press, Stanford, Calif., pp. 73–97.

Rall, W. (1967). Distinguishing theoretical synaptic potentials computed for different soma-dendritic distributions of synaptic input. *J. Neurophysiol.* 30, 1138–1168.

Rall, W. (1969). Time constants and electrotonic length of membrane cylinders and neurons. *Biophys. J.* 9, 1483–1508.

Rall, W. (1970). Dendritic neuron theory and dendrodendritic synapses in a simple cortical system. In *The Neurosciences: Second Study Program* (ed. F. O. Schmitt). Rockefeller University Press, New York, pp. 552–565.

Rall, W. (1977). Core conductor theory and cable properties of neurons. In *Handbook of Physiology, Cellular Biology of Neurons* (ed. E. R. Kandel). American Physiological Society, Bethesda, Md., pp. 39–97.

Rall, W., Burke, R. E., Smith, T. G., Nelson, P. G., and Frank, K. (1967) Dendritic location of synapses and possible mechanisms for the monosynaptic EPSP in motoneurons. *J. Neurophysiol.* 30, 1169–1193.

Rall, W., and Hunt, C. C. (1956). Analysis of reflex variability in terms of partially correlated excitability fluctuations in a population of motoneurons. *J. Gen. Physiol.* 39, 397–422.

Rall, W., and Segev, I. (1985). Space-clamp problems when voltage clamping branched neurons with intracellular microelectrodes. In *Voltage and Patch Clamping with Microelectrodes* (T. G. Smith, Jr., H. Lecar, S. J. Redman, and P. W. Gage). American Physiological Society, Bethesda, Md., pp. 191–215.

Rall, W., and Segev, I. (1987). Functional possibilities for synapses on dendrites and on dendritic spines. In *Synaptic Function.* (ed. G. M. Edelman, W. E. Gall, and W. M. Cowan). Wiley, New York, pp. 605–636.

Rall, W., and Segev, I. (1988). Synaptic integration and excitable dendritic spine clusters: Structure/function. In *Intrinsic Determinants of Neuronal Form and Function* (ed. R. J. Lasek, and M. M. Black) Alan R. Liss, New York, pp. 263–282.

Rall, W., and Shepherd, G. M. (1968). Theoretical reconstruction of field potentials and dendrodendritic synaptic interactions in olfactory bulb. *J. Neurophysiol.* 31, 884–915.

Rinzel, J., and Rall, W. (1974). Transient response in a dendritic neuron model for current injected at one branch. *Biophys. J.* 14, 759–790.

Rosenblueth, A., Wiener, N., Pitts, W., and Garcia-Ramos, J. (1949). A statistical analysis of synaptic excitation. *J. Cell. Comp. Physiol.* 34, 173–205.

Segev, I., Fleshman, J. W., Miller, J. P., and Bunow, B. (1985). Modeling the behavior of anatomically complex neurons using a network analysis program: Passive membrane. *Biol. Cybern.* 53, 27–40.

Segev, I., and Rall, W. (1983). Theoretical analysis of neuron models with dendrites of unequal electrical lengths. *Soc. Neurosci. Abst.* 9, 102.20.

Segev, I., and Rall, W. (1988). Computational study of an excitable dendritic spine. *J. Neurophysiol.* 60, 499–523.

Shepherd, G. M., Brayton, R. K., Miller, J. P., Segev, I., Rinzel, J., and Rall, W. (1985). Signal enhancement in distal cortical dendrites by means of interaction between active dendrite spines. *Proc. Nat. Acad. Sci.* 82, 2192–2195.

8

Does the Size Principle Give Insight into the Energy Requirements of Motoneurons?

V. R. EDGERTON, R. R. ROY, AND
G. R. CHALMERS

Given the wealth of physiological and anatomical information about motor units (Burke, 1981; Henneman and Mendell, 1981), the motoneuron may be an ideal model for studying the sources of energy drive for neurons throughout the central nervous system. Also, given the size principle that has evolved primarily from work published over the last 25–30 years, there is a basis on which metabolic hypotheses that are readily testable can be proposed. The reason that the motoneurons provide such a useful strategic basis for studying the metabolic characteristics of neurons in general is that many of the motor unit properties that may be related to the motoneuron's energy drive are reasonably well understood. On the other hand, the relative importance of these different functions in motoneurons, or any other neuron, as a driver of its energy needs is poorly understood.

Our present knowledge about the metabolism of the central nervous system is fragmented at best. The metabolism of the whole brain has been studied by measuring the rate of oxygen uptake and the selective uptake of substrate, e.g., 2-deoxyglucose (Sokoloff, 1984). Based on these studies, it is clear that blood glucose is the most important substrate, probably representing at least 90% of the brain's total substrate utilization (Balazs, 1970; Siesjo, 1978). It is also clear that oxidative phosphorylation is the principal pathway by which ATP is synthesized, and that without a continuous supply of adequate oxygen, neurons will be irreversibly damaged within minutes (Gelfan and Tarlov, 1963; Siesjo et al., 1974; Siesjo, 1978; Rothman and Olney, 1987). Although glycogen is stored in the brain, it is used at high rates only when there is ischemia. Further, the amount stored is depleted shortly after the onset of an oxygen deficiency (Guth and Watson, 1968). It is also known that the metabolic rate, as measured by 2-deoxyglucose uptake (Sandler and Tator, 1976) and blood flow (Rawe, et al., 1981) in the gray matter of the spinal cord, is about twice that of the white matter. In addition, numerous studies have attempted to demonstrate active regions of the brain during a variety of tasks and have shown that with an increase in neuronal activity, glucose uptake increases proportionately (Sokoloff, 1975). These tasks ranged from the selective activation of single whiskers of the rat (Durham and Woolsey, 1977) to forelimb movement (Matsunami et al., 1981; Shimamura et al., 1987). One major disadvantage of studying 2-deoxyglucose uptake, or any other metabolic analogue, using available autoradiographic or imaging techniques is that these measurements are not quantitatively reliable indices of the metabolic responses of individual neurons. This limitation in localization of the metabolic properties to a single neuron can be overcome, in part, by measuring enzyme activities.

Although the issue can be raised of whether the activity of an enzyme of a neuron reflects its acute metabolic capabilities, there are numerous cases that demonstrate that the concentrations of enzymes associated with oxidative phosphorylation are directly related to the metabolic requirments of the specific cell (Padykula, 1952). For example, the chronic metabolic demands of a muscle fiber seem closely matched with enzymes of the citric acid cycle and of the electron transport chain (Holloszy, 1967). Given this supposition, it would be useful to determine the activity of a marker enzyme of oxidative metabolism of single motoneurons, while also determining the size of the motoneuron. Consequently, the hypothesis that one or more aspects of the size principle largely dictates the relative energy need of a motoneuron within a given motor pool, and that this energy need will be reflected in an oxidative marker enzyme, can be examined. The purposes of this chapter, therefore, are to identify the motoneuronal functions that require energy, to provide evidence suggesting which of these functions are most important, and finally, to point out how the size principle of recruitment provides the basis for understanding the energy-requiring functions of the motoneuron.

ENERGY REQUIREMENTS OF MOTONEURONS RELATIVE TO INTRANEURONAL SPECIALIZATION IN FUNCTION

One of the neuronal functions that seems to have great metabolic impact is the maintenance of a stable resting membrane potential. One reason for this may be the widely varying conditions under which the potential must be maintained. Neural inputs can vary by orders of magnitude in quantity and can range from those that hyperpolarize to those that depolarize. A second function of neurons is to maintain homeostasis among the cytoplasmic components. The soma of a motoneuron is the initial site of regulation of most proteins, although it can represent only a small percentage of the total volume of the motoneuron (Fig. 8–1). In motoneurons that innervate a large number of muscle fibers, we have

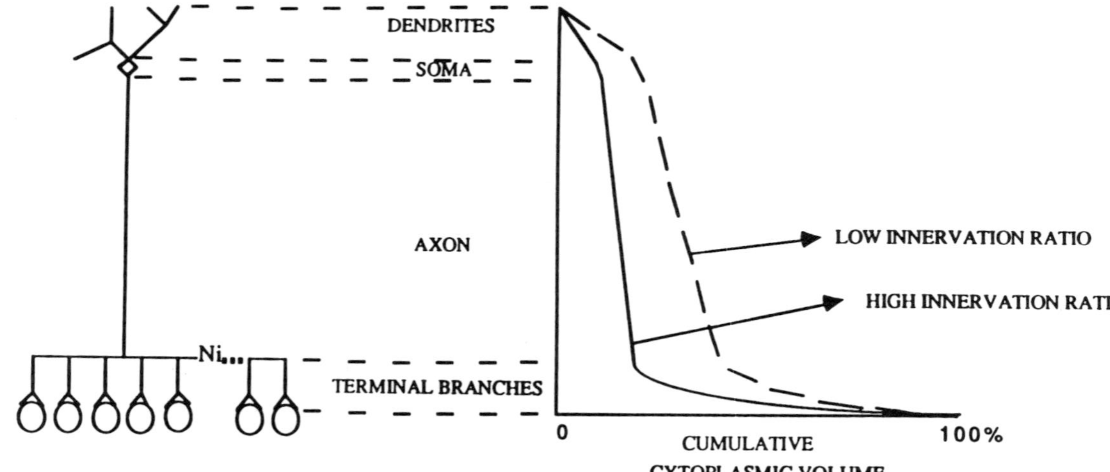

Fig. 8–1. Graphic illustration of estimated cumulative cytoplasm in a motoneuron, beginning at the tip of the dendrites and ending at the terminal axons. Note particularly the relatively small volume of the soma and the large proportion of the cytoplasm that is located in the axonal tree. Two alternatives are shown at the level of the axon, which illustrate the importance of the size of the axonal tree (innervation ratio) in determining cell volume.

estimated that as much as 90% of the axoplasm is probably located in the axon projection and its many branches. This estimate is based on the total dendritic lengths derived from anatomical reconstructions of intracellularly labeled motoneurons and the size of motoneurons, as reviewed by Stuart and Enoka (1983), and the estimated lengths of axons to the distal musculature of the hindlimbs of cats. A third function of neurons is to transmit signals at the postsynaptic sites i.e., the neuromuscular junctions.

Maintenance of the Membrane Potential

Suprathreshold

Repolarization of the membrane following an action potential requires energy, but the energy cost is generally thought to be small. For example, based on a variety of assumptions regarding the energy cost of an action potential (i.e., the number and frequency of action potentials that are thought to occur, the length of axons, and the number of neurons and glial cells in the cortex), spike activity has been estimated to require only 0.3–3% of cortical energy consumption (Creutzfeldt, 1975). It has been estimated that the combined energy required for extruding Na^+ and assimilating K^+ is 12.6 kJ $\cdot$ mole^{-1}. The hydrolysis of one ATP molecule provides a change in energy of -50 kJ $\cdot$ mole^{-1}. A number of experiments have suggested that three Na^+ are transported per ATP (Siesjo, 1978). In spite of this theoretically specific value of free energy change (ΔG), it remains unclear how much energy is required to propagate an action potential in a motoneuron based on its diameter, myelination, number and length of nodes, degree of axonal branching, and many other factors. With respect to the impact of the energy demands of an action potential, the surface area (a square function) to cytoplasmic volume (a cubic function) must be taken into account as well. Therefore, a larger neuron could have a relatively lower concentration of mitochondria to support ionic exchange than might be the case for smaller cells.

Another means of assessing the metabolic impact of action potentials has been the measurement of changes in oxygen consumption in response to nerve stimulation. These studies show that the resting metabolism can be doubled in the frog sciatic nerve by stimulating at a rate of 280 shocks per second (Gerard, 1927). But these responses vary significantly, depending on the experimental conditions, e.g., ionic concentrations (Ritchie, 1967). Further, it may not be appropriate to assume that the elevated oxygen consumption immediately following nerve stimulation is necessarily due to the generation of action potentials. In effect, it is not possible to make a reasonably precise estimate of the energy cost of generating and propagating action potentials in motoneurons in vivo. In regard to the metabolic consequences of action potentials in axons, it is interesting that there is little difference in the volume of mitochondria located in the cytoplasm of an axon at the node of Ranvier compared to the internodal regions of the axoplasm. However, there is a higher concentration in the volume of mitochondria in the cytoplasm of the Schwann cell at the nodal and paranodal regions than in the axon (Berthold, 1968; Landon and Williams, 1963). These results alert one to the possible role of the glia, the Schwann cells in this case, as a cell type that has a metabolically interactive function with a neuron (Berthold, 1965; Landon and Williams, 1963; Hyden, 1967; Varon and Somjen, 1979).

Although it is not feasible to estimate the quantity of energy needed to generate and propagate action potentials, it is clear that this function must have some metabolic impact on the motoneuron. Further, based on the specialized regions of a motoneuron, i.e., dendrites, soma, initial segment, axon, nodes of Ranvier, and axon terminals, it seems likely that suprathreshold events will require the most energy in the axonal projection. More specifically, the energy demands will probably be highest at the nodes of Ranvier, given the saltatory nature of impulse propagation (Fig.8–2).

Subthreshold

Maintenance of the "resting" membrane potential at -70 to -90 mV even in the absence of action potentials requires ATP since the polarized state is dependent on active transport of Na^+ and K^+. Subthreshold fluctuations in the resting membrane potential are due to the constant bombardment of the dendrites and soma (Fig.8–2) by neurotransmitters at thousands of synaptic terminals on their surfaces. Even though the amplitude of a single excitatory postsynaptic potential (EPSP) produced by stimulation of a single Ia afferent is inversely related to the size of the soma (Burke, 1981; Henneman and Mendell, 1981), the actual amount of current, i.e., the ionic flux, may be independent of soma size. If this is the case, there would be a similar energy cost in the large and small motoneurons for each EPSP. However, the impact of the EPSP on the smaller motoneurons would be larger because of the higher energy requirements per unit tissue. Consequently, the smaller motoneurons would be expected to require relatively greater amounts of energy than the larger motoneurons to maintain their membrane potential. The net effect of these metabolic requirements may be an inverse relationship between the concentration of mitochondria and soma size.

To preserve the appropriate excitability of motoneurons, it is essential that the resting membrane potential be maintained within rather narrow limits. The energy required to maintain a stable membrane potential undoubtedly depends, to a large degree, on the quantity of subthreshold synaptic input that is localized principally in the dendrites and soma. In contrast, action potentials are generated in the initial segment and are subsequently propagated down the axonal tree. Thus, one might expect more mitochondria to be localized in the dendrites and soma if subthreshold membrane fluctuations are major energy drivers (Fig. 8–2).

Maintenance of Cytoplasmic Components

If it is assumed that the turnover rates of cytoplasmic components are similar in all motoneurons, then the number of cytoplasmic components to be synthesized and regulated must be proportional to the size of the motoneuron. Since these processes require energy, and if they are a dominating element in driving

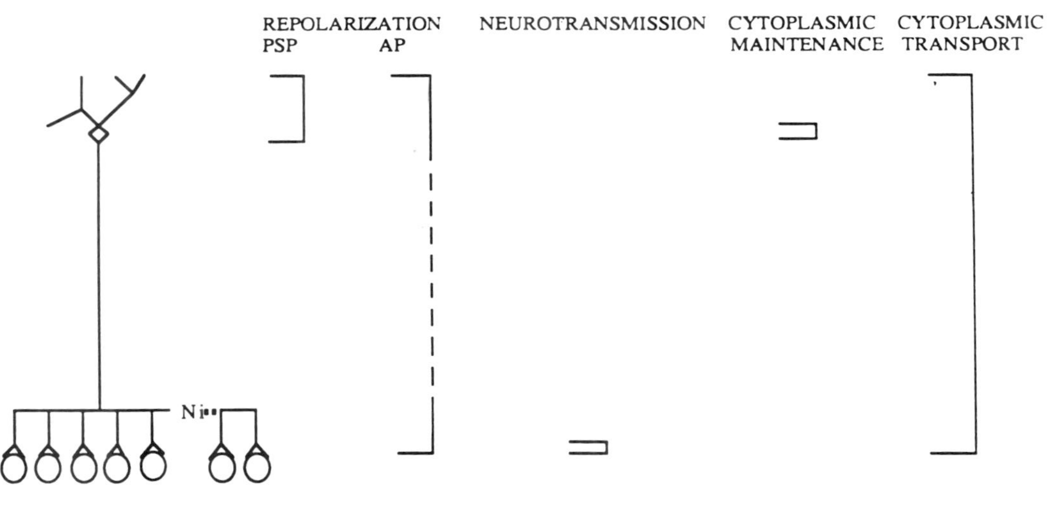

Fig. 8–2. The sites at which various cellular functions are likely to be localized are shown, with brackets on the right. The dashed line along the length of the axon emphasizes the potential localization of the metabolic drive of saltatory propagation of action potentials along myelinated axons. PSP, postsynaptic potential; AP, action potential.

the energy needs of the motoneuron, then the oxidative potential should be directly related to motoneuron size.

The energy required for maintenance of cytoplasmic components is likely to be localized in the soma (Fig. 8–2). Although it is known that there is some intrinsic protein synthesis within mitochondria, most proteins are regulated by nuclear DNA (Grivell, 1983; Hay et al., 1984). While some of the cytochromes are partially coded by mitochondrial DNA, all citric acid cycle enzymes appear to be coded by nuclear DNA, with synthesis occurring in the cytoplasm (Grivell, 1983). Therefore, if the cost of maintaining cytoplasmic components is large, one would expect the mitochondrial concentration in the soma to reflect this requirement, even though the soma may represent as little as 1% of the total cytoplasm of a motoneuron (Fig. 8–1).

Cytoplasmic Transport

Anterograde and retrograde has transport of a wide variety of materials have been shown to occur in motoneurons (Kreutzberg and Schubert, 1981; Ochs, 1982). This process occurs in axons as well as dendrites, and the rates of transport for most cellular components can be identified as either being part of a fast or a slow transport system. Although the energy cost of cytoplasmic transport is unknown, it appears that the mechanisms involved require high-energy phosphates. In fact, this process has been compared to the contractile process in muscle (Hill, 1987). The rate of cytoplasmic transport and the consequent energy requirements may be proportional to the cell volume. There is also evidence that the cytoplasmic transport rate increases with neuronal activity (Dahlstrom et al., 1978; Jasmin et al., 1987). This activity dependence would have the opposite effect on energy needs based on the volume of the cytoplasm alone. Thus, the interactive effects of cell volume and the amount of neuronal activity on cytoplasmic transport may make it difficult to define the energy costs of cytoplasmic transport as a function of the size principle.

Neurotransmission

All neurons secrete one or more substances that serve as neurotransmitters or modulators. A significant amount of the energy requirements of motoneurons may be associated with neurotransmission and related functions, i.e., the incorporation of vesicular membranes within the terminal membrane, the release of acetycholine, the reuptake of acetyl CoA and choline into the terminals, the formation of vesicles for repackaging acetylcholine, the repackaging of acetylcholine in vesicles, and the resynthesis of acetylcholine from the precursors. This may be the case particularly in the larger motoneurons (Fig. 8–1).

The energy requirements of neurotransmission may be accommodated by the large number of mitochondria located in the terminals (Saito and Zacks, 1969). If these energy demands are met by mitochondria within the terminals, the soma will not necessarily reflect the metabolic impact of neurotransmission. On the other hand, it seems likely that such a complex function will have some metabolic influence on the soma because most mitochondrial protein synthesis is regulated by nuclear DNA.

The potential metabolic impact of neurotransmission may reflect the number of action potentials generated per day per motoneuron (Hennig and Lomo, 1985) and the number of axonal projections per motoneuron (Herrera and Grinnell, 1985). Based on the work of Hennig and Lomo (1985), it appears that up to about 500,000 impulses per day may be generated in the slow oxidative motor units of the rat soleus whereas as few as 3000 impulses per day may be generated in the less active, probably fast glycolytic, units of the rat tibialis anterior muscle. If similar unit characteristics are exhibited in respiratory muscles such as the diaphragm and posterior cricoarytenoid, given the respiratory rates and burst durations in rats (Mortola and Noworaj, 1985), some of the lower threshold units of these muscles could produce up to 1,000,000 impulses per day. In the case of the posterior cricoarytenoid, which has about five muscle fibers (i.e., neuromuscular junctions) per motor unit (Hinrichsen and Ryan, 1982), this would result in about 5,000,000 action potentials at the synaptic terminals per day. In contrast, a large motor unit in the diaphragm innervating 300 muscle fibers and generating 3000 impulses per day would result in 900,000 action potentials at the synaptic terminals per day. Consequently, the metabolic cost of neurotransmission would be reflected in the size of the motor unit, i.e., the number of muscle fibers per motoneuron, as well as the susceptibility of the neuron to excitability.

BIOCHEMICAL INTERACTIONS BETWEEN GLIA CELLS AND MOTONEURONS

The idea that there is biochemical interaction between glia and motoneurons was suggested by the early work of Hyden (1964). This author reported an inverse relationship in the RNA concentrations and oxidative enzyme activities of glia and surrounding motoneurons. Following vestibular stimulation for 25 min per day for 7 days, Deiters' nerve cells of the lateral vestibular nucleus demonstrated an increase in RNA content and in succinate dehydrogenase and cytochrome oxidase activities. There was a decrease in these measures in adjacent glial cells. Also, Hyden (1964) reported a 25% increase in RNA in ventral horn cells in the barracuda 4 hr after a 30-min bout of exhaustive swimming. Although little can be stated with certainty about the potential contributions of glial cells to the energy demands of motoneurons, there is general agreement that the glia and associated neurons are interdependent metabolically (Hyden, 1967; Berthold, 1968; Varon and Somjen, 1979; Katoh-Semba et al., 1988).

ADAPTABILITY OF MOTONEURONS TO VARYING LEVELS OF ACTIVITY

The literature detailing the morphologic response of a motoneuron to increased activity levels is contradictory and often confusing (see Geinismann et al., 1971, and Gilliam et al., 1977, for discussion). The most striking evidence that activity affects motoneurons was reported by Edstrom (1957), who demonstrated that a single bout of exercise results in a swelling of the soma and a slight chromophilic state in the cytoplasm, indicating a loss of nucleoproteins. In contrast, chronic exercise of moderate intensity results in no change in the volume of the soma or nucleus but a dramatic increase in the volume of the nucleolus (Edstrom, 1957). In addition, there was an elevated nucleoprotein content, indicating a high rate of protein synthesis associated with this level of chronic activity (Hyden, 1964, 1967). More recently, Gilliam et al. (1977) showed that more intense training regimens result in decreased soma and nucleus diameters. These changes in soma properties are accompanied by a decrease in the axonal diameter of a corresponding peripheral nerve (Roy et al., 1983). Thus, the morphological adaptation of the motoneuron to increased activity appears to be intensity and duration dependent, confounding variables that are often ignored and may explain the contradictory results reported in the literature. Some types of chronic exercise (e.g., running but not swimming) also result in an enhanced rate of fast axonal transport of certain materials, e.g., acetylcholinesterase (Jasmin et al., 1987) and acetylcholine (Dahlstrom et al., 1978).

The adaptations in the metabolic properties of the motoneurons following increased neuromuscular activity are also conflicting. Chronic exercise training has been shown to result in an enhanced oxidative potential, as measured by malate dehydrogenase staining intensity if the intensity of training was not too severe (Gerchman et al., 1975). These data were consistent with the metabolic adaptations observed in the muscles of the same animals (Edgerton et al., 1969). However, in other models of increased activity, the results have been equivocal. Following 8 weeks of chronic stimulation of a peripheral nerve, a population of the associated motoneurons showed no alterations in succinate dehydrogenase activity or soma size (Donselaar et al., 1986). However, in the associated musculature, the fibers were significantly atrophied and demonstrated elevated oxidative enzyme staining properties (Kernell et al., 1987). Pearson and Sickles (1987) showed a concomitant decrease in the nicotinamide adenine dinucleotide tetrazolium reductase (NADH-tetrazolium reductase) activity in motoneurons and muscle fibers 60 days after overloading the neuromuscular unit by removing its major synergists. Unfortunately, no morphological data were reported. Sickles et al. (1987) also reported that in hyperthyroid rats the NADH-tetrazolium reductase activity of motoneurons and muscle fibers of a slow muscle were elevated, whereas this metabolic marker was unchanged in either cell type in a predominantly fast muscle. The metabolic response of motoneurons to reduced activity levels has also been studied (Chalmers et. al., 1988). After 6 months of virtual electrical silence induced by surgically eliminating supraspinal and peripheral input to lumbar motoneurons, succinate dehydrogenase activity and soma size were unchanged in the lumbar motoneurons.

Together, these data indicate that motoneurons have the ability to adapt, but it remains unclear as to what stimuli (or lack of stimuli) may induce these changes. The motoneurons seem to be extremely responsive to some perturbations while remaining resistant to others. These apparent contradictions reflect our incomplete understanding of the mechanisms that drive the energy requirements of a neuron, as well as the factors that regulate their response to altered energy demands.

EVIDENCE THAT THE OXIDATIVE POTENTIAL OF MOTONEURONS IS LINKED TO THE SIZE PRINCIPLE

The first papers to draw significant attention to the metabolic properties of motoneurons in relation to their size were by Campa and Engel (1970, 1971). Although these papers were not quantitative with respect to metabolic parameters, they concluded that the larger neurons had lower staining intensities for oxidative enzymes, e.g., succinate dehydrogenase (SDH), and higher staining intensities for glycogenolytic enzymes, e.g., phosphorylase, than the smaller neurons. However, it is likely (as they stated) that the smaller neurons were gamma, rather than alpha, motoneurons.

Subsequent studies by Penny and collaborators (1975) on motoneuron succinate and isocitrate dehydrogenase activities, using a quantitative histochemical method of enzyme analysis, examined the relationship between soma volume and enzyme activity. Their data illustrated that small motoneurons may have a range of oxidative enzyme levels, while larger motoneurons have consistently low activities. However, there was little relationship between malate and lactate dehydrogenase activities and motoneuron soma volume. More recently, Wong-Riley and Kageyama (1986) studied the relationship between soma size and cytochrome oxidase activity in a combined population of ventral horn cells in the cervical, thoracic, and lumbar regions of the spinal cord of a primate. They clearly demonstrated that there was some upper limit for the combination of soma size and enzyme activity. For example, no large neurons demonstrated high cytochrome oxidase activity, whereas small neurons expressed a larger range of activities. Donselaar and co-workers (1986) reported a negative correlation between SDH activity and soma diameter in cat lumbar motoneurons. The relationships between enzyme activity and soma size found by Penny et al. (1975), Wong-Riley and Kageyama (1986), and Donselaar et al. (1986) are remarkably similar, showing a wide range in the oxidative capacities of smaller cells, while larger cells are limited to only low oxidative capacities. Some recent results differ from these findings. For example, Ishihara et al. (1988) did not observe any small cells that demonstrated low oxidative capacities. They found an inverse relationship with a high correlation ratio between soma size and SDH activity. In contrast, a positive relationship between soma size and cytochrome oxidase activity was reported by Van Raamsdonk et al. (1987), while SDH activity was inversely related to cell size. Finally, Mjaatvedt and Wong-Riley (1986) reported that the cytochrome oxidase activity of motoneurons, identified for a specific motor pool using a radioactive label, was not directly related to soma size.

In each of the previous studies, one or more technical limitations temper the significance of the results. Perhaps most importantly, only in the work of Penny et al. (1975) was there reasonable evidence that the enzyme assays used were quantitative. The cytochrome oxidase activities reported by Wong-Riley and Kageyama (1986) and Mjaatvedt and Wong-Riley (1986) are quantitative only in that photometric readings were taken, but the tissues were fixed chemically. Therefore, the enzyme activities had to be inhibited to some unknown and, perhaps, variable level (Chalmers and Edgerton, in press a). The SDH assay employed by Donselaar et al. (1986) was not validated in neural tissue. In addition, in only one of these studies (Mjaatvedt and Wong-Riley, 1986) was the enzyme activity of a muscle-specific motor pool examined.

Sickles and McLendon (1983) quantified the activity of NADH-tetrazolium reductase in rat lumbar alpha-motoneurons. Interestingly, they found a size–activity relationship that was remarkably similar to that reported by Penny et al. (1975), Wong-Riley and Kageyama (1986), and Donselaar et al. (1986). Sickles and Oblak (1984) were the first to report a quantitative analysis of an oxidative enzyme in motoneurons linked to a specific pool. Using horseradish peroxidase injected into the muscle, they showed that the NADH-tetrazolium reductase activity was highest in the motoneurons that innervated the soleus muscle, moderate in the tibialis anterior, and lowest in the tensor fascia latae motoneurons of the rat. The relative activity levels corresponded to the types of muscle fibers innervated by each pool, with the soleus fibers being the most fatigue resistant, the tibialis anterior moderately fatigable, and the tensor fascia latae the most fatigable (Sickles and Oblak, 1984). Since soma size was not measured in this study, a more detailed conclusion regarding the relevance of the size principle to motoneuronal metabolic properties is precluded.

We have recently begun to examine the relationship between soma size and SDH activity in cat lumbar motoneurons (Chalmers et. al., in press b). We have found a large range in SDH activities in the smaller motoneurons, while most of the larger motoneurons have the lowest enzyme activities (Fig. 8–3). However, it is apparent that the relevance of quantitative enzyme activ-

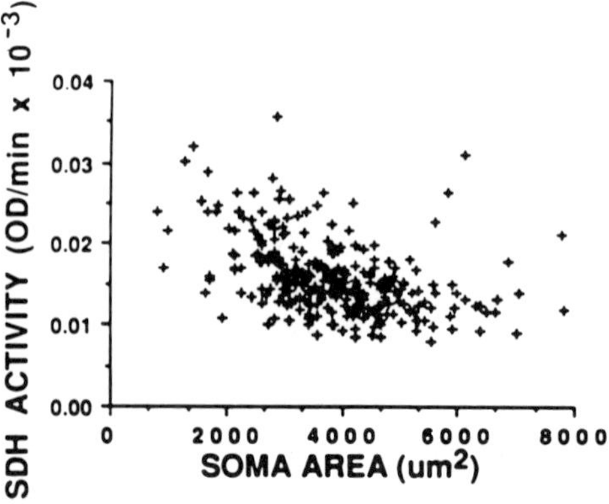

Fig. 8–3. The cross-sectional area sectioned through the nucleus and the SDH activity of motoneurons of the lumbar region of six adult normal cats are shown. Note that the region with the highest density of data points suggests an inverse relationship. There appears to be a sparsity of data points in the upper right quadrant of the graph. All of the data points that fall above the area of highest density are from one cat. SDH activity was determined by the technique of Chalmers and Edgerton (in press b).

ities and the "size" of the motoneurons of identified motor pools to the physiological phenomenon of recruitment order remain undefined.

In summary, although the relative importance of the various cellular functions that drive the oxidative potential of neurons is unknown, there is substantial experimental and theoretical evidence indicating that several factors play important roles. Maintenance of a resting membrane potential, maintenance of cytoplasmic components and their intraneuronal transport, and neurotransmission and neurotransmitter reuptake are among those functions that may influence the metabolic needs of motoneurons. Further, there are reasons to believe that the quantitative importance of each of these neuronal functions reflects the size principle of motor unit recruitment. Finally, it is predicted that the morphological and physiological bases of the size principle of motor unit recruitment will be manifested as a predictable relationship between SDH activity and the combined effects of these size principle–related properties.

Acknowledgment

This work was funded in part by NIH Grant NS-16333. Gordon R. Chalmers was funded by the Natural Sciences and Engineering Research Council of Canada.

REFERENCES

Balazs, R. (1970). Carbohydrate metabolism. In *Handbook of Neurochemistry*, Vol. II. (ed. A. Lajtha). Plenum Press, New York, pp. 1–36.

Berthold, C.-H. (1965). Ultrastructure and histochemistry of the developing node of Ranvier in the hindlimb nerves of the cat. *Acta Societatis Medicorum Upsaliensis* 70, 287–293.

Berthold, C.-H. (1968). Ultrastructure of the nodal-paranode region of mature feline ventral lumbar spinal root fibers. *Acta Societatis Medicorum Upsaliensis* 73, Suppl. 9, 37–70.

Burke, R. E. (1981). Motor units: Anatomy, physiology, and functional organization. In *Handbook of Physiology—The Nervous System*, Vol. II, Part 1 (ed. V. B. Brooks). American Physiological Society, Bethesda, Md., pp. 345–422.

Campa, J. F., and Engel, W. K. (1970). Histochemistry of motor neuron and interneurons in the cat lumbar spinal cord. *Neurology* 20, 559–568.

Campa, J. F., and Engel, W. K. (1971). Histochemical and functional correlations in anterior horn cells of the cat spinal cord. *Science* 171, 198–199.

Chalmers, G. R., and Edgerton, V. R. (In press a). Marked and variable inhibition by chemical fixation of cytochrome oxidase and succinate dehydrogenase in single motoneurons. *J. Histochem. Cytochem.*

Chalmers, G. R., and Edgerton, V. R. (In press b). Single motoneuron succinate dehydrogenase activity. *J. Histochem. Cytochem.*

Chalmers, G. R., Roy, R. R., and Edgerton, V. R. (In press). Normal succinate dehydrogenase activity in motoneurons six months after spinal isolation. *Soc. Neurosci. Abstr.*

Creutzfeldt, O. D. (1975). Neurophysiological correlates of different functional states of the brain, In *Brain Work* (ed. D. H. Ingvar and N. A. Lassen). Academic Press, New York, pp. 21–46.

Dahlstrom, A., Heiwall, P.-O., Booj, S., and Dahllof, A.-G. (1978). The influence of supraspinal impulse activity on the intra-axonal transport of acetylcholine, choline acetyltransferase and acetylcholinesterase in rat motor neurons. *Acta Physiol. Scand.* 103, 308–319.

Donselaar, Y., Kernell, D., and Eerbeek, O. (1986). Soma size and oxidative enzyme activity in normal and chronically stimulated motoneurons of the cat's spinal cord. *Brain Res.* 385, 22–29.

Durham, D., and Woolsey, T. A. (1977). Barrels and columnar cortical organization: Evidence from 2-deoxyglucose (2-DG) experiments. *Brain Res.* 137, 169–179.

Edgerton, V. R., Gerchman, L., and Carrow, R. (1969). Histochemical changes in rat skeletal muscle after exercise. *Exp. Neurol.* 24, 110–123.

Edstrom, J. (1957). Effects of increased motor activity on the dimensions and staining properties of the neuron soma. *J. Comp. Neurol.* 107, 295–304.

Geinismann, Y. Y., Larina, V. N., and Mats, V. N. (1971). Changes of neurones' dimensions as a possible morphological correlate of their increased functional activity. *Brain Res.* 26, 247–257.

Gelfan, S., and Tarlov, I. M. (1963). Altered neuron population in L7 segment of dogs with experimental hind-limb rigidity. *Am. J. Physiol.* 205, 606–616.

Gerard, R. W. (1927). Studies on nerve metabolism II. Respiration in oxygen and nitrogen. *Am. J. Physiol.* 82, 381–404.

Gerchman, L. B., Edgerton, V. R., and Carrow, R. E. (1975). Effects of physical training on the histochemistry and morphology of ventral motor neurons. *Exp. Neurol.* 49, 790–801.

Gilliam, T. B., Roy, R. R., Taylor, J. F., Heusner, W. W., and Van Huss, W. D. (1977). Ventral motor neuron alterations in rat spinal cord after chronic exercise. *Experientia* 33, 665–667.

Grivell, L. A. (1983). Mitochondrial DNA. *Sci Am* 248, 78–89.

Guth, L., and Watson, P. K. (1968). A correlated histochemical and quantitative study on cerebral glycogen after brain injury in the rat. *Exp. Neurol.* 22, 590–602.

Hay, R., Bohni, P., and Gasser, S. (1984). How mitochondria import proteins. *Acta Biochim. Biophys.* 779, 65–87.

Henneman, E., and Mendell, L. M. (1981). Functional organization of motoneuron pool and its inputs. In *Handbook of Physiology—The Nervous System*, Vol. II, Part 1 (ed. V. B. Brooks). American Physiological Society, Bethesda, Md., 423–507.

Hennig, R., and Lomo, T. (1985). Firing patterns of motor units in normal rats. *Nature* 314, 164–166.

Hill, T. L. (1987). Use of muscle contraction formalism for kinesin in fast axonal transport. *Proc. Natl. Acad. Sci. USA* 84, 474–477.

Hinrichsen, C. F. L., and Ryan, A. (1982). The size of motor units in the laryngeal muscles of the rat. *Experientia* 38, 360–361.

Herrera, A. A., and Grinnell, A. D. (1985). Effects of changes in motor unit size on transmitter release at the frog neuromuscular junction. *J. Neurosci.* 5, 1896–1900.

Holloszy, J. O. (1967). Biochemical adaptations in muscle: Effect of exercise on mitochondrial oxygen uptake and respiratory enzyme activity in skeletal muscle. *J. Biol. Chem.* 242, 2278–2282.

Hyden, H. (1964). Biochemical and functional interplay between neuron and glia. *Rec. Adv. Biol. Psych.* 6, 31–53.

Hyden, H. (1967). Dynamic aspects on the neuron–glia relationship. In *The Neuron* (ed. H. Hayden). Elsevier, New York, pp. 179–219.

Ishihara, A., Araki, H., Nishihira, Y., and Naitoh, H. (1988). A histochemical study of the relationship between soma size and the oxidative enzyme activity of motoneurons innervating the rat soleus muscle. *J. Health Phy. Ed. U. Tokushima* 21, 27–32.

Jasmin, B. J., Lavoie, P. A., and Gardiner, P. F. (1987). Fast axonal transport of acetylcholinesterase in rat sciatic motoneurons is enhanced following prolonged daily running, but not following swimming. *Neurosci. Lett.* 78, 156–160.

Katoh-Semba, R., Keino, H., and Kashiwamata, S. (1988). A possible contribution of glial cells to neuronal energy production: Enzyme-histochemical studies in the developing rat cerebellum. *Cell Tissue Res.* 252, 133–139.

Kernell, D., Donselaar, Y., and Eerbeek, O. (1987). Effects of physiological amounts of high- and low-rate chronic stimulation on fast-twitch muscle of the cat hindlimb. II. Endurance-related properties. *J. Neurophysiol.* 58, 614–627.

Kreutzberg, G. W., and Schubert, P. (1981). Intraneuronal transport as demonstrated by histochemical, cytochemical and autoradiographic methods. *Acta Histochem.* Suppl. 24, 27–32.

Landon, D. N., and Williams, P. L. (1963). Ultrastructure of the node of ranvier. *Nature* 199, 575–577.

Matsunami, K., Kageyama, T., and Kubota, K. (1981). Radioactive 2-deoxy-D-glucose incorporation into the prefrontal and premotor cortex of the monkey performing a forelimb movement. *Neurosci. Lett.* 26, 37–41.

Mjaatvedt, A. E., and Wong-Riley, M. T. T. (1986). Double-labeling of rat alpha-motoneurons for cytochrome oxidase and retrogradely transported [3H]WGA. *Brain Res.* 368, 178–182.

Mortola, J. P., and Noworaj, A. (1985). Breathing pattern and growth: Comparative aspects. *J. Comp. Physiol.* 155, 171–176.

Ochs, S. (1982). *Axoplasmic Transport and Its Relation to Other Nerve Functions.* Wiley, New York.

Padykula, H. A. (1952). The localization of succinate dehydrogenase in tissue sections of the rat. *Am. J. Anat.* 91, 107–145.

Pearson, J. K., and Sickles, D. W. (1987). Enzyme activity changes in rat soleus motoneurons and muscle after synergist ablation. *J. Appl. Physiol.* 63, 2301–2308.

Penny, J. E., Kukums, J. R., Tyrer, J. H., and Eadie, M. J. (1975). Quantitative oxidative enzyme histochemistry of the spinal cord. 2. Relation of cell size and enzyme activity to vulnerability to ischaemia. *J. Neurol. Sci.* 26, 187–192.

Rawe, S. E., Lee, W. A., and Perot, P. H. (1981). Spinal cord glucose utilization after experimental spinal cord injury. *Neurosurgery* 9, 40–47.

Ritchie, J. M. (1967). The oxygen consumption of mammalian non-myelinated nerve fibres at rest and during activity. *J. Physiol. (Lond.)* 188, 309–329.

Rothman, S. M., and Olney, J. W. (1987). Excitotoxicity and the NMDA receptor. *TINS* 10, 299–302.

Roy, R. R., Gilliam, T. B., Taylor, J. F., and Heusner, W. W. (1983). Activity-induced morphologic changes in rat soleus nerve. *Exp. Neurol.* 80, 622–632.

Saito, A., and Zacks, S. I. (1969). Fine structure of neuromuscular junctions after nerve section and implantation of nerve in denervated muscle. *Exp. Mol. Pathol.* 10, 256–273.

Sandler, A. N., and Tator, C. H. (1976). Review of the measurement of normal spinal cord blood flow. *Brain Res.* 118, 181–198.

Shimamura, M., Edgerton, V. R., and Kogure, I. (1987). Application of autoradiographic analysis of 2-deoxyglucose in the study of locomotion. *J. Neurosci. Methods* 21, 303–310.

Sickles, D. W., and McLendon, R. E. (1983). Metabolic variation among rat lumbosacral alpha motoneurons. *Histochemistry* 79, 205–217.

Sickles, D. W., and Oblak, T. G. (1984). Metabolic variation among alpha motoneurons innervating different fiber types. I. Oxidative enzyme activity. *J. Neurophysiol.* 51, 529–537.

Sickles, D. W., Oblak, T. G., and Scholer, J. (1987). Hyperthyroidism selectively increases oxidative metabolism of slow-oxidative motor units. *Exp. Neurol.* 97, 90–105.

Siesjo, B. K. (1978). *Brain Energy Metabolism*. Wiley, New York.

Siesjo, B. K., Johannsson, H., Ljunggren, B., and Norberg, K. (1974). Brain dysfunction in cerebral hypoxia and ischemia. In *Brain Dysfunction in Metabolic Disorders* (ed. F. Plum). Raven Press, New York, pp. 75–112.

Sokoloff, L. (1975). Influence of functional activity on local cerebral glucose utilization. In *Brain Work* (ed. D. H. Ingvar and N. A. Lassen). Academic Press, New York, pp. 385-388.

Sokoloff, L. (1984). *Metabolic Probes of Central Nervous System Activity in Experimental Animals and Man*. Sinauer Associates, Sunderland, Mass.

Stuart, D. G., and Enoka, R. M. (1983). Motoneurons, motor units, and the size principle. In *The Clinical Neurosciences*, Sect. 5, *Neurobiology* (ed. R. N. Rosenburg). Churchill Livingstone, New York, pp. 471–517.

Van Raamsdonk, W., Smit-Onel, M., Donselaar, Y., and Diegenbach, P. (1987). Quantitative cytochemical analysis of cytochrome oxidase and succinate dehydrogenase activity in spinal neurons. *Acta Histochem.* 81, 129–141.

Varon, S. S., and Somjen, G. G. (1979). Neuron–glia interactions. *Neurosci. Res. Bull.* 17, 1–239.

Wong-Riley, M. T., and Kageyama, G. H. (1986). Localization of cytochrome oxidase in the mammalian spinal cord and dorsal root ganglia, with quantitative analysis of ventral horn cells in monkeys. *J. Comp. Neurol.* 245, 41–61.

9

The Role of Motoneuron Membrane Properties in the Determination of Recruitment Order

MARTIN J. PINTER

In 1965, Elwood Henneman and co-workers published an important series of papers that continue to influence spinal cord research and theories about motor control. These papers were concerned with the manner in which motor units are recruited during muscle activation (see Henneman and Mendell, 1981, for a detailed review). Henneman and his co-workers uncovered what appeared to be a fairly stereotyped recruitment pattern. Using recordings obtained from small numbers of motor axons in ventral root filaments, they found that motoneurons with low-amplitude axonal action potentials were recruited first in response to muscle stretch in decerebrate cats (Henneman et al., 1965a). As the amount of stretch was increased, these units increased their firing frequency as other motoneurons possessing larger-amplitude action potentials were recruited. As the amount of stretch was decreased, motor axons showing the lowest-amplitude action potentials were the last to be silenced. Thus, recruitment occurred according to the amplitude of the motor axon action potential. Other studies revealed that such recruitment could be observed under a variety of different stimulus conditions (Henneman et al., 1965b).

The mechanisms underlying this type of recruitment have since been the subject of much attention (Zucker, 1973; Stein and Bertoldi, 1981; Stuart and Enoka, 1983). It was originally suggested that the size of a motoneuron played a key role in determining its recruitment position (Henneman et al., 1965a). This suggestion was based on the direct relationship between axonal action potential amplitude and recruitment position observed in decerebrate cats. The amplitude of the extracellularly recorded axonal action potential was interpreted as a direct index of the axon size, and it was further assumed that larger motoneurons possessed larger axons. The hypothesis that emerged from these results thus held that motoneuron size and factors that correlate with motoneuron size determine recruitment position; smaller motoneurons innervating those muscle units producing the least tension output would be recruited first, with larger motoneurons and their greater tension output units being recruited successively thereafter. This hypothesis has been termed the "size principle." Recruitment of motor units in the order of increasing tension output has been termed "orderly recruitment" (Henneman et al., 1965a, 1965b; Zajac and Faden, 1985; Chapter 5, this volume).

In emphasizing the role of motoneurons size, Henneman called attention to the possibility that factors inherent in the motoneurons themselves may provide the mechanism underlying orderly recruitment (see Chapter 10, this volume). The purpose of this chapter is to explore this possibility in detail, making use of recent experimental findings.

THE REQUIREMENTS OF ORDERLY RECRUITMENT

In principle, it is possible to specify what is needed of the motoneuron pool and its synaptic input in order to accomplish orderly recruitment. A threshold spectrum needs to be developed in which those motoneurons that innervate muscle units developing the least tension possess the lowest thresholds, with those motoneurons innervating progressively larger muscle units possessing progressively larger thresholds. In other words, a monotonic relationship needs to be established between motoneuron threshold and the tension of the associated muscle unit. In this way, motor units producing the lowest-tension outputs would be recruited first.

There are certain strategies with which this structuring of the excitability profile of the motoneuron pool can be accomplished. First, the temporal and spatial patterns of synaptic input organization to the motoneuron pool can be appropriately arranged. Second, the properties of the motoneurons themselves can be arranged to provide the needed threshold spectrum. An obvious third possibility is that both of these mechanisms contribute to the required excitability pattern, and given the weight of present knowledge, this seems most likely (Burke, 1981). The contributions made to recruitment by those properties that determine the intrinsic excitability of the motoneurons themselves will now be considered.

DETERMINATION OF INTRINSIC EXCITABILITY

The term "intrinsic excitability" generally refers to the responsiveness of a motoneuron to excitatory current injected either via synaptic mechanisms or through an intracellular electrode. Experimentally, this responsiveness is usually assessed by measuring the amount of current that needs to be injected through an intracellular electrode in order to elicit a single action potential or a train of action potentials (Kernell, 1966; Fleshman et al., 1981; Gustafsson and Pinter, 1984b). The various factors that can influence the amount of current needed to elicit an action potential will now be considered, since this provides a useful framework for discussing experimental results.

The first item to be considered is the amount of depolarization required to elicit an action potential. There is evidence that under normal conditions the process of cat motoneuron spike generation is initiated in the axon initial segment (Gustafsson and Jankowska, 1976), so this depolarization is likely to be equivalent to the voltage threshold for spike initiation at the initial segment. For any particular voltage threshold, there is also a collection of interactive properties that can influence the amount of current that is needed for depolarizing the membrane to the voltage threshold. Some of these properties are conveniently illustrated by considering longer-duration stimulus pulses in a uniformly depolarized spherical neuron with linear membrane properties in subthreshold membrane potential regions. In this case, the current threshold (I_{TH}) is related to the voltage threshold (V_{TH}) by Ohm's law. Thus,

$$V_{TH} = I_{TH} \times R_{IN}$$

where R_{IN} equals the input resistance. For the spherical neuron, the input resistance is equal to the specific membrane resistivity $(\Omega - cm^2)$ divided by the membrane surface area. Variation in either of these properties can thus alter the amount of current needed to reach a particular voltage threshold by virtue of its effect on input resistance. It is also useful to keep in mind that the duration of the current stimulus itself plays an important role in determining the current threshold. Because of increasing capacitative losses, increasingly brief current pulses require a larger amplitude to reach voltage threshold than do pulses of longer duration (see Noble and Stein, 1966).

The situation with regard to real motoneurons is more complex because of the presence of an elaborate dendritic tree. In contrast to uniformly depolarized case, not all of the current injected through an electrode lodged in the soma, for example, is available for depolarizing the initial segment to its voltage threshold. As the current injection commences, substantial voltage gradients develop within the neuron that act to drive current out of the soma through the relatively low-resistance pathways formed by the internal cores of the dendrites. These gradients diminish as the injection continues and deposits more charge in these distal regions. Progressively more current is thus made available for depolarization of the initial segment. Despite this complexity, the steady-state relationship between the current and voltage thresholds defined for the uniformly depolarized (spherical) case is still valid for neurons with dendritic trees, provided that the membrane behaves linearly at voltages leading up to threshold.

Membrane conductance systems that are voltage dependent and active in subthreshold regions of the membrane potential ("nonlinear" systems) may also influence excitability. Such systems may or may not be directly involved in the generation of action potentials. Among cat motoneurons, there are several possible mechanisms that fall into this category. For example, there is some evidence for accommodation among cat motoneurons (Burke and Nelson, 1971).

Assuming that the underlying mechanism is similar to that in the squid axon (Hodgkin and Huxley, 1952) and is localized in the initial segment, accommodation acts by decreasing the maximum available inward current in the initial segment. In order to reach the initial segment threshold, more injected current is thus required. The "overshoot, undershoot" phenomenon first described by Ito and Oshima (1965) represents another "active" membrane process that may influence cat motoneuron excitability. Still another is an inward current described by Schwindt and Crill (1980) that is thought to be carried by calcium and appears to be activated in the region of the initial segment voltage threshold. There are undoubtedly other mechanisms that remain to be uncovered. The common denominator among such systems, however, is their ability to influence motoneuron excitability by either adding to or subtracting from the amount of injected current needed to evoke an action potential.

EVIDENCE FROM CAT MOTONEURONS

Systematic variation of any or all of the properties just described within pools of motoneurons could conceivably contribute to the excitability profile required for orderly recruitment. Several recent reports have been concerned with establishing (1) whether the variations in these properties are indeed sufficient to establish the requirements of orderly recruitment and (2) which of those properties are most important. Some of these recent experimental findings will now be considered (Fleshman et al., 1981; Gustafsson and Pinter, 1984a, 1984b, 1985a, 1985b).

Current Thresholds

Because the measurement of current threshold in cat motoneurons is feasible, a number of studies have analyzed the relationships between current thresholds and other motoneuron properties (Kernell, 1966, Fleshman et al., 1981; Gustafsson and Pinter, 1984b). Figure 9–1 is taken from Gustafsson and Pinter (1984b) and shows a plot of thresholds for 50-ms current pulses (rheobase current) versus input conductance $(1/R_{IN})$ for 153 normal cat hindlimb motoneurons. It is apparent from this plot that there is a very systematic relationship between these parameters. However, it may be observed that the overall range of rheobase current exceeds that of input conductance by a factor of 2 (see also Fleshman et al., 1981). This indicates that rheobase and input conductance are not linearly related, as in the simple cases considered earlier, and that factors (e.g., voltage threshold and active membrane properties) in addition to those that determine input conductance are important in determining rheobase current. The contributions of these other factors will be considered.

Despite the fact that other parameters are apparently involved in setting the rheobase, the correlation between rheobase and input conductance in Figure 9–1 $(r^2 = 0.81)$ indicates that much of the variation in rheobase current among these motoneurons can be explained by a corresponding variation in input con-

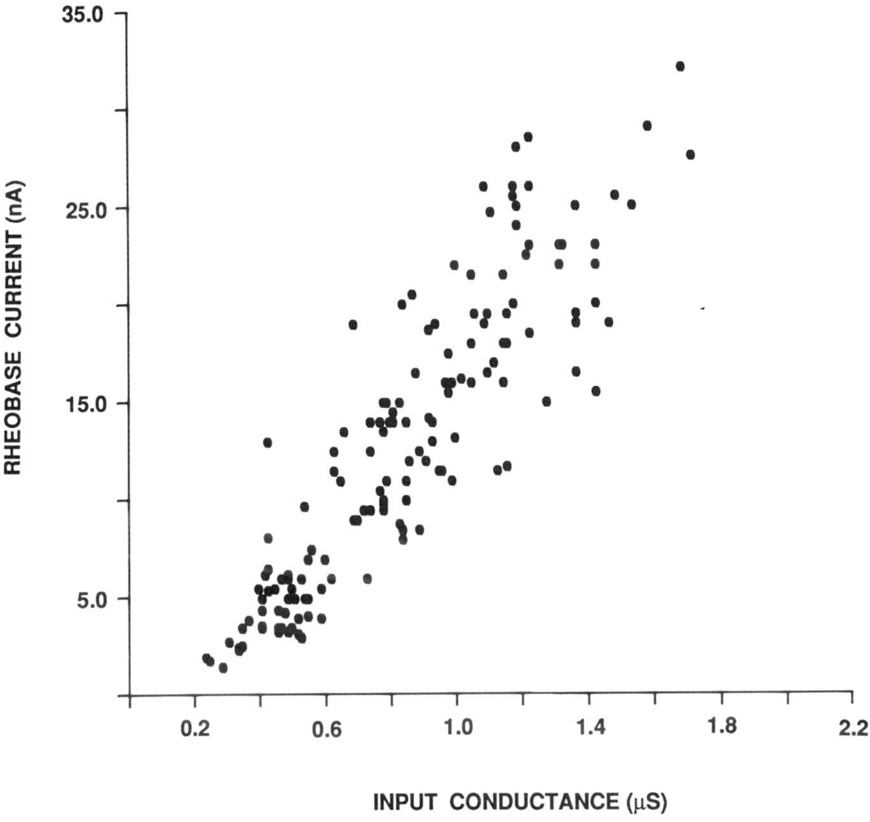

Fig. 9–1. Plot of rheobase current versus input conductance for normal cat hindlimb motoneurons. The linear correlation coefficient was 0.91. (Adapted from Gustafsson and Pinter, 1984b, with permission.)

ductance. As noted earlier, two of the chief determinants of input conductance are the specific membrane conductivity ($G_M = 1/R_M$) and the membrane surface area (A_N) of the motoneuron. Unfortunately, neither of these properties can be measured directly using only electrophysiological methods. Gustafsson and Pinter (1984a, 1984b), however, used electrophysiological measurements to estimate these parameters. The method for estimating A_N will be described. For an index of resting membrane conductivity Gustafsson and Pinter (1984a, 1984b) used the inverse of the longest time constant measured from the voltage decay following brief (0.5 ms) current pulses. The rationale for this practice derives from linear cable theory (Rall, 1977); after the charge delivered from the micropipette has been redistributed such that all areas of the cell are isopotential, the final voltage decay time constant is equal to the quotient of specific membrane capacitance and resting membrane conductivity. This relationship depends, however, on a number of assumptions concerning the structure of the motoneuron and the spatial uniformity of membrane properties such as resistivity (Rall, 1977). Since there have been questions concerning the validity of some of these assumptions (particularly the uniformity of membrane resistivity; see Fleshman et al., 1983; Ulfhake and Kellerth, 1984), it is probably best to view the measurement obtained from voltage transients as the "effective" membrane time constant and its inverse as the "effective" rate constant.

Figure 9–2 shows the relationship between the effective membrane rate constant and rheobase current for a subset of the data in Figure 9–1. As with the relationship shown in Figure 9–1, it is evident that this index of effective resting conductivity is well correlated with rheobase current, the correlation coefficient being 0.88. It should be noted, however, that the range of rheobase exceeds that of the effective rate constant, again indicating the likely existence of a nonlinear relationship. Nevertheless, the strength of the correlation between rheobase and the effective rate constant clearly parallels that between rheobase and input conductance, and illustrates the importance of the effective membrane conductivity in determining input conductance and, hence, rheobase current (see Kernell and Zwaagstra, 1981).

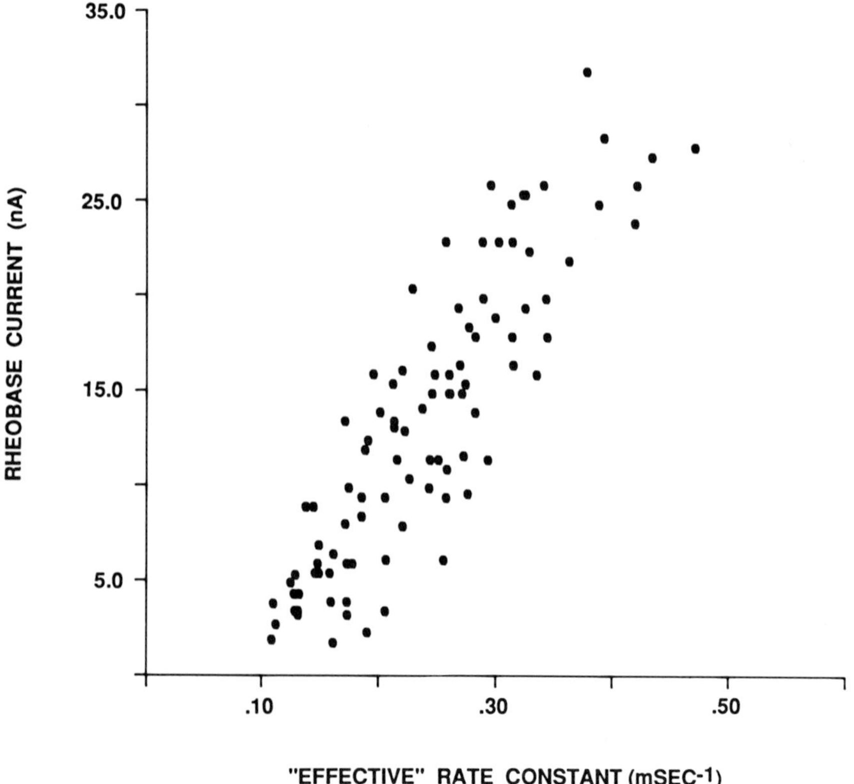

Fig. 9–2. Plot of rheobase current versus the effective rate constant for normal cat hindlimb motoneurons. The effective rate constant is equivalent to the inverse of the effective membrane time constant. The linear correlation coefficient in this case was 0.88. (Adapted from Gustafsson and Pinter, 1984b, with permission.)

The Role of Cell Size

If cell size (or any other parameter used as an index of cell size) were the chief determinant of recruitment order among motoneurons, then one might reasonably suppose that cell size itself or a correlated parameter should exhibit a clearcut, systematic relationship with a measure of cell excitability such as rheobase. In the past, axonal conduction velocity was used as an index of cell size (Henneman et al., 1965a; Clamann and Henneman, 1976; Bawa et al., 1984). The lower panel of Figure 9–3 illustrates the relationship between axonal conduction velocity and rheobase current for the cells shown in Figures 9–1 and 9–2. Clearly, the relationship shown in Figures 9–1 and 9–2 is not evident in this plot (cf. Fleshman et al., 1981). This indicates that axonal conduction velocity is not a good overall indicator of motoneuron excitability as reflected by rheobase current.

Establishing the direct relationship between rheobase current and cell size is a very difficult experimental proposition. It requires the comparison of a reasonably sized sample of motoneuron rheobase currents with cell surface area measurements obtained from the same cells. Although intracellular injections of horseradish peroxidase (HRP) would allow such a comparison, this hercu-

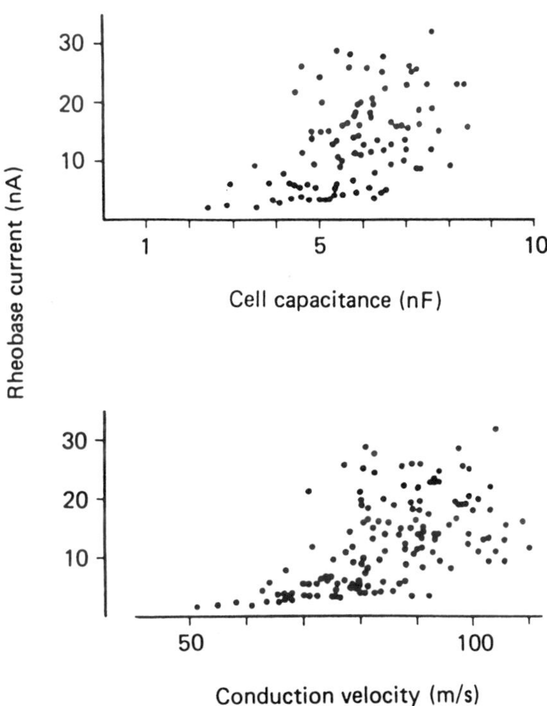

Fig. 9–3. *Upper panel*: plot of rheobase current versus CTOT for normal cat hindlimb motoneurons. As noted in text, CTOT is an electrophysiological estimate of total cell surface area. *Lower panel*: plot of rheobase current versus motor axonal conduction velocity for the same data set shown in the upper panel. (Adapted from Gustafsson and Pinter, 1984b, with permission.)

lean task has yet to be performed. Meanwhile, more indirect methods of addressing the issue of cell excitability and its relation to cell size must be employed. Gustafsson and Pinter (1984a) approached this issue using estimates of total cell capacitance obtained with electrophysiological measurements. Given estimates of electrotonic length (L), the effective membrane time constant (γ_M), and cell input resistance (R_IN), total cell capacitance (C_TOT) is calculated according to the following formula based upon the equivalent cylinder representation developed by Rall (1977):

$$C_\mathrm{TOT} = \frac{\gamma_\mathrm{M}\, L}{R_\mathrm{IN}\, \tanh(L)}$$

If one assumes that specific membrane capacitance (C_M) is identical for all motoneurons (as it seems to be among many different cell types; Cole, 1968), then C_TOT can provide an estimate of the total cell surface area (see Gustafsson and Pinter, 1984a). It must be emphasized that this calculation requires not only data from well-impaled cells, but also that the motoneurons meet or at least approximate the requirements of the equivalent cylinder model as outlined by Rall. As mentioned earlier, there have been questions about some of the assumptions embodied in this model. The problem concerning the effective membrane time constant and spatial uniformity of membrane resistivity is an example. Another potential problem with equivalent cylinder assumptions is raised by evidence indicating that the electrotonic lengths of individual motoneuron dendrites may differ significantly (Ulfhake and Kellerth, 1984). These indications serve as warnings of the potential danger associated with the unqualified use of formulations based upon the equivalent cylinder model.

Despite these potential problems with the equivalent cylinder assumptions, calculations of C_TOT (assuming a specific membrane capacitance of 1 μF/cm^2) provided estimates of motoneuron surface area that were consistent with surface area estimates obtained from HRP-filled motoneurons (Gustafsson and Pinter, 1984a; see Ulfhake and Kellerth, 1982, and Burke et al., 1982). More recent estimates of motoneuron surface area obtained from completely reconstructed, HRP-filled motoneurons are also quite consistent with the C_TOT area estimates (Cullheim et al., 1987). A full discussion of the reasons that may underlie the apparent agreement between C_TOT and anatomical estimates of motoneuron surface area is beyond the scope of this chapter. The possibility should be considered, however, that the departures from the mathematical idealizations of the equivalent cylinder model indicated by recent evidence are not sufficient to limit significantly the overall usefulness of the model.

The upper panel of Figure 9–3 illustrates a plot of C_TOT against rheobase current. It can be seen that there is no clear relationship between these parameters, suggesting that motoneuron surface area is as poor an indicator of cell excitability as axon conduction velocity. The overall similarity of the plots in Figure 9–3 is noteworthy in view of the positive correlation between HRP-estimates of motoneuron surface area and axonal conduction velocity demonstrated by Burke et al. (1982). This similarity thus seems to provide indirect support for the usefulness of C_TOT as an estimate of motoneuron surface area.

Other Membrane Properties

There is indirect evidence of a net inward rectification process in cat motoneurons that may operate in the region of the voltage threshold for spike initiation (Gustafsson and Pinter, 1984b). This was revealed as a consistent discrepancy between the rheobase current–input resistance product and estimated
threshold depolarizations for spike initiation. In virtually all cases, the estimates of threshold depolarization were greater than the rheobase–input resistance product, suggesting the presence of an additional net inward current. This
current could conceivably be equivalent to the conductance process termed I_i
by Schwindt and Crill (1980), which is believed to be a Ca^{2+} current. The
difference between these parameters showed a clear tendency to increase with
effective membrane time constant and with afterhyperpolarization (AHP) duration (Gustafsson and Pinter, 1984a). However, it is not clear whether this
apparent inward rectifier provides an additional mechanism for differential excitability among motoneurons (Gustafsson and Pinter, 1984b).

There is some information concerning possible differences in voltage
thresholds among motoneurons. Pinter et al. (1983) measured both threshold
depolarization and absolute voltage thresholds (resting potential minus threshold depolarization) for orthodromic action potentials evoked by large group Ia
excitatory postsynaptic potentials (EPSPs). These authors found no clear tendency for these measures of excitability to covary with parameters such as AHP
duration or the twitch contraction time of associated muscle units. Gustafsson
and Pinter (1984a) obtained similar threshold estimates from hindlimb motoneurons activated with intracellular current pulses used to measure rheobase
current. Among these cells, there was a clear tendency for the estimated threshold depolarization to decrease with AHP duration and input resistance. This
suggests that motoneurons innervating slower muscle units may possess lower
threshold depolarizations, at least for longer duration current pulses. Further
analysis of the data indicated, however, that these trends may have been due
to differences in the way voltage thresholds of slow and fast motoneurons (distinguished by the AHP durations) react to the variable resting potentials inev-
itably imposed by impalement with intracellular electrodes. Such reactions might
be consistent with differences in accommodation among fast and slow motoneurons (Burke and Nelson, 1971) or may be a response to impalement injury.
In either case, it is important to note that the effect of the underlying mechanism clearly covaries with parameters such as input conductance and may represent a means by which the threshold spectrum among motoneurons can be
expanded in response to steady conditioning currents from any source.

A final membrane property to consider is the overshoot, undershoot phenomenon of Ito and Oshima (1965). The important issues here are whether the
effect of this phenomenon covaries with parameters such as AHP duration and
the potential significance of such a variation. Burke and Nelson (1971) examined this issue and found no evidence of a systematic relationship between
the extent of overshoot, undershoot and other motor unit parameters. More
recently, however, Gustafsson and Pinter (1984b) have demonstrated a clear
inverse relationship between the extent of this "sag" process and AHP duration.

This relationship is also suggested in Figure 3 of Zengel et al. (1985), where the responses of three medial gastrocnemius motoneurons of different motor unit type to intracellularly injected 1-nA current pulses are illustrated. The potential significance of this systematic variation of the sag process has been considered by Gustafsson and Pinter (1985a). In particular, results generated with the use of mathematical models suggest that the variation in sag among motoneurons may contribute importantly to the associated variation of the AHP duration. Further support for this possibility derives from results obtained from axotomized motoneurons. In these cells, an overall increase in AHP duration is associated with a decrease in the extent of sag (Figure 2 of Gustafsson and Pinter, 1985a; Pinter and Vanden Noven, unpublished findings). The sag process may also affect the frequency required of afferent firing to provide adequate summation of postsynaptic potentials (PSPs) by hastening the decay phase of these potentials (Zengel et al., 1985). The available evidence thus indicates that the overshoot, undershoot phenomenon plays an important role in the overall variation of motoneuron excitability. The mechanism underlying this process, however, remains unknown.

RECRUITMENT MODELS

The evidence previously reviewed suggests that the variation in intrinsic excitability among motoneurons, as reflected by rheobase current measurements, is largely determined by a systematic variation in membrane properties. Moreover, it appears that this variation in membrane properties is poorly related to the overall variation in cell size. Support for these views comes from a consideration of the correlations of rheobase with the effective rate constant and with C_{TOT} estimates of cell surface area. In the latter case, the linear correlation coefficient was 0.51, while in the former case it was 0.88 (Gustafsson and Pinter, 1984b). It is thus likely that the variance in rheobase current among the investigated motoneurons is better explained by covariance with effective membrane conductivity (and its correlates) than by covariance with size (and its correlates) by a factor of 3. Because of this, it seems justifiable to emphasize the role of intrinsic membrane properties in establishing the gradation of excitability within motoneuron pools (see also Kernell and Zwaagstra, 1981).

This mechanism for organizing the excitability profile of motoneuron pools has implications for the manner in which motoneurons are recruited. It is useful to consider this issue in the context of the various schemes that have been proposed to account for the recruitment order of motor units. There are essentially three such schemes: (1) size-related recruitment (Henneman, 1979); (2) recruitment according to motor unit type (Fleshman et al., 1981; Sypert and Munson, 1981; Zengel et al., 1985); and (3) recruitment according to the force output of muscle units (Henneman et al., 1965a; Zajac and Faden, 1985).

Size-Related Recruitment

As noted earlier, systematic relationships have not been observed between rheobase current and estimated cell surface area (Gustafsson and Pinter, 1984b) or between rheobase current and axonal conduction velocity (Fleshman et al., 1983; Gustafsson and Pinter, 1984b). Such findings argue against a significant role for cell size in the determination of either recruitment position or intrinsic excitability. Recently, however, Bawa et al. (1984) have clearly demonstrated that among motoneurons recruited during stretch reflexes in decerebrate cats, these cells with lower conduction velocities invariably begin to fire their action potentials first. This was observed in both mixed-type and homogeneous hind-limb muscles. This observation suggests that recruitment may be size dependent under these circumstances and is not consistent with the relationships shown in Figure 9–3. However, it seems likely that recruitment during the stretch reflex in decerebrate cats selects a subpopulation of the motoneuron pool. Burke (1968) has noted that many type F medial gastrocnemius motoneurons cannot be made to fire action potentials during the stretch reflex in the decerebrate cat. A clear indication of such selective recruitment in decerebrate cats is provided in Figure 9–4. This figure shows conduction velocity data from medial gastrocnemius motoneurons recruited during the stretch reflex (dashed line; data

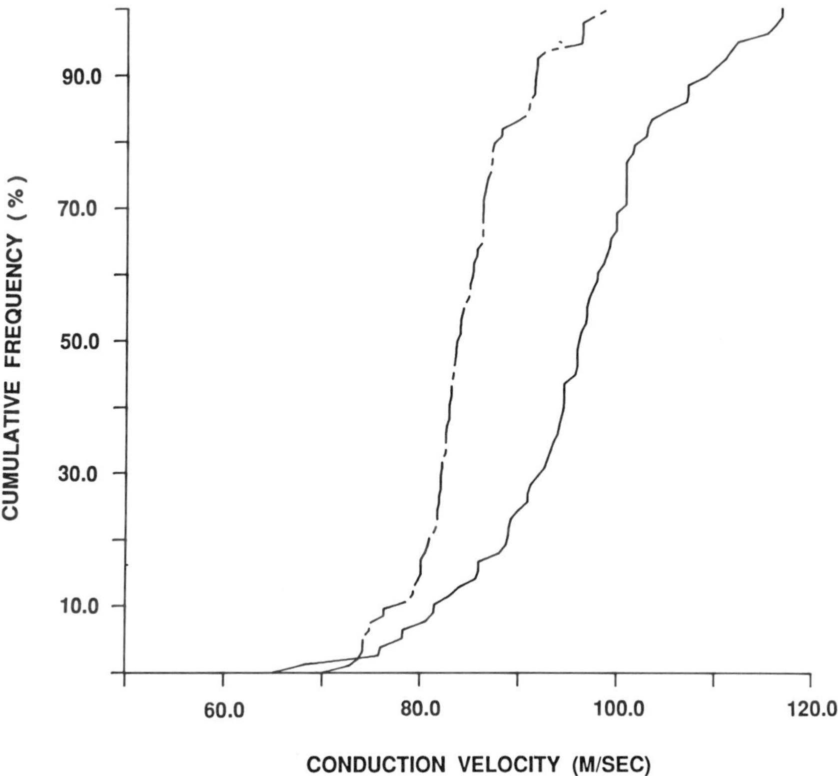

Fig. 9–4. Cumulative histograms of conduction velocity data from cat medial gastrocnemius motoneurons. The dashed line represents data from Bawa et al. (1985) that were sampled from motoneurons recruited during the stretch reflex in decerebrate cats. The solid line represents conduction velocity data obtained by intracellular sampling from normal motoneurons (Zengel et al., 1985). Note that the point at which the sample of Bawa et al. is virtually complete corresponds to only approximately the 50th percentile of Zengel et al. (Data used with permission.)

from Bawa et al., 1984) and sampled by intracellular recording in normal cats (solid line; data from Zengel et al., 1985) plotted in cumulative histogram form. It can be seen that the 95th percentile of the data from the decerebrate preparation corresponds to less than the 50th percentile of the data from the normal preparation. Assuming that the sample of Zengel et al. is representative of the entire motoneuron pool, Figure 9–4 indicates a clear sampling bias in the decerebrate preparation toward motoneurons with slower conduction velocities. Zajac and Faden (1985) have also made this point based upon recruitment studies in decerebrate cats in which conduction velocity and muscle unit tension were measured for each motor unit.

Even though it seems clear that the sampling of Bawa et al. (1984) is biased, their data support the conclusion that motoneurons were recruited in a conduction-velocity-dependent manner and indicate that a size principle of recruitment may operate among these motoneurons. One way to reconcile these conclusions with the data shown in Figure 9–3 is to consider the possibility that the mechanisms that determine intrinsic excitability may vary somewhat within motoneuron pools. Gustafsson and Pinter (1984b) found that the correlation between rheobase current and estimated surface area (C_{TOT}) was higher for motoneurons with long-duration AHPs (>80-ms, "slow" motoneurons) than in motoneurons with briefer AHP durations (<55-ms, "fast" motoneurons). The opposite was observed when rheobase was correlated with the effective membrane rate constant in the same groups. It thus seems possible that size may be of some importance in determining intrinsic excitability among motoneurons that possess slow conduction velocities. This suggestion does not, however, weaken the conclusion that membrane properties are the chief determinants of excitability when the entire motoneuron pool is considered. What seems likely is that size and membrane properties covary to a greater extent among slow than among fast motoneurons. A fuller discussion of these issues can be found in Gustafsson and Pinter (1984a, 1984b).

Recruitment by Motor Unit Type

This scheme views the motoneuron pool as being composed of separate groups that share the same motor unit type designation defined by the mechanical properties of the associated muscle units (Burke, 1981). These groups are recruited in sequence in the order types S > FR > FF. The basis for viewing the motoneuron pool as a collection of discrete functional groups is the failure to find clear-cut relationships such as those illustrated in Figures 9–1 and 9–2 when the comparisons are confined to data from the separate groups. For example, Fleshman et al. (1981) found a significant negative correlation between rheobase current and input resistance when all data from normal cat medial gastrocnemius motoneurons were pooled, but failed to find such correlations within motor unit types. These authors thus suggested that the good correlation between rheobase and input resistance observed in the entire data set was the consequence of pooling data from the separate groups. The data reviewed earlier (Gustafsson and Pinter, 1984b) cannot be used to deal directly with this proposition, since motor unit type was not determined. However, Gustafsson and Pinter (1984b) did demonstrate significant correlations between rheobase and input conductance in two groups of motoneurons that had average rheobase currents corresponding to types S and FF medial gastrocnemius motoneurons of Fleshman et al. (1981). A significant correlation was not observed in the intermediate group, which had an average rheobase corresponding to type FR. Detailed analysis of this latter result indicated the presence of a sampling problem in the intermediate group that was not present in the other groups. It is conceivable that such problems could exist in the data of Fleshman et al. (1981), although correlations between other parameters such as AHP duration and twitch contraction time are also absent within motor unit types while being significant overall (Zengel et al., 1985). Evaluation of this recruitment scheme is difficult because it is based on negative results. One possibility that should be considered is that extracting data subsets according to motor unit type might provoke a situation wherein the variance of the sampled parameters becomes a substantial fraction of the overall range of the data subsets. Such a situation could conceivably obscure relationships, especially when dealing with such potentially labile measurements as rheobase current (see Gustafsson and Pinter, 1984b).

Recruitment by Motor Unit Force

In this final scheme to be considered, recruitment proceeds in the order of increasing force output of the motor unit, as originally suggested by Henneman and co-workers. As noted earlier, this scheme is termed "orderly recruitment" and, from a mechanical point of view, has great appeal, since it can optimize the smoothness of force development in individual muscles and thus minimize higher rotational or translational time derivatives around the associated joints (see Hatze, 1979). Zajac and Faden (1985) have provided compelling evidence for this type of recruitment in the hindlimb muscle of decerebrate cats during the stretch reflex. Among pairs of motor units that included *all types of units,* the one generating the least tetanic tension was always recruited first. It should be noted that posttetanic potentiation of monosynaptic Ia EPSPs was used to ensure that recruitment of higher-strength type F units could be studied.

Recruitment by motor unit force appears to be most consistent with evidence that the excitability spectrum of motoneuron pools is organized around a variation of intrinsic membrane properties. The motoneuron threshold study of Gustafsson and Pinter (1984b) did not include investigation of muscle unit properties, so this point must be addressed indirectly, as shown in Figure 9–5. An index of excitability that can be attributed to intrinsic membrane properties was obtained by normalizing rheobase currents to the associated estimates of cell surface area (C_{TOT}). These data (in units of nA/nF) are shown in histogram form in Figure 9–5A. It is noteworthy that this normalization only reduced the rheobase range from 15-fold to 11-fold, illustrating that much of the overall variation in rheobase current is likely to be independent of size. Figure 9–5B shows a histogram of cat medial gastrocnemius muscle unit tetanic tension from Burke (1981). As can be seen, both of these histograms show a similar skew, consistent with evidence that unnormalized rheobase current and muscle unit force are correlated (Fleshman et al., 1981; Zengel et al., 1985)

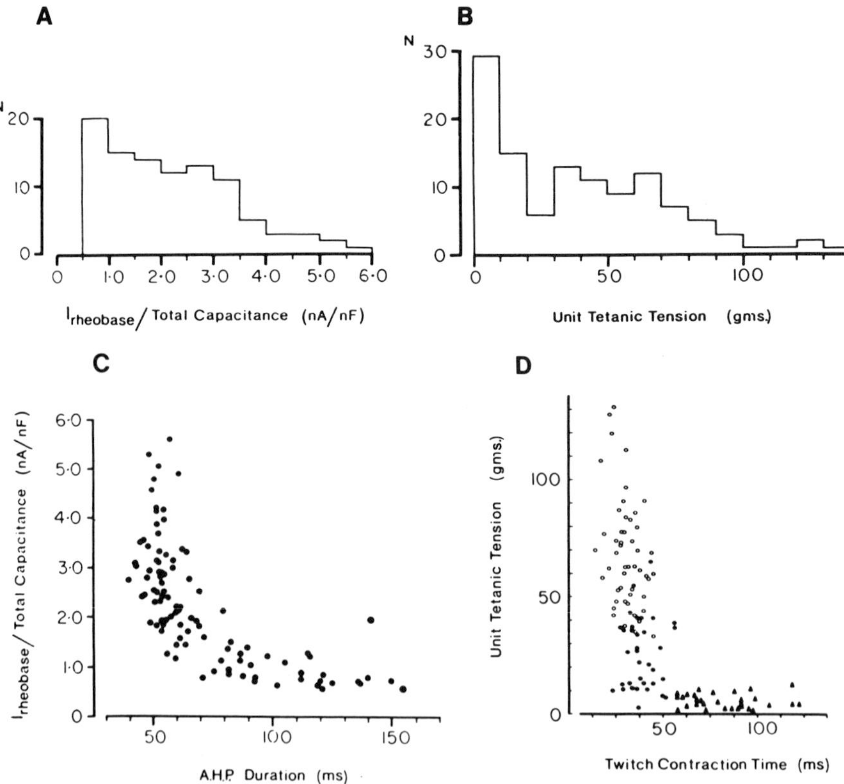

Fig. 9–5. Comparison of motoneuron and muscle unit properties. (A) Histogram of rheobase currents normalized to corresponding CTOT values from normal cat hindlimb motoneurons. (B) Histogram of tetanic tensions from cat medial gastrocnemius muscle units. (C) Plot of normalized rheobase currents versus AHP duration. (D) Plot of muscle unit tetanic tensions versus twitch contraction time. Data in (A) and (C) from Gustafsson and Pinter (1984b). Data in (B) and (D) from Burke (1981). (Adapted from Gustafsson and Pinter, 1985b, with permission.)

and with the notion that intrinsic excitability and muscle unit force covary. This latter point is illustrated further in Figures 9–5C and 9–5D. Normalized rheobase currents from Gustafsson and Pinter (1984b) are plotted against AHP duration in Figure 9–5C, and Figure 9–5D shows a plot of motor unit tetanic tension versus twitch contraction time from Burke (1981). In view of the strong correlation known to exist between AHP duration and twitch contraction time (Pinter et al., 1983; Zengel et al., 1985), the comparison of Figures 9–5C and 9–5D supports the view that the variation in excitability among motoneurons that is established by variations in membrane properties is exquisitely matched to the mechanical properties of the associated muscle units.

FINAL CONSIDERATIONS

This chapter has focused on how the properties of the motoneurons themselves may contribute to the order of recruitment. The evidence reviewed indicates that the distribution of membrane properties among motoneurons may impose orderly recruitment as a default mode. It must be emphasized, however, that this view does not relegate the role of the organization of synaptic input to motoneuron pools to a subsidiary position (see Chapters 10 and 17, this volume). The precise control of motoneuron pools is obviously the net outcome of many pre- and postsynaptic factors. Indeed, the organization of synaptic input and the properties of the synapses themselves serve the vital function of integrating the motoneuron pool into the larger context of whole animal behavior. Nevertheless, it seems fair to suggest that orderly recruitment may be a built-in feature of motoneuron pools and that this feature is a consequence of the distribution of intrinsic membrane properties.

Interesting questions concerning how these properties are regulated in the adult remain for future investigation. A number of studies have shown that the normal range of motoneuron properties is altered considerably following axotomy (Kuno et al., 1974; Gustafsson, 1979; Gustafsson and Pinter, 1984c; Foehring et al., 1986). What remains is a more homogeneous collection of cells whose properties seem to resemble normal slow motoneurons (Gustafsson and Pinter, 1984c). As a consequence, it has been argued that axotomy may provoke a "dedifferentiation" of motoneuron properties (Kuno et al., 1974; Gustafsson and Pinter, 1984c). Other findings have also suggested the possible existence of trophic interactions between motoneuron and muscle that may play a role in maintaining adult motoneuron properties (Kuno, 1984; Foehring et al., 1987). The questions raised by the effects of axotomy on motoneuron properties represent basic issues in neuroscience and illustrate the continuing importance of the conceptual framework established by Elwood Henneman.

Acknowledgments

The author wishes to thank Dr. J. B. Munson for kindly providing data for Figure 9–4 and Dr. S. Vanden Noven for criticisms of the manuscript. Work in the author's laboratory is supported by NIH grants NS 24000 and NS 24707.

REFERENCES

Bawa, P., Binder, M. D., Ruenzel, P., and Henneman, E. (1984). Recruitment order of motoneurons in stretch reflexes is highly correlated with their conduction velocity. *J. Neurophysiol.* 52, 410–420.

Burke, R. E. (1968). Firing patterns of gastrocnemius motor units in the decerebrate cat. *J. Physiol. (Lond.)* 196, 631–654.

Burke, R. E. (1981). Motor units: Anatomy, physiology and functional organization. In *Handbook of Physiology. The Nervous System, Motor Control*, Vol. II, Sect. 1, Part 1 (ed. V. B. Brooks). American Physiological Society, Bethesda, Md., pp. 345–422.

Burke, R. E., and Nelson, P. G. (1971). Accommodation to current ramps in motoneurons of fast and slow twitch motor units. *Int. J. Neurosci.* 1, 347–356.

Burke, R. E., Dum, R. P., Fleshman, J. W., Glenn, L. L., Lev-Tov, A., O'Donovan, M. J., and Pinter, M. J. (1982). An HRP study of the relation between cell size and motor unit type in cat ankle extensor motoneurons. *J. Comp. Neurol.* 209, 17–28.

Burke, R. E., and Ten Bruggencate, G. (1971). Electrotonic characteristics of α-motoneurons of varying size. *J. Physiol. (Lond.)* 212, 1–20.

Clamann, H. P., and Henneman, E. (1976). Electrical measurements of axon diameter and its use in relating motoneuron size to critical firing level. *J. Neurophysiol.* 39, 844–851.

Cullheim, S., Fleshman, J. W., Glenn, L. L., and Burke, R. E. (1987). Membrane area and dendritic structure in type-identified triceps surae alpha motoneurons. *J. Comp. Neurol.* 255, 68–81.

Fleshman, J. W., Munson, J. B., Sypert, G. W., and Friedman, W. A. (1981). Rheobase, input resistance and motor unit type in medial gastrocnemius in the cat. *J. Neurophysiol.* 46, 1326–1338.

Fleshman, J. W., Segev, I., Cullheim, S., and Burke, R. E. (1983). Matching electrophysiological with morphological measurements in cat α-motoneurons. *Soc. Neurosci. Abstr.* 9:341.

Foehring, R. C., Sypert, G. W., and Munson, J. B. (1986). Properties of self-reinnervated motor units of medial gastrocnemius of cat: II. Axotomized motoneurons and time course of recovery. *J. Neurophysiol.* 55, 947–965.

Foehring, R. C., Sypert, G. W., and Munson, J. B. (1987). Motor unit properties following self-reinnervation of cat lateral gastrocnemius and soleus muscles with medial gastrocnemius nerve. II. Influence of muscle on motoneuron. *J. Neurophysiol.* 57, 1227–1245.

Gustafsson, B. (1979). Changes in motoneurone electrical properties following axotomy. *J. Physiol. (Lond.)* 293, 197–215.

Gustafsson, B., and Jankowska, E. (1976). Direct and indirect activation of nerve cells by electrical pulses applied extracellularly. *J. Physiol. (Lond.)* 258, 33–61.

Gustafsson, B., and Pinter, M. J. (1984a). Relations among passive electrical properties of lumbar α-motoneurons of the cat. *J. Physiol. (Lond.)* 356, 401–431.

Gustafsson, B., and Pinter, M. J. (1984b). An investigation of threshold properties among cat spinal motoneurons. *J. Physiol. (Lond.)* 357, 453–483.

Gustafsson, B., and Pinter, M. J. (1984c). Effects of axotomy on the distribution of passive electrical properties of cat motoneurones. *J. Physiol. (Lond.)* 356, 433–442.

Gustafsson, B., and Pinter, M. J. (1985a). Factors determining the variation of the afterhyperpolarization duration in cat lumbar α-motoneurons. *Brain Res.* 326, 392–395.

Gustafsson, B., and Pinter, M. J. (1985b). Factors determining orderly recruitment of motor units: The role of intrinsic membrane properties. *Trends Neurosci.* 8, 431–433.

Hatze, H. A. (1979). A teleological explanation of Weber's law and the motor unit size law. *Bull. Math. Biol.* 41, 407–425.

Henneman, E. (1979). Functional organization of motoneuron pools: The size principle. In *Integration in the Nervous System* (ed. H. Asanuma and V. J. Wilson). Igaku-Shoin, Tokyo, pp. 13–25.

Henneman, E., and Mendell, L. M. (1981). Functional organization of motoneuron pool and its input. In *Handbook of Physiology. The Nervous System,* Vol. II, Sect. 1, part 1 (ed. V. B. Brooks). American Physiological Society, Bethesda, Md., pp. 423–507.

Henneman, E., Somjen, G., and Carpenter, D. O. (1965a). Functional significance of cell size in spinal motoneurons. *J. Neurophysiol.* 28, 560–580.

Henneman, E., Somjen, G., and Carpenter, D. O. (1965b). Excitability and inhibitability of motoneurons of different size. *J. Neurophysiol.* 28, 599–620.

Hodgkin, A. L., and Huxley, A. F. (1952). The dual effect of membrane potential on sodium conductance in the giant axon of Loligo. *J. Physiol. (Lond.)* 116, 497–506.

Ito, M., and Oshima, T. (1965). Electrical behavior of the motoneurone membrane during intracellularly applied current steps. *J. Physiol. (Lond.)* 180, 607–637.

Kernell, D. (1966). Input resistance, electrical excitability and cell size of ventral horn cells in cat spinal cord. *Science* 152, 1637–1640.

Kernell, D., and Zwaagstra, B. (1981). Input conductance, axonal conduction velocity and cell size among hindlimb motoneurons of the cat. *Brain Res.* 204, 311–326.

Kuno, M. (1984). A hypothesis for neural control of the speed of muscle contraction in the mammal. *Adv. Biophys.* 17, 69–95.

Kuno, M., Miyata, Y., and Munoz-Martinez, E. J. (1974). Differential reaction of fast and slow α-motoneurones to axotomy. *J. Physiol. (Lond.)* 240, 725–739.

Noble, D., and Stein, R. B. (1966). The theoretical conditions for initiation of action potentials by excitable cells. *J. Physiol. (Lond.)* 187, 129–162.

Pinter, M. J., Curtis, R. L., and Hosko, M. J. (1983). Voltage threshold and excitability among variously sized cat hindlimb motoneurons. *J. Neurophysiol.* 50, 644–657.

Rall, W. (1977). Core conductor theory and cable properties of neurons. In *Handbook of Physiology. The Nervous System*, Vol. I, Sect. 1, Part 1 (ed. E. R. Kandel). American Physiological Society, Bethesda, Md., pp. 39–97.

Schwindt, P. C., and Crill, W. E. (1980). Properties of a persistent inward current in normal and TEA-injected motoneurons. *J. Neurophysiol.* 43, 1700–1724.

Stein, R. B., and Bertoldi, R. (1981). The size principle: A synthesis of neurophysiological data. In *Motor Units, Recruitment and Plasticity in Health and Disease. Progress in Clinical Neurophysiology*, Vol. 9 (ed. J. E. Desmedt). Karger, Basel, pp. 85–96.

Stuart, D. G., and Enoka, R. M. (1983). Motoneurons, motor units and the size principle. In *The Clinical Neurosciences, Sect. 5: Neurobiology* (ed. R. G. Grossman; section ed., W. D. Willis). Churchill Livingstone, New York, pp. 471–518.

Sypert, G. W., and Munson, J. B. (1981). Basis of segmental control: Motoneuron size or type? *Neurosurgery* 8, 1700–1724.

Ulfhake, B., and Kellerth, J.-O. (1982). Does α-motoneuron size correlate with motor unit type in cat triceps surae? *Brain Res.* 251, 201–209.

Ulfhake, B., and Kellerth, J.-O. (1984). Electrophysiological and morphological measurements in cat gastrocnemius and soleus α-motoneurons. *Brain Res.* 307, 167–179.

Zajac, F. E., and Faden, J. S. (1985). Relationship among recruitment order, axonal conduction velocity, and muscle-unit properties of type-identified motor units in cat plantaris. *J. Neurophysiol.* 53, 1303–1322.

Zengel, J. E., Reid, S. A., Sypert, G. W., and Munson, J. B. (1985). Membrane electrical properties and prediction of motor-unit type of medial gastrocnemius motoneurons in the cat. *J. Neurophysiol.* 53, 1323–1344.

Zucker, R. (1973). Theoretical implications of the size principle of motoneuron recruitment. *J. Theor. Biol.* 38, 557–596.

10

Neural Mechanisms Underlying the Orderly Recruitment of Motoneurons

C. J. HECKMAN AND MARC D. BINDER

The neural mechanisms underlying orderly motoneuron recruitment have been a preeminent issue in motor systems physiology since the publication of Elwood Henneman's seminal description of the phenomenon nearly 25 years ago (Henneman et al., 1965a). While it is generally agreed that orderly recruitment reflects the presence of a strict hierarchy in the recruitment thresholds of the constituents of a motoneuron pool, the determinants of motoneuron recruitment threshold and the extent to which it can be modified have been the subject of considerable debate (Burke, 1981; Henneman and Mendell, 1981; Enoka and Stuart, 1984; Gustafsson and Pinter, 1985; Chapter 9, this volume).

In this chapter, we present a theoretical framework for considering the contributions of both the intrinsic properties of motoneurons and the organization of their synaptic inputs to the establishment of recruitment thresholds. Further, we champion Henneman's original thesis that the normal sequence of motoneuron recruitment is primarily determined by the intrinsic properties of the motoneurons themselves.

DETERMINANTS OF RECRUITMENT THRESHOLD

The recruitment threshold of a motoneuron is generally thought to depend on both the magnitude of its synaptic inputs and the processing of these inputs by the neuron's intrinsic electrophysiological properties (Burke, 1981; Henneman and Mendell, 1981; Chapter 9, this volume). Therefore, systematic variance in recruitment thresholds within a motoneuron pool must arise from differences in the relative distribution of the synaptic input to motoneurons, differences in the intrinsic properties of motoneurons, or differences in both factors. In theory, this issue could be settled by comparing all of the synaptic inputs and all of the intrinsic electrophysiological properties to actual recruitment thresholds measured during the execution of a variety of movements. However, in practice, the formidable technical difficulties inherent in such experiments make the acquisition of these definitive data unlikely at present or in the immediate future. To date, only the properties of muscle units and motor axons have been quantitatively compared to recruitment order (Henneman, 1957; Henneman et al., 1965a, 1965b; Clamann et al., 1974; Binder et al., 1983; Bawa et al., 1984; Zajac and Faden, 1985; reviewed in Burke, 1981).

In the absence of a complete description of the intrinsic properties, synaptic inputs, and recruitment order of the motoneurons within a pool, we can still make some rather strong inferences regarding the determinants of recruitment order by formulating a simple model. Constructing a model requires that the sources of variance in both the synaptic input distributions and the intrinsic electrophysiological properties of motoneurons be clearly defined, permitting subsequent evaluation of their contributions to systematic variance in the recruitment thresholds within the motoneuron pool. This approach requires a thorough understanding of the theoretical framework that underlies the interrelationships among the various factors that influence recruitment thresholds. To this end, we begin with the simplest possible model system in order to clearly formulate the basic concepts.

The motoneurons in our model are spherical, and the synapses on them act like current sources. Further, all conditions are steady-state (see Burke, 1968a). Thus, for our model motoneurons, there are only three factors that determine their recruitment thresholds: the total amount of synaptic current entering the cells, the total resistance of the cells, and the voltage threshold for action potential initiation. The total synaptic current entering the cell (I_{TOT}) from the activation of a particular source of synaptic input is equal to the number of synapses from that source (N_S) times the average current produced by each of those synapses (I_S). In equation form:

$$I_{TOT} = N_S \times I_S \tag{10-1}$$

In a spherical cell with uniform membrane properties, the total resistance of the cell (i.e., its input resistance, R_N) is equal to the resistance per unit area of membrane (i.e., the specific membrane resistance or membrane resistivity, R_m) divided by the size of the neuron, expressed in terms of total surface area of the soma (A_N). In equation form:

$$R_N = \frac{R_m}{A_N} \tag{10-2}$$

The voltage threshold of a motoneuron depends upon the properties of the spike-generating conductances. The crucial factor for recruitment order is the relative voltage threshold, which is the difference between the absolute voltage threshold and the resting potential. For the discussion that follows, the term "voltage threshold (V_T)" will solely refer to relative voltage threshold. Since there do not appear to be any systematic differences in the level of the resting potential in motoneurons (Kuno, 1959; Pinter et al., 1983), any differences in the relative voltage threshold will actually be due to differences in the absolute voltage threshold.

In the model system presented here, the roles of pre- and postsynaptic factors in the determination of recruitment order can be clearly separated. The inputs (i.e., the presynaptic factors) are completely contained in I_{TOT}. The motoneuron's recruitment threshold, then, depends upon the processing of this input by two intrinsic properties of the motoneurons, R_N and V_T. The essential theoretical link between these three parameters is, of course, Ohm's law.

One way of viewing the processing of the input by the intrinsic properties is to combine the synaptic current and the input resistance to form a synaptic potential. From Ohm's law, it is apparent that the amplitude of the synaptic potential (PSP_{SS}; the subscript emphasizes the restriction to steady-state conditions) is the product of these two parameters:

$$PSP_{SS} = I_{TOT} \times R_N \tag{10-3}$$

If the amplitude of the synaptic potential is large enough to reach the voltage threshold (V_T), the cell is recruited. One important point that emerges from this analysis is that synaptic potentials are clearly a combination of the presynaptic factors contained in I_{TOT} and the postsynaptic factors that determine R_N (cf., Burke, 1968a, 1981). Again, expressed in equation form:

$$PSP_{SS} = (N_S \times I_S) \times \frac{R_m}{A_N}. \tag{10-4}$$

This formula emphasizes that the amplitude of a synaptic potential is clearly not an appropriate measure of the synaptic input because of its dependence on the intrinsic properties of the motoneuron.

Ohm's law also allows the synaptic potential to be expressed as the product of the synaptic current density and the membrane resistivity. In equation form:

$$PSP_{SS} = I_m \times R_m, \tag{10-5}$$

where I_m is the current per unit membrane area and is, therefore, equal to I_{TOT}/A_N. By expanding the definition of I_{TOT} according to Equation (10-1), it is easy to show that the two formulations of Ohm's law (Eqs. 10-3 and 10-5) are simply two different algebraic rearrangements of the same basic set of parameters:

$$PSP_{SS} = I_m \times R_m$$

$$= \frac{I_{TOT}}{A_N} \times R_m \tag{10-5}$$

$$= I_{TOT} \times \frac{R_m}{A_N}$$

$$= I_{TOT} \times R_N \tag{10-3}$$

The two formulas for the synaptic potential (Eqs. 10–4 and 10–5) really only differ in where they place the cell size factor (A_N). Burke and colleagues (Burke, 1968a; Lev-Tov et al., 1983; Burke, 1987) have chosen to combine cell size and total synaptic current in order to emphasize the role of synaptic input in determining recruitment order (Eq. 10–5), pointing out that synaptic current density is an inverse function of cell size. In our formula (Eq. 10–4), the cell size factor has been placed with R_m, so that synaptic potentials are viewed as a product of total current and total resistance (Eq. 10–3). This arrangement has the heuristic advantage inherent in the clear separation of pre- and postsynaptic factors.

An additional simplification of the analysis of the factors that determine recruitment threshold is achieved by combining the intrinsic properties of the motoneurons into a single parameter, the current threshold for spike initiation (usually referred to as rheobase, I_R). Using a rearrangement of Ohm's law, it can be seen that I_R is simply equal to the voltage threshold (V_T) divided by R_N:

$$I_R = \frac{V_T}{R_N} \qquad (10-6)$$

Thus, we can conveniently express recruitment solely in current terms (i.e., a motoneuron will be recruited when $I_{TOT} > I_R$). This formula has the clear advantage of containing only a single presynaptic factor and a single postsynaptic factor.

While our simple model permits a conceptual separation of the synaptic input and a motoneuron's intrinsic properties, it is not clear that this will be true when real motoneurons are considered. A spherical cell is isopotential such that current, resistance and potential are the same everywhere (assuming that the resistivity of cytoplasm is small and uniform throughout the cell). This is clearly not the case in a real motoneuron, where all three parameters (resistance, current, and potential) vary with location in the cell. A major cause of this variance is the extensive and complex dendritic arborizations of motoneurons. As a result of this morphological factor, even if the membrane resistivity were uniform throughout the cell, the input resistance of distal dendrites could be 100 times that of the soma (Barrett and Crill, 1974; Rall, 1977).

Another crucial distinction between our simple spherical model and a real motoneuron lies in the location of synapses. For example, most Ia synapses are located on the dendrites rather than on the soma (Burke et al., 1980; Brown and Fyffe, 1981). The synaptic current entering the cell at one of these dendritic synapses will undergo attenuation by current loss through the cell membrane (and will interact with whatever active dendritic conductances are present) before it reaches other parts of the cell such as the soma (Barrett and Crill, 1974; Rall, 1977). It is also important to note that real synapses are not current sources, as in our model, but instead are conductances. Thus, the current flow into the cell at a particular synapse depends upon the magnitude of the conductance change and the driving force across this conductance. Therefore, the total synaptic current reaching the soma of the cell depends on the number of synapses that are active, the conductance change at each synapse, the driving force at each synapse, and the extent to which synaptic current is attenuated en route from the synapse to the soma. In our recent work (Heckman and Binder, 1985, 1986, 1988; Heckman et al., 1986; Lindsay and Binder, 1987), we have referred to the total current at the soma as the "effective synaptic current (I_N)." One reason we have done so is to emphasize that I_N is not equivalent to the I_{TOT} of the spherical model; the major difference is that I_N subsumes all the factors that influence current transfer to the soma.

In a real motoneuron, Ohm's law must be referred to a specific locus. At the soma, which is the presumed site of intracellular recordings, the amplitude of a synaptic potential is the product of the total synaptic current reaching the soma (I_N) and the total resistance at the soma (R_N). As is the case for the current term (I_N), the total resistance of a motoneuron (R_N) is a much more complex parameter than its counterpart in the simplified spherical model. R_N depends not only on the membrane resistivity and cell surface area, but also on the details of the cell's geometry (Burke and Rudomin, 1977; Rall, 1977). Furthermore, it has been hypothesized that membrane resistivity may not be uniform within the cell (Fleshman et al., 1983; Iansek and Redman, 1973).

Do the complexities of R_N and I_N in a real motoneuron invalidate the recruitment threshold concepts established earlier for the simplistic spherical cell model? We would respond with a qualified "no." R_N in a motoneuron is still determined only by intrinsic cellular properties, so it remains a purely postsynaptic factor, as in the model system. The same is true for V_T, so that I_R still summarizes the purely intrinsic factors that influence recruitment threshold. However, unlike I_{TOT} in the model, I_N is clearly not determined solely by properties of the presynaptic neurons. The driving force at each synapse and the attenuation of current from dendritic synapses are definitely interactions between the pre- and postsynaptic cells (see Burke, 1981). Note that even if the total synaptic current entering a motoneuron could somehow be measured, it would still not provide a purely presynaptic measurement. This is because of the unavoidable influence of the driving force at each synapse, which is highly dependent on the geometry and specific membrane properties of the motoneuron. Thus, it is very difficult, even in theory, to distinguish clearly the synaptic input to a cell from the intrinsic properties of the cell that transform the current input at the synapses to a frequency output at the initial segment. However, this conceptual uncertainty can be circumvented, and the essential concepts of our model system retained, if the transformation of synaptic input to motoneuron output is considered from a functional standpoint, as will be outlined.

The spike-generating conductances that form each motoneuron's output are located in the soma and initial segment of the axon (Fuortes et al., 1957; Burke and Rudomin, 1977). Since only the synaptic current that actually reaches these conductances (by definition, I_N) directly affects the motoneuron's recruitment threshold, I_N is the functionally relevant or effective synaptic current in motoneurons. Thus, in a real motoneuron, recruitment threshold is determined by the processing of the effective synaptic input current, I_N, by the intrinsic cellular properties that determine I_R. If the total I_N received by a motoneuron from all active inputs exceeeds I_R, the cell will be recruited. However, it is important to keep in mind that the recruitment threshold is derived from an interaction between the functional input current and the intrinsic current threshold. For example, if motoneuron A receives precisely one-half as much I_N from the overall synaptic drive as is received by motoneuron B, and if these two motoneurons have the same rheobase, then the recruitment threshold of A is effectively twice that of B.

The foregoing theoretical analysis demonstrates that the hierarchy of recruitment thresholds within a motoneuron pool must be due to systematic variance in I_R, I_N, or both. Before proceeding to an examination of the available experimental data on these two parameters, it should be noted that our theoretical framework advocates a crucial departure from the traditional approach of inferring the contribution of the synaptic input from analyses of the synaptic potentials generated by various input sources. Since the amplitude of a steady-state synaptic potential recorded at the soma of a motoneuron (PSP_{SS}) is the product of I_N and R_N, the amplitudes of synaptic potentials are very strongly dependent on the intrinsic properties of the cell they are recorded in. The effect of R_N on the amplitude of the synaptic potential will be profound because the experimental data clearly show that R_N has a very wide range of systematic variance within the motoneuron pool. Fortunately, direct measurements of I_N can be used to avoid the confounding effect of the wide variance of R_N inherent in analyses of the amplitudes of synaptic potentials, and thus provide a more direct measure of the contribution of a synaptic input to the recruitment threshold of a motoneuron than does the PSP. By measuring I_N, R_N is separated from the input and placed where it properly belongs, with the intrinsic cellular factors that influence recruitment threshold.

Expressing recruitment thresholds in terms of I_N and I_R (instead of PSP amplitude and V_T) has more than just the heuristic advantage of allowing the factors that determine recruitment threshold to be specified in terms of the functionally relevant synaptic input versus the intrinsic cellular properties. It has a practical experimental value as well. I_R has been frequently measured in motoneurons by injection of current into the soma (Fleshman et al., 1981; Lucas and Binder, 1984; Gustafsson and Pinter, 1984b; Powers and Binder, 1985; Zengel et al., 1985). Furthermore, our recent studies have demonstrated that I_N from a particular synaptic input source is, in fact, relatively easy to measure under steady-state conditions (Heckman and Binder, 1985, 1988; Heckman et al., 1986; Lindsay and Binder, 1987). Armed with these data, one can make strong inferences regarding the roles of intrinsic properties and synaptic inputs in generating orderly recruitment.

INTRINSIC CELLULAR PROPERTIES

To evaluate the role of intrinsic cellular properties in determining recruitment order (see also Chapter 9, this volume), we begin with a consideration of rheobase, which, as emphasized in the previous section, is a direct measure of steady-state intrinsic cellular properties that influence the recruitment threshold of the motoneuron. One of the most striking features of the organization of the motoneuron pool is the wide range of rheobase values within it. In the cat medial gastrocnemius (MG) motoneuron pool, for example, there is at least a 10-fold range of rheobase values (Fleshman et al., 1981; Gustafsson and Pinter, 1984b; Lucas and Binder, 1984; Powers and Binder, 1985; Zengel et al., 1985). This wide range of variance must exert a major influence on the recruitment thresholds of the motoneuron pool. In the simplest case in which the synaptic input is uniform (i.e., homogeneously distributed within the pool), one would find a 10-fold range of recruitment thresholds attributable solely to rheobase.

We can extend the analysis of intrinsic properties by factoring rheobase into two components, input resistance (R_N) and voltage threshold (V_T; see Eq 10–6). Numerous studies have shown that R_N, like rheobase, also varies widely within the MG pool, with an approximately 8 to 10-fold range (Kernell, 1966; Burke, 1967, 1968a, 1968b; Burke and Ten Bruggencate, 1971; Fleshman et al., 1981; Lucas and Binder, 1984; Gustafsson and Pinter, 1984a, 1984b; Powers and Binder, 1985; Zengel et al., 1985). Thus, it is not surprising that more than 80% of the variance in rheobase values is attributable to variance in R_N (Gustafsson and Pinter, 1984b). This implies that differences in voltage threshold account for the residual 20% of the variance in rheobase, which has been confirmed by direct measurement (Gustafsson and Pinter, 1984b).

> The differences in the voltage threshold presumably reflect systematic variance in the properties of the active conductances in motoneurons. For example, differences in the degree of accommodation of putative low-threshold and high-threshold motoneurons to slowly rising ramp-injected currents have been reported (Burke and Nelson, 1971). However, Gustafsson and Pinter (1984b) have pointed out that impalement injury may play a significant role in producing the differences in voltage threshold. Thus, the possible role of systematic variance of active conductances in the generation of the hierarchy of recruitment thresholds within a motoneuron pool remains uncertain.

To proceed further, we must evaluate the extent to which each of the factors that determine R_N contributes to its wide range of variance within a motoneuron pool. As noted earlier, R_N is determined by cell surface area, cell geometry, and membrane resistivity. One of these factors, cell size, was the basis of Henneman's "size principle" hypothesis, wherein it was proposed that if all other factors were constant; the variation in cell size would determine recruitment order via its effect on R_N (Henneman et al., 1965a, 1956b). Although it is clear that the size of motoneurons, whether measured in terms of soma diameter or total surface area, has at least a two- to threefold range within the MG motoneuron pool (Kernell and Zwaagstra, 1981; Burke et al., 1982; Ulfhake and Kellerth, 1982), it appears that size alone cannot be responsible for the 8- to 10-fold differences in R_N values within the pool. Thus, systematic differences in membrane resistivity (R_m) and cell geometry must also contribute to the variance in R_N.

A considerable body of data indicates that R_m does vary systematically within the motoneuron pool (Kernell and Zwaagstra, 1981; Burke et al., 1982; Gustafsson and Pinter, 1984a). Even though R_m may not be uniform within each cell (Fleshman et al., 1983; Iansek and Redman, 1973), the average membrane resistivity appears to be greater in motoneurons with high R_N values than in those with low R_N values. The range of the putative differences in "average" membrane resistivity is approximately two- to threefold, which, coupled with the range in cell sizes, could account for the complete range in R_N values. In this light, it is interesting to note that the equivalent electrotonic length (L) of motoneurons, which is determined by the combination of membrane resistivity, cell size, and cell geometry, shows little (Gustafsson and Pinter, 1984a) or no (Barrett and Crill, 1974; Burke and ten Bruggencate, 1971; Lux et al., 1970) systematic variance within the motoneuron pool. Since cell size and membrane resistivity appear to covary (cf. Burke et al., 1982; Gustafsson and Pinter, 1984a), it follows that either the assumptions and cumulative measurement errors associated with the values obtained for R_m and L obscure the correlation between R_N and L or else that the differences in average membrane resistivity and cell size are offset by differences in cell geometry.

Considering all of the uncertainties inherent in the requisite measurements and their underlying assumptions, the contributions of cell size and membrane resistivity in determining R_N and rheobase remains an open question. Cell surface area has been measured directly via reconstruction of horseradish peroxidase (HRP) filled motoneurons (e.g., Burke et al., 1982), but these experiments are exceedingly laborious and hence the available data base is quite restricted. Axonal conduction velocity, while relatively easy to measure, may not be a very precise indicant of cell size (Barrett and Crill, 1974; Kernell and Zwaagstra, 1981; Burke et al., 1982). Total cell capacitance would provide a measure of cell size, but only if specific membrane capacitance is the same in all motoneurons (Gustafsson and Pinter, 1984a, 1985b), as is generally assumed (Rall, 1977), However, at present, total cell capacitance cannot be measured directly and instead must be calculated from equivalent cylinder representations of motoneurons (Gustafsson and Pinter, 1984a, 1984b), which involves a number of additional assumptions (Rall, 1977).

Measurements of membrane resistivity also require full histological reconstructions of motoneuron morphologies. Estimating membrane resistivity from measurements of time constant (Gustafsson and Pinter, 1984a, 1984b) involves two critical assumptions: (1) that specific membrane capacitance is constant, for which, as mentioned earlier, no direct evidence exists (Barrett and Crill, 1974), and (2) that membrane resistivity is uniform throughout each cell, which appears not to be true (Iansek and Redman, 1973; Fleshman et al., 1983). Additionally, measurements of time constants are invariably contaminated by active conductances (Burke and ten Bruggencate, 1971; Gustafsson and Pinter, 1984a, 1984b; Zengel et al., 1985).

> Gustafsson and Pinter (1984a, 1984b, 1985; see also Chapter 9, this volume) have argued that membrane resistivity is considerably more important than cell size in determining R_N and rheobase. The data in support of this conclusion are chiefly their finding that rheobase has a higher degree of correlation with the inverse of the membrane time constant than with conduction velocity. One problem with this interpretation is that the active conductances that influence time constant measurements may also participate directly in the generation of voltage thresholds and, thereby, rheobases. This common source of variance would be expected to increase the rheobase–time constant correlation independently of the

membrane resistivity factor in the time constant. Thus, it is not clear that mean membrane resistivity is better correlated with rheobase than is cell size (as inferred from axonal conduction velocity). This reservation is further supported by the relationships between R_N, time constant, and conduction velocity. As noted earlier, differences in R_N account for fully 80% of the variance in rheobase (Gustafsson and Pinter, 1984b). In the data of Gustafsson and Pinter (1984a), R_N appears to us to be as well correlated with conduction velocity (their Fig. 9) as it is with the time constant (their Fig. 3A). Furthermore, membrane time constant and conduction velocity clearly covary in their data (Fig. 8D; Gustafsson and Pinter, 1984a), which implies the presence of covariance between cell size and membrance resistivity.

At this stage, our tentative conclusion is that membrane resistivity and cell size are equally important in the determination of R_N and rheobase. This conclusion is based on the approximately equal ranges of these two variables (two- to threefold) and by the approximately similar relationships of R_N to conduction velocity and time constant (Gustafsson and Pinter, 1984a).

In view of the considerable degree of covariance among the intrinsic properties of motoneurons, it is possible that an underlying process that is not explicitly measured by any one of these properties in isolation causes the covariance among all of them. For example, the wide range of variance in cell size and in membrane resistivity (and many other motoneuron and muscle unit properties) could be independent consequences of whatever evolutionary, developmental, or trophic processes produce the distinct motor unit types (Burke et al., 1973a; Burke, 1981; Sypert and Munson, 1981). Alternatively, the covariance in these intrinsic parameters might be the consequence of the very phenomenon that they promote, namely, orderly recruitment.

While there is considerable information available about the development and differentiation of mammalian motor units (reviewed in Burke, 1981), little is known regarding the development of recruitment order within a motoneuron pool. We can only speculate that a recruitment order appears as soon as there are adequate synaptic inputs to activate the motoneurons. The initial recruitment order should be governed by the same factors that determine it in the adult motoneuron pool, that is, a hierarchy of recruitment thresholds will emerge from a combination of rheobase and the amount of effective synaptic currents the different cells receive. One need not specify either the initial values of the intrinsic properties of the neonatal motoneurons or the initial pattern of the synaptic inputs. As long as there is some variance in either of these two factors within the pool, a recruitment order will ensue.

The stability of the initial recruitment order will depend on how the intrinsic properties of the motoneurons and the synaptic input patterns change during the neonatal period. However, it seems reasonable to suppose that the initial recruitment sequence itself will strongly influence the developmental expression of the motoneurons' intrinsic properties. Motoneurons with low initial recruitment thresholds will be activated more frequently than motoneurons with higher recruitment thresholds. By analogy to the influence that motoneurons exert on the muscle fibers they innervate, it is possible that as a consequence of their increased usage, motoneurons with low initial recruitment thresholds develop higher membrane resistivities, express higher levels of oxidative enzyme activity, and develop less extensive dendritic trees than the motoneurons with higher initial recruitment thresholds.

One interesting feature of this speculative scenario is that an initial random combination of intrinsic properties and synaptic inputs establishes a rough "rank order" for each motoneuron that is subsequently reinforced and solidified by muscle activation. Another interesting feature is that the covariance between motoneuron intrinsic properties, including size, develop in part as a consequence of their recruitment history. Likewise, the correlations between the properties of the motoneurons and the mechanical properties of their muscle units could be attributed in part to the initial recruitment order and the pattern of usage it imparts. One might also envision that the efficacies and patterns of the different synaptic input systems within the pool are shaped by the pattern of motoneuron utilization that arises from the initial recruitment order.

SYNAPTIC INPUTS

Regardless of the origin of differences in intrinsic motoneuron properties, the wide range of variance in R_N and I_R must exert a profound influence on the recruitment thresholds of motoneurons. What roles, then, do the synaptic inputs play in shaping the output of the pool? Three distinct possibilities can be envisioned for any particular input source. For excitatory inputs, these possibilities can be stated in terms of effective synaptic current (I_N) as follows: (1) If a synaptic input generates the same I_N in all motoneurons, it would serve merely as a uniform drive to the pool without altering the differences in recruitment thresholds already generated by the intrinsic cellular properties; (2) if a synaptic input generates more I_N in low-rheobase, high-input-resistance motoneurons, it would tend to enhance the range of recruitment thresholds conferred on the pool by the motoneurons' intrinsic properties; and (3) if a synaptic input generates more I_N in high-rheobase, low-input-resistance motoneurons, it could mediate the types of deviations from the normal output pattern that have been reported (Burke, 1981).

It should be emphasized at this juncture that uniform I_N within the pool is not produced by an equal density of synapses on all motoneurons. As Kernell (1983) has pointed out, if all other factors that determine I_N are equal, constant synaptic density will result in high-rheobase motoneurons receiving three times as much effective synaptic current as low-rheobase motoneurons. This is because they have a threefold greater surface area and therefore, require three times as many synapses to achieve a constant density. Uniform I_N would only be generated by inputs that have the same number of synapses on each motoneuron, again assuming that all other factors (e.g., location, efficacy) are equal.

Recently, we developed a technique to measure I_N under steady-state conditions (Heckman and Binder, 1985, 1986, 1988). We focused first on the input from homonymous Ia afferents onto MG motoneurons, since this is the best studied of all synaptic inputs to the motoneuron pool. Previously, it had been shown that the amplitudes of transient Ia excitatory postsynaptic potentials

(EPSPs) covaried with R_N values (Burke, 1968a; Luscher et al., 1983). This finding has been interpreted as indicating that the number of Ia synapses is about the same on all motoneurons and that the differences in transient Ia EPSP amplitude are simply due to differences in the input resistances of the motoneurons (Burke, 1968a; Stein and Bertoldi, 1981). We thus expected to find that under steady-state conditions, I_N from Ia afferents (Ia I_N) would be approximately the same in all MG motoneurons. Instead, the results showed that Ia I_N is systematically related to R_N. In fact, high-R_N motoneurons tended to receive about twice as much Ia I_N as low-R_N motoneurons (Fig. 10–1A). Therefore, the Ia steady-state input is an example of the second pattern of synaptic input (see earlier), one that enhances the hierarchy of recruitment thresholds generated by the motoneurons' intrinsic properties (see Chapter 17, this volume). This unexpected finding illustrates the difficulties inherent in indirect evaluation of I_N from measurements of synaptic potentials. In this case, even though the steady-state Ia EPSP directly covaries with R_N (Fig. 10–1B), Ia I_N is not uniformly distributed to the motoneurons of the MG pool.

Our results for homonymous Ia afferent input prompted us to examine the distributions of other synaptic input systems within a motoneuron pool. To study the reciprocal Ia inhibitory pathway, we generated steady-state Ia inhibitory postsynaptic potentials (IPSPs) in cat tibialis anterior and extensor digitorum longus motoneurons by activating Ia afferents in the antagonist triceps surae muscles (Heckman et al., 1986). In our initial motoneuron sample, we found that the amplitudes of the steady-state Ia IPSPs covary with motoneuron R_N (Fig. 10–2B), as had been reported previously for transient Ia IPSPs (Burke et al., 1976; Dum and Kennedy, 1980). However, although the range and mean values for the Ia inhibitory effective synaptic currents (-Ia I_N) were similar to those for the Ia excitatory currents (Ia I_N), they did not vary systematically with motoneuron R_N or rheobase (Fig. 10–2A).

We obtained a similar result from our preliminary analysis of the distribution of synaptic input within a motoneuron pool generated by Renshaw interneurons. In these experiments, steady-state, recurrent IPSPs were produced in MG motoneurons by stimulating the synergist lateral gastrocnemius and soleus muscle nerves with the ipsilateral dorsal roots cut. We found that the amplitudes of the steady-state, recurrent IPSPs covary with motoneuron R_N (Lindsay and Binder, unpublished data; Fig. 10–3B), as had been reported previously for transient recurrent IPSPs (Friedman et al., 1981). However, as was the case for Ia inhibition, the effective synaptic currents from the Renshaw cells (RC I_N) were uniformly distributed within the motoneuron pool, displaying no systematic variance with motoneuron parameters (Fig. 10–3A). These results again illustrate the problem inherent in making inferences about the magnitude of synaptic inputs based on synaptic potential amplitudes: If one were to measure only the amplitudes of the recurrent IPSPs, one might erroneously infer that MG motoneurons with high R_N values receive more input from Renshaw cells that those with low R_N values.

Although the distributions of I_N from other synaptic inputs have not yet been studied, it is likely that many will be nonuniform, particularly those that display striking qualitative differences in the types of synaptic potentials they

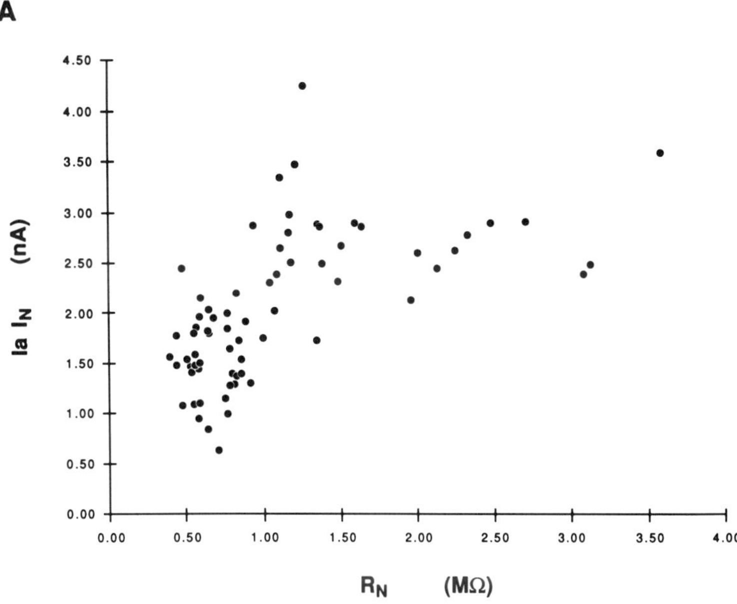

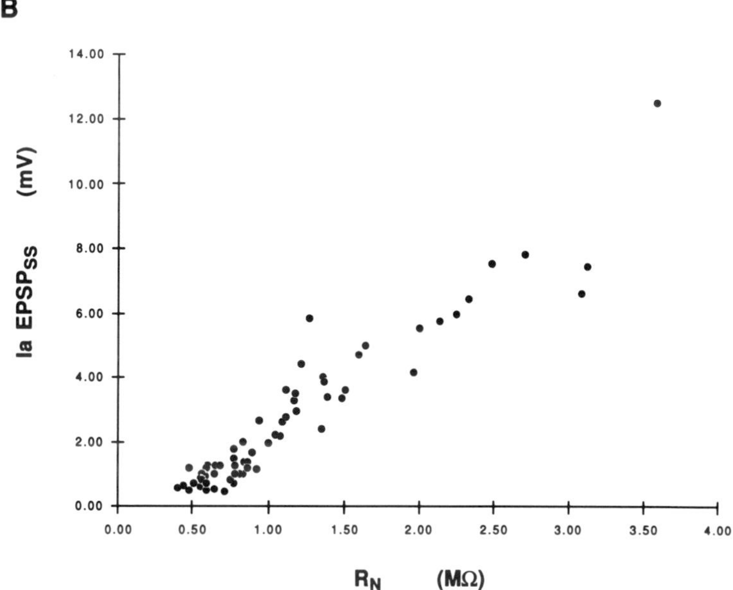

Fig. 10–1. The distribution of synaptic input from homonymous Ia afferents in the cat medial gastrocnemius motoneuron pool. Steady-state Ia EPSPs were generated by subjecting the triceps surae muscles (lateral gastrocnemius and soleus nerves cut) to longitudinal vibration (150 μm peak-to-peak) at 200 Hz. In (A), the effective synaptic currents (Ia I_N), measured by voltage clamp, are plotted versus motoneuron input resistance (R_N). Curvilinear regression, assuming a power function: $r = 0.64$, $n = 70$, Ia $I_N = 1.96 \times R_N^{0.45}$, $p < 0.001$. In (B), the amplitudes of the steady-state synaptic potentials (Ia $EPSP_{ss}$) are plotted versus R_N (linear regression: $r = 0.95$, $p < 0.001$). (Data from Heckman and Binder, 1988.)

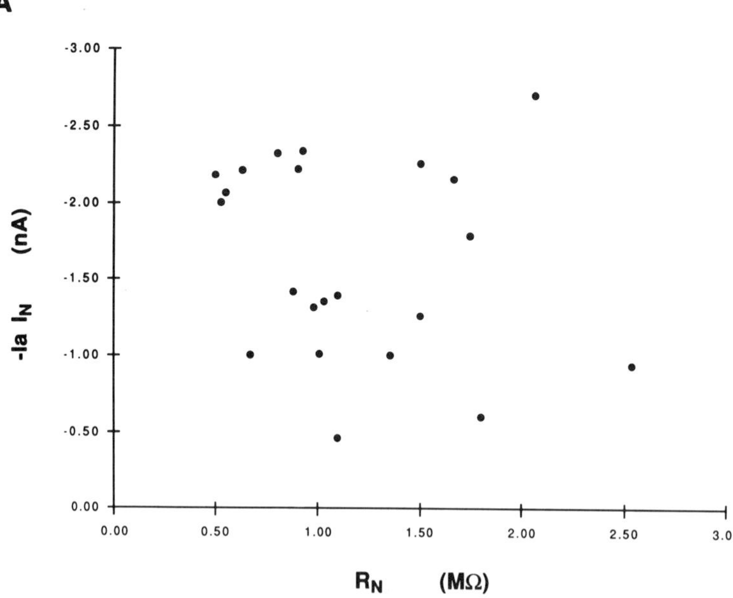

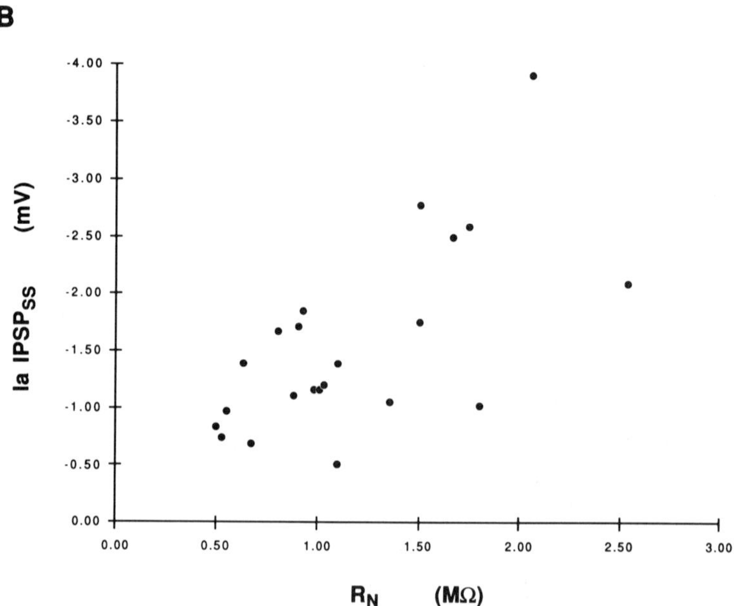

Fig. 10–2. The distribution of synaptic input to tibialis anterior and extensor digitorum longus motoneurons from Ia inhibitory interneurons. The Ia inhibitory interneurons were activated by subjecting the triceps surae muscles (lateral gastrocnemius and soleus nerves cut) to longitudinal vibration (150 μ peak-to-peak) at 200 Hz. In (A), the effective synaptic currents ($-$Ia I_N), measured by voltage clamp, are plotted versus motoneuron input resistance (R_N). Notice that while $-$Ia I_N appears to be uniformly distributed to the motoneurons, as shown in (B), the amplitude of the steady-state Ia IPSPs is correlated with R_n (linear regression: $r = 0.66$, $n = 22$, $p < 0.05$). (Data from Heckman et al., 1986.)

194

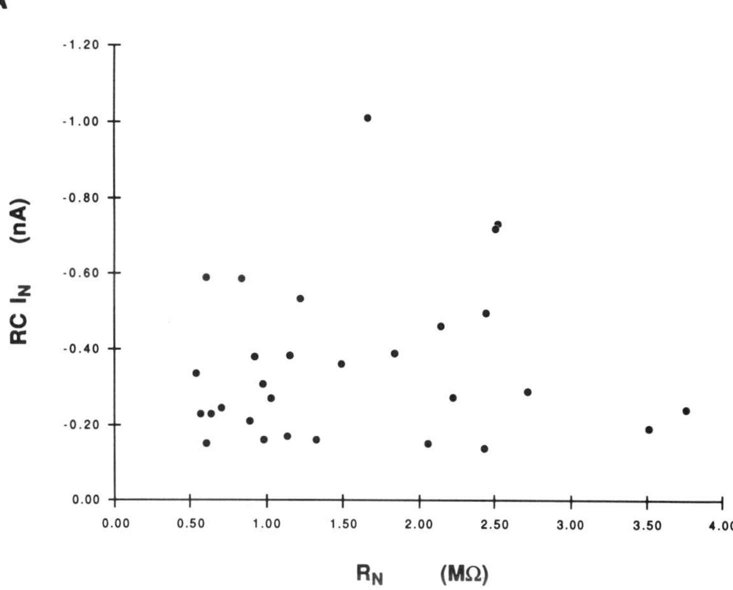

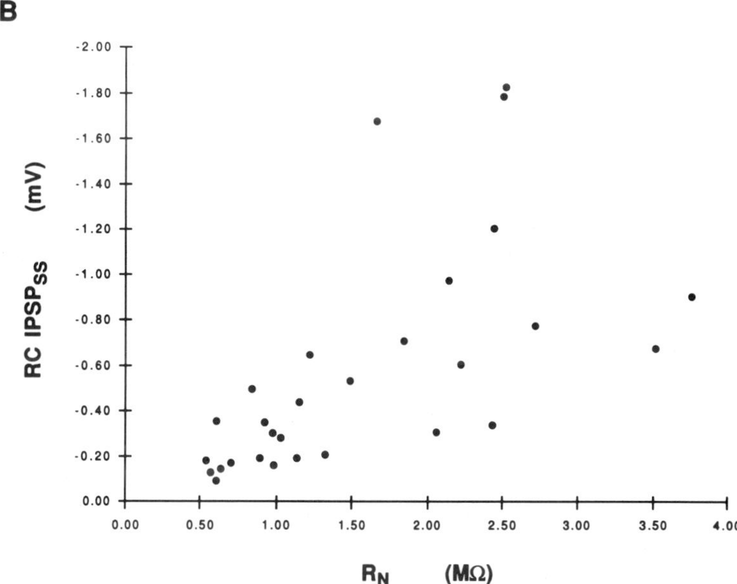

Fig. 10–3. The distribution of synaptic input from Renshaw cells within the cat medial gastrocnemius motoneuron pool. The Renshaw input was activated by stimulating the lateral gastrocnemius and soleus muscle nerves at 100 Hz with the ipsilateral dorsal roots cut. The relationship between the effective synaptic currents (RCI_N) generated by the Renshaw cells versus motoneuron input resistance (R_N) is plotted in (A). As was the case for Ia inhibitory input (cf. Fig. 10–2), the synaptic input from the Renshaw cells does not appear to vary systematically in the MG motoneuron pool, although the amplitudes of the steady-state recurrent IPSPs are correlated with R_N, as shown in (B) (linear regression: $r = 0.61$; $n = 29$; $p < 0.01$). (From Lindsay and Binder, unpublished data.)

evoke in different motoneurons within the same pool (Burke, et al., 1970, 1976; Powers and Binder, 1985). These inputs, of course, are more difficult to evaluate quantitatively (see Powers and Binder, 1985) and may not prove amenable to steady-state analysis.

MECHANISMS OF ORDERLY RECRUITMENT

How can orderly recruitment persist under the concurrent influences of non-uniform synaptic inputs from a number of different sources? It seems reasonable to speculate that the 8- to 10-fold range in rheobase values that is largely attributable to differences in R_N strongly biases the output of the pool toward the normal pattern of recruitment documented in numerous studies (reviewed in Burke, 1981; Henneman and Mendell, 1981). One might even define "normal recruitment" as that recruitment pattern produced by differences in R_N. Although there is no direct evidence supporting this hypothesis, R_N has been compared to the firing patterns of cat motoneurons recruited by stretch reflex activation (Burke, 1968b). Motoneurons that fired tonically to the imposed muscle stretch tended to have higher R_N values and lower conduction velocities and to generate smaller muscle unit forces than those of motoneurons that fired in phasic bursts. Since cat motor units with low conduction velocities and low force outputs tend to have low recruitment thresholds (Binder et al., 1983; Bawa et al., 1984; Zajac and Faden, 1985), one can infer from the Burke study (1968b) that the tonically firing motoneurons with high R_N values had lower recruitment thresholds than the motoneurons with lower R_N values that fired only in bursts. In further support of this hypothesis are other studies of cat motoneurons demonstrating that R_N is inversely correlated with both conduction velocity (Kernell, 1966; Burke, 1967, 1968b; Gustafsson and Pinter, 1984a) and muscle unit force (Fleshman et al., 1981).

We propose that in most instances the normal recruitment sequence is manifested even when some of the active input systems do not support it. This view is based on a consideration of the magnitude of the nonuniformity in synaptic input that would be required to generate a major alteration in the recruitment order based on the cells' intrinsic properties. For example, the extreme case of reversed recruitment, where all the high-force type FF units are recruited before any low-force type S units, would require that the net effective synaptic current from all active inputs be more than 10 times larger in high-I_R motoneurons than in low-I_R ones. Thus, a completely inverse recruitment pattern probably occurs only rarely, if ever. Nonetheless, clear changes in recruitment order, involving neurons with similar recruitment thresholds, should be relatively easy to produce. It has, in fact, been shown that activation of some inputs, such as the cutaneous afferents in the sural nerve, can produce unequivocal alterations in recruitment order (Kanda et al., 1977).

Although the functional advantages of the normal recruitment sequence, including smooth force gradation and optimal fatigue resistance, have long been recognized (Henneman and Olson, 1965), there are probably instances in which a motor task would be better served by subtly changing the sequence. For example, Burke (1981) has suggested that the distribution of synaptic input from the sural nerve (i.e., predominant inhibition of low-threshold motoneurons and predominant excitation of high-threshold motoneurons) might play a role in increasing the "gain" of the whole motoneuron pool input-output function by increasing the participation of motor units with high-force outputs in certain motor tasks.

What, then, is the function of synaptic input systems that enhance the normal recruitment order? Our analysis of homonymous Ia input (Heckman and Binder, 1988) suggests that it expands the range of recruitment thresholds generated by intrinsic cellular properties; thus, a tonic background of homonymous Ia input could potentially compensate for the heterogeneous input distributions from other sources. Perhaps a major role of Ia input is the preservation of the normal orderly recruitment under a wide variety of input combinations (Harrison and Taylor, 1981; Stein and Bertoldi, 1981; see Clamann et al., 1983).

In addition, Ia input appears to favor strongly recruitment of the low-threshold type S units (Heckman and Binder, 1988). Two advantages might stem from this. First, the usage of fatigue-resistant units would be maximized; second, the gain of the motoneuron pool input-output function would be reduced by emphasizing the activation of low-force type S units while limiting, to some extent, the activation of high-force type FF units. This provides a mechanism for a gain control that is precisely the opposite of that possibly offered by sural input (Burke, 1981). A lower input-output gain should be advantageous in movements requiring a high degree of precision (Hultborn et al., 1979). Since the contraction speed of type S units is slow, an obvious corollary of this idea is that Ia input may be important in slow movements. Together these ideas suggested to us the hypothesis that the Ia input is particularly important in the control of vernier movements (Binder and Stuart, 1980), i.e., precisely controlled movements executed at low force levels and slow speeds.

The foregoing discussion also reveals some potential liabilities of the Ia input. During movements requiring high speed or large forces, overemphasis on type S unit activation is, at best, superfluous. Furthermore, the Ia input would be expected to accentuate greatly the "overstimulation problem" for type S units when the input becomes large enough to recruit type FF units (Kernell, 1983). One way to avoid these problems is to alter the composition of the synaptic input as the overall level of drive to the pool increases. The Ia input and other inputs with similar distributions could be dominant at low levels of recruitment, whereas other synaptic inputs could become increasingly prominent when higher forces and speeds are required. Type FR and especially type FF units would be recruited with the addition of synaptic inputs distributed like those from the sural nerve, while simultaneously limiting further increases in the Ia type input pattern. This hypothesis stands in contrast to the ideas of Kernell (1983) and Harrison and Taylor (1981), who have assumed that the combination of synaptic inputs remains constant as the overall level of drive to the pool is increased.

DETERMINANTS OF FREQUENCY MODULATION

As Kernell (1976, 1983; Chapter 2, this volume) has emphasized, frequency modulation of motoneuron discharge can be reduced to the same terms used to quantify recruitment threshold: the intrinsic properties of the motoneurons and the distribution of synaptic inputs. The work of Granit, Kernell, and colleagues (Granit et al., 1963a, 1963b; Kernell, 1965a, 1965b, 1965c) demonstrated that, under steady-state conditions, the properties of the synaptic spike-generating conductances are such that the transformation of injected current into a spike frequency output is remarkably simple. This current-to-frequency "gain" function consists of two linear ranges: a relatively low-slope, primary range starting at threshold and a higher-slope, secondary range manifested at higher current levels (Kernell, 1965a, 1965b, 1965c).

The slopes of the primary range vary from 1 to 2 Hz per nA of injected current, but this variance appears to be random, since it is not systematically related to the contraction times of muscle units (Kernell, 1979). In contrast, the limits of the primary range definitely vary systematically within the MG pool. The current at which the cell begins to fire at a steady frequency (the rhythmic firing threshold) is closely related to the single spike threshold (i.e., rheobase) and also has an approximately 10-fold range in the MG pool (Kernell and Monster, 1981). The frequencies at these rhythmic firing thresholds are correlated with both the duration of the afterhyperpolarization and the contraction time of the muscle unit, factors thought to be important for the appropriate matching of motoneuron and muscle unit properties (Kernell, 1965c, 1979).

It has been demonstrated that currents generated by synaptic inputs sum linearly with injected currents over the primary range (Granit et al., 1966; Kernell, 1969; Schwindt and Calvin, 1973a, 1973b), indicating that injected and synaptic currents appear to be equivalent with respect to their actions on the spike-generating conductances in the soma and initial segment of a motoneuron. This equivalence means that the descriptions obtained with injected current are valid representatives of how the motoneurons transform synaptic inputs into frequency outputs. Obviously, this information on the input–output transformations of motoneurons requires that the synaptic inputs be expressed in terms of I_N instead of the standard measurement, the synaptic potential. This again emphasizes the functional relevance of I_N. While synaptic potentials can be used for assessment of recruitment thresholds, once threshold is attained, it is necessary to deal with the effective synaptic current-to-frequency transforms because the spike-generating conductances obscure the underlying synaptic potentials.

The effect of nonuniform distributions of synaptic input within the motoneuron pool on frequency modulation can be clearly understood with the example of the Ia input distribution discussed in the previous section. The fact that low-R_N motoneurons receive about half as much Ia I_N as high-R_N motoneurons means that the recruitment threshold of low-R_N cells is increased by a factor of 2 in comparison to the recruitment thresholds of high R_N cells. Obviously, the rhythmic firing threshold is similarly affected. Exactly the same principle applies to the slope between I_N and frequency. The frequency-current gain (f–I) of a motoneuron is determined by the slope of its intrinsic I_N to frequency function and the relative proportion of the I_N the cell receives (cf. Kernell, 1976, 1983). Since the low-R_N motoneurons receive 50% less Ia I_N, the slopes of their I_N to frequency transformations are halved relative to those of high-R_N cells. This means the Ia input tends to decrease dramatically the effective frequency gains of high-R_N motoneurons, thereby providing an additional mechanism through which the Ia input will tend to reduce the overall gain of the pool.

CONCLUSIONS

Hypotheses like the ones discussed in this chapter about the detailed functional roles of different synaptic inputs on recruitment order and frequency modulation are very difficult to address with the presently available experimental techniques and limited data on the effective synaptic currents (I_N). It seems likely that a synthetic approach that combines additional experimental data with computer modeling will be necessary to achieve further progress in our understanding of the recruitment and frequency modulation of the motoneuron pool. We are presently developing a computer model of the motoneuron pool input–output function that uses effective synaptic currents as inputs. A particular advantage of measurements of effective synaptic currents over synaptic potentials for a modeling approach is that currents can be summated and applied to the intrinsic cellular properties that determine each neuron's threshold and frequency output. As discussed earlier, these intrinsic properties have been thoroughly studied under steady-state conditions. As more information becomes available about the quantitative distribution of I_N from various input sources, it should eventually become possible to model the detailed behavior of the motoneuron pool when subjected to realistic combinations of synaptic inputs.

There are still many uncertainties regarding the neural mechanisms of orderly recruitment. Our viewpoint, which is admittedly highly speculative due to a lack of direct experimental evidence, can be summarized in the following way. The intrinsic properties of motoneurons such as R_N strongly predispose the motoneuron pool to orderly recruitment. One can, in fact, define the normal pattern of orderly recruitment as that sequence determined solely by these intrinsic properties. Synaptic inputs have heterogeneous distribution patterns within the pool and, thus, may modify this normal pattern to a significant degree. The modified recruitment patterns have clear functional advantages. We hypothesize that the composition of the synaptic drive varies according to the activation level of the pool in order to ensure appropriate functional usage of the motor unit population. The Ia input pattern (I_N decreases from low-threshold to high-threshold motoneurons) appears to be desirable in vernier movements at low levels of activation to the pool, whereas the sural nerve input pattern appears to be optimal for control of high-speed, higher-force movements. Nonetheless, it needs to be emphasized that these modifications of the normal orderly recruitment pattern are usually rather modest and that, as Henneman originally proposed (Henneman et al., 1965, Henneman and Olson, 1965), the design of the segmental motor system is centered on the orderly recruitment of motoneurons.

Acknowledgments

We wish to thank Drs. Martin J. Pinter, Randall K. Powers, Lorne M. Mendell and Amy D. Lindsay for their comments on the manuscript. The experimental work on effective synaptic currents was supported by NIH grants NS 22417 and NS 26840.

REFERENCES

Barrett, J. N., and Crill, W. E. (1974). Influence of dendritic location and membrane properties on the effectiveness of synapses in cat motoneurons. *J. Physiol.* 239, 325–345.

Bawa, P., Binder, M. D., Ruenzel, P., and Henneman, E. (1984). Recruitment order of motoneurons in stretch reflexes is highly correlated with their axonal conduction velocity. *J. Neurophysiol.* 52, 410–420.

Binder, M. D., Bawa, P., Ruenzel, P., and Henneman, E. (1983). Does orderly recruitment of motoneurons depend on the existence of different types of motor units? *Neurosci. Lett.* 136, 55–58.

Binder, M. D., and Stuart, D. G. (1980). Motor unit–muscle receptors interactions: Design features of the neuromuscular control system. In *Spinal and Supraspinal Mechanisms of Voluntary Motor Control and Locomotion. Progress in Neurophysiology*, Vol. 8 (ed. J. E. Desmedt). Karger, Basel, pp. 72–98.

Brown, A. G., and Fyffe, R. E. (1981). Direct observations on the contacts made between Ia afferent fibres and alpha motoneurons in the cat's lumbosacral spinal cord. *J. Physiol.* 313, 121–140.

Burke, R. E. (1967). Motor unit types of cat triceps surae muscle. *J. Physiol.* 193, 141–160.

Burke, R. E. (1968a). Group Ia synaptic input to fast and slow twitch motor units of cat triceps surae. *J. Physiol.* 196, 605–630.

Burke, R. E. (1968b). Firing patterns of gastrocnemius motor units in the decerebrate cat. *J. Physiol.* 196, 631–654.

Burke, R. E. (1981). Motor units: Anatomy, physiology, and functional organization. In *Handbook of Physiology, The Nervous System, Motor Control*, (ed. V. B. Brook). American Physiological Society, Vol. II, Sect. 1, Part 1, Bethesda, Md, pp. 345–422.

Burke, R. E. (1987). Synaptic efficacy and the control of neuronal input-output relations. *Trends Neurosci.* 10, 42–45.

Burke, R. E., Dum, R. P., Fleshman, J. W., Glenn, L. L., Lev-Tov, A., O'Donovon, M. J., and Pinter, M. J. (1982). An HRP study of the relation between cell size and motor unit type in cat ankle extensor motoneurons. *J. Comp. Neurol.* 209, 17–28.

Burke, R. E., Jankowska, E., and Ten Bruggencate, G. (1970). A comparison of peripheral and rubrospinal input to slow and fast twitch motor units of triceps surae. *J. Physiol.* 1207, 709–732.

Burke, R. E., Levine, D. N., Tsairis, P., and Zajac, F. E. (1973a). Physiological types and histochemical profiles in motor units of the cat gastrocnemius. *J. Physiol.* 234, 723–748.

Burke, R. E., and Nelson, P. G. (1971). Accommodation to current ramps in motoneurons of fast and slow twitch motor units. *Int. J. Neurosci.* 1, 347–356.

Burke, R. E., Pinter, M. J., Lev-Tov, A., and O'Donovon, M. J. (1980). Anatomy of monosynaptic contacts from group Ia afferents to defined types of extensor alpha-motoneurons in the cat. *Soc. Neurosci. Abstr.* 6, 713.

Burke, R. E., and Rudomin, P. (1977). Spinal neurons and synapses. In *Handbook of Physiology, The Nervous System, Cellular Biology of Neurons*, Vol. I, Sect. 1, Part 2 (ed. E. Kandel). American Physiological Society, Bethesda, Md., pp. 877–994.

Burke, R. E., Rymer, W. Z., and Walsh, J. V., Jr. (1973b). Functional specialization in the motor unit population of cat medial gastrocnemius muscle. In *Control of Posture and Locomotion* (ed. R. B. Stein, K. G. Pearson, R. S. Smith, and J. B. Redford). Plenum, New York, pp. 29–44.

Burke, R. E., Rymer, W. Z., and Walsh, J. V., Jr. (1976). Relative strength of synaptic input from short-latency pathways to motor units of defined type in cat medial gastrocnemius. *J. Neurophysiol.* 39, 447–458.

Burke, R. E., and Ten Bruggencate, G. (1971). Electrotonic characteristics of alpha motoneurones of varying size. *J. Physiol.* 212, 1–20.

Clamann, H. P., Gillies, J. D., Skinner, R. D., and Henneman, E. (1974). Quantitative measures of output of a motoneuron pool during monosynaptic reflexes. *J. Neurophysiol.* 37, 1328–1337.

Clamann, H. P., Ngai, A. C., Kukulka, C. G., and Goldberg, S. J. (1983). Motor pool organization in monosynaptic reflexes: Responses in three different muscles. *J. Neurophysiol.* 50, 725–742.

Dum, R. P., and Kennedy, T. T. (1980). Synaptic organization of defined motor unit types in cat tibialis anterior. *J. Neurophysiol.* 43, 1631–1644.

Enoka, R. M., and Stuart, D. G. (1984). Henneman's "size principle": Current issues. *Trends Neurosci.* 7, 226–228.

Fleshman, J. W., Munson, J. B., Sypert, G. W., and Friedman, W. A. (1981). Rheobase, input resistance, and motor-unit type in medial gastrocnemius motoneurons in the cat. *J. Neurophysiol.* 46, 1326–1338.

Fleshman, J. W., Segev, I., Cullheim, S., and Burke, R. E., (1983). Matching electrophysiological with morphological measurements in cat spinal alpha-motoneurons. *Soc. Neurosci. Abstr.* 3, 341.

Friedman, W. A., Sypert, G. W., Munson, J. B., and Fleshman, J. W. (1981). Recurrent inhibition in type-identified motoneurons. *J. Neurophysiol.* 46, 1349–1359.

Fuortes, M. G., Frank, K., and Becker, M. C. (1957). Steps in the production of motoneuron spikes. *J. Gen. Physiol.* 40, 735–752.

Granit, R., Kernell, D., and Lamarre, Y. (1966). Algebraical summation in synaptic activation of motoneurons firing within the "primary range" to injected currents. *J. Physiol.* 187, 379–399.

Granit, R., Kernell, D., and Shortess, G. K. (1963a). Quantitative aspects of repetitive firing of mammalian motoneurones caused by injected currents. *J. Physiol.* 169, 743–754.

Granit, R., Kernell, D., and Shortess, G. K. (1963b). The behavior of mammalian motoneurones during long-lasting, antidromic and trans-membrane stimulation. *J. Physiol.* 168, 911–931.

Gustafsson, B., and Pinter, M. J. (1984a). Relations among passive electrical properties of lumbar alpha-motoneurones of the cat. *J. Physiol.* 356, 401–431.

Gustafsson, B., and Pinter, M. J. (1984b). An investigation of threshold properties among cat spinal alpha-motoneurons. *J. Physiol.* 357, 453–483.

Gustafsson, B., and Pinter, M. J. (1985). On factors determining orderly recruitment of motor units: a role for intrinsic membrane properties. *Trends Neurosci.* 8, 431–433.

Harrison, P. J., and Taylor, A. (1981). Individual excitatory post-synaptic potentials due to muscle spindle Ia afferents in cat triceps surae motoneurones. *J. Physiol.* 312, 455–470.

Heckman, C. J., and Binder, M. D. (1985). Analysis of steady-state synaptic currents generated in cat motoneurons by homonymous Ia afferents. *Soc. Neurosci. Abstr.* 11, 402.

Heckman, C. J., and Binder, M. D. (1986). Analysis of steady-state Ia synaptic potentials and synaptic currents in cat motoneurons. *Proc. Int. Union Physiol. Sci.* 16, 512.

Heckman, C. J., and Binder, M. D. (1988). Analysis of steady-state effective synaptic currents generated by homonymous Ia afferent fibers in motoneurons of the cat. *J. Neurophysiol.*, 60, 1946–1966.

Heckman, C. J., Lindsay, A. D., and Binder, M. D. (1986). Analysis of steady-state inhibitory synaptic potentials and currents generated in cat motoneurons by activating Ia afferent fibers. *Soc. Neurosci. Abstr.* 12, 247.

Henneman, E. (1957). Relation between size of neurons and their susceptibility to discharge. *Science* 126, 1345–1346.

Henneman, E., and Mendell, L. M. (1981). Functional organization of motoneuron pool and its inputs. In *Handbook of Physiology, The Nervous System, Motor Control,*Vol. II, Sect. 1, Part 1 (ed. V. B. Brooks). American Physiological Society, Bethesda, Md., pp. 423–507.

Henneman, E., and Olson, C. B. (1965). Relations between structure and function in the design of skeletal muscle. *J. Neurophysiol.* 28, 581–598.

Henneman, E., Somjen, G., and Carpenter, D. O. (1965a). Functional significance of cell size in spinal motoneurons. *J. Neurophysiol.* 28, 560–580.

Henneman, E., Somjen, G., and Carpenter, D. O. (1965b). Excitability and inhibitibility of motoneurons of different sizes. *J. Neurophysiol.* 28, 599–620.

Hultborn, H., Lindstrom, S., and Wigstrom, H. (1979). On the function of recurrent inhibition in the spinal cord. *Exp. Brain Res.* 37, 399–403.

Iansek, R., and Redman, S. J. (1973). The amplitude, time course and charge of unitary excitatory post-synaptic potentials evoked in spinal motoneurone dendrites. *J. Physiol.* 234, 665–688.

Kanda, K., Burke, R. E., and Walmsley, B. (1977). Differential control of fast and slow twitch motor units in the decerebrate cat. *Exp. Brain Res.* 29, 57–74.

Kernell, D. (1965a). The adaptation and relation between discharge frequency and current strength of cat lumbosacral motoneurones stimulated by long-lasting injected currents. *Acta Physiol. Scand.* 65, 65–73.

Kernell, D. (1965b), High-frequency repetitive firing of cat lumbosacral motoneurones stimulated by long-lasting injected currents. *Acta Physiol. Scand.* 65, 74–86.

Kernell, D. (1965c). The limits of firing frequency in cat lumbosacral motoneurones possessing different time course of afterhyperpolarization. *Acta. Physiol. Scand.* 65, 87–100.

Kernell, D. (1966). Input resistance, electrical excitability, and size of ventral horn cells in cat spinal cord. *Science* 152, 1637–1640.

Kernell, D. (1969). Synaptic conductance changes and the repetitive impulse discharge of spinal motoneurones. *Brain Res.* 15, 291–294.

Kernell, D. (1976). Recruitment, rate modulation and the tonic stretch reflex. *Prog. Brain Res.* 44, 257–265.

Kernell, D. (1979).Rhythmic properties of motoneurones innervating muscle fibers of different speed in m. gastrocnemius medialis of the cat. *Brain Res.* 160, 159–162.

Kernell, D. (1983). Functional properties of spinal motoneurons and gradation of muscle force. In *Motor Control Mechanisms in Health and Disease* (ed. J. E. Desmedt). Raven Press, New York, pp. 213–226.

Kernell, D., and Monster, A. W. (1981). Threshold current for repetitive impulse firing in motoneurones innervating muscle fibres of different fatigue sensitivity in the cat. *Brain Res.* 229, 193–196.

Kernell, D., and Zwaagstra, B. (1981). Input conductance, axonal conduction velocity and cell size among hindlimb motoneurones of the cat. *Brain Res.* 204, 311–326.

Kuno, M. (1959). Excitability following antidromic activation in spinal motoneurons supplying red muscles. *J. Physiol.* 149, 374–393.

Lev-Tov, A., Miller, J. P., Burke, R. E., and Rall, W. (1983). Factors that control the amplitude of EPSPs in dendritic neurons. *J. Neurophysiol.* 50, 399–412.

Lindsay, A. D., and Binder, M. D. (1987). Analysis of steady-state recurrent IPSPs and their underlying effective synaptic currents in cat motoneurons. *Soc. Neurosci. Abstr.* 13, 1695, 1987.

Lucas, S. M., and Binder, M. D. (1984). Topographic factors in distribution of homonymous group Ia-afferent input to cat medial gastrocnemius motoneurons. *J. Neurophysiol.* 51, 50–63.

Luscher, J.- R., Ruenzel, P., and Henneman, E. (1983). Composite EPSPs in motoneurons of different sizes before and during PTP: implications for transmission failure and its relief in Ia projections. *J. Neurophysiol.* 49, 269–289.

Lux, H. D., Schubert, P., and Kreutzberg, G. W. (1970). Direct matching of morphological and electrophysiological data in cat spinal motoneurons. In *Excitatory Synaptic Mechanisms* (ed. P. Anderson and J. K. S. Jansen). Universitetsforlaget, Oslo, pp. 189–198.

Pinter, M. J., Curtis, R. L., and Hosko, M. J. (1983). Voltage threshold and excitability among variously sized cat hindlimb motoneurons. *J. Neurophysiol.* 50, 644–657.

Powers, R. K., and Binder, M. D. (1985). Distribution of oligosynaptic input to the cat medial gastrocnemius motoneuron pool. *J. Neurophysiol.* 53, 497–517.

Rall, W. (1977). Core conductor theory and cable properties of neurons. In *Handbook of Physiology, The Nervous System, Cellular Biology of Neurons* Vol. 1, Sect. 1, Part 1 (ed. by E. Kandel). American Physiological Society, Bethesda, Md., pp. 39–97.

Schwindt, P. C., and Calvin, W. H. (1973a). Equivalence of synaptic and injected current in determining the membrane potential trajectory during rhythmic firing. *Brain Res.* 59, 389–394.

Schwindt, P. C., and Calvin, W. H. (1973b). The nature of the conductances underlying rhythmic firing in cat spinal motoneurons. *J. Neurophysiol.* 36, 955–973.

Smith, T. G., Wuerker, R. B., and Frank, K. (1967). Membrane impedance changes during synaptic transmission in cat spinal motoneurons. *J. Neurophysiol.* 30, 1072–1096.

Stein, R. B., and Bertoldi, R. (1981). The size principle: A synthesis of neurophysiological data. In *Motor Unit Types, Recruitment and Plasticity in Health and*

Disease, Progress in Clinical Neurophysiology, (ed. J. E. Desmedt). Karger, Basel, pp. 85–96.

Sypert, G. W., and Munson, J. B. (1981). Basis of segmental motor control: motoneuron size or motor unit type? *Neurosurgery* 8, 608–621.

Ulfhake, B., and Kellerth, J.- O. (1983). A quantitative morphological study of HRP-labelled cat alpha-motoneurones supplying different hindlimb muscles. *Brain Res.* 264, 1–19.

Zajac, F. E., and Faden, J. S. (1985). Relationship among recruitment order, axonal conduction velocity, and muscle-unit properties of type-identified motor units in cat plantaris muscle. *J. Neurophysiol.* 53, 1303–1322.

Zengel, J. E., Reid, S. A., Sypert, G. W., and Munson, J. B. (1985). Membrane electrical properties and prediction of motor-unit type of medial gastrocnemius motoneurons in the cat. *J. Neurophysiol.* 53, 1323–1344.

IV
PROPERTIES OF MOTOR UNITS AND MUSCLE FIBERS

11

Motor Unit Types: Some History and Unsettled Issues

R. E. BURKE

A LITTLE HISTORY

The phenomenon of orderly motor unit recruitment and its relation to mechanical muscle properties was described by Derek Denny-Brown (1929) in pioneering animal experiments done while he was working with Sir Charles Sherrington and later amplified in electromyographic studies of voluntary contraction in normal human subjects and in patients with neuromuscular diseases (Denny-Brown and Pennybacker, 1938; Denny-Brown, 1949; see also Creed et al., 1932; Norris and Gasteiger, 1955). Denny-Brown and Pennybacker (1938, p. 324) state that

> a particular voluntary movement appears to begin always with discharge of the same motor unit. More intense contraction is secured by the addition of more and more units added in a particular sequence. This "recruitment" of motor units into willed contraction is identical with that occurring in certain reflexes . . . early motor units in normal graded voluntary contraction are always in our experience small ones. The larger and more powerful motor units, each controlling many more muscle fibres, enter contraction late.

On another front, there was growing interest during the late 1940s in the possible coexistence of "fast" and "slow" motor units in mammalian muscles (Gordon and Holbourn, 1949; Gordon and Phillips, 1953; see also Andersen and Sears, 1964). However, the first report of the entire spectrum of mechanical properties of individual motor units in a single muscle (the cat lumbrical), and their relation to motor axon conduction velocity, appeared in 1963 in a paper by Bessou et al. (1963). Thus, the stage was set for the appearance of Elwood Henneman's seminal papers in the *Journal of Neurophysiology* in 1965. Three of these papers (Henneman et al., 1965a, 1965b; Somjen et al.,

1965) elaborated on Henneman's earlier (Henneman, 1957) idea that motoneuron size controls the orderly recruitment of alpha-motoneurons, inferring motoneuron size from the amplitude of extracellular action potentials recorded in ventral root filaments. Henneman and his colleagues reported that excitation from a variety of afferent and supraspinal sources recruited motor axons in a more or less fixed order, with a direct correlation between functional threshold and motor axon spike size.

Two other papers (McPhedran et al., 1965; Wuerker et al., 1965) reported extensive surveys of the mechanical properties of individual motor units in two large cat limb muscles, the medial gastrocnemius (MG) and the soleus, that were familiar to all students of motor control. The authors demonstrated a wide range of twitch contraction times, tension outputs, and relative fatigability in motor units of the MG and a much narrower range, skewed to the slow-twitch end of the spectrum, in the soleus. As in the cat lumbrical, there was a direct correlation between motor axon conduction velocity and force output, but this was more precise in the homogeneous soleus population than in the MG.

The sixth paper, by Henneman and Olson (1965), put all of these data together with newly emerging observations in the histochemical characteristics of different muscle fiber types into a single frame of reference—a coordination of motor unit properties from motoneuron to muscle unit such that

> the size of the cell dictates its excitability, its excitability determines the degree of use of the motor unit, and its "usage," in turn, specifies or influences the type of muscle fiber required. (Henneman and Olson, 1965, p. 598)

These six papers on the "size principle" became instant classics and have, for more than two decades, influenced research and ideas on the mechanisms present in the spinal segment by which the central nervous system (CNS) controls movement at the level of the final common path. They pulled together a large body of information into a coherent, easily grasped picture that suggested a single factor, motoneuron size, as the organizing principle.

The idea that cell size somehow provides intrinsic control of the functional threshold was intuitively appealing and, in principle, testable—the *sine qua non* of a good scientific hypothesis. Over the years, the term "size principle" has been used in two contexts: (1) as a description of motor unit organization and (2) as a proposed mechanism for the control of functional thresholds. It has been enormously useful as a shorthand description, but it seems safe to say that there is still no consensus about the role of motoneuron size, per se, in producing orderly recruitment (see Chapters 9 and 10, this volume). There is, however, no doubt that the size principle hypothesis has stimulated a great deal of research that might otherwise have been much less focused.

After reading Henneman's remarkable papers in 1965, I became intensely interested in the interrelations between the mechanical, morphological, and biochemical characteristics of mammalian muscle fibers, the intrinsic properties of motoneurons that innervate them, and the synaptic organizations impinging upon the motoneurons that produce and control movement. Other chapters in this volume provide a variety of views about these issues, on which I have already had ample opportunity to comment (e.g., Burke, 1968a, 1968b, 1973,

1975, 1981, 1987). I will therefore limit my remarks to a few unsettled issues related to the notion of motor unit "types."

MOTOR UNIT TYPES

The imprecision inherent in language often distorts communication. For example, the size principle hypothesis postulates a continuous gradation of functional thresholds among the motoneurons that make up a given motor pool, yet the idea of a continuum tends to get lost in the inevitable descriptions of "small" versus "large" or "low" versus "high" threshold motoneurons. This is also true when discussing the mechanical properties of muscle units. The actual distributions of isometric twitch contraction times and tetanic force outputs are essentially continuous for mixed motor unit populations (e.g., Bessou et al., 1963; Wuerker et al., 1965; Burke, 1967; Close, 1967; Burke et al., 1973; Kugelberg, 1973; Dum and Kennedy, 1980), but we are forced by the limitations of language into drawing contrasts between "fast" and "slow" and between "large" and "small" motor units.

A taxonomy of motor units is essential for communication but, to be meaningful, it must be based on features that permit clear and reliable distinctions between different categories. It is also desirable that the categories have functional correlates and that the taxonomy is strengthened, rather than weakened, by new information (see Burke, 1975). Although motoneuron "size" is, in principle, an appealing classification feature, it is in practice a very difficult thing to measure (e.g., Ulfhake and Kellerth, 1984; Cullheim et al., 1987). Studies of motor control have, for practical reasons, relied on features of the peripheral portions of the motor unit—the motor axon or, more frequently, the muscle unit. The notion of defined motor unit "types" based on characteristics of muscle units has thus had considerable appeal for studies of motor control at the spinal segmental level.

FAST VERSUS SLOW MUSCLE UNITS: THE SAG PROPERTY

In my own initial work on motor units (Burke, 1967, 1968a, 1968b), it appeared possible to use isometric twitch contraction times to separate MG motor units into fast-twitch (F) and slow-twitch (S) types. However, the isometric twitch contraction of individual muscle units can exhibit quite marked changes, usually prolongation, during and after repetitive activation (e.g., Burke et al., 1971, 1973; Dubose et al., 1987; see Bagust et al., 1974). Figure 11–1 illustrates the magnitude of this change in cat gastrocnemius motor units and shows the essentially continuous distribution of isometric twitch contraction times, both before ("initial" twitch; abscissa) and after maximal posttetanic potentiation (ordinate). As different motor unit populations were studied, it also became clear that the range in twitch contraction times, and the line between "fast" and "slow" units, vary markedly from one muscle to another even within the

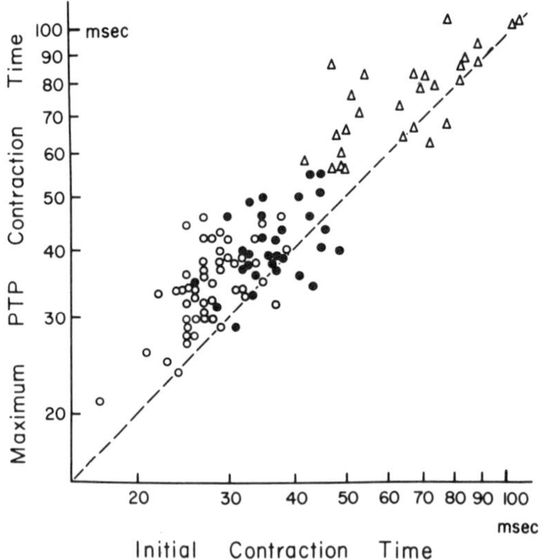

Fig. 11–1. Scatter plot of isometric contraction times for initial (unpotentiated) twitches (abscissa) and twitches during maximal PTP (ordinate) in a sample of 109 cat gastrocnemius motor units, showing prolongation of most twitch times during PTP. The dashed line represents no change, and the logarithmic axes permit assessment of the percentage of change, which did not differ with the unit type. Motor unit types denoted by symbols: open circles, type FF; filled circles, type FR; open triangles, type S. (Data from Burke et al., 1973.)

same species. Clearly, no fixed contraction time criterion can be guaranteed to separate F and S muscle units unambiguously. Some other feature is needed.

In 1969, Pablo Rudomin, Felix Zajac, and I were looking at force production by individual motor units in unfused tetanic contractions. We noted that stimulation at relatively low frequencies gave two types of tension envelope. In units with relatively fast twitch contractions, the tension rose to an early maximum and then "sagged" to a lower plateau with input frequencies over a rather wide range. In units with slower twitch contractions, this "sag" occurred only at very low input frequencies, while at slightly higher frequencies the tension envelope rose monotonically to reach a constant level late in the response. The difference in sag behavior was obvious in most units, but in a few, it was necessary to define a critical frequency for the test. By trial and error, we found that an interpulse interval about 1.25 times the twitch contraction time of the first twitch component gave the cleanest separation of units into two groups—those with sag and those without.

A large sample of units showed that there was a good correlation between the presence or absence of sag and other muscle unit characteristics, notably twitch contraction time and tetanic force output (Burke et al., 1971, 1973; their text, Fig. 5). A smaller sample of physiologically characterized and glycogen-depleted muscle units (Burke et al., 1973; their text, Fig. 7) indicated that sag was present in units with histochemical type II fibers (both IIA and IIB), all of which exhibited fast twitch contractions, but was absent at and near the criterion input frequency in muscle units with type I fibers, all of which had slow twitch contractions. Moreover, muscle units in the homogeneous cat soleus, which is composed overwhelmingly of type I muscle fibers, do not exhibit sag (Burke et al., 1974). It seemed to us more appropriate to rely on the all-or-none sag property to categorize units as fast (F) or slow (S), rather than to use an essentially arbitrary contraction time criterion.

In subsequent studies of a variety of motor unit populations in the cat (e.g., Proske and Waite, 1974; Dum and Kennedy, 1980; McDonagh et al., 1980; Fleshman et al., 1981; Dum et al., 1982; Jami et al., 1982; Kernell et al., 1983; Bodine et al., 1987; Foehring et al., 1986) and rat (Kanda et al., 1986; Bennett and Ho, 1988), the sag property (or some variant thereof; see Botterman, et al., 1985) has proven to be useful for unit classification. A number of authors, however, have encountered problems in applying the sag criterion in a minority of units (see, e.g., Reinking et al., 1975; Kernell et al., 1983; Botterman et al., 1985). In our experience (Burke et al., 1976; see also McDonagh et al., 1980), the sag property, like other mechanical properties of individual muscle units (e.g., Fig. 11–1), is quite sensitive to the detailed time history of activation. This factor may explain some of the differences among laboratories. The available evidence suggests that the sag property (or the quantitative variant introduced by Botterman et al., 1985), despite its oddity and occasional failures, is an appropriate criterion to use in separating F and S unit types. The type F group can then be subdivided into three categories [types FF, F(int), and FR] on the basis of the muscle unit's relative resistance to fatigue during a standardized stimulation regimen (Burke et al., 1971, 1973; Burke, 1981). The issue of fatigue is discussed elsewhere in this volume.

I believe that the sag property is not a laboratory curiosity but rather a reflection of intrinsic muscle properties that are related to excitation–contraction (E–C) coupling. It is certainly not a manifestation of fatigue, since high-frequency tetani superimposed after the development of sag produce the same plateau force, often rather more quickly, than similar tetani in isolation (Fig. 11–2). The electromyographic signals do not display any corresponding change, making neuromuscular transmission failure an unlikely explanation (Burke et al., 1976; see also Fig. 11–4). The fact that F and S muscle units intermingled within the same muscle systematically exhibit different sag behaviors argues that it cannot be due to differences in passive mechanical properties (e.g., ten-

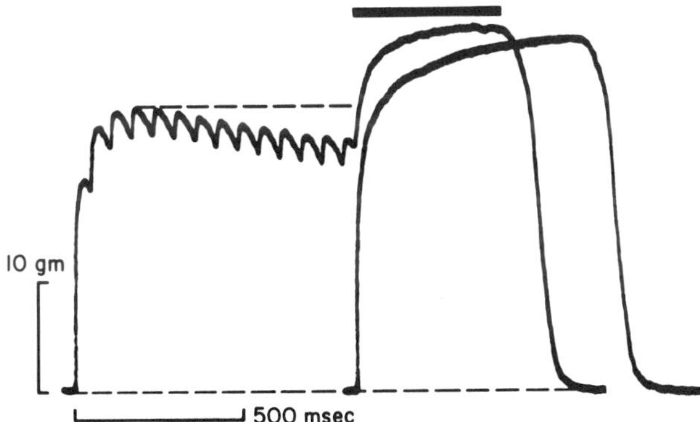

Fig. 11–2. Records of isometric force production from a type F cat gastrocnemius motor unit, showing similar maximum force levels during brief 200-Hz tetanization (bar) when superimposed following the development of sag in an unfused tetanus, versus an isolated 200-Hz tetanus in the same unit. (Unpublished records from experiments of Burke et al., 1976.)

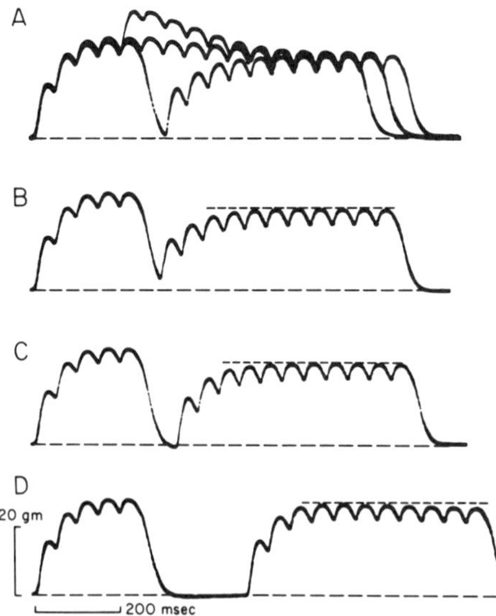

Fig. 11–3. Unfused tetani from a type F gastrocnemius motor unit showing persistence of the sag phenomenon during interrupted stimulus trains. (A) Two tetani with altered fifth intervals superimposed on an unfused tetanus with constant interpulse intervals, showing return to the same late plateau force whether the fifth interval was shorter or longer than the basic train. (B, C) Tetani with long fifth intervals showing lack of sag during force redevelopment. The dashed line indicates the force plateau of the basic unfused tetanus, as in (A), even though force had returned to baseline in (C). (D) Prolongation of the fifth interval to about 300 ms produced a slight sag during tension redevelopment (dashed line denotes peak early force in the second tetanus). Unpublished records from work reported by Burke, Rudomin and Zajac (1976).

don elasticity). This conclusion is amplified by the fact that sag persists for several hundred milliseconds after its development when low-frequency tetani are interrupted, even when the isometric force returns to baseline (Fig. 11–3). Most telling, however, is the observation that the individual component responses that make up the unfused tetanus shorten in the time needed to peak as sag develops, when compared to earlier components with the same peak force (Fig. 11–4). This strongly suggests that the duration of intrinsic fiber activation that occurs during low-frequency tetanization varies over a wide range of input frequencies in type F units and over a narrower range in type S (Burke et al., 1976). The resulting subtle change in the shape of component "twitches" apparently reduces tension summation during the later parts of unfused tetani, producing the sag.

The mechanism underlying the sag phenomenon is unknown (at least to me), but it seems quite likely to be related to the kinetics of intrafiber Ca^{2+} movement during E–C coupling—i.e., release from the sarcoplasmic reticulum (SR), binding to the regulatory proteins that initiate contraction, release from these binding sites, and reuptake into the SR. In such a multicompartmental system, the complexity of interactions seem quite capable of producing the change shown in Figure 11–4. In amphibian twitch fibers, the signals produced by free sarcoplasmic Ca^{2+} (using Ca^{2+}-sensitive indicators such as aequorin or Arsenazo-III; see Blinks et al., 1978; Miledi et al., 1982) during repetitive activation exhibit changes in amplitude and decay time course that are compatible with a multicompartmental system. There are significant quantitative differences between the SR in mammalian type II (fast-twitch) and type I (slow-twitch) fibers (reviewed by Eisenberg, 1983). Furthermore, the drug Dantrolene sodium, which inhibits Ca^{2+} release from the SR, markedly reduces twitch and unfused tetanic responses in FF and FR units in the cat peroneus tertius muscle, with little depression of fused tetanic tension, but affects type S units

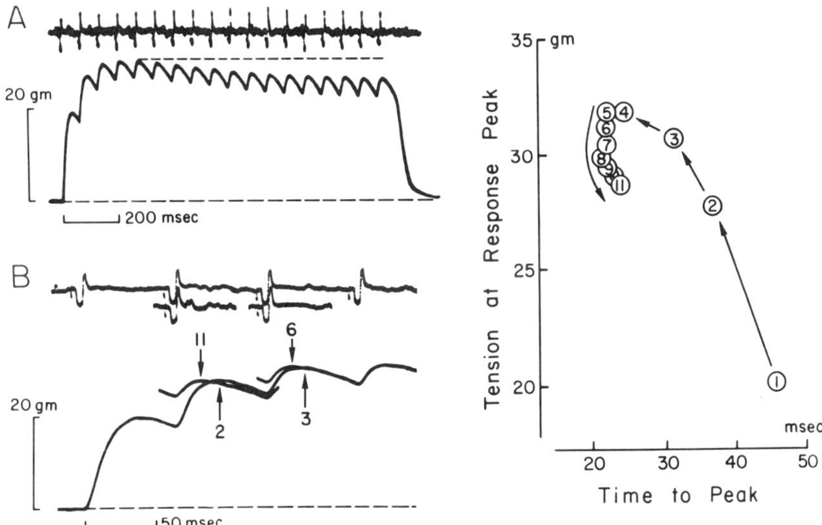

Fig. 11–4. Decrease in the time to peak of unfused tetanus components after development of sag in an unfused tetanus. (A) Unfused tetanus to constant frequency input in a type F gastrocnemius motor unit (upper trace is the EMG recorded from the muscle surface). (B) Fast sweep record of the initial components of the response shown in (A), compared to photographically superimposed records of later components that reached the same peak force. When aligned on the EMG responses (upper traces), the 11th component exhibited a shorter time to peak than the 2nd, as did the 6th when compared to the 3rd. The graph on the right shows a plot of time to peak (abscissa) versus peak force (ordinate) in the first 11 responses (number symbols). (From Fig. 8 in Burke et al., 1976; reproduced with permission.)

much less markedly (Jami et al., 1983). There is also evidence from mechanically skinned rat muscle fibers studied in vitro that the relation between steady-state force and Ca^{2+} concentration is quite different for fast-twitch (extensor digitorum longus) and slow-twitch (soleus) fibers (Stephenson and Williams, 1982). It seems quite likely that the sag phenomenon tells us something important about differences in E–C coupling mechanisms in fast- and slow-twitch muscle fibers, but, to my knowledge, there are no systematic studies of this issue.

FACTORS THAT CONTROL FORCE POPULATION BY INDIVIDUAL MOTOR UNITS

The second unresolved issue that I wish to discuss concerns the factors that produce the remarkable range (over two orders of magnitude) in maximum isometric tetanic force (P_0) that have been observed in many heterogeneous motor unit populations (reviewed by Burke, 1981; see Chapter 15, this volume). There are also systematic differences related to motor unit type. For example, in cat MG the type FF units have an average P_0 of about 71 g, while that of type FR is about 29 g and that of type S is about 8 g (Burke et al., 1973).

Differences in P_0 for individual motor units have often been attributed solely to differences in the number of muscle fibers belonging to individual motor units (the "innervation ratio," or *IR*; e.g., Denny-Brown, 1949; Henneman and Olson, 1965). Although there is no doubt that variation in *IR* is a major factor producing force variation among individual motor units, it is important to consider that P_0 is determined by two factors:

$$P_0 = A_{act} \cdot F_{sp} \tag{11-1}$$

where A_{act} is the total cross-sectional area of the active unit muscle fibers and F_{sp} is the specific force output of the active fibers measured in units of force per unit area. In turn, A_{act} can be estimated as the product of the average cross-sectional area (A_{av}) of the muscle unit fibers multiplied by *IR*:

$$A_{act} = A_{av} \cdot IR \tag{11-2}$$

In principle, the glycogen depletion technique (Edstrom and Kugelberg, 1968) is appropriate to assess A_{av} and *IR* directly, but F_{sp} can only be derived from Equations 11–1 and 11–2, knowing P_0, A_{av}, and *IR*.

Despite significant technical problems (see, e.g., Bodine et al., 1987), A_{av} can, with suitable care, be measured from glycogen-depleted muscle unit material. Unfortunately, it is much more difficult to determine *IR* directly by counting depleted fibers in frozen sections. This difficulty is due, in part, to the complex internal architecture (e.g., fiber pinnation) of many muscles, which limits the number of unit fibers that appear at any level of muscle cross section, and partly because it is difficult to be sure that *all* muscle unit fibers are indeed recognizably depleted of glycogen (Burke and Tsairis, 1973). Barker and co-workers (1977; see also Bodine et al., 1987) have provided direct evidence that some muscle fibers, especially type I fibers of S muscle units, display irregular glycogen depletion, making muscle fiber counts from serial sections problematic. Toop et al. (1982) used 2-deoxyglucose autoradiography as an alternative marking method for single muscle unit fibers and found fibers in type S units that were labeled by this metabolic uptake tracer but not recognizably depleted of glycogen.

Because of such problems, Peter Tsairis and I (Burke and Tsairis, 1973) resorted to an indirect approach to determine *average* values for *IR* (*IR*$_{av}$) for each motor unit type. The *overall* average *IR* for any muscle is simply the total number of muscle fibers in it, *M*, divided by the total number of alpha motoneurons, *N*, in its motor nucleus (Eccles and Sherrington, 1930; Clark, 1931). For the *i*th motor unit type;

$$IR_{av,i} = \frac{M}{N} \cdot \frac{p_i}{q_i} \tag{11-3}$$

where p_i and q_i are, respectively, the relative frequencies of the *i*th histochemical fiber type and the motor unit type associated with it (see Burke, 1981). The ratio p_i/q_i (the "relative innervation ratio," or *RIR*) determines whether, for example, the hypothetical *average* type S muscle unit has more or fewer fibers than the overall average for the muscle. This calculation obviously requires reliable estimates of p_i and q_i, and it furthermore depends critically on the ability to associate a given histochemical fiber type with a particular physiological motor unit type.

As shown in Table 11–1, indirect data from seven studies of six cat hindlimb motor unit populations (using Eqs. 11–1 to 11–3) suggest that the *RIR* of type S muscle units, as a class, is not systematically smaller than that of FF and FR unit groups, despite the large differences in mean force output among these groups (Burke and Tsairis, 1973; McDonagh et al., 1980; Dum and Kennedy, 1980; Dum et al., 1982; Foehring et al., 1986; see Table 1). When $A_{av,i}$ values are taken into account, these studies also suggest that F_{sp} must be two to as much as six times smaller in type S muscle units in heterogeneous unit

Table 11–1 Summary of data from six cat hindlimb muscles giving tetanic forces (P_0), mean fiber areas (A_{av}), motor unit frequencies (q_i), relative innervation ratios (*RIR*), and specific force outputs (F_{sp}), all normalized by the values for type S units

Muscle	Type	P_0	A_{av}	q_i	*RIR*	F_{sp}
MG[a]	FF	9.39	2.27	.52	1.10	3.76
	FR	3.78	1.20	.23	.91	3.49
	S	1.00	1.00	.25	1.00	1.00
MG[b]	FF	8.26	1.96	.52	1.21	3.47
	FR	1.86	1.15	.24	1.08	1.50
	S	1.00	1.00	.24	1.00	1.00
FDL[c]	FF	27.27	2.57	.32	1.83	5.80
	FR	4.87	1.37	.56	.73	4.80
	S	1.00	1.00	.12	1.00	1.00
TP[d]	FF	9.78	2.35	.38	1.28	3.25
	FR	3.19	1.35	.20	.91	2.58
	S	1.00	1.00	.42	1.00	1.00
FHL[e]	F*	2.45	1.31	.84	.87	2.16
	S	1.00	1.00	.16	1.00	1.00
PerL[f]	F*	4.68	2.00	.79	1.21	1.93
	S	1.00	1.00	.21	1.00	1.00
TA[g]	FF	8.14	2.98	.39	1.33	2.05
	FR	2.39	1.74	.50	.52	2.64
	S	1.00	1.00	.11	1.00	1.00
TA[h]	FF	5.57	1.33		2.74	1.45
	FR	2.52	.98		2.12	1.23
	S	1.00	1.00		1.00	1.00

[a]MG = medial gastrocnemius; from Burke et al. (1973).

[b]From Foehring et al. (1986).

[c]FDL = flexor digitorum longus; from Dum et al. (1982).

[d]TP = tibialis posterior; from McDonagh et al. (1980).

[e]FHL = flexor hallucis longus; (mean fiber areas given only for type I and type II fibers (*) from Westerman et al. (1979).

[f]PerL = peroneus longus; physiological data from Kernell et al. (1983); fiber area data (type I and II fibers only) from Donselaar et al. (1987).

[g]TA = tibialis anterior; physiological data from Dum and Kennedy (1980); fiber area data from Mayer (1973).

[h]TA data from glycogen-depleted motor units, with *IR* directly determined; from Bodine et al. (1987).

populations than in either FF or FR units (see also Table 2 in Burke, 1981, and Table 4 in Bodine et al., 1987). This conclusion has been disputed (e.g., Edjtehadi and Lewis, 1979; Bodine et al., 1987; Lucas et al., 1987) and does not fit well with estimates of F_{sp} for homogeneous muscles like cat soleus (e.g., Close, 1972; Murphey and Beardsley, 1974), which are made up almost exclusively of type S units and type I muscle fibers (Burke et al., 1974).

Two recent studies have reevaluated the F_{sp} of fast and slow twitch fibers in heterogeneous cat muscles. Lucas et al. (1987) measured force production by chemically skinned single muscle fibers dissected from the cat MG in relation to their diameter and ATPase histochemistry. These authors found essentially no difference in mean F_{sp} (about 2.4 kg/cm^2) for histochemical type II and type I fibers, although individual fibers in both groups displayed wide ranges in calculated F_{sp}. Lucas and co-workers also found a similar average F_{sp} value (2.3 kg/cm^2) for cat soleus fibers, which is comparable to that found in whole muscle studies (Murphey and Beardsley, 1974). They noted, however, that the conditions under which skinned fibers can be studied in vitro are very different from those in living fibers in situ. The F_{sp} values derived from skinned fiber that are completely activated by exogenous ATP do not necessarily reflect the forces produced by those same fibers when activated by physiological mechanisms involved in E–C coupling. On the other hand, there is no obvious reason why type I fibers in heterogeneous muscle should be less completely activated during fused tetani *in situ* than their fast-twitch brethren.

Bodine and co-workers (1987) used the glycogen-depletion approach in the cat tibialis anterior (TA) to assess *IR* directly and to investigate its relation to P_0, physiological motor unit type, and fiber histochemistry in individual motor units. These authors argued that the architecture of the cat TA, in contrast to the highly pinnate MG muscle studied by Burke and Tsairis (1973), permits accurate enumeration of *IR* in the individual muscle units studied. Bodine et al. (1987) estimated that F_{sp} values for FF and FR units were similar (means: 2.5 kg·cm^2 and 2.1 kg/cm^2, respectively), while the value for type S units was only 20–30% less (mean: 1.7 kg/cm^2). There is thus an unresolved discrepancy between these results and the series of indirect estimates of F_{sp} in type S units of mixed muscles discussed earlier (Table 11–1).

The reasons for this discrepancy are not immediately obvious. Although the differences in average P_0 for FF, FR, and S units found by Bodine and colleagues were comparable to those reported by others (Dum and Kennedy, 1980), their differences in A_{av} for the three unit types were less than those found in another study of the TA (Mayer, 1973) and of other cat hindlimb muscles (Table 11–1; cf. Bodine et al., 1987, Table 4). This may, in part, reflect differences in technical factors (Bodine et al., 1987). Although they had no independent confirmation that *all* fibers in their type S units were recognizably depleted of glycogen, Bodine et al. showed that the motor unit territories of the S units were smaller than those of the fast units, and they excluded units that showed evidence of incomplete depletion along the length of some fibers. This careful study clearly pushes the glycogen depletion approach to its limits in assessing *IR*, but its interpretation depends critically on the reliability of *IR* estimates in the three type S muscle units studied.

There are many sources of potential error in the indirect estimation of F_{sp} for a given motor unit type using Equations 11–1 to 11–3. The first consideration is whether the association between physiological motor unit types and histochemical fiber types is secure. To date, published evidence on this issue is unequivocal—muscle units in normal or self-reinnervated muscles that exhibit the FF physiological profile have histochemical type IIB fibers, FR units have type IIA fibers, and S units have type I muscle fibers (Burke et al., 1971, 1973; Dum and Kennedy, 1980; McDonagh et al., 1980; Dum et al., 1982, 1983; Gauthier et al., 1983; Foehring et al., 1986; Bodine et al., 1987). This is also true in the rat (Bennett and Ho, 1988; see also Edstrom and Kugelberg, 1968; Kugelberg, 1973, 1976; Kugelberg and Lindegren, 1979). The available evidence thus provides very strong support for the assumption that there is a systematic and predictable match between muscle unit mechanical properties and histochemistry.

With respect to the factors required to calculate F_{sp} using Equations 11–1 to 11–3, technical issues complicate assessment of A_{av} and the relative frequency of histochemical fiber types, p_i. However, it seems likely that the major source of variability and potential error is the sampling of motor unit populations to determine $P_{0,i}$ and the relative frequency, q_i, of the different motor unit types. Most of the published data result from different animals, since the available methods make it difficult to generate a large sample from any individual animal. This factor probably accounts for much of the variation in relative F_{sp} values shown in Table 11–1, but the agreement among the indirect studies that at least a twofold difference exists between F_{sp} in type F and S muscle units is difficult to explain by random sampling errors.

In summary, there seems to be general agreement from studies of motor units in situ that F_{sp} is smaller in type S muscle units than in either type FF or FR—it is only the magnitude of the difference that is in doubt. This seemingly small point has been vexatious because the extent of the difference originally proposed (Burke and Tsairis, 1973) was so large and unexpected. The weight of evidence that has accumulated since that paper was published suggests that the difference may well be on the order of two- to threefold, rather than four- to fivefold, but it seems unlikely that we have heard the last word on the issue.

REFERENCES

Andersen, P., and Sears, T. A. (1964). The mechanical properties and innervation of fast and slow motor units in the intercostal muscles of the cat. *J. Physiol. (Lond.)* 173, 114–129.

Bagust, J., Lewis, D. M., and Luck, J. C. (1974). Post-tetanic effects in motor units of fast and slow twitch muscle of the cat. *J. Physiol. (Lond.)* 237, 115–121.

Barker, D., Emonet-Denand, F., Harker, D. W., Jami, L., and Laporte, Y. (1977). Types of intra- and extrafusal muscle fibre innervated by dynamic skeletofusimotor axons in cat peroneus brevis and temissimus muscles as determined by the glycogen depletion method. *J. Physiol. (Lond.)* 266, 713–726.

Bennett, M. R., and Ho, S. (1988). The formation of topographical maps in developing rat gastrocnemius muscle during synapse elimination. *J. Physiol. (Lond.)* 396, 471–496.

Bessou, P., Emonet-Denand, F., and Laporte, Y. (1963). Relation entre le vitesse de conduction des fibres nerveuses motrices et le tempe de contraction de leurs unites motrices. *Compt. Rend. Acad. Sci. (Paris)* 256, 5626–5627.

Blinks, J. R., Rudel, R., and Taylor, S. R. (1978). Calcium transients in isolated amphibian skeletal muscle fibres: Detection with Aequorin. *J. Physiol. (Lond.)* 277, 291–323.

Bodine, S. C., Roy, R. R., Eldred, E., and Edgerton, V. R. (1987). Maximal force as a function of anatomical features of motor units in the cat tibialis anterior. *J. Neurophysiol.* 57, 1730–1745.

Botterman, B. R., Iwamoto, G. A., and Gonyea, W. J. (1985). Classification of motor units in flexor carpi radialis muscle of the cat. *J. Neurophysiol.* 54, 676–690.

Burke, R. E. (1967). Motor unit types of cat triceps surae muscle. *J. Physiol. (Lond.)* 193, 141–160.

Burke, R. E. (1968a). Group Ia synaptic input to fast and slow twitch motor units of cats triceps surae. *J. Physiol. (Lond.)* 196, 615–631.

Burke, R. E. (1968b). Firing patterns of gastrocnemius motor units in the decerebrate cat. *J. Physiol. (Lond.)* 196, 631–654.

Burke, R. E. (1973). On the central nervous system control of fast and slow twitch motor units. In *New Developments in Electromyography and Clinical Neurophysiology*, Vol. 1, (ed. J. E. Desmedt). Karger, Basel, pp. 69–94.

Burke, R. E. (1975). A comment on the existence of motor unit "types." In *The Nervous System*, Vol. I: *The Basic Neurosciences*, (ed. R. O. Brady). Raven Press, New York, pp. 611–619.

Burke, R. E. (1981). Motor units: Anatomy, physiology and functional organization. In *Handbook of Physiology*, Sect. I, *The Nervous System*, Vol. II. *Motor Systems* (ed. V. B. Brooks). American Physiological Society: Bethesda, Md., pp. 345–422.

Burke, R. E. (1987). Synaptic efficacy and the control of neuronal input-output relations. *Trends Neurosci.* 10, 42–45.

Burke, R. E., Levine, D. N., Salcman, M., and Tsairis, P. (1974). Motor units in cat soleus muscle: Physiological, histochemical and morphological characteristics. *J. Physiol. (Lond.)* 238, 503–514.

Burke, R. E., Levine, D. N., Tsairis, P., and Zajac, F. E. (1973). Physiological types and histochemical profiles in motor units of the cat gastrocnemius. *J. Physiol. (Lond.)* 234, 723–748.

Burke, R. E., Levine, D. N., Zajac, F. E., Tsairis, P., and Engel, W. K. (1971). Mammalian motor units: Physiological–histochemical correlation in three types in cat gastrocnemius. *Science* 174, 709–712.

Burke, R. E., Rudomin, P., and Zajac, F. E. (1976). The effect of activation history on tension production by individual muscle units. *Brain Res.* 109, 515–529.

Burke, R. E., and Tsairis, P. (1973). Anatomy and innervation ratios in motor units of cat gastrocnemius. *J. Physiol. (Lond.)* 234, 749–765.

Clark, D. A. (1931). Muscle counts of motor units: A study in innervation ratios. *Am. J. Physiol.* 96, 296–304.

Close, R. (1967). Properties of motor units in fast and slow skeletal muscles of the rat. *J. Physiol. (Lond.)* 193, 45–55.

Close, R. (1972). Dynamic properties of mammalian skeletal muscles. *Physiol. Rev.* 52, 129–197.

Creed, R. S., Denny-Brown, D., Eccles, J. C., Liddell, E. G. T., and Sherrington, C. S. (1932). *Reflex Activity of the Spinal Cord.* Oxford University Press, London.

Cullheim, S., Fleshman, J. W., Glenn, L. L., and Burke, R. E. (1987). Membrane area and dendritic structure in type-identified triceps surae alpha motoneurons. *J. Comp. Neurol.* 255, 68–81.

Denny-Brown, D. (1929). On the nature of postural reflexes. *R. Soc. Proc. B.* 104, 252–301.

Denny-Brown, D. (1949). Interpretation of the electromyogram. *Arch. Neurol. Psychiatry (Chicago)* 61, 99–128.

Denny-Brown, D., and Pennybacker, J. B. (1938). Fibrillation and fasciculation in voluntary muscle. *Brain* 61, 311–344.

Donselaar, Y., Eerbeek, O., Kernell, D., and Verhey, B. A. (1987). Fibre size and histochemical staining characteristics in normal and chronically stimulated fast muscle of cat. *J. Physiol. (Lond.)* 382, 237–254.

Dubose, L., Schelhorn, T. B., and Clamann, H. P. (1987). Changes in contractile speed of cat motor units during activity. *Muscle Nerve.* 10, 744–752.

Dum, R. P., Burke, R. E., O'Donovan, M. J., Toop, J., and Hodgson, J. A. (1982). Motor unit organization in the flexor digitorum longus muscle of the cat. *J. Neurophysiol.* 47, 1108–1125.

Dum, R. P., and Kennedy, T. T. (1980). Physiological and histochemical characteristics of motor units in cat tibialis anterior and extensor digitorum longus muscles. *J. Neurophysiol.* 43, 1615–1630.

Dum, R. P., O'Donovan, M. J., Toop, J., and Burke, R. E. (1983). Cross-reinnervated motor units in cat muscle. I. Flexor digitorum longus muscle units reinnervated by soleus motoneurons. *J. Neurophysiol.* 54, 818–836.

Eccles, J. C., and Sherrington, C. S. (1930). Numbers and contraction values of individual motor units examined in some muscles of the limb. *Proc. R. Soc. Series B* 106, 326–357.

Edjtehadi, G. D., and Lewis, D. M. (1979). Histochemical reactions of fibres in a fast twitch muscle of the cat. *J. Physiol. (Lond.)* 287, 439–453.

Edström, L., and Kugelberg, E. (1968). Histochemical composition, distribution of fibres and fatigability of single motor units. Anterior tibial muscle of the rat. *J. Neurol. Neurosurg. Psychiatry* 31, 424–433.

Eisenberg, B. (1983). Quantitative ultrastructure of mammalian skeletal muscle. In *Handbook of Physiology*, Sect. 10: *Skeletal Muscle* (ed. L. D. Peachey). American Physiological Society, Bethesda, Md., pp. 73–112.

Fleshman, J. W., Munson, J. B., Sypert, G. W., and Friedman, W. A. (1981). Rheobase, input resistance, and motor-unit type in medial gastrocnemius motoneurons in the cat. *J. Neurophysiol.* 46, 1326–1338.

Foehring, R. C., Sypert, G. W., and Munson, J. B. (1986). Properties of self-reinnervated motor units of medial gastrocnemius of cat. I. Long-term reinnervation. *J. Neurophysiol.* 55, 931–946.

Gauthier, G. F., Burke, R. E., Lowey, S., and Hobbs, A. W. (1983). Myosin isozymes in normal and cross-reinnervated cat skeletal muscle fibers. *J. Cell Biol.* 97, 756–771.

Gordon, G., and Holbourn, A. (1949). The mechanical activity of single motor units in reflex contraction of skeletal muscles. *J. Physiol. (Lond.)* 110, 26–35.

Gordon, G., and Phillips, C. G. (1953). Slow and rapid components in a flexor muscle. *Q. J. Exp. Physiol.* 38, 35–45.

Henneman, E. (1957). Relations between size of neurons and their susceptibility to discharge. *Science* 126, 1345–1346.

Henneman, E., and Olson, C. B. (1965). Relations between structure and function in the design of skeletal muscles. *J. Neurophysiol.* 28, 581–598.

Henneman, E., Somjen, G., and Carpenter, D. O. (1965a). Functional significance of cell size in spinal motoneurons. *J. Neurophysiol.* 28, 560–580.

Henneman, E., Somjen, G., and Carpenter, D. O., (1965b). Excitability and inhibitability of motoneurons of different sizes. *J. Neurophysiol.* 28, 599–620.

Jami, L., Murthy, K. S. K., Petit, J., and Zytnicki, D. (1982). Distribution of physiological types of motor units in the cat pertoneus tertius muscle. *Exp. Brain Res.* 48, 177–184.

Jami, L., Murthy, K. S. K., Petit, J., and Zytnicki, D. (1983). Action of Dantrolene sodium on single motor units of cat muscle in vivo. *Brain Res.* 261, 285–294.

Kanda, K., Hasizume, K., Nomoto, E., and Asaki, S. (1986). The effects of aging on physiological properties of fast and slow twitch motor units in the rat gastrocnemius. *Neurosci Res.* 3, 242–246.

Kernell, D., Eerbeek, O., and Verhey, B. A. (1983). Motor unit categorization on basis of contractile properties: An experimental analysis of the composition of the cat's M. peroneus longus. *Exp. Brain Res.* 50, 211–219.

Kugelberg, E. (1973). Histochemical composition, contraction speed and fatigability of rat soleus motor units. *J. Neuro. Sci.* 20, 177–198.

Kugelberg, E. (1976). Adaptive transformation of rat soleus motor units during growth. Histochemistry and contraction speed. *J. Neuro. Sci.* 27, 269–289.

Kugelberg, E., and Lindegren, B. (1979). Transmission and contraction fatigue of rat motor units in relation to succinate dehydrogenase activity of motor unit fibres. *J. Physiol. (Lond.)* 288, 285–300.

Lucas, S. M., Ruff, R. L., and Binder, M. D. (1987). Specific tension measurements in single soleus and medial gastrocnemius muscle fibers of the cat. *Exp. Neurol.* 95, 142–154.

Mayer, R. F. (1973). Observations on motor units in cat anterior tibial muscle. In *New Developments in Electromyography and Clinical Neurophysiology*, Vol. 1. (ed. J. E. Desmedt). Karger, Basel, pp. 31–34.

McDonagh, J. C., Binder, M. D., Reinking, R. M., and Stuart, D. G. (1980). Tetrapartite classification of motor units of cat tibialis posterior. *J. Neurophysiol.* 44, 696–712.

McPhedran, A. M., Wuerker, R. B., and Henneman, E. (1965). Properties of motor units in a homogeneous red muscle (soleus) of the cat. *J. Neurophysiol.* 28, 71–84.

Miledi, R., Parker, I., and Zhu, P. H. (1982). Calcium transients evoked by action potentials in frog twitch muscle fibres. *J. Physiol. (Lond.)* 333, 655–679.

Murphy, R. A., and Beardsley, A. C. (1974). Mechanical properties of the cat soleus muscle in situ. *Am. J. Physiol.* 227, 1008–1013.

Norris, F. H., and Gasteiger, E. L. (1955). Action potentials of single motor units in normal muscle. *Electroenceph. Clin. Neurophysiol.* 7, 115–126.

Proske, U., and Waite, P. M. E. (1974). Properties of types of motor units in the medial gastrocnemius muscle of the cat. *Brain Res.* 67, 89–102.

Reinking, R. M., Stephens, J. A., and Stuart, D. G. (1975). The motor units of cat medial gastrocnemius: Problems of their categorisation on the basis of mechanical properties. *Exp. Brain Res.* 23, 301–313.

Somjen, G., Carpenter, D. O., and Henneman, E. (1965). Responses of motoneurons of different sizes to graded stimulation of supraspinal centers of the brain. *J. Neurophysiol.* 28, 958–965.

Stephenson, D. G., and Williams, D. A. (1982). Effects of sarcomere length on the force–pCa relation in fast- and slow-twitch skinned muscle fibres from the rat. *J. Physiol. (Lond.)* 333, 637–653.

Toop, J., Burke, R. E., Dum, R. P., and O'Donovan, M. J. (1982). 2-Deoxy-$[^{14}C]$ glucose autoradiography of motor units: Labeling of individual acutely active muscle fibers. *J. Neurosci. Meth.* 5, 283–289.

Ulfhake, B., and Kellerth, J. -O. (1984). Electrophysiological and morphological measurements in cat gastrocnemius and soleus α-motoneurones. *Brain Res.* 307, 167–179.

Wuerker, R. B., McPhendran, A. M., and Henneman, E. (1965). Properties of motor units in a heterogeneous pale muscle (M. gastrocnemius) of the cat. *J. Neurophysiol.* 28, 85–99.

12

Mechanical Properties of Extraocular Motor Units

STEPHEN J. GOLDBERG

This chapter represents a departure from most of the other chapters in the book in that it discusses the motor units that move the eye rather than the limbs. The work on classifying extraocular motor units has a relatively short history, but the same rigorous and detailed study that has been commonplace in the spinal cord is now being applied to the eye movement motor control system. It is important to examine this fast, precise system at the level of the motor unit to see if the organizational patterns observed in the spinal cord are generally applicable to the brain stem.

Most animals have six muscles in each orbit to move the eye (Baker, 1986). The lateral rectus is innervated by the principal abducens nucleus, and the superior oblique is innervated by the trochlear nucleus. The medial, superior, and inferior recti are innervated by the oculomotor nucleus, as is the inferior oblique. The retractor bulbi muscle, which often consists of four muscle slips attached to the meridian of the globe, is found in animals with a nictitating membrane and serves to retract the eye into the orbit (Hutson et al., 1979; Spencer et al., 1980; Crandall et al., 1981). This seventh extraocular muscle is innervated primarily by the accessory abducens nucleus, which lies ventrolateral to the principal abducens nucleus. Accessory abducens motoneuron axons course through the principal abducens nucleus and join the abducens nerve.

Extraocular muscle fiber morphology has been examined in some detail (Mayr, 1971; Peachey et al., 1974; Alvarado and Van Horn, 1975; Mayr et al., 1975; Lennerstrand and Nichols, 1977; Alvarado-Mallart and Pincon-Raymond, 1979; Chiarandini and Davidowitz, 1979; Spencer and Porter, 1981; Pachter, 1982, 1983, 1984; Pachter and Colbjornsen, 1983). Each of the six main muscles can be divided into distinct orbital and global layers. At least three types of singly innervated (i.e., one motor end plate per fiber) muscle fibers (comprising 70% of the muscle fibers) can be found in the global muscle layer. The smallest-diameter, singly innervated type is also found in the orbital layer. There are two types of multiply innervated (i.e., more than one end plate per fiber) fibers (Hess, 1961), both of small diameter, with one type in the orbital and one type in the global layer (Chiarandini and Davidowitz, 1979; Bondi and Chiarandini, 1983).

There have also been studies of extraocular motoneurons (see Sasaki, 1963; Baker et al., 1969; Robinson, 1970, 1986; Baker and Precht, 1972; Barmack, 1974, 1976; Goldberg et al., 1974; Naito et al., 1974; Baker and Highstein, 1975; Remmel and Marrocco, 1975; Grantyn et al., 1977; Grantyn and Grantyn, 1978; Grant et al., 1979a, 1979b; Destombes et al., 1983; Fuchs et al., 1985; Baker, 1986; Delgado-Garcia et al., 1986; Gomez et al., 1986; McCrea et al., 1986; Nelson et al., 1986) and muscle fiber physiology (see Hess and Pilar, 1963; Bach-y-Rita and Ito, 1966; Pilar, 1967; Chiarandini, 1976; Hansen and Lennerstrand, 1977; Bondi and Chiarandini, 1979, 1983; Chiarandini and Davidowitz, 1979; Chiarandi and Stefani, 1979), as well as anatomical examinations of the brain stem motor nuclei making up the eye movement control system (see Tarlov and Tarlov, 1971; Gacek, 1974, 1979; Tredici et al., 1976; Spencer and Sterling, 1977; Steiger and Buttner-Ennever, 1978; Grant et al., 1979b; Hutson et al., 1979; Kerns, 1980; Spencer et al., 1980; Goldberg et al., 1981; Meredith et al., 1981; Highstein et al., 1982; McClung et al., 1983; Miyanzaki, 1985; McCrea et al., 1986). But this chapter focuses on the properties of mammalian extraocular motor units and their relation to our ideas of motor unit recruitment as delineated by Henneman (Henneman and Mendell, 1981). Motoneuron properties including size, location within the nucleus, and axonal conduction velocity will be compared with the mechanics (i.e., contraction time, fusion frequency, tension, and fatigue) of the muscle fibers.

INITIAL EXTRAOCULAR MOTOR UNIT STUDIES

The first studies of extraocular motor unit mechanics (Bach-y-Rita and Ito, 1966; Lennerstrand, 1972) focused on the delineation of motor unit types. Lennerstrand (1974a) examined cat retractor bulbi motor units in some detail by recording the forces produced in a single retractor muscle slip in response to extracellular stimulation of single motoneuron cell bodies or their axons in the principal abducens nucleus. He found that the retractor bulbi motor units were all of the singly innervated type and were generally fatigable. No correlations among contraction time, tension, and fatigability were observed in this unit population.

Lennerstrand (1974b) also studied cat inferior oblique motor units by stimulating single axons in teased nerve filaments. He reported three distinct populations of motor units. Singly innervated (SI) units, like skeletal muscle motor units, exhibited the fastest contraction times. Multiply innervated conducting

(MIC) units showed intermediate contraction times. Multiply innervated non-conducting (MINC) units did not exhibit twitch contractions or propagated action potentials and produced tension only in response to tetanic stimulation. ("Conducting" fibers propagate action potentials along the muscle membrane, while "nonconducting" fibers show a depolarization only in the vicinity of the neuromuscular junction.) The MINC motor units were probably equivalent to the slow extraocular units described by Hess and Pilar (1963). Recent studies (Mayr et al., 1975; Chiarandini and Davidowitz, 1979; Pachter, 1983) have not confirmed the existence of MIC units and therefore "twitch" or "non-twitch" motor units might be more appropriate terminology. Although fatigue was not studied in detail, it was noted that the slower units were generally more fatigue resistant.

At about the same time, Close and Luff (1974) examined some rat inferior rectus motor units. While they did not observe slow units, the contraction speed of their fast units was generally comparable to that of fast units found by Lennerstrand (1974b) in the cat.

EARLY EXTRAOCULAR MOTOR UNIT SIZE PRINCIPLE-RELATED STUDIES

In another study of the cat inferior oblique muscle and nerve, Lennerstrand and Bach-y-Rita (1974) questioned the applicability of the size principle to the eye movement system. They found slower-contracting, fatigue-resistant motor units innervated by large-diameter axons. Smaller-diameter axons should have innervated such units in a rigorous application of the size principle.

In 1976 we used intracellular stimulation of single motoneurons to activate motor units in the cat lateral rectus muscle (Goldberg et al., 1976). Lateral rectus motor units were mechanically similar to the inferior oblique units previously studied (Lennerstrand, 1974b). Although our axonal conduction velocity measurements were relatively imprecise due to a short conduction distance, we noted that the slower-contracting units with lower fusion frequencies exhibited slower axonal conduction velocities and generally weaker twitch tensions. However, the faster-contracting units with higher fusion frequencies had a wide range of conduction times. These data also indicated that axonal conduction velocity was apparently not closely related to muscle unit contraction speed and strength.

Barmack (1977) observed a reasonably linear size-related recruitment order in the rabbit inferior rectus muscle, although axonal conduction velocity was not examined. He used spike-triggered averaging to define motor unit size as the isometrically recorded twitch tension that was time locked to the discharge of one extraocular muscle fiber. Recruitment threshold followed a size principle when size was defined operationally as the twitch amplitude of the motor unit. In addition, suprathreshold frequency modulation (Barmack, 1977) of single extraocular muscle fibers was also correlated with size.

MOTONEURON "POOLS" IN THE CAT EXTRAOCULAR SYSTEM

Spinal cord motoneuron pools (arranged in columns) apparently provide a good target for uniform afferent inputs that are important for a size-related recruitment order (Burke et al., 1977; Burke, 1981; Henneman and Mendell, 1981; Clamann et al., 1983; Henneman, 1985). In 1981 we examined some aspects of the organization of extraocular motoneuron pools. Intracellular studies of cell bodies and axons in the principal abducens nucleus revealed motor units whose muscle fibers were divided among the retractor bulbi muscle slips, as well as units whose muscle fibers were found in both the retractor bulbi and lateral rectus muscles (Crandall et al., 1981). The use of intracellular horseradish peroxidase (HRP) injections revealed that some motoneurons that innervated only the retractor bulbi muscle had their motoneuron cell bodies in the principal abducens nucleus, along with the lateral rectus motoneurons. We also confirmed electrophysiologically (Meredith et al., 1981) the anatomical finding (Spencer et al., 1980) that some motoneurons that innervate the retractor bulbi muscle can be found in the oculomotor nucleus and that those axons are included in the oculomotor nerve. These findings illustrate that the retractor bulbi motoneuron pool is located in three separate brain stem nuclei with axons carried in two cranial nerves. Could such a motoneuron "pool" receive a uniform afferent input? In what "pool" do motoneurons belong whose innervated muscle fibers are contained in two separate muscles?

We also found that some motoneurons that innervated only the lateral rectus muscle were located in the oculomotor nucleus and that their axons were carried in the third cranial nerve (McClung et al., 1983). This finding further compounds the dilemma of anatomically defining extraocular motoneuron pools. The concept of "one muscle, one motoneuron pool" (Hoffer et al., 1987; Stuart et al., 1988) does not appear to fit here.

In a study of lateral rectus motoneurons located in the principal abducens nucleus (Goldberg et al., 1981) we confirmed an earlieir observation (Goldberg et al., 1976) that the motoneurons tend to be organized within the nucleus with regard to the twitch contraction speed and fusion frequency of the innervated motor units. Motoneurons innervating faster-contracting units tend to be located more dorsally than those innervating slower-contracting muscle units. We also clearly identified two units that, based on mechanical criteria, were similar to the multiply innervated units with nonpropagated electrical activity (MINC units) seen in the inferior oblique muscle.

EXTRAOCULAR MOTONEURON SIZE AND MOTOR UNIT MECHANICS

Three motor units with unusually large (over 100 mg) twitch tensions were observed in the study (Goldberg et al., 1981) of principal abducens nucleus lateral rectus motor units. Similar powerful units have also been seen in the medial rectus (Meredith and Goldberg, 1986) and superior oblique (Nelson et al., 1986) muscles. However, intracellular HRP injections showed that while these powerful contractors were innervated by large motoneurons (40–50 μm), units with more normal twitch tensions could also be innervated by large cell bodies. In additional studies (Goldberg and McClung, 1982) of lateral rectus motoneurons, we labeled nine cells intracellularly with HRP. In this population of nine cells, we did note a tendency for larger motoneuron cell bodies to innervate motor units with stronger twitch contractions. However, three cell bodies, each with an average diameter close to 40 μm, were found that innervated a weak nontwitch unit, a unit of average twitch tension, and an unusually strong unit (Fig. 12–1). If the size principle applies, then such motoneurons with nearly equal cell sizes ought to be recruited at about the same time in a movement, even though they feed such divergent motor unit types.

This apparent contradiction of the size principle could be explained by differently sized dendritic trees associated with similarly sized cell bodies. We therefore carefully measured the dendritic trees of lateral rectus motoneurons (Russell-Mergenthal et al., 1986). In this effort, modeled after a study by Ulfhake and Kellerth (1984), we developed a formula whereby a measurement of the diameter of a proximal dendrite could be used to predict reliably the surface area of the entire dendritic tree. The application of this formula to the previously studied (Goldberg and McClung, 1982) HRP-labeled lateral rectus motoneurons did not significantly alter our estimate of their relative sizes.

We have obtained accurate measures of actual motoneuron size in relation to the motor units' mechanical characteristics and have observed discrepancies in size-related correlations (Goldberg and McClung, 1982). But Henneman's size principle is primarily based on correlations with axonal conduction velocity (Wuerker et al., 1965; Henneman and Mendell, 1981; Zajac and Faden, 1985).

A RETURN TO AXONAL CONDUCTION VELOCITY AND A LEAP INTO FATIGUE

While it is generally accepted that cell size, axon diameter, and therefore conduction velocity should be directly related, we still felt that a critical shortcoming of the studies discussed earlier is that axonal conduction velocity measurements were either equivocal or absent. Studies of the lateral rectus and retractor bulbi muscles were done by antidromically identifying the motoneurons by stimulation of the abducens nerve within the brain stem at a site some 4–5 mm from the motoneurons. The longer conduction distance that would be afforded by stimulating the muscle nerve in the orbit was rejected in order to preserve the structural integrity of the muscles for mechanical recording. The short brain stem conduction distance and the convolutions often observed in motoneuron axons near the cell body made accurate conduction velocity assessments difficult.

We turned to the cat trochlear nucleus and superior oblique muscle (Nelson et al., 1986) because their anatomy enabled us to stimulate the muscle nerve in the orbit while preserving the functional integrity of the muscle. A total of

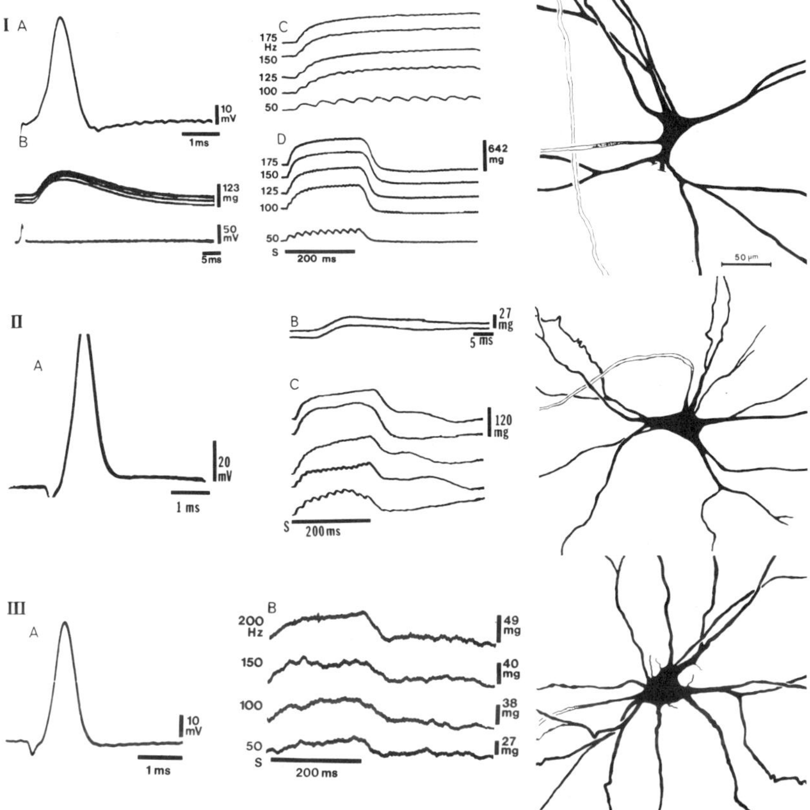

Fig. 12–1. Cat lateral rectus muscle motor units and cell body sizes of the innervating moto-neurons. (IA) Antidromic response recorded intracellularly. (IB) Five superimposed twitches of a powerful unit (top) and intracellular activation of a motoneuron (bottom). (IC) Tetanic stimuli delivered to motoneuron, with fusion occurring at about 150 Hz. (ID) Same sequence as in (IC), but at a slower sweep speed to illustrate the full 200-ms time course. The 200-ms bar in (ID) is 80 ms in (IC). Vertical bar in (ID) applies to (IC). (IIA) Antidromic response of another cell recorded intracellularly. (IIB) Two sweeps of this slower and weaker motor unit's twitch re-sponses. (IIC) Tetanic stimuli delivered to motoneuron, with fusion occurring at about 125 Hz. Sequence of tetanic frequencies in (IIC) is 50, 75, 100, 125, and 150 Hz from bottom to top. (IIIA) Antidromic response of a third cell recorded intracellularly. (IIIB) Tetanic stimuli delivered to motoneuron of this weak, non-twitch motor unit. Note the increase in tetanic tension with increasing stimulation frequency, even though the unit is always fused. The camera lucida draw-ing to the right of each (I, II, and III) mechanical illustration shows the motoneuron cell body sizes drawn to scale. (The unfilled line represents the axon in each drawing.) These HRP-injected motoneurons are all about 40 μm in diameter. The 50-μm bar in the top drawing applies to the bottom two drawings.

101 superior oblique motor units were studied with intracellular recording. Nontwitch units ($n = 5$) generally had slow conduction velocities, produced weak tetanic tensions, and were fatigue resistant. Their conduction velocities, however, did overlap with those of the twitch units. Twitch motor units ex-hibited a wide range of properties. Motoneuron rheobase and axon conduction velocity were directly related to muscle unit contraction speed and tension and

inversely related to input resistance. The linearity of these relationships was not perfect, but the trends were clear and consistent with relationships observed in limb muscle motor units (Wuerker et al., 1965; Stephens and Stuart, 1975; Fleshman et al., 1981; Burke et al., 1982).

In addition, this study, Nelson et al. (1986) incorporated an analysis of the fatigue properties of extraocular motor units. The equivalents of fast fatigable (FF), fast fatigue resistant (FR), and slow (S) units were observed (Burke, 1967, 1981; Burke et al., 1971, 1973). However, our attempts to subdivide the population of twitch units in a manner similar to that employed in Burke's (1981) studies did not yield convincing results. The superior oblique twitch motor unit population appeared as a continuum, and no single unit property or combination of properties permitted the units to cluster as in limb motor units.

The superior oblique conduction velocity study (Nelson et al., 1986) showed the best agreement, of the extraocular muscle studies, with Henneman's size principle. However, even the trochlear nucleus motoneuron pool exhibits an anatomical complexity. Some of the motoneurons that innervate the superior oblique muscle are present in the ipsilateral rather than the contralateral trochlear nucleus (Miyazaki, 1985), and we did not study those ipsilateral motoneurons or their muscle units.

The complexities of the lateral rectus and retractor bulbi innervation patterns (see the earlier discussion) led us to examine (Gurahian and Goldberg, 1987) whether these motor units exhibit a continuous distribution of fatigue indices similar to those of superior oblique motor units. All pure retractor bulbi motor units found in one or more of the four retractor bulbi muscle slips were readily fatigable. If the unit involved more than one slip, the muscle fibers in each slip exhibited similar fatigue properties. This finding (Gurahian and Goldberg, 1987) confirmed and extended Lennerstrand's (1974a) results on the cat retractor bulbi muscle, in which he studied one slip only. Although the number of pure lateral rectus motor units studied was not large, they were heterogeneous in their fatigue properties, as was seen in the superior oblique. The most interesting finding was that motor units split between the retractor bulbi and lateral rectus muscles did not exhibit uniform fatigue properties (Gurahian and Goldberg, 1987). The lateral rectus components of such units were heterogeneous in their fatigue properties, like their pure lateral rectus counterparts, while the retractor bulbi components were all fatigable, like their pure retractor bulbi counterparts. We do not feel that this finding negates the fact that motoneuron activity is involved in muscle fiber type differentiation (Close, 1965; Salmons and Vrbova, 1969; Vrbova et al., 1978), but it does suggest that other factors may also be involved in their determination (Edgerton et al., 1980; Dum et al., 1985). (See Fig. 12–2 for examples of fatigue.)

CONJUGATE HORIZONTAL EYE MOVEMENTS AT THE MOTOR UNIT LEVEL

Our studies of the mechanical properties of extraocular muscle units were extended to obtain information regarding the coordination of eye movements.

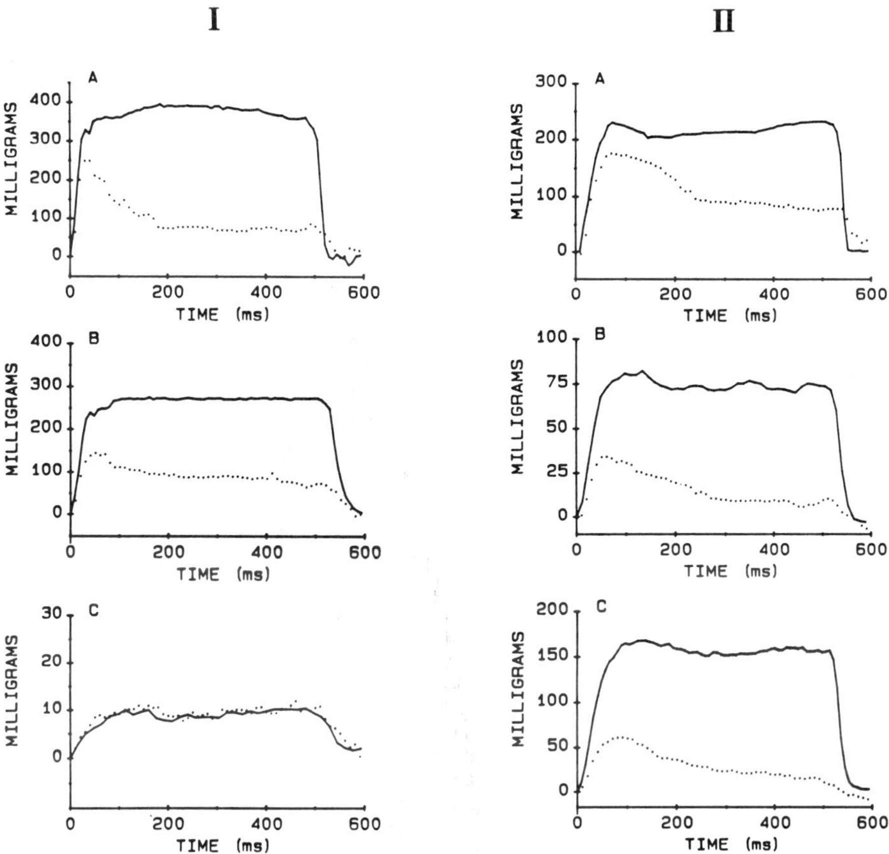

Fig. 12–2. Muscle mechanical response of three separate lateral rectus motor units to a 150-Hz fatigue test in column I. Solid line in each trace is tetanic tension of first stimulus train, and dotted line is tension after 1.5 min (same for column II). (IA) Fatigue index = 0.18. (IB) Fatigue index = 0.30. (IC) Fatigue index = 1.0. Muscle mechanical response of a single motor unit divided between the lateral rectus muscle (IIA) and two slips of the retractor bulbi muscle (IIB—superior lateral, IIC—inferior lateral). (IIA) Fatigue index = 0.3. (IIB) Fatigue index = 0.11. (IIC) Fatigue index = 0.1.

Motor units in different extraocular muscles that must act in precise synergy should have the same mechanical characteristics. We examined the motor units of both the lateral and medial rectus muscles under similar experimental conditions (Meredith and Goldberg, 1986). Previous studies had indicated that the inputs to the medial rectus subdivision of the oculomotor nucleus and the principal abducens nucleus were not identical (Baker and Highstein, 1978) and that the morphology of the motoneurons of the two nuclei was different (Evinger et al., 1979), e.g., medial rectus motoneurons possess axon collaterals that ramify in the nucleus (Evinger et al., 1979), while lateral rectus motoneurons do not possess such collaterals.

We were surprised to find significant differences in the speed-related and tension-related contractile properties between medial and lateral rectus twitch motor units (Meredith and Goldberg, 1986). Medial rectus units exhibited significantly faster twitch contractions and the rate of stimulation at which these units reached fused tetany was significantly higher than that of lateral rectus motor units. However, medial rectus units had significantly weaker maximum tetanic tensions and lower tetanus-to-twitch ratios than lateral rectus units. These findings indicate that different motoneuron discharge rates are needed to effect similar contractile conditions in the medial and lateral rectus muscles (see Fig. 12–3). Indeed, higher rate/position coefficients were observed for oculomotor as opposed to abducens motoneurons in behaving monkeys (Mays and Porter, 1984). A complex interaction of central and peripheral factors is probably needed to preserve the conjugacy of eye movements generated by agonist muscles with different inputs and contractile properties.

In summary, we have compiled a substantial amount of information about the mechanical characteristics of cat extraocular motor units. There have been studies of retractor bulbi, inferior, and superior oblique, as well as lateral and medial rectus motor units. Less exhaustive (and as yet unpublished) studies of both the cat superior and inferior rectus muscles have also been performed (Meredith, 1981). Table 12–1 indicates some mechanical properties of cat twitch motor units revealed by our studies. It includes data from muscles innervated by the abducens and oculomotor nerves. Cat superior oblique motor unit mechanics (trochlear nerve) are generally similar to those of units innervated by the oculomotor nerve.

It is interesting that the motor units innervated by midbrain nuclei are generally faster than either the pontine lateral rectus or retractor bulbi units. The retractor twitch units are clearly the slowest and, paradoxically, are uniformly fatigable.

SOME UNANSWERED QUESTIONS

Two related questions raised by our previous studies are: (1) Why did one of the first studies of extraocular motor unit mechanics (Lennerstrand, 1974b) yield a bimodal distribution of twitch motor unit speed–related properties, while more recent studies did not? (2) Have our fatigue tests been appropriately chosen to permit subdivision of extraocular motor units into fatigue-related categories, as Burke's (1981) tests have done for hindlimb motor units?

We have initiated studies on the cat inferior oblique muscle and nerve (Sorg et al., 1986) in order to answer these questions. One study has shown that the lateral (orbital) division of the inferior oblique muscle nerve contains fibers that innervate more slowly contracting twitch motor units than the medial (global) half of the nerve. This is in agreement with earlier findings (Sas and Schab, 1952) on this muscle nerve. HRP retrogradely transported in each nerve division revealed that the motoneurons in the inferior oblique subdivision of the oculomotor nucleus were not spatially segregated within the nucleus. However, smaller motoneurons were retrogradely labeled when HRP was applied to the lateral branch of the nerve. The 5-μm average difference in motoneuron

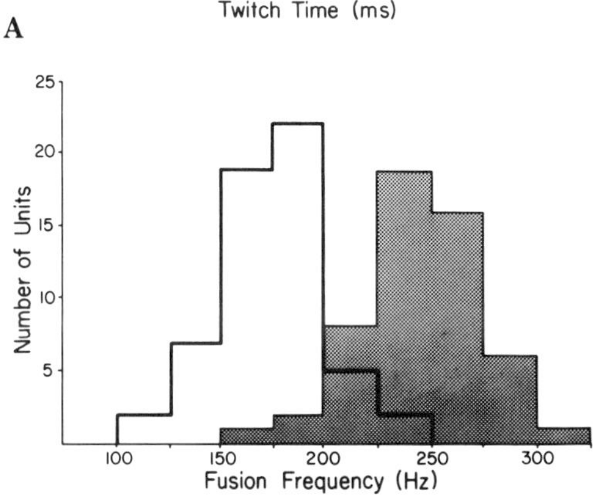

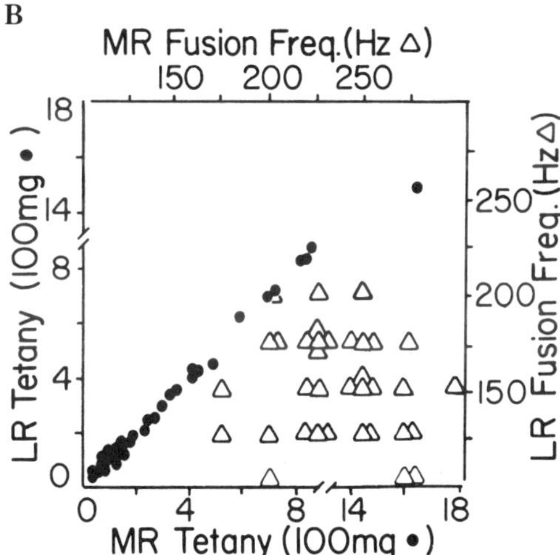

Fig. 12–3. (A) Distribution of lateral rectus (open bars) and medial rectus (shaded bars) fusion frequencies. (B) Medial rectus (MR) ($n = 34$) and lateral rectus (LR) ($n = 34$) motor units with similar (0–9% difference, mean = 2.4%) maximum tetanic tensions were paired, and the relationship of their tension to their rate-related properties was compared. A strong correlation between the tetanic tensions of the medial rectus–lateral rectus unit pairs is evident (filled circles), but there is no correlation of fusion frequencies among the same pairs (open triangles).

cell body size between medial and lateral branches of the nerve was statistically significant. These findings indicate that the inferior oblique muscle nerve appears to be "compartmentalized" (English and Weeks, 1984; Richmond et al., 1985; Weeks and English, 1987; Stuart et al., 1988), while the motor nucleus is not. In fact, Lennerstrand's (1974b) use of teased filaments from the medial and lateral divisions of the physiologically compartmentalized inferior oblique muscle nerve could well have yielded a bimodal speed-related motor unit distribution that would not have been evident if motoneurons had been sampled randomly from the nucleus.

The search for an appropriate fatigue test should be continued in the ex-

Table 12–1 Cat extraocular motor unit properties (averages)

	Contraction time (ms)	Fusion frequency (pps)	Twitch tension (mg)	Maximum tetanic tension (mg)
Retractor bulbi	9.6	170	50	450 (single slips)
Lateral rectus	6.5	165	40	375
Medial rectus	5.5	230	43	262
Superior rectus	5.9	235	45	309
Inferior rectus	5.9	240	40	224
Inferior oblique	5.4	260	20	142

Note: This table incorporates information from several studies to produce the average mechanical characteristics listed. Data from Goldberg et al. (1974, 1982), Lennerstrand (1974a, 1974b), Crandall et al., (1981), Goldberg et al. (1981), Meredith (1981), Meredith and Goldberg (1986), and Gurahian and Goldberg (1987) are included. Neither lateral rectus nor retractor bulbi motor units innervated by motoneurons in the oculomotor nucleus are included in the table.

traocular system because fatigue has proved to be an important factor in distinguishing limb muscle motor units. Fatigue typing might facilitate the examination of recruitment and rate coding in extraocular muscle, as it has in skeletal muscles. It might also allow a comparison of histochemical, mechanical, and axonal conduction velocity data in extraocular muscles, as well as provide information on the function of the nontwitch muscle fibers that are found almost exclusively in these muscles.

The phenomenon of muscle hysteresis might also be useful, alone or together with fatigue, in differentiating motor units. Hysteresis exists in extraocular motoneurons (Eckmiller, 1974; Goldstein and Robinson, 1986) and spinal cord innervated (Partridge, 1966, 1979) skeletal muscles: (1) this makes the systems unpredictable because one stimulus frequency can produce many levels of force, depending on activation history; (2) we know neither the form of such hysteresis loops nor the degree of hysteresis in extraocular muscle. What are the differences in hysteresis parameters that are dependent on motor unit type, and can those parameters help define motor unit type in conjunction with fatigue?

Our studies of cat extraocular motor units have revealed discrepancies from strict size-related correlations, as well as some novel features pertaining to motoneuron pools. Actual motoneuron size (Burke et al., 1982; Ulfhake and Kellerth, 1982; Cullheim et al., 1987) does not appear to be closely related to muscle unit contraction strength or speed. In contrast, axonal conduction velocity, motoneuron input resistance, and rheobase are correlated with muscle unit mechanics (Fleshman et al., 1981; Munson et al., 1984; Nelson et al., 1986). Motoneuron pools for the lateral rectus, superior oblique, and retractor bulbi muscles are certainly not in discrete brain stem locations. In what motoneuron pool do the motor units divided between the lateral rectus and retractor bulbi muscles belong? The nature of the nontwitch extraocular motor units, which are not found in spinal cord–innervated units, also needs further elucidation as to structure and function.

But even with the distinctions mentioned, it should now be clear that the important questions of motor unit recruitment, the size principle, and the nature of motoneuron pools are as relevant to our understanding of the extraocular motor control system as they are to our understanding of other motor systems. That studies of extraocular motor units have benefited from these basic ideas attests to their general applicability and usefulness. There is little doubt that these constructs will provide a background for future developments in the neuroscience of motor control.

Acknowledgments

Most of the students who have earned degrees in this laboratory have contributed to the information contained in this chapter. They include, in chronological order, Drs. J. S. Wilson, W. F. Crandall, M. A. Meredith, J. S. Nelson, S. A. Gurahian, and P. J. Sorg. My colleague in much of this work has been Dr. J. R. McClung, and technical assistance has been supplied by R. E. Revels, Jr., and A. J. Goldberg. My current student, M. A. Snyder, has given me invaluable assistance throughout the writing of this chapter.

These investigations were supported, in part, by NSF grant BNS-8507610.

REFERENCES

Alvarado, J., and Van Horn, C. (1975). Muscle cell types of the cat inferior oblique. In *Basic Mechanisms of Ocular Motility and Their Clinical Implications* (ed. Lennerstrand and P. Bach-y-Rita). Pergamon Press, Oxford, pp. 15–45.

Alvarado-Mallart, R. M., and Pincon-Raymond, M. (1979). The palisade endings of cat extraocular muscles: A light and electron microscopic study. *Tissue Cell* 11, 567–584.

Bach-y-Rita, P., and Ito, F. (1966). In vivo studies of fast and slow muscle fibers in cat extraocular muscles. *J. Gen. Physiol.* 49, 1177–1198.

Baker, R. (1986). Brainstem neurons are peculiar for oculomotor organization. *Prog. Brain Res.* 64, 257–271.

Baker, R., and Highstein, S. M. (1975). Physiological identification of interneurons and motoneurons in the abducens nucleus. *Brain Res.* 91, 292–298.

Baker, R., and Highstein, S. M. (1978). Vestibular projections to medial rectus subdivision of oculomotor nucleus. *J. Neurophysiol.* 41, 1629–1646.

Baker, R., and Precht, W. (1972). Electrophysiological properties of trochlear motoneurons as revealed by IVth nerve stimulation. *Exp. Brain Res.* 14, 127–157.

Baker, R. G., Mano, N., and Shimazu, H. (1969). Intracellular recording of antidromic responses from abducens motoneurons in the cat. *Brain Res.* 15, 573–576.

Barmack, N. H. (1974). Saccadic discharges evoked by intracellular stimulation of extraocular motoneurons. *J. Neurophysiol.* 37, 395–412.

Barmack, N. H. (1976). The relationship of afterhyperpolarizations of extraocular motoneurons to membrane potential. *J. Neurosci. Res.* 2, 433–438.

Barmack, N. H. (1977). Recruitment and suprathreshold frequency modulation of single extraocular muscle fibers in the rabbit. *J. Neurophysiol.* 40, 779–790.

Bondi, A. Y., and Chiarandini, D. J. (1979). Ionic basis for electrical properties of tonic fibres in rat extraocular muscles. *J. Physiol.* 295, 273–281.

Bondi, A. Y., and Chiarandini, D. J. (1983). Morphologic and electrophysiologic identification of multiply innervated fibers in rat extraocular muscles. *Invest. Ophthalmol.* 24, 517–519.

Burke, R. E. (1967). Motor unit types of cat triceps surae muscle. *J. Physiol.* 193, 141–160.

Burke, R. E. (1981). Motor units: Anatomy, physiology and functional organization. In *Handbook of Physiology*, Vol. II, Sect. 1, Part 1: *The Nervous System: Motor Control* (ed V. B. Brooks). American Physiological Society, Bethesda, Md., pp. 345–422.

Burke, R. E., Dum, R. P., Fleshman, J. W., Glenn, L. L., Lev-Tov, A., O'Donovan, M. J., and Pinter, M. J. (1982). An HRP study of the relation between cell size and motor unit type in cat ankle extensor motoneurons. *J. Comp. Neurol.* 209, 17–28.

Burke, R. E., Levine, D. N., Tsairis, P., and Zajac, F. E. (1973). Physiological types and histochemical profiles in motor units of the cat gastrocnemius. *J. Physiol.* 234, 723–748.

Burke, R. E., Levine, D. N., Zajac, F. E., Tsairis, P., and Engel, W. K. (1971). Mammalian motor units: Physiological–histochemical correlation in three types in cat gastrocnemius. *Science* 174, 709–712.

Burke, R. E., Strick, P. L., Kanda, K., Kim, C. C., and Walmsley, B. (1977). Anatomy of medial gastrocnemius and soleus motor nuclei in cat spinal cord. *J. Neurophysiol.* 40, 667–680.

Chiarandini, D. J. (1976). Activation of two types of fibers in rat extraocular muscles. *J. Physiol.* 259, 199–212.

Chiarandini, D. J., and Davidowitz, J. (1979). Structure and function of extraocular muscle fibers. *Curr. Topics Eye Res.* 1, 91–142.

Chiarandini, D. J., and Stefani, E. (1979). Electrophysiological identification of two types of fibers in rat extraocular muscles. *J. Physiol.* 290, 453–465.

Clamann, H. P., Ngai, A. C., Kukulka, C. G., and Goldberg, S. J. (1983). Motor pool organization in monosynaptic reflexes: Responses in three different muscles. *J. Neurophysiol.* 50, 725–742.

Close, R. (1965). Effects of cross-union of motor nerves to fast and slow skeletal muscles. *Nature* 206, 831–832.

Close, R. I., and Luff, A. R. (1974). Dynamic properties of inferior rectus muscle of the rat. *J. Physiol.* 236, 259–270.

Crandall, W. F., Goldberg, S. J., Wilson, J. S., and McClung, J. R. (1981). Muscle units divided among retractor bulbi muscle slips and between the lateral rectus and retractor bulbi muscles in cat. *Exp. Neurol.* 71, 251–260.

Cullheim, S., Fleshman, J. W., Glenn, L. L., and Burke, R. E. (1987). Membrane area and dendritic structure in type-identified triceps surae alpha motoneurons. *J. Comp. Neurol.* 255, 68–81.

Delgado-Garcia, J. M., del Pozo, F., and Baker, R. (1986). Behavior of neurons in the abducens nucleus of the alert cat—I. Motoneurons. *Neuroscience* 17, 929–952.

Destombes, J., Durand, J., Gogan, P., Gueritaud, J. P., Horcholle-Bossavit, G., and Tyc-Dumont, S. (1983). Ultrastructural and electrophysiological properties of accessory abducens nucleus motoneurons: An intracellular horseradish peroxidase study in the cat. *Neuroscience* 10, 1317–1332.

Dum, R. P., O'Donovan, M. J., Toop, J., and Burke, R. E. (1985). Cross-reinnervated motor units in cat muscle. I. Flexor digitorum longus muscle units reinnervated by soleus motor neurons. *J. Neurophysiol.* 54, 818–836.

Eckmiller, R. (1974). Hysteresis in the static characteristics of eye position coded in the alert monkey. *Pflugers Arch.* 350, 249–258.

Edgerton, B. R., Goslow, G. E., Rasmussen, S. A., and Spector, S. A. (1980). Is resistance of a muscle to fatigue controlled by its motoneurons? *Nature* 285, 589–590.

English, A. W., and Weeks, O. I. (1984). Compartmentalization of single muscle units in cat lateral gastrocnemius. *Exp. Brain Res.* 56, 361–368.

Evinger, C., Baker, R., and McCrea, R. (1979). Axon collaterals of the cat medial rectus motoneurons. *Brain Res.* 174, 153–160.

Fleshman, J. W., Munson, J. B., Sypert, G. W., and Friedman, W. A. (1981). Rheobase, input resistance, and motor-unit type in medial gastrocnemius motoneurons in the cat *J. Neurophysiol.* 46, 1326–1338.

Fuchs, A. F., Kaneko, C. R. S., and Scudder, C. A. (1985). Brainstem control of saccadic eye movements. *Ann. Rev. Neurosci.* 8, 307–337.

Gacek, R. R. (1974). Localization of neurons supplying the extraocular muscles in kitten using horseradish peroxidase. *Exp. Neurol.* 44, 381–403.

Gacek, R. R. (1979). Location of abducens afferent neurons in the cat. *Exp. Neurol.* 64, 342–353.

Goldberg, S. J., Clamann, H. P., and McClung, J. R. (1981). Relation between motoneuron position and lateral rectus motor unit contraction speed: An intracellular study in the cat abducens nucleus. *Neurosci. Lett.* 23, 49–54.

Goldberg, S. J., Hull, C. D., and Buchwald, N. A. (1974). Afferent projections in the abducens nerve: An intracellular study. *Brain Res.* 68, 205–214.

Goldberg, S. J., Lennerstrand, G., and Hull, C. D. (1976). Motor unit responses in the lateral rectus muscle of the cat: Intracellular current injection of abducens nucleus neurons. *Acta Physiol. Scand.* 96, 58–63.

Goldberg, S. J., and McClung, J. R. (1982). Lack of firm relation between motoneuron size and muscle unit mechanical characteristics in cat extraocular motor units. *Soc. Neurosci. Abst.* 8, 959.

Goldstein, H. P., and Robinson, D. A. (1986). Hysteresis and slow drift in abducens unit activity. *J. Neurophysiol.* 55, 1044–1056.

Gomez, C., Torres, B., Jimenez-Ridruejo, G., and Delgado-Garcia, J. M. (1986). A quantitative analysis of abducens motoneuron behavior during saccadic eye movements in the alert cat. *Neurosci Res.* 3, 345–350.

Grant, K., Gueritaud, J. P., Horcholle-Bossavit, G., and Tyc-Dumont, S. (1979a). Morphological characteristics of lateral rectus motoneurones shown by intracellular injection of HRP. *J. Physiol.* 75, 513–519.

Grant, K., Gueritaud, J. P., Horcholle-Bossavit, G., and Tyc-Dumont, S. (1979b). Anatomical and electrophysiological identification of motoneurons supplying the cat retractor bulbi muscle. *Exp. Brain Res.* 34, 541–550.

Grantyn, R., and Grantyn, A. (1978). Morphological and electrophysiological properties of cat abducens motoneurons. *Exp. Brain Res.* 31, 249–274.

Grantyn, R., Grantyn, A., and Schaaf, P. (1977). Conduction velocity, input resistance and size of cat ocular motoneurons stained with procion yellow. *Brain Res.* 135, 167–173.

Gurahian, S. M., and Goldberg, S. J. (1987). Fatigue of lateral rectus and retractor bulbi motor units in cat. *Brain Res.* 415, 281–292.

Hanson, J., and Lennerstrand, G. (1977). Contractile and histochemical properties of the inferior oblique muscle in the rat and in the cat. *Acta Ophthalmol.* 55, 88–102.

Henneman, E. (1985). The size-principle: A deterministic output emerges from a set of probabilistic connections. *J. Exp. Biol.* 115, 105–112.

Henneman, E., and Mendell, L. M. (1981). Functional organization of motoneuron pool and its inputs. In *Handbook of Physiology*, Vol. II, Sect. 1, Part 1: *The*

Nervous System: Motor Control. (ed. V. B. Brooks). American Physiological Society, Bethesda, Md., pp. 423–507.

Hess, A. (1961). The structure of slow and fast extrafusal muscle fibers in the extraocular muscles and their nerve endings in guinea pigs. *J. Cell Comp. Physiol.* 58, 63–80.

Hess, A., and Pilar, G. (1963). Slow fibers in the extraocular muscles of the cat. *J. Physiol.* 169, 780–798.

Highstein, S. M., Karabelas, A., Baker, R., and McCrea, R. A. (1982). Comparison of the morphology of physiologically identified abducens motor and internuclear neurons in the cat: A light microscopic study employing the intracellular injection of horseradish peroxydase. *J. Comp. Neurol.* 208, 369–381.

Hoffer, J. A., Loeb, G. E., Sugano, N., Marks, W. B., O'Donovan, M. J., and Pratt, C. A. (1987). Cat hindlimb motoneurons during locomotion. III. Functional segregation in sartorius. *J. Neurophysiol.* 57, 554–562.

Hutson, K. A., Glendenning, K. K., and Masterton, R. B. (1979). Accessory abducens nucleus and its relationship to the accessory facial and posterior trigeminal nuclei in cat. *J. Comp. Neurol.* 188, 1–16.

Kerns, J. M. (1980). Postnatal differentiation of the rat trochlear nerve. *J. Comp. Neurol.* 189, 291–306.

Lennerstrand, G. (1972). Fast and slow units in extrinsic eye muscles of cat. *Acta Physiol. Scand.* 86, 285–288.

Lennerstrand, G. (1974a). Mechanical studies on the retractor bulbi muscle and its motor units in the cat. *J. Physiol.* 236, 43–55.

Lennerstrand, G. (1974b). Electrical activity and isometric tension in motor units of the cat's inferior oblique muscle. *Acta Physiol. Scand.* 91, 458–474.

Lennerstrand, G., and Bach-y-Rita, P. (1974). Activation of slow motor units by threshold stimulation of cat eye muscle nerves. *Invest. Ophthalmol.* 13, 879–882.

Lennerstrand, G., and Nichols, K. C. (1977). Morphology of motor units in cat extraocular muscle. *Acta Ophthalmol.* 55, 913–918.

Mayr, R. (1971). Structure and distribution of fibre types in the external eye muscles of the rat. *Tissue Cell,* 3, 433–462.

Mayr, R., Gottschall, J., Gruber, H., and Neuhuber, W. (1975). Internal structure of cat extraocular muscle. *Anat. Embryol.* 148, 25–34.

Mays, L. E., and Porter, J. D. (1984). Neural control of vergence eye movements: Activity of abducens and oculomotor neurons. *J. Neurophysiol.* 52, 743–761.

McClung, J. R., Goldberg, S. J., Nelson, J. S., and Fowlkes, C. H. (1983). Oculomotor nucleus innervation of the lateral rectus muscle in the cat. *Soc. Neurosci. Abst.* 9, 13.

McCrea, R. A., Strassman, A., and Highstein, S. M. (1986). Morphology and physiology of abducens motoneurons and internuclear neurons intracellularly injected with horseradish peroxidase in alert squirrel monkeys. *J. Comp. Neurol.* 243, 291–308.

Meredith, M. A. (1981). Contractile responses of extraocular motor units controlled by the oculomotor nucleus in the cat: An intracellular stimulation study. Ph.D. thesis, Virginia Commonwealth University.

Meredith, M. A., and Goldberg, S. J. (1986). Contractile differences between motor units in the medial rectus and lateral rectus muscles in the cat. *J. Neurophysiol.* 56, 50–61.

Meredith, M. A., McClung, J. R., and Goldberg, S. J. (1981). Retractor bulbi muscle responses to oculomotor nerve and nucleus stimulation in the cat. *Brain Res.* 211, 427–432.

Miyazaki, S. (1985). Bilateral innervation of the superior oblique muscle by the trochlear nucleus. *Brain Res.* 348, 52–56.

Munson, J. B., Fleshman, J. W., Zengel, J. E., and Sypert, G. W. (1984). Synaptic and mechanical coupling between type-identified motor units and individual spindle afferents of medial gastrocnemius muscle of the cat. *J. Neurophysiol.* 51, 1268–1283.

Naito, H., Tanimura, K.-I., Taga, N., and Hosoya, Y. (1974). Microelectrode study on the subnuclei of the oculomotor nucleus in the cat. *Brain Res.* 81, 215–231.

Nelson, J. S., Goldberg, S. J., and McClung, J. R. (1986). Motoneuron electrophysiological and muscle contractile properties of superior oblique motor units in cat. *J. Neurophysiol.* 55, 715–726.

Pachter, B. R. (1982). Fiber composition of the superior rectus extraocular muscle of the rhesus macaque. *J. Morphol.* 174, 237–250.

Pachter, B. R. (1983). Rat extraocular muscle. 1. Three dimensional cytoarchitecture, component fiber populations and innervation. *J. Anat.* 137, 143–159.

Pachter, B. R. (1984). Rat extraocular muscle. 3. Histochemical variability along the length of multiply-innervated fibers of the orbital surface layer. *Histochemistry* 80, 535–538.

Pachter, B. R., and Colbjornsen, C. (1983). Rat extraocular muscle. 2. Histochemical fibre types. *J. Anat.* 137, 161–170.

Partridge, L. D. (1966). Signal-handling characteristics of load-moving skeletal muscle. *Am. J. Physiol.* 210, 1178–1191.

Partridge, L. D. (1979). Muscle properties: A problem for the motor controller physiologist. In *Posture and Movement* (ed. R. F. Talbot and D. P. Humphreys). Raven Press, New York, pp. 189–229.

Peachey, L., Takeichi, M., and Nag, A. C. (1974). Muscle fiber types and innervation in adult cat extraocular muscles. In A. T. Milhorst (ed.), *Exploratory Concepts in Muscular Dystrophy,* Vol. II (ed. A. T. Milhorst). Elsevier, New York, pp. 246–257.

Pilar, G. (1967). Further study of the electrical and mechanical responses of slow fibers in cat extraocular muscles. *J. Gen. Physiol.* 50, 2289–2300.

Remmel, R. S., and Marrocco, R. T. (1975). Impulse generation properties of abducens motoneurons. *Vision Res.* 15, 1039–1043.

Richmond, F. J. R., MacGillis, D. R. R., and Scott, D. A. (1985). Muscle-fiber compartmentalization in cat splenius muscles. *J. Neurophysiol.* 53, 868–885.

Robinson, D. A. (1970). Oculomotor unit behavior in the monkey. *J. Neurophysiol.* 33, 393–404.

Robinson, D. A. (1986). The systems approach to the oculomotor system. *Vision Res.* 26, 91–99.

Russell-Mergenthal, H., McClung, J. R., and Goldberg, S. J. (1986). The determination of dendrite morphology on lateral rectus motoneurons in cat. *J. Comp. Neurol.* 245, 116–122.

Salmons, S., and Vrbova, G. (1969). The influence of activity on some contractile characteristics of mammalian fast and slow muscles. *J. Physiol.* 201, 535–549.

Sas, J., and Schab, R. (1952). Die sogenannten "Palisaden-Endigungen" der Augenmuskeln. *Acta Morphol. Acad. Sci. Hung.* 2, 259–266.

Sasaki, K. (1963). Electrophysiological studies on oculomotor neurons of the cat. *Jpn. J. Physiol.* 13, 287–302.

Sorg, P. J., Goldberg, S. J., and McClung, J. R. (1986). Mechanical properties of the cat inferior oblique muscle with respect to the anatomy of the nerve and nucleus. *Soc. Neurosci. Abst.* 12, 1419.

Spencer, R. F., Baker, R., and McCrea, R. A. (1980). Localization and morphology of cat retractor bulbi motoneurons. *J. Neurophysiol.* 43, 754–770.

Spencer, R. F., and Porter, J. D. (1981). Innervation and structure of extraocular muscles in the monkey in comparison to those of the cat. *J. Comp. Neurol.* 198, 649–665.

Spencer, R. F., and Sterling, P. (1977). An electron microscope study of motoneurons and interneurons in the cat abducens nucleus identified by retrograde intraaxonal transport of horseradish peroxidase. *J. Comp. Neurol.* 176, 65–86.

Steiger, H. J., and Buttner-Ennever, J. A. (1978). Relationship between motoneurons and internuclear neurons in the abducens nucleus: A double retrograde tracer study in the cat. *Brain Res.* 148, 181–188.

Stephens, J. A., and Stuart, D. G. (1975). The motor units of cat medial gastrocnemius: Speed–size relations and their significance for the recruitment order of motor units. *Brain Res.* 91, 177–195.

Stuart, D. G., Hamm, T. M., and Vanden Noven, S. (1988). Partitioning of mono-synaptic Ia EPSP connections with motoneurons according to neuromuscular to-pography: Generality and functional implications. *Prog. Neurobiol.* 30, 437–447.

Tarlov, E., and Tarlov, S. R. (1971). The representation of extraocular muscles in the oculomotor nuclei: Experimental studies in the cat. *Brain Res.* 34, 37–52.

Tredici, G., Pizzini, G., and Milanesi, S. (1976). The ultrastructure of the nucleus of the oculomotor nerve (somatic efferent portion) of the cat. *Anat. Embryol.* 149, 323–346.

Ulfhake, B., and Kellerth, J. O. (1982). Does α-motoneurone size correlate with motor unit type in cat triceps surae? *Brain Res.* 251, 201–209.

Ulfhake, B., and Kellerth, J. O. (1984). Electrophysiological and morphological mea-surements in cat gastrocnemius and soleus α-motoneurones. *Brain Res.* 307, 167–179.

Vrbova, G., Gordon, T., and Jones, R. (1978). *Nerve–Muscle Interaction.* Chapman and Hall, London, pp. 133–144.

Weeks, O. I., and English, A. W. (1987). Cat triceps surae motor nuclei are organized topologically *Exp. Neurol.* 96, 163–177.

Wuerker, R. B., McPhedran, A. M., and Henneman, E. (1965). Properties of motor units in a heterogeneous pale muscle (m. gastrocnemius) of the cat. *J. Neuro-physiol.* 28, 85–99.

Zajac, F. E., and Faden, J. S. (1985). Relationship among recruitment order, axonal conduction velocity, and muscle-unit properties of type-identified motor units in cat plantaris muscle. *J. Neurophysiol.* 53, 1303–1322.

13

Changes That Occur in Motor Units During Activity
Causes and Amelioration of Fatigue

H. PETER CLAMANN

> Skeletal muscles and the motoneurons that control them are the products of evolution. Survival placed a premium on speed of movement to capture prey or escape predators, on the capacity to resist fatigue, on a favorable ratio between the weight and strength of muscle, and, perhaps above all, on efficient use of energy. (Henneman, 1980, p. 674)

The idea of fatigue is not unlike the idea of quality: We all know what it is when we see it, but it is very difficult to define. Fatigue can take many forms, and the intensity of each is graded from the imperceptible to the incapacitating. Its many forms and its very familiarity make the discussion of fatigue a problem. This chapter attempts to simplify that problem by limiting consideration to neuromuscular fatigue. It will be restricted to physical and chemical changes that occur in the motor unit: the motoneuron and all the muscle fibers it innervates. Activation and inhibition of motoneurons, fatigue of neural circuits, central drive, and motivation are beyond the scope of the discussion.

Attempts are often made to define fatigue by introducing the notion that fatigue is a delayed result of physical activity; first, there is fresh activity, and then, after a definable interval, fatigue sets in. The contrast between the two states can then define fatigue. But this does not work; the onset of fatigue is as difficult to define as fatigue itself. It is best to discard the idea that fatigue occurs when some process crosses a definable threshold or that it has an onset at all. There is probably no such thing as an unfatigued state. Bigland-Ritchie et al. (1986a, p. 137) have stated it well:

> Fatigue is an integral part of all forms of physical activity, and the factors responsible for it start to appear immediately after the onset of exercise. When one

makes a sustained maximal effort the force that can be developed starts to fall at once. . . . Fatigue has often been defined as an inability to maintain the expected force or power output (Edwards, 1981). This implies that it is in some way different from normal exercise. We prefer Simonson and Weiser's (1976) definition: a transient loss of work *capacity* resulting from preceding work regardless of whether or not the current performance is affected.

The continuous nature of fatigue can be illustrated by two quite different examples. A single motor unit known to be fatigable may be stimulated continually over an extended period. When this is done, the force never reaches a plateau; fatigue probably develops from the first stimulus, and the loss of contractile capacity increases even as force builds up. The electrical activity (electromyogram, EMG) changes throughout the test as well, although the change may be small. These effects are seen when stimuli are delivered continuously at a high stimulus frequency (100 pps; Wuerker et al., 1965; Clamann and Robinson, 1985) and at lower discharge rates produced by steady current injection into the motoneuron (Kernell and Monster, 1982).

Such stimulation may be considered unphysiological, so a less stressful pattern of stimuli may be used: the one introduced by Burke (Burke et al., 1973) to define a standard fatigue test for motor units. A fatigable motor unit is stimulated with a train of 13 pulses lasting for 330 ms; these trains are delivered once per second. The frequency is much lower than in the previous test, and the unit is allowed to "rest" two-thirds of the time. Single twitches may be elicited during the rest periods to measure twitch force and speed (Dubose et al., 1987). In these circumstances, force also changes continuously, as many published records illustrate (Burke et al., 1973; Kernell et al., 1975; Reinking et al., 1975). Figure 13–1 illustrates such a record. Motor unit speed, as judged by the twitch contraction time, changes continuously as well. The time to peak of the twitches may increase to over 50 ms before the twitches become so small that measurement can no longer be made. The half-relaxation time shows similar continuous changes.

These examples readily show that muscle undergoes many changes during activity and that the changes are continuous. Some, such as force loss, are obviously related to fatigue; others, such as contractile slowing, are not. In fact, it may be possible to take advantage of contractile slowing to forestall muscle fatigue: Since a slowly contracting muscle requires a lower discharge frequency to produce maximum force than does a rapidly contracting one, a lower, less fatiguing stimulus rate can produce high levels of force as muscle contraction slows.

I begin by examining some mechanisms by which fatigue occurs. I then consider how the control and design of muscles are related to fatigue. Although fatigue has long fascinated physiologists (Mosso, 1915), a full understanding of its effects was not possible until the pioneering work of Henneman and his co-workers provided an explanation for the way a muscle is organized to produce reflex and voluntary movements (Henneman et al., 1965a, 1965b) and revealed the range of motor units, strong and weak, fatigable and fatigue resistant, that subserve those movements (Henneman and Olson, 1965). Finally,

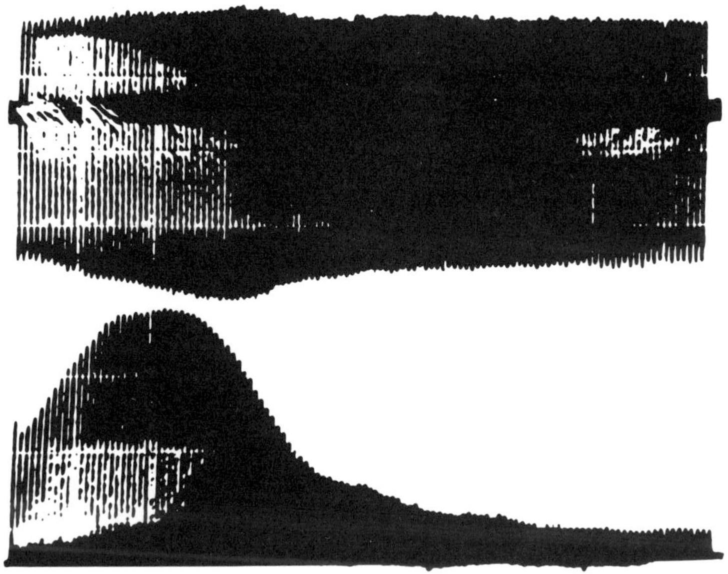

Fig. 13–1. EMG waveforms (above) and force (below) of an FF motor unit subjected to Burke's fatigue test. Observe that neither EMG amplitude nor force reaches a plateau level; rather, they change continuously. Calibration: EMG, 500 μV; force: 5 g; time, 25 sec.

some changes occurring in muscle will be described that may be used to postpone or minimize fatigue.

CHANGES PRODUCING FATIGUE IN ACTIVE MUSCLE

The signal that commands a muscle contraction begins as the discharge of a motoneuron and is carried to the muscle in a chain of events illustrated in Figure 13–2. Each link in that chain is susceptible to changes produced by repeated activity, and each link may alter the signal or fail to transmit it further. Loss of muscle force may occur from transmission failure in the nerve axon, at the neuromuscular junction, or in the muscle fiber. Once the muscle fiber has propagated the signal, it may fail to complete the process of excitation–contraction coupling or provide the chemical-mechanical reaction that generates force (Clamann, 1987). Let us examine these steps in detail.

Nerve axons and muscle fibers share a common property: Both are bounded by excitable membranes, so that both conduct action potentials by similar ionic mechanisms. Hence both are subject to similar limitations, resulting in fatigue: Repeated activation results in the flow of K^+ ions out of the fiber and into the extracellular space. The consequent progressive depolarization of the fiber can lead to conduction block (Smith and Hatt, 1976). In the nerve fiber this is most

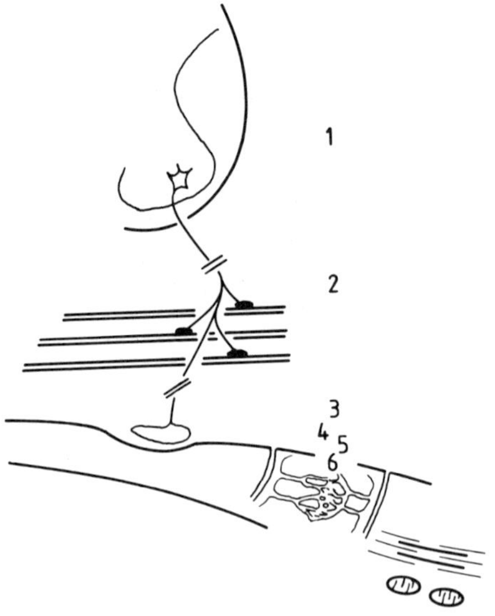

Fig. 13–2. Diagrammatic representation of a motor unit, showing (1) location of a motoneuron in the spinal cord; (2) part of the muscle unit with myoneural junctions at greater magnification; (3,4) the presynaptic bouton and muscle fiber membrane; (5,6) the sarcoplasmic reticulum and t-tubule system; and (7,8) the contractile system and mitochondria. Sites 1–4 are sites of electrical fatigue that may be recognized by EMG changes, sites 5 and 6 are sites of electrical fatigue that is not reflected in the EMG, and sites 7 and 8 are sites of contractile or metabolic fatigue. (From Clamann, 1987.)

likely to occur at axonal branch points, where the safety factor for propagation is lowest to begin with. It has been shown that high-frequency stimulation can lead to such block in motor units (Krnjevic and Miledi, 1958; Smith, 1980; Clamann and Robinson, 1985). The block begins most distally in the axon (Smith, 1980) and probably involves only one or a few muscle fibers at first, but then progressively larger groups of muscle fibers fail to receive a signal as more proximal nerve branches are blocked (Clamann and Robinson, 1985). It is not clear if motor units normally discharge fast enough for a long enough period of time to produce such nerve conduction blocks. Although electrical failure is a known cause of muscle fatigue, it probably occurs at or beyond the neuromuscular junction.

One possible fatigue mechanism may be eliminated immediately. The neuromuscular junction does not run out of transmitter in normal activity. Krnjevic and Miledi (1958) showed long ago that after transmission across the neuromuscular junction was no longer possible, miniature endplate potentials continued to appear with normal frequency and size, showing that spontaneous release of transmitter continued normally.

The muscle fiber membrane is a complex structure that is particularly vulnerable to electrical block. The surface of the muscle fiber is indented by the t-tubular system; the "insides" of the t-tubules are effectively part of the extracellular space. To activate the sarcomeres in the interior of the muscle fiber, the action potential must reach into their vicinity by fully invading the t-tubules (Adrian et al., 1969; Adrian and Peachey, 1973). In effect, the surface area of the muscle fiber is much larger than that of an equivalent cylinder. As a result, conduction is much slower than the size of the muscle fiber would lead one to expect (Adrian, 1983), and the shape of the action potential is altered by ionic changes in the t-tubules (Adrian et al., 1969; Adrian and Peachey, 1973). Depolarizing currents still exist in these tubules after the action potential at the surface has decayed; the result is a prolonged afterdepolarization following the action potential recorded at the surface of the muscle fiber (Adrian and Peachey, 1973). Both the amplitude and the duration of this afterpotential are positively correlated with muscle fiber diameter, as might be expected (calculated from Fig. 8 in Adrian and Peachey, 1973).

The complex geometry of the muscle fiber membrane offers numerous opportunities for electrical fatigue. It is well known that the motor unit action potential increases in duration and decreases in amplitude with repetitive activity (Krnjevic and Miledi, 1958; Grabowski et al., 1972; Bigland-Ritchie, 1981; Bigland-Ritchie et al., 1983; Clamann and Robinson, 1985). This has been attributed to accumulation of ions in the t-tubular system and in the extracellular space. This extracellular space is small, being approximately 10% the size of the intracellular space (Sjøgaard and Saltin, 1982). This is very different from the classical "squid giant axon environment," in which the extracellular space is effectively infinite, and only changes in intracellular concentration can affect conduction. Accumulation of K^+ is known to occur in the extracellular space of muscle (Bigland-Ritchie et al., 1979; Jones et al., 1979; Jones, 1981; Jennische et al., 1982; Sjøgaard, 1983), and Ca^{2+} accumulation (Bianchi and Narayan, 1982) and shifts of other ions and water have been demonstrated as well (Sjøgaard and Saltin, 1982; Sjøgaard, 1983; Sjøgaard et al., 1985). These ions can easily interfere with propagation of the action potential along the fiber and into the t-tubular system (Grabowski et al., 1972; Lüttgau and Spiecker, 1979; Jones, 1981; Jennische et al., 1982; Noma and Shibasaki, 1985). In this way, graded fatigue can occur when not all sarcomeres of a muscle fiber are activated (Adrian et al., 1969; Adrian and Peachey, 1973; Peachey, 1985). Electrical fatigue can thus occur by a graded decline of the muscle fiber action potential, and may produce incomplete activation of individual muscle fibers or activation of only some of the fibers of a motor unit. It must be noted that a large safety factor exists in excitation–contraction coupling (Katz, 1966; Carlson and Wilkie, 1976), so that the muscle fiber action potential can decline considerably before a fall in force occurs (Clamann and Robinson, 1985).

We have seen that the action potential may fail to penetrate all of the branches of a motor axon or, having reached the neuromuscular junction, may fail to excite a certain number of muscle fibers. These events result in partial activation of motor units and are recognized as electrical fatigue, since they produce a decline in average electrical activity (integrated electromyogram, or IEMG). An experimental model of such partial activation was presented some years ago by Locke and Henneman (1960). If the failure is axonal, step-like fluctuations in both EMG and force may result (Clamann and Robinson, 1985).

The final source of fatigue is a depletion of metabolic substrates necessary for force generation. Although it is possible to deplete muscle fibers of glycogen completely (Edstrom and Kugelberg, 1968; Burke et al., 1973), it is not clear that substrate depletion is actually a cause of fatigue. If ATP is fully depleted, the fatigued muscle should go into rigor, and rigor is not seen in fatigue. Subjects exercised to exhaustion show some remaining glycogen in the exhausted muscles (Gollnick et al., 1974; Vollestad et al., 1984; Vollestad and

Blom, 1985). Interestingly, it is the slow-twitch muscle fibers that are most thoroughly depleted. Bigland-Ritchie and co-workers have recently argued that exhaustion is not due to metabolic depletion. They asked volunteer subjects to produce submaximal contractions at regular intervals to exhaustion. While both the maximum force a subject could produce and the maximum force elicited by tetanic stimulation fell to 50% or less of the initial values, the EMG remained normal. In addition, biopsies revealed considerable glycogen depletion in type I muscle fibers and far less in types IIa and IIb. The authors concluded that adequate stores of glycogen remained to sustain further contractions. The cause of "metabolic" fatigue was attributed to failure of excitation–contraction coupling (Bigland-Ritchie et al., 1986a). EMG records would not show this, since it can be assumed that the muscle fiber action potential need not be severely distorted at the muscle surface by blockage in the t-tubular system or by later events, and only force would fall. This is corroborated indirectly by the observation that recovery from fatigue, particularly from fatigue produced by sustained contractions or stimulations, is usually very rapid. Recovery from metabolic fatigue might be expected to take many minutes or hours as metabolites are replenished. Instead, recovery of force production often occurs in much less than a second. Two examples of fatigue and rapid recovery are shown in Figure 13–3. A motor unit may be stimulated with a train of pulses whose instantaneous frequency rises from near zero to above the unit's tetanic fusion frequency and then declines linearly back to zero. If the unit is of type FF, three cycles of such "triangular stimulation" are sufficient to produce fatigue. This is seen as a decline in force and EMG amplitude (Fig. 13–3, top). Force decline probably occurs first and is not a result of electrical failure in these units, since force is known to decline before EMG when FF motor units are stimulated continuously at high frequencies (Clamann and Robinson, 1985) or intermittently at lower frequencies (Burke et al., 1973; see also Fig. 13–1).

The striking thing about the recovery from such fatigue is its speed. Force may actually rise as stimulus frequency declines below about 40 pps, showing that the "rest" periods produced by interpulse intervals of 25 ms are sufficient for recovery. A similar recovery is seen when fatigable motor units are subjected to Burke's fatigue test (Burke et al., 1973). Stimulation at 40 pps for 330 ms, repeated every second, produces a fall in force to below 25% of its initial value in under 2 min. As force falls, inspection of the force and EMG output during individual trains shows marked fatigue *within* each train (Fig. 13–3, bottom). Thus, there is recovery in the 670-ms rest period between trains. The first stimuli of the next train produce a high force and EMG, which falls again during the train. This may be seen in Figure 13–3, bottom.

Although recovery from fatigue may be very rapid after strong effort, recovery of endurance is not. It takes much less time to exhaust a motor unit a second time than a first time (Petrofsky et al., 1980). Recovery of endurance after the fatigue induced by Burke's fatigue test can take 45 min or longer (Clamann and Robinson, 1985).

A remarkable feature of motor units, whether fatigable of fatigue resistant, is how well their components (motor axon, neuromuscular junction, muscle fiber) are matched in their respective resistance to fatigue. Fatigable motor units

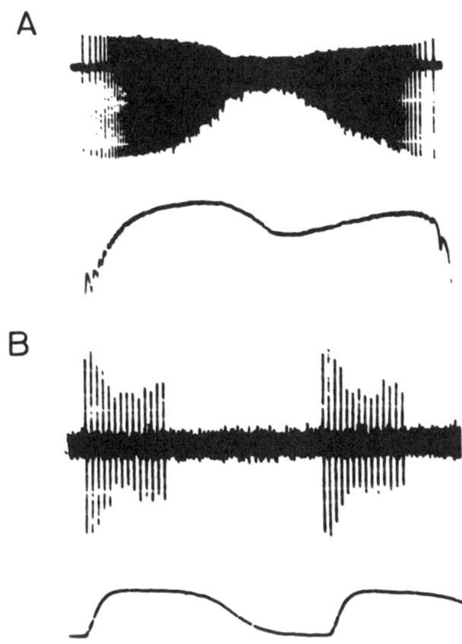

Fig. 13–3. Two examples of rapid recovery from fatigue. (A) A motor unit was stimulated with a train of pulses that varied linearly from 0 to 100 pps and back to 0. The top trace shows EMG pulses; the lower trace, force output of the unit. Note that EMG and force fall off during high-frequency stimulation, and both recover as stimulus frequency slows. (B) Burke's fatigue test carried out on an FF motor unit. EMG pulses above, force below. Note that EMG amplitude falls during each 330-ms train and has recovered at the onset of the next train. This record also illustrates motor unit slowing. The force record is fully fused during 40 pps stimulation, although the initial fusion frequency was 70 pps. Calibration: (A) EMG, 400 μV; force 4 g; time, 1 sec. (B) EMG, 100 μV; force, 10 g; time, 2.5 sec.

readily show a decline in EMG as well as force after brief stimulation; fatigue-resistant units show both electrical and mechanical endurance (McPhedran et al., 1965; Wuerker et al., 1965; Burke et al., 1973, Henneman, 1980; Clamann and Robinson, 1985). It has often been suggested that failure at some stage of action potential transmission protects subsequent elements from fatigue; with the possible exception of the failure in excitation–contraction coupling, this is unlikely to be true. It has recently been shown that during sustained contractions produced under identical conditions, different motor unit types fail for different reasons (Clamann and Robinson, 1985; Clamann, 1987). This would suggest that a protective element, if one exists, differs among motor units of different fatigability.

Normal muscle use involves bursts of activity interspersed with pauses, allowing some recovery. Fatigable motor units seem designed to take advantage of this situation. The one element that may act as a protective device is excitation–contraction coupling, since failure at this point may be induced in all motor unit types by appropriately chosen intermittent stimulation. It would seem reasonable to protect the contractile elements from total metabolic depletion, which could induce rigor and actual tissue damage. The existence of K^+ channels controlled by ATP concentration and so suited for this purpose has been reported (Noma and Shibasaki, 1985).

MUSCLE CONTROL AND MUSCLE FATIGUE

Muscle fatigue can reduce the effectiveness of movements or prevent their execution entirely; clearly, this should be avoided if at all possible. In a review article in 1922, Forbes suggested a way to avoid fatigue: perhaps a group of muscle fibers could be active for a while and then, by some reflex mechanism, excite a different group of fibers while they themselves fell silent to recover. The second group could similarly activate a third, "and so the fiber groups may take up the load in rotation and, for some reason, by this means attain an economy otherwise impossible" (Forbes, 1922). With the discovery of motor units (Liddell and Sherrington, 1925), the idea acquired greater appeal, although there was no direct evidence for it. The notion of motor unit rotation persisted in the literature for many years. It stimulated careful studies of human motor units in the next two decades, and it was clearly shown that, at least in human voluntary contractions, motor units had fixed recruitment thresholds and motor unit rotation could not be demonstrated (Smith, 1934; Lindsley, 1935; Gilson and Mills, 1941; Kugelberg and Skoglund, 1946). Gilson and Mills (1941) succeeded in recording from pairs of motor units and showed that the first recruited unit of the pair was always the last to fall silent. This suggested the remarkable precision of the recruitment order, a precision that would be quantified much later (Henneman et al., 1974; Clamann and Henneman, 1976). Lindsley (1935) reported the fact, puzzling to him, that "a motor unit during fatigue shows a progressive diminution of amplitude, whereas a motor unit during sustained contraction, which does not cause fatigue, shows no variation in amplitude or frequency of response, although it discharges at the same rate and for a longer period of time." An understanding of the enormous range of fatigability of motor units of different thresholds still lay 30 years in the future.

Henneman first showed clearly (Henneman et al., 1965a, 1965b, 1974) that motor units have relatively fixed thresholds and, as force is graded in most reflex and voluntary contractions, are recruited in the same order. It is hard to imagine a scheme worse suited to the prevention of fatigue. With a fixed order of recruitment, low-threshold units are almost perpetually active, while high-threshold units are rarely used at all. The size principle initially met with some resistance because of just this argument. Of course, further analysis of the size principle (Henneman and Olson, 1965) reveals that motor units are designed for just such disparity of use, and their enormous range of strength and fatigue resistance have been repeatedly documented (McPhedran et al., 1965; Wuerker et al., 1965; Burke et al., 1973; for review, see Burke, 1981). It is with good reason that Henneman could refer to muscle as "the servant of the nervous system" (Henneman, 1980).

The early studies on single human motor units produced a curious result: During sustained contractions, motor units tended to discharge at rates that rarely exceeded about 30 pps (Smith, 1934; Lindsley, 1935; Creed et al., 1972 [1932]). These authors pointed out that it was difficult to record the activity of single motor units at high force levels, and that during near-maximal contractions, higher rates of discharge might be seen. Later studies, however, confirmed the original observations of low discharge rates (Bigland and Lippold, 1954; Clamann, 1969, 1970; Monster and Chan, 1977; DeLuca et al., 1982).

There were some exceptions. Merton and co-workers (Marsden et al., 1983) reported instantaneous frequencies above 150 pps for pairs of impulses or for very short trains. Others (Grimby et al., 1981a, 1981b; Borg et al., 1983) have also reported rates above 50 pps, but again, these were not sustained. Additionally, these records were obtained from muscles in which lesions had reduced the number of motor units (Grimby et al., 1981b; Borg et al., 1983) or in which a few motor units of a muscle were innervated by a branch of an aberrant nerve (Marsden et al., 1983). It has been suggested that such motor units may not be subjected to normal inhibitory influences because of their isolation (Kukulka and Clamann, 1981) and that their high discharge rates are thus exceptional. In these cases also, motor unit discharges fell to rates of 20–30 pps during sustained contractions.

It is important to distinguish between instantaneous frequency, the reciprocal of the interspike interval of a single pair of discharges, and the average frequency produced by a motor unit during a sustained contraction. Motor units sometimes begin their discharges with a high-frequency burst or a single high-frequency doublet (Andreassen and Rosenfalck, 1980; Marsden et al., 1983; Hoffer et al., 1987), and such irregularities may persist. Such high-frequency discharge is never sustained, as we have seen. Even during the burst-like discharges accompanying locomotion or other rhythmic movements, motor units rarely discharge at rates above 40 pps in animals (Hoffer et al., 1981, 1987) or in humans (Grimby, 1984).

It has now become possible to record from motor units during maximum voluntary contractions. During a sustained contraction in which the force is the maximum a subject can produce, the mean discharge rate of motor units is 30 pps in the fast biceps and 11 pps in the slow soleus (Bellemare et al., 1983). The range of discharge rates of motor units is thus quite narrow, and the maximum rate, about 30 pps, is well below the 50–100 pps that would be expected from the known mechanical properties of muscles or their motor units.

HIGH FORCE AT LOW DISCHARGE RATES: CHANGES IN ACTIVE MUSCLES

We have seen that sustained high-frequency discharge produces the most fatiguing contractions (e.g., Fig. 13–4, bottom) and that brief pauses, or even stimulation at low frequencies, will permit recovery from or postponement of fatigue. Recent work (Bigland-Ritchie et al., 1983, 1986b; Marsden et al., 1983), has shown that motor unit discharge rates actually decrease during sustained contractions in humans, where such measurements can be made. What is not clear is how these diminished discharge rates can continue to produce high levels of force. Marsden and colleagues (1983) reported that 100 pps of stimulation increased force in the human adductor pollicis muscle by about 10% over that produced by 50 pps stimulation. Rates of 50–60 pps are said to be

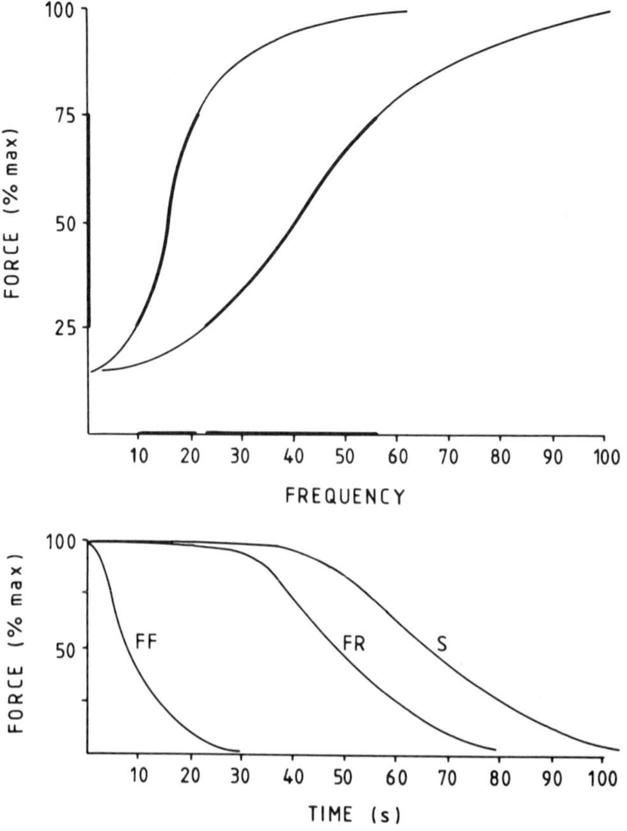

Fig. 13–4. *Above*: hypothetical force–frequency relation for a fast motor unit (right curve) and a slow motor unit (left curve). (Curves based on data of Cooper and Eccles, 1930; Kernell, 1983, 1984; Kernell et al., 1983b) *Below:* Force–time relation of motor units of the three types identified by Burke when they are subjected to continuous stimulation at 80 pps. (Data from Clamann and Robinson, 1985.)

required to produce maximum force in small muscle of the hand (Bigland-Ritchie et al., 1983) or of the foot (Borg et al., 1983), and single motor units in human gastrocnemius produce maximum force at similar rates (Garnett et al., 1979). Experiments with animal muscles (Dryer and Sherrington, 1918; Cooper and Eccles, 1930) or motor units (McPhedran et al., 1965; Burke et al., 1973; Kernell et al., 1983a, 1983b; Reinking et al., 1975) suggest that discharge rates of 60 pps and above are needed for full activation of a muscle, and rates of 30–60 pps are needed for even partial activation to levels above 30% of maximum. Instead, discharge rates of 30 pps are rarely exceeded in sustained contractions (Bellemare et al., 1983; Marsden et al., 1983; Hoffer et al., 1987). How is this possible?

Two possibilities suggest themselves. The first is that a maximum voluntary contraction does not produce the maximum force of which the muscle is capable; that is, the low frequencies seen are not sufficient to fully activate a muscle. This possibility may be eliminated since several workers have shown that a muscle may be fully activated voluntarily (Bigland and Lippold, 1954; Merton, 1954; Naess and Storm-Mathisen, 1955; Bigland-Ritchie, 1981; Bigland-Ritchie et al., 1983). This is done by showing that supramaximal stimuli applied to a muscle undergoing maximum voluntary contraction produce no additional force. The second possibility is that the properties of a muscle change during activity, and that stimulus frequencies of around 30 pps are indeed sufficient to produce the maximum force of an active or a fatiguing muscle. The continuous process of change in an active muscle includes some features that lead to fatigue and others that may be used to advantage to forestall fatigue.

Two important changes take place in motor units when they are stimulated. The contractions of active muscles slow down, as judged by their twitch half-relaxation times (Mosso, 1915; Bigland-Ritchie et al., 1983; Kukulka et al., 1986), and muscle displays a memory or hysteresis allowing it to sustain high forces at low stimulus frequencies after being stimulated at a higher frequency. We will examine these mechanisms and show that the CNS appears to take advantage of both.

It has been known for over a century that when a muscle is fatigued, twitch duration increases; that is, muscle contraction becomes slower (Mosso, 1915). During fatigue tests, the tetanic fusion frequency of FF motor units in the cat gastrocnemius falls from above 80 pps to below 40 pps (Burke et al., 1973, Fig. 1). Curiously, this observation has been largely neglected. It has been noted, however, that human motor units slow their discharge rates during isometric contractions of constant force (Bigland-Ritchie et al., 1983, 1986b; Marsden et al., 1983), and this slowing of discharge has been invoked to explain the unexpected fatigue resistance of human muscles. An electrically stimulated muscle fatigues much more rapidly than it does when a voluntary exertion produces the same force. Apparently, the CNS is able to take advantage of muscle slowing in order to postpone fatigue. (How this occurs is still disputed.) This raises a question: Are all motor units equally susceptible to contractile slowing?

A study has recently been undertaken to examine speed changes in cat motor units subjected to Burke's fatigue test (Dubose et al., 1987). The twitch durations of fatigable motor units were shown to increase continuously throughout the test. Motor unit contractile slowing, like some electrical changes, thus appears to begin with the onset of motor unit activation. These experiments ended when twitch amplitude became too low to continue making the measurements, at which time twitch duration was still increasing. Twitch contraction time increased to more than 50 ms in some FF units; they could then easily have been classified as slow units.

In contrast, slowly contracting units actually became faster, while fast, fatigue-resistant motor units showed little change in contractile speed during several minutes of measurement. Both the twitch contraction time and the half-relaxation time of slow units decreased markedly during the first few tetani and then remained constant. Twitch contraction times of slow units typically fell from above 70 ms to around 50 ms. The time course of these changes was quite different from that of fast units, in which contractile speed decreased continuously.

There is a curious discrepancy between these studies and some recent ones in humans. In several human experiments, only the half-relaxation time of fatigued muscles increased, while the twitch contraction time appeared to remain the same (Bigland-Ritchie, 1981; Bigland-Ritchie et al., 1983; Kukulka et al., 1986). The measurements of Dubose et al. (1987) in cats clearly showed increases in twitch contraction times as well. The figures in Mosso (1915) on whole frog muscles show increases in both the rise and fall times of twitches. The difference is thus unlikely to be attributable to species differences or to an artifactual difference between studies on single motor units versus whole muscles.

For many years, it has been accepted that there is a unique relationship between the frequency with which a muscle or a motor unit is stimulated and the resulting force output (Cooper and Eccles, 1930; Kernell, 1983; Bigland-Ritchie et al., 1983; Kernell et al., 1983b). Figure 13–4 illustrates a force–frequency relation for fast (right curve) and slow (left curve) units based on the data of these workers. The heavy lines indicate the region where rate coding, the grading of force by means of frequency changes, should be most effective. Barring fatigue, a given stimulus frequency should always result in a given force output. This contradicts the change in discharge frequency seen during sustained human contractions (Bigland-Ritchie et al., 1983; Marsden et al., 1983). Contractile slowing was thought to account for this discrepancy. As the work of Dubose et al. (1987) has shown, however, it is only fatigable motor units that slow during activity. This contractile slowing does not progress rapidly enough to account fully for the observed force–frequency relation. Another mechanism must be sought, one that applies to all motor unit types equally.

It is known that muscle force depends on stimulus frequency and on prior stimulus history in a complex, nonlinear way. Stein and Parmiggiani (1979) showed that a second twitch following closely on a first contributed more to the total force–time integral than the first twitch did. Burke (Burke et al., 1976) and Zajac (Zajac and Young, 1980) demonstrated that a single twitch interpolated in a steady train of twitches would raise the force level, which then would remain high for many seconds. It was as if that one twitch had in effect increased the stimulus frequency for many subsequent pulses. This work suggested that a train of pulses whose frequency varied, and in particular decreased, would produce more force than a train of constant frequency, even if the constant frequency was higher on average. This was appealing for the reasons given earlier: It is known that motor units discharge that way in voluntary contractions and when injected with constant currents.

The results from recent experiments from my laboratory (Clamann and Binder-Macleod, 1985; Binder-Macleod and Clamann, 1987) have shown that there is no unique relation between force and frequency in motor units. Instead, the force is dependent on both the current stimulus frequency and the immediate past frequency. The force–frequency relation exhibits a marked hysteresis, as illustrated in Figure 13–5. This hysteresis is equally prominent in all

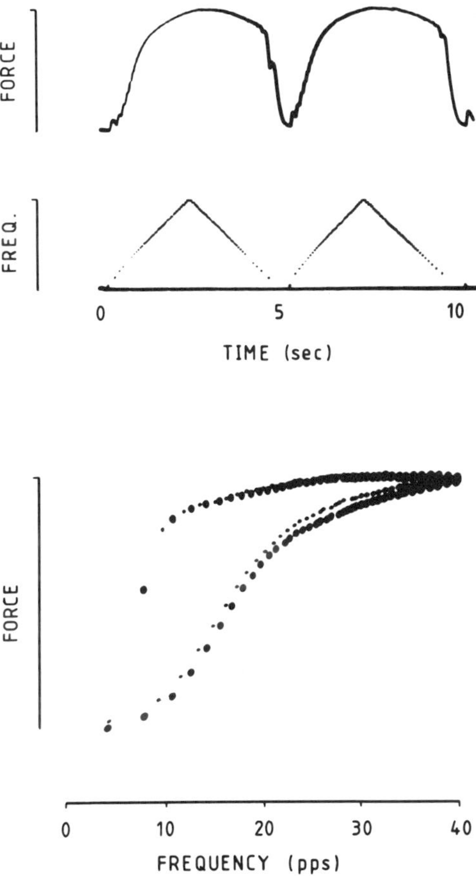

Fig. 13–5. A slow motor unit exhibiting force hysteresis. Two cycles of triangular stimulation are shown. *Above;* force in response to two cycles of stimulation in which a continuous train increased in frequency linearly from 0 to 40 pps and back to 0; frequency of the train is graphed on the middle trace. *Below:* a plot of force versus frequency for these two cycles of stimulation. Heavy dots are the first cycle, light dots the second. Force bars, 30 g.

motor unit types. Although it is strongly modified by posttetanic potentiation and muscle slowing, it possesses a component independent of these phenomena.

The hysteresis allows a motor unit to produce very close to its maximum force when it is stimulated at 30 pps or less, as Figure 13–5 shows. In fact, stimulus or discharge rates below 30 pps are sufficient to elicit near-maximum force from any unit, regardless of type. A surprising result of this work, in light of the marked differences among different motor units, is how homogeneously they respond when stimulated at a high frequency, which is then reduced to about 20 pps. The frequency required to produce 80% of the maximum force under these conditions is largely independent of the unit's fusion frequency, unit type, or most other motor unit characteristics. A subset of slow motor units can produce 80% of maximum force at still lower frequencies, around 10 pps. This is characteristic of soleus motor units in voluntary movements as well.

The properties of motor unit force-frequency hysteresis allow two important observations to be made. First, it is clear that by taking advantage of this property, it is possible to elicit unexpectedly high force levels from motor units while their discharge rates remain rather low. This postpones the effects of fatigue. It makes it clear why voluntary contractions can be sustained longer than the same force levels produced by nerve or muscle stimulation. Second, since hysteresis is rather similar for all motor units, it can now be understood why motor units cannot be clearly distinguished by their discharge properties in human voluntary contractions. As we have noted, all motor units in the same muscle appear to discharge at similar frequencies; there are no clearly definable, rapidly discharging and slowly discharging motor units. I suggest, as others have (Bigland Ritchie et al., 1983, 1986; Marsden et al., 1983), that the CNS drives motor units at frequencies that are optimal for the task at hand. This requires continuous frequency modulation, even during the production of constant force. Whether this modulation is a result of properties of the motoneuron (Kernell, 1965, 1984) or a result of feedback (Bigland-Ritchie et al., 1986b) is not yet fully established.

SUMMARY

Fatigue as a phenomenon is difficult to define and may include far more than merely a loss of force. It is also a continuous process, beginning with the onset of neuromuscular activity. The components of fatigue, changes in electrical activity, electrical propagation, excitation–contraction coupling, and the diverse elements of the contraction process all act together. Yet one process may be especially vulnerable to change in response to a particular discharge pattern. Stimulus patterns may thus be chosen to maximize "electrical" or "mechanical" changes. It is remarkable, however, how well matched all of these changes are. One can reliably predict that a motor unit classified as rapidly fatigable will show early prominent changes in all of the previously mentioned responses, while few changes of any kind will be visible in a slowly fatiguing unit.

Changes that predict or are involved in fatigue may be utilized to postpone fatigue. Prominent among these is motor unit contractile slowing, which allows motor units to be driven at low frequencies and still produce high levels of tension. Changes in active muscle must be added to the list of properties that make muscle such a good servant of the nervous system.

Acknowledgments

Supported in part by a grant from the Foote and Levy Fund.

REFERENCES

Adrian, R. H. (1983). Electrical properties of striated muscle. In *Handbook of Physiology, Sect. 10: Skeletal Muscle* (ed. L. D. Peachey). American Physiological Society, Bethesda, Md., pp. 275–300.

Adrian, R. H., Constantin, L. L., and Peachey, L. D. (1969). Radial spread of contraction in frog muscle fibres. *J. Physiol.* 204, 231–257.

Adrian, R. H., and Peachey, L. D. (1973). Reconstruction of the action potential of frog sartorius muscle. *J. Physiol.* 235, 103–131.

Andreassen, S., and Rosenfalck, A. (1980). Regulation of the firing pattern of single motor units. *J. Neurol. Neurosurg. Psychiatry* 43, 897–906.

Bellemare, F., Woods, J. J., Johansson, R., and Bigland-Ritchie, B. (1983). Motor-unit discharge rates in maximal voluntary contractions of three human muscles. *J. Neurophysiol.* 50, 1380–1392.

Bianchi, P. C., and Narayan, S. (1982). Muscle fatigue and the role of transverse tubules. *Science* 215, 295–296.

Bigland, B., and Lippold, O. C. J. (1954). Motor unit activity in voluntary contraction of human muscle. *J. Physiol.* 125, 322–335.

Bigland-Ritchie, B. (1981). EMG/force relations and fatigue of human voluntary contractions. *Exerc. Sports Sci. Rev.* 9, 75–117.

Bigland-Ritchie, B., Cafarelli, E., and Vollestad, N. K. (1986a). Fatigue of submaximal static contractions. *Acta Physiol. Scand.* 128 (Suppl. 556), 137–148.

Bigland-Ritchie, B. R., Dawson, N. J., Johansson, R. S., and Lippold, O. C. J. (1986b). Reflex origin for the slowing of motoneurone firing rates in fatigue of human voluntary contractions. *J. Physiol.* 379, 451–459.

Bigland-Ritchie, B. R., Johansson, R., Lippold, O. C. J., and Woods, J. J. (1983). Contractile speed and EMG changes during fatigue of sustained maximal voluntary contractions. *J. Neurophysiol.* 50, 313–324.

Bigland-Ritchie, B., Jones, D. A., and Woods, J. J. (1979). Excitation frequency and muscle fatigue: Electrical responses during human voluntary and stimulated contractions. *Exp. Neurol.* 64, 414–427.

Binder-Macleod, S. A., and Clamann, H. P. (1987). Force hysteresis of single motor units during frequency-varying stimulation. *Neurosci. Abstr.* 13, 1212.

Borg, J., Grimby, L., and Hannerz, J. (1983). The fatigue of voluntary contraction and the peripheral electrical propagation of single motor units in man. *J. Physiol.* 340, 435–444.

Burke, R. E. (1981). Motor units: Anatomy, physiology, and functional organization. In: *Handbook of Physiology*, Vol. I, Sect. 1: *The Nervous System*, Part 1: *Motor Control* (ed. V. B. Brooks). American Physiological Society, Bethesda, Md., pp. 345–422.

Burke, R. E., Levine, D. N., Tsairis, P., and Zajac, F. E., III. (1973). Physiological types and histochemical profiles in motor units of the cat gastrocnemius. *J. Physiol.* 234, 723–748.

Burke, R. E., Rudomin, P., and Zajac, F. E. (1976). The effect of activation history on tension production by individual muscle units. *Brain Res.* 109, 515–529.

Carlson, F. D., and Wilkie, D. G. (1974). *Muscle Physiology.* Prentice-Hall, Englewood Cliffs, N.J., p. 170.

Clamann, H. P. (1969). Statistical analysis of motor unit firing patterns in a human skeletal muscle. *Biophys. J.* 9, 1233–1251.

Clamann, H. P. (1970). Activity of single motor units during isometric tension. *Neurology* 20, 254–260.

Clamann, H. P. (1987). Fatigue mechanisms and contractile changes in motor units of the cat hindlimb. *Can. J. Sport Sci.* 12 (Suppl 1), 20–25.

Clamann, H. P., and Binder-Macleod, S. A. (1985). Force-frequency relations of cat motor units during different patterns of stimulation. *Neurosci. Abstr.* 11, 408.

Clamann, H. P., and Henneman, E. (1976). Electrical measurement of axon diameter and its use in relating motoneuron size to critical firing level. *J. Neurophysiol.* 39, 844–851.

Clamann, H. P., and Robinson, A. J. (1985). A comparison of electromyographic and mechanical fatigue properties in motor units of the cat hindlimb. *Brain Res.* 327, 203–219.

Cooper, S., and Eccles, J. C. (1930). The isometric responses of mammalian muscles. *J. Physiol.* 69, 377–385.

Creed, R. S., Denny-Brown, D., Eccles, J. C., Liddell, E. G. T., and Sherrington, C. S. 1972 [1932]. *Reflex Activity of the Spinal Cord.* Clarendon Press, Oxford.

DeLuca, C. J., LeFever, R. S., McCue, M. P., and Xenakis, A. P. (1982). Behaviour of human motor units in different muscles during linearly varying contractions. *J. Physiol.* 329, 113–128.

Dreyer, N. B., and Sherrington, C. S. (1918). Brevity, frequency of rhythm, and amount of reflex nervous discharge, as indicated by reflex contractions. *Proc. R. Soc.* Series B (Biology) 90, 270–282.

Dubose, L., Schelhorn, T. B., and Clamann, H. P. (1987). Changes in contractile speed of cat motor units during activity. *Muscle Nerve* 10, 744–752.

Edstrom, L., and Kugelberg, E. (1968). Histochemical composition, distribution of fibres and fatigability of single motor units. Anterior tibial muscle of the rat. *J. Neurol. Nurosurg. Psychiatry* 31, 424–433.

Edwards, R. H. T. (1981). Human muscle function and fatigue. In: *CIBA Foundation Symposium 82. Human Muscle Fatigue: Physiological Mechanisms* (ed. R. Porter and J. Whelan). Pitman Medical, London, pp. 1–18.

Forbes, A. (1922). The interpretation of spinal reflexes in terms of present knowledge of nerve conduction. *Physiol. Rev.* 2, 361–414.

Garnett, R. A. F., O'Donovan, M. J., Stephens, J. A., and Taylor, A. (1979). Motor unit organization of human medial gastrocnemius. *J. Physiol.* 287, 33–43.

Gilson, A. S., Jr., and Mills, W. B. (1943). Activities in single motor units in man during slight voluntary efforts. *Am. J. Physiol.* 133, 658–669.

Gollnick, P. D., Piehl, K., and Saltin, B. (1974). Selective glycogen depletion pattern in human muscle fibres after exercise of varying intensity and at varying pedalling rates. *J. Physiol.* 241, 45–57.

Grabowski, W., Lobsiger, E. A., and Lüttgau, H. C. (1972). The effect of repetitive stimulation at low frequencies upon the electrical and mechanical activity of single muscle fibres. *Pfluegers Arch.* 334, 222–239.

Grimby, L. (1984). Firing properties of single human motor units during locomotion. *J. Physiol.* 346, 195–202.

Grimby, L., Hannerz, J., Borg, J., and Hedman, B. (1981a). Firing properties of single human motor units on maintained maximal voluntary effort. In: *CIBA Foundation Symposium 82. Human Muscle Fatigue: Physiological Mechanisms* (ed. R. Porter and J. Whelan). Pitman Medical, London, pp. 157–165.

Grimby, L., Hannerz, J., and Hedman, B. (1981b). The fatigue and voluntary discharge properties of single motor units in man. *J. Physiol.* 316, 545–554.

Henneman, E. (1980). Skeletal muscle. The servant of the nervous system. In: *Medical Physiology*, 14th ed. (ed. V. B. Mountcastle). C. V. Mosby, St. Louis, pp. 674–702.

Henneman, E., Clamann, H. P., Gillies, J. D., and Skinner, R. D. (1974). Rank order of motoneurons within a pool: Law of combination. *J. Neurophysiol.* 37, 1338–1349.

Henneman, E., Somjen, G., and Carpenter, D. O. (1965a). Functional significance of cell size in spinal motoneurons. *J. Neurophysiol.* 28, 560–580.

Henneman, E., Somjen, G., and Carpenter, D. O. (1965b). Excitability and inhibitability of motoneurons of different sizes. *J. Neurophysiol.* 28, 599–620.

Henneman, E., and Olson, C. B. (1965). Relation between structure and function in the design of skeletal muscles. *J. Neurophysiol.* 28, 581–598.

Hoffer, J. A., O'Donovan, M. J., Pratt, C. A., and Loeb, G. E. (1981). Discharge pattern of hindlimb motoneurons during normal cat locomotion. *Science* 213, 466–468.

Hoffer, J. A., Sugano, N., Loeb, G. E., Marks, W. B., O'Donovan, and M. J., and Pratt, C. A. (1987). Cat hindlimb motoneurons during locomotion. II. Normal activity patterns. *J. Neurophysiol.* 57, 530–553.

Jennische, E., Hagberg, H., and Haljamae, H. (1982). Extracellular potassium concentration and membrane potential in rabbit gastrocnemius muscle during tourniquet ischemia. *Pfluegers Arch.* 392, 335–339.

Jones, D. A. (1981). Muscle fatigue due to changes beyond the neuromuscular junction. In *CIBA Foundation Symposium 82. Human Muscle Fatigue: Physiological Mechanisms*, (ed. R. Porter and J. Whelan). Pitman Medical, London, pp. 178–192.

Jones, D. A., Bigland-Ritchie, B., and Edwards, R. H. T. (1979). Excitation frequency and muscle fatigue: Mechanical responses during voluntary and stimulated contractions. *Exp. Neurol.* 64, 401–413.

Katz, B. (1966). *Nerve, Muscle and Synapse*. McGraw-Hill, New York.

Kernell, D. (1965). The adaptation and the relation between discharge frequency and current strength of cat lumbosacral motoneurons stimulated by long-lasting injected currents. *Acta Physiol. Scand.* 65, 65–73.

Kernell, D. (1983). Functional properties of spinal motoneurons and gradation of muscle force. In *Advances in Neurology*, Vol. 39: *Motor Control Mechanisms in Health and Disease* (ed. J. E. Desmedt). Raven Press, New York, pp. 213–226.

Kernell, D. (1984). The meaning of discharge rate: Excitation-to-frequency transduction as studied in spinal motoneurones. *Arch. Ital. Biol.* 122, 5–15.

Kernell, D., Ducati, A., and Sjöholm, H. (1975). Properties of motor units in the first deep lumbrical muscle of the cat's foot. *Brain Res.* 98, 37–55.

Kernell, D., Eerbeek, O., and Verhey, B. A. (1983a). Motor unit categorization on basis of contractile properties: An experimental analysis of the composition of the cat's M. peroneus longus. *Exp. Brain Res.* 50, 211–219.

Kernell, D., Eerbeek, O., and Verhey, B. A. (1983b). Relation between isometric force and stimulus rate in cat's hindlimb motor units of different twitch contraction time. *Exp. Brain Res.* 50, 220–227.

Kernell, D., and Monster, A. W. (1982). Motoneurone properties and motor fatigue. An intracellular study of gastrocnemius motoneurones of the cat. *Exp. Brain Res.* 46, 197–204.

Krnjevic, K., and Miledi, R. (1958). Failure of neuromuscular propagation in rats. *J. Physiol.* 140, 440–461.

Kugelberg, E., and Skoglund, C. R. (1946). Natural and artificial activation of motor units, a comparison, *J. Neurophysiol.* 9, 399–412.

Kukulka, C. G., and Clamann, H. P. (1981). Comparison of the recruitment and discharge properties of motor units in human brachial biceps and adductor pollicis during isometric contractions. *Brain Res.* 219, 45–55.

Kukulka, C. G., Russel, A. G., and Moore, M. A. (1986). Electrical and mechanical changes in human soleus muscle during sustained maximum isometric contractions. *Brain Res.* 362, 47–54.

Liddell, E. G. T., and Sherrington, C. S. (1925). Recruitment and some other features of reflex inhibition. *Proc. R. Soc. B.* 97, 488–518.

Lindsley, D. B. (1935). Electrical activity of human motor units during voluntary contraction. *Am. J. Physiol.* 114, 90–99.

Locke, S., and Henneman, E. (1960). Fractionation of motor units by curare. *Exp. Neurol.* 2, 638–651.

Lüttgau, H. Ch., and Spiecker, W. (1979). The effects of calcium deprivation upon mechanical and electrophysiological parameters in skeletal muscle fibers of the frog. *J. Physiol.* 296, 411–429.

Marsden, C. D., Meadows, J. C., and Merton, P. A. (1983). "Muscular wisdom" that minimizes fatigue during prolonged effort in man: Peak rates of motoneuron discharge and slowing of discharge during fatigue. In *Advances in Neurology*, Vol. 39 (ed. J. E. Desmedt). Raven Press, New York, pp. 169–212.

McPhedran, A. M., Wuerker, R. B., and Henneman, E. (1965). Properties of motor units in a homogeneous red muscle (soleus) of the cat. *J. Neurophysiol.* 28, 71–84.

Merton, P. A. (1954). Voluntary strength and fatigue. *J. Physiol.* 123, 553–564.

Monster, A. W., and Chan, H. (1977). Isometric force production by motor units of extensor digitorum communis muscle in man. *J. Neurophysiol.* 40, 1432–1443.

Mosso, A. (1915). *Fatigue.* Allen & Unwin, London.

Naess, K., and Storm-Mathisen, A. (1955). Fatigue of sustained tetanic contractions. *Acta Physiol. Scand.* 34, 351–366.

Noma, A., and Shibasaki, T. (1985). Membrane current through adenosine-triphosphate-regulated potassium channels in guinea pig ventricular cells. *J. Physiol.* 363, 463–480.

Peachey, L. D. (1985). Excitation–contraction coupling: The link between the surface and the interior of the muscle cell. *J. Exp. Biol.* 115, 91–98.

Petrofsky, J. S., Weber, C., and Phillips, C. A. (1980). Mechanical and electrical correlates of isometric muscle fatigue in skeletal muscle in the cat. *Pflueggers Arch.* 387, 33–38.

Reinking, R. M., Stephens, J. A., and Stuart, D. G. (1975). The motor units of cat medial gastrocnemius: Problem of their categorisation on the basis of mechanical properties. *Exp. Brain Res.* 23, 301–313.

Simonson, E., and Weiser, P. (1976). *Physiological Aspects and Physiological Correlates of Work Capacity and Fatigue.* Charles C. Thomas, Springfield, Ill.

Sjøgaard, G. (1983). Electrolytes in slow and fast muscle fibers of human at rest and with dynamic exercise. *Am. J. Physiol.* 245, R25–R31.

Sjøgaard, G., Adams, R. P., and Saltin, B. (1985). Water and ion shifts in skeletal muscle of humans with intense dynamic knee extension. *Am. J. Physiol.* 248, R190–R196.

Sjøgaard, G., Saltin, B. (1982). Extra- and intracellular water spaces in muscles of man at rest and with dynamic exercise. *Am. J. Physiol.* 243, R271–280.

Smith, D. O. (1980). Mechanisms of action potential propagation failure at sites of axon branching in the crayfish. *J. Physiol.* 301, 243–259.

Smith, D. O., and Hatt, H. (1976). Axon conduction block in a region of dense connective tissue in crayfish. *J. Neurophysiol.* 39, 794–801.

Smith, O. J. (1934). Action potentials from single motor units in voluntary contraction. *Am. J. Physiol.* 108, 629–638.

Stein, R. B., and Parmiggiani, F. (1979). Optimal motor patterns for activating mammalian muscle. *Brain Res.* 175, 373–376.

Vollestad, N. K., and Blom, P. (1985). Effect of varying exercise intensity on glycogen depletion in human muscle fibres. *Acta Physiol. Scand.* 125, 395–405.

Vollestad, N. K., Vaage, O., and Hermansen, L. (1984). Muscle glycogen depletion patterns in type I and subgroups of type II fibres during prolonged severe exercise in man. *Acta Physiol. Scand.* 122, 433–441.

Wuerker, R. B., McPhedran, A. M., and Henneman, E. (1965). Properties of motor units in a heterogeneous pale muscle (m. gastrocnemius) of the cat. *J. Neurophysiol.* 28, 85–99.

Zajac, F. E., Young, J. L. (1980). Properties of stimulus trains producing maximum tension-time area per pulse from single motor units in medial gastrocnemius muscle of the cat. *J. Neurophysiol.* 43, 1206–1220.

14

Metabolic Fiber Types and Influences on Their Transformation

PATTI M. NEMETH

Refinements in biochemical techniques have enhanced our knowledge of the metabolic and contractile proteins of muscle. A high degree of specialization among individual muscle fibers has been revealed, yet the motor unit stands as a functionally homogeneous alliance of cells. The metabolic properties of muscle fibers are not fixed, but adjust to changing physical demands encountered during development, as well as to various perturbations of mature muscle. This phenomenon of adaptability challenges the meaning of fiber types and questions the intrinsic nature of muscle and the limits of its mutability. This chapter addresses the criteria for defining metabolic fiber types and some of the major influences capable of altering these properties.

METABOLIC FIBER TYPES

The concept of metabolic specialization among individual muscle fibers evolved from classical observations in whole muscle. In 1865, Kuehne proposed that an intracellular factor was responsible for the intensity of the red color of muscle. The functional significance of muscle color was recognized at about the same time, and experimental evidence showed that certain red muscles contracted more slowly than white ones, with the corollary that slow-contracting muscles were always red but that not all red muscles were slow (see Close, 1972). Kuehne's intracellular factor is now known to be the cytosolic oxygen-binding protein myoglobin. High myoglobin levels, together with an enrichment of capillaries and iron-containing mitochondrial cytochromes, give the characteristic deep red color to muscles that rely on oxygen for energy metabolism. This high aerobic capacity permits continuous contractile activity without fatigue. A relative paucity of oxidative apparatus gives a white appearance to muscles that obtain energy primarily from glycolytic metabolism. This metabolism supplies ATP at a faster rate than oxidative metabolism, permitting a faster contraction speed, but with rapid fatigue. A third form of metabolic specialization combines both high oxidative and glycolytic potential, and affords more continuous bouts of high-frequency contractions.

It is now apparent that the same differences observed in whole muscle persist at the cellular level. The physiological, structural, and biochemical properties that differentiate muscle fibers have been elucidated by motor unit studies (see Burke, 1981; Chapters 11 and 12, this volume) and have given rise to a classification system for mammalian skeletal muscle fibers incorporating contractile speed and energy-generating metabolic pathways (Peter et al., 1972): slow-twitch oxidative (SO), fast-twitch oxidative glycolytic (FOG), and fast-twitch glycolytic (FG). If these physical–biochemical relationships are strict, then fiber types can be identified by relative amounts of aerobic and anaerobic enzyme concentrations.

The application of microanalytical biochemistry to muscle has made it possible to characterize precisely the metabolic profiles of single fibers (Lowry and Passonneau, 1972; Essén et al., 1975). Aerobic capacity can be judged by relative concentrations of enzymes of the tricarboxylic acid cycle, fatty acid metabolism, and ketone oxidation, and anaerobic metabolism can be assessed by levels of enzymes representing glycolysis, gluconeogenesis, and glycogenolysis. Several representative enzymes have wide activity ranges across muscle fiber populations, with sufficient discontinuity between fast and slow fiber groups to be useful for enzymatic typing.

In addition to aerobic and anaerobic enzymes, enzymes of high-energy phosphate metabolism are exceptionally useful for fiber typing. For example, adenylokinase has an extremely wide range of activity across fiber types, up to 12-fold in human muscles (Lowry et al., 1978). The role of this enzyme in muscle is presumably related to the enhancement of free energy via ADP–ATP transfer, which may account for its close correlation with the myofibrillar ATPase staining reaction (Hintz et al., 1984) and with calcium-dependent myofibrillar ATPase activity (Nemeth, unpublished observations). Its advantage is one of resolution: Whereas adenylokinase activity varies substantially among and within fiber types, myofibrillar ATPase activity varies only two- to threefold across the major fiber types (Essén et al., 1975). Values for enzyme activities of various energy-generating pathways are given in Table 14–1.

The most significant contribution of quantitative single-fiber biochemistry is the disclosure of the wide variation of enzyme activities within a given fiber type. In a review of their work, Pette and Spamer (1986) reported threefold variations in oxidative enzyme activities in type SO fibers (referred to as "type I") of rabbit soleus and fourteenfold variations in FOG (referred to as "type IIA") fibers of rabbit psoas. Others have shown wide ranges within fiber types for a variety of enzymes, including a sixfold range in lactate dehydrogenase activity and a fourfold range in adenylokinase activity (Nemeth and Turk, 1984), as well as a ninefold range in malate dehydrogenase activity (Hintz et al., 1980) in fast fibers of rat tibialis anterior.

Table 14–1 Comparison of average enzyme activities in muscle fiber types from different species

	SO	FOG	FG
Malate dehydrogenase			
Rat	11	16	9
Human	8	- 5 -	
Rabbit	27	32	7
Cat	16	14	5
Snake	10[a]	11	3
Fumarate hydrotase			
Rat	8	16	7
Human	5	4	3
Beta-hydroxyacyl CoA dehydrogenase			
Rat	5	5	1
Human	2	2	1
Cat	10	9	2
Lactate dehydrogenase			
Rat	19	54	109
Human	10	37	49
Rabbit	30	146	240
Cat	36	251	213
Snake	95[a]	171	236
Glycogen phosphorylase			
Rat	2	3	7
Human	3	- 5 -	
Phosphofructokinase			
Rat	0.3	2	3
Human	1	2	3
Rabbit	1	- 3 -	
Pyruvate kinase			
Rat	5	15	33
Human	11	27	30
Fructose-bisphosphatase			
Rat	1	14	30
Human	55	150	201
Creatine kinase			
Rat	177	242	420
Human	206	198	237
Adenylokinase			
Rat	40	99	149
Human	21	71	132
Rabbit	56	120	223
Cat	33	182	225
Snake	12[a]	43	118

Source: Data compiled from Hintz et al. (1980), Nemeth et al. (1986), and unpublished data of Nemeth.

Note: Activities are in moles per kilogram of dry weight per hour at 21°C, except that fructose-bisphosphatase is in millimoles per kilogram of dry weight per hour. Muscles are rat soleus and tibialis anterior, human biceps, rabbit soleus and extensor digitorum longus, cat tibialis posterior, and snake transversus abdominis.

[a]SO refers to tonic fibers in the snake.

Given the tremendous range of enzyme activities, it is not surprising that levels of a single enzyme can overlap, so as to obscure the boundaries between fiber types (Lowry et al., 1978; Hintz et al., 1980; Nemeth and Pette, 1981). Therefore, concomitant measurement of aerobic and anaerobic enyzme activities has proven beneficial for clearer definition of metabolic types. Because the quantitative biochemical technique permits analysis of multiple enyzmes on a single muscle fiber, the interrelationship of two or more enzymes can separate fibers into groups. In Figure 14–1A, for example, the tibials anterior type FG and FOG fiber populations are indistinguishable by lactate dehydrogenase activities, but are separable if this enzyme is assayed in combination with malate dehydrogenase. In contrast, type SO and FOG fibers overlap in malate dehydrogenase activities but are distinct with lactate dehydrogenase activities. Figure 14–1A illustrates another point: that SO fibers are not necessarily the same in different muscles. The SO and FOG fibers of tibialis anterior are intermediate with respect to both lactate dehydrogenase and malate dehydrogenase compared to those same fiber types in soleus.

Despite characteristic enyzmatic domains, there is a metabolic spectrum within each fiber type. Some FG fibers are very similar in the activity levels

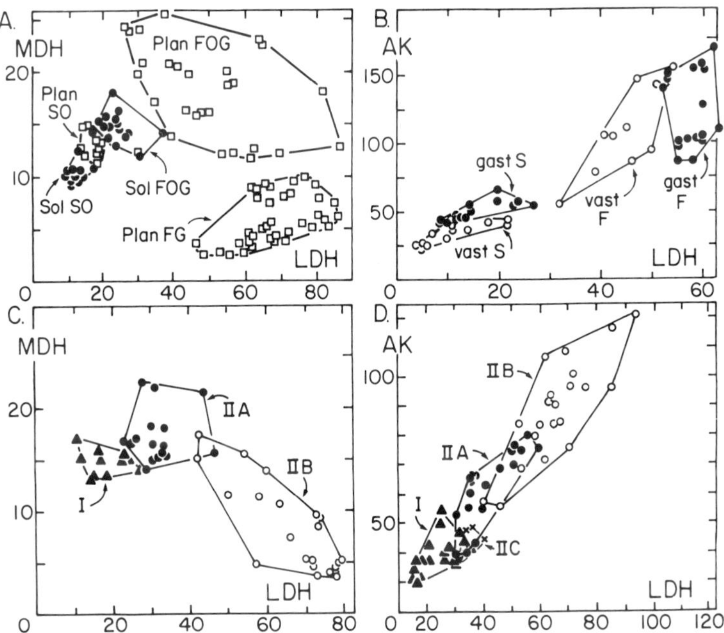

Fig. 14–1. Fiber type domains produced by plotting activities of two enzymes on the same individual fiber; each symbol represents a separate fiber. (A) Rat soleus (sol) and plantaris (plan) muscle fibers. (Modified with permission from Hintz et al., 1982.) (B) Human gastrocnemius (gast) and vastus lateralis (vast) muscle fibers. (Modified with permission from Chi et al., 1983.) (C) Rat plantaris muscle fibers typed by myosin ATPase staining intensities. (Reproduced with permission from Hintz et al., 1984.) (D) Rat extensor digitorum longus muscle fibers typed by myosin ATPase. (Modified from Nemeth and Turk, 1984.) Enzymes are malate dehydrogenase (MDH), lactate dehydrogenase (LDH), and adenylokinase (AK). Activities are in moles per kilogram of dry weight per hour at 21°C.

of multiple enzymes to FOG fibers, as are FOG to SO fibers, suggesting that a functional continuum exists across a given fiber population.

Variation in energy-generating capacity undoubtedly reflects differences in the specific ability to sustain contractile work. This might vary in different muscles within a species or in the same muscle from separate species. Fibers from human gastrocnemius and vastus lateralis (Fig. 14–1B) illustrate this point. Slow fibers differ in adenylokinase but not lactate dehydrogenase activity, while fast fibers differ in lactate dehydrogenase but not adenylokinase. Table 14–1 further emphasizes cross-species enzyme differences.

Metabolic Uniformity of the Motor Unit

Despite the diversity among muscle fibers and fiber types, the fiber constituents of a motor unit are uniform in metabolic capacity. This was recognized by Kugelberg and Edström (1968) and Burke and colleagues (1973) from histochemical analyses. A quantitative test of this important principle was made for malate dehydrogenase in individual motor units of the rat (Nemeth et al., 1981). Uniformity for enzymes representing all major energy pathways has been confirmed in cat hindlimb motor units using single-cell biochemistry combined with in situ histochemistry (Nemeth et al., 1986) and with quantitative 2-deoxyglucose 6-phosphate determinations (Nemeth et al., 1988). Further support for metabolic homogeneity comes from microphotometric enzyme determinations (Vetter et al., 1984) and quantitative biochemistry (Nemeth and Turk, 1984) of newly assembled motor units of reinnervated muscles.

Consistency in energy metabolism among the fibers of the motor unit, limited only by minor subcellular fluctuation, supports its role as the functional unit of muscle. One would predict that the homogeneity principle would extend to functionally associated properties. Although this has not been directly confirmed, the idea is strengthened by reports that numerous aspects of muscle biochemistry and structure vary coordinately from muscle to muscle and from cell to cell. These include isozymes of energy-related enzymes, mitochondrial volume, myoglobin, sarcoplasmic reticulum volume and calcium-uptake capacity, width of z-bands, fiber size, and isozymes of structural and regulatory contractile proteins (Pette and Vrbová, 1985). The premise underlying functional myology is that these properties will ultimately be correlated with the correspondingly wide spectrum of physiological properties observed in motor units (Burke, 1981; Stuart et al., 1983).

Contractile Proteins

Myofibrillar proteins are of particular interest in the study of cellular diversity because their hydrolysis of ATP is a primary determinant of twitch contraction speed (Barany, 1967). Myosin, the predominant contractile protein, is a hexamer of two heavy chains noncovalently associated with four light chains. The light chains were of initial interest because different combinations of isoforms in fast and slow muscle suggested their involvement in the regulation of ATPase activity. Subsequent studies showed the enzymatic activity to reside in the heavy chain meromyosin head, shifting the emphasis to the polymorphism of myosin heavy chains. Amino acid sequencing and specific cDNA probes have identified a seven-member family of myosin heavy chain genes (Mahdavi et al., 1986).

The functional roles of the three major adult myosin heavy chain genes can be extrapolated from whole muscle studies (Izumo et al., 1986). Cardiac beta heavy chain dominates muscles containing predominantly slow fibers (e.g., rat soleus); skeletal fast IIA heavy chain is found primarily in muscles containing high proportions of FOG fibers (e.g., diaphragm); skeletal fast IIB is found exclusively in pure FG muscle (e.g., tensor fascia lata, masseter); and coexpression of the latter two genes is found in mixed muscle (e.g., extensor digitorum longus, EDL). The heavy chain isoforms have been directly correlated with the shortening velocity of the fiber (Reiser et al., 1985) and appear to be responsible for the specific myofibrillar ATPase activity (Billeter et al., 1981; Staron and Pette, 1986).

Thus, histochemical staining for myofibrillar ATPase is justifiably employed as a means of fiber typing. Three major myosin ATPase fiber types are readily obtainable (Brooke and Kaiser, 1970), with the limitation that many factors, including incubation time, temperature, pH, type of buffer, and ionic composition of the assay medium, can markedly influence the reaction product (Gollnick and Hodgson, 1986).

Despite the wide use of myosin ATPase fiber typing, several studies show an incomplete homology between it and metabolic typing, as indicated in Figures 14–1C and 14–1D. Specifically, ATPase reactivity is not a reliable indicator of a fiber's oxidative capacity (Nemeth et al., 1979; Nemeth and Pette, 1981). In fact, the myosin IIB subgroup of rabbits has been shown to have a spectrum of oxidative enzyme values as wide as that of the entire fiber population (Pette and Spamer, 1986).

It stands to reason, however, that properties of myosin and energy metabolism should be coupled. This might not be visualized by myosin histochemistry, in which only two or three types are resolved, compared to the spectrum of metabolic properties. The mismatch between myosin staining and aerobic capacity could be a consequence of the coexpression in the same fiber of different myosin isoforms (Betto et al., 1986). The next two sections of this chapter deal with influences on cellular remodeling, in which the expression of metabolic and contractile proteins is considered.

POSTNATAL DEVELOPMENT

Developmental modifications of prospective fast and slow muscles in the rat involve the sequential expression of embryonic, neonatal, and adult slow and fast myosin heavy chains (Whalen et al., 1981; Lyons et al., 1983; Periasamy et al., 1984; Mahdavi et al., 1986; Narusawa et al., 1987). Metabolic energy systems also show early differentiation (Hudlicka et al., 1973; Dangain et al., 1987). The relationship between metabolic and myosin transitions is fundamental to an understanding of the control of the synthesis of proteins underlying muscle function.

Quantitative single-fiber biochemistry has provided a precise picture of metabolic changes during the postnatal development of rat hindlimb muscles. Fiber type- and enzyme-specific changes, as well as the relationship between metabolic and myosin proteins, have been recognized as the animal adapts to changing environmental and hormonal conditions (Nemeth et al., in press).

The metabolic diversification of prospective fast EDL and slow soleus muscles proceeds in two phases. The early phase can be characterized by differences in the activities of lactate dehydrogenase and adenylokinase, two enzymes correlated with contractile function in the adult muscle (Hamm et al., 1988), while levels of key oxidative enzymes are not divergent. There is, even at birth, significant variability among fibers of both the EDL and soleus, indicating that the relatively pure slow adult soleus muscle develops from a tissue with a potential as diverse as that of the EDL. Differences in adenylokinase and lactate dehydrogenase separating the two muscles progressively expand by amplification of the activities of these enzymes in the EDL but not in the soleus.

The increased lactate dehydrogenase activity in the EDL results exclusively from accumulation of the M isozyme (Margreth, 1970). By contrast, a qualitative change occurs in the soleus as the H subunit progressively replaces the M subunit. This switch can be detected in the rat soleus by 5 days of age. Hudlická et al. (1973) have reported a similar switch in the soleus of 4-day-old kittens. Therefore, differential regulation of genes encoding the M and H isozymes of lactate dehydrogenase ensues very early. Equally early modifications have been reported in mRNAs for aldolase isozymes (Schweighoffer et al., 1986).

The second phase of metabolic diversity occurs between 10 and 21 days, when fast fibers display an abrupt rise in adenylokinase activity and begin to specialize into oxidative and glycolytic phenotypes. In the EDL, lactate dehydrogenase activity rises and expands in range so that distinct populations of fibers with high and low values can be recognized. At the same time, pronounced increases and differentiation of oxidative enzymes occur. Together the enzyme distribution gives rise to the fast FOG and FG fiber types (Fig. 14–2). The third week is also eventful in the development of the soleus (Fig. 14–2). Enzyme activities of high energy and high glycolytic metabolism have an abrupt and transient rise. Because high levels of adenylokinase activity correlate with fast fiber types by myosin ATPase staining (Hintz et al., 1984), its pattern of activity in the adolescent soleus can be attributed to the temporary presence of a significant population of fast (myosin IIA) fibers. These comprise 40% of the population at 21 days, but less than 15% remain in the adult (Kugelberg, 1976).

Although some metabolic diversity of fast and slow muscles is established prior to functional demands, remodeling of metabolic programs continues into adulthood. Muscle-specific aldolase, phosphorylase, and creatine kinase RNA concentrations increase steadily up to the 30th day of postnatal development (Schweighoffer et al., 1986).

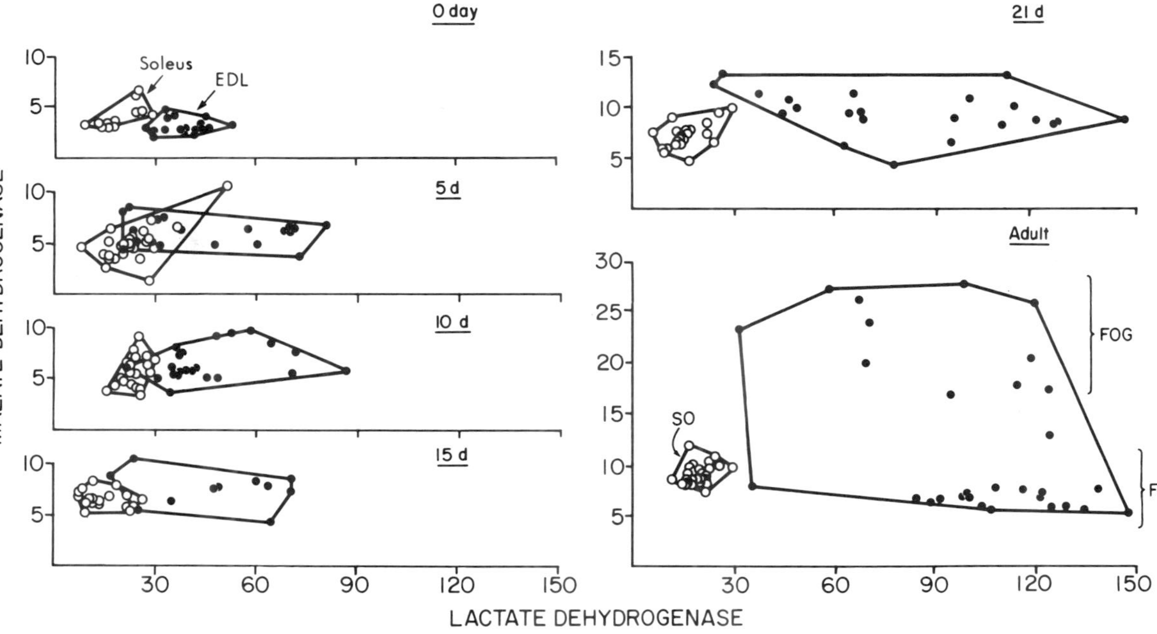

Fig. 14–2. Developmental profiles of fiber types determined by MDH and LDH activities on individual fibers of extensor digitorum longus (EDL) and soleus muscles of rat siblings on successive days of neonatal life. Enzyme activities are as in Figure 14–1. (Modified from Nemeth et al., in press.)

Energy Metabolism and Contractile Function

Neonatal muscle has only a modest ability to generate ATP. In both EDL and soleus, oxidative and glycolytic enzymes are low at birth (Nemeth et al., in press). Both muscles have prolonged velocities of shortening and relaxation (Close, 1972), are activated phasically at low rates, and can sustain contractions for only short periods (Vrbová et al., 1985). There is an early expression of the slow adult myosin isozyme in fetal and neonatal muscle (Narusawa et al., 1987). Since slow myosin has a low energy cost per unit force production (Crow and Kushmerick, 1982), it appears that the contractile machinery of the newborn rat is adapted to make economical use of restricted energy supplies, so that fatigue does not inhibit their modest but essential capacity.

Thus, while it is widely accepted that neurally imposed contractile activity regulates the metabolic enzyme levels in mature muscle (see the following section), the role of nerves in regulating enzyme levels of developing muscle appears to be different. There is evidence to suggest that the early diversity is not due to the nerve. For example, several energy-generating enyzmes differ considerably among single myotubes dissected from 7- and 14-day aneural primary cultures of rat hindlimb muscle (Nemeth et al., 1985). Diversity of myosin isozymes among early myotubes also precedes innervation (Miller et al., 1985) and, therefore, is also presumably a result of intrinsic fiber type programming (Wilkinson and Lichtman, 1985; Vogel and Landmesser, 1987). In fact, the onset of postural activity follows the accumulation of adult slow myosin, as this isozyme has been detected in significant amounts in fetal rat muscle (Kelly and Rubinstein, 1980; Narusawa et al., 1987). Therefore, induction of slow myosin synthesis in fetal rats is not dependent upon imposed tonic impulse traffic, suggesting that the early myosin gene transitions represent a progressive cellular specialization that emerges in advance of specific functional demands.

During the period of early diversity, the nerve appears to assume progressive control over the contractile and metabolic properties of muscle. Enzyme data indicate that neural activity plays a role in tailoring enzyme levels to specific functional needs after the second postnatal week. Here metabolic transitions in suckling and adolescent rats coincide with development of adult locomotor behavior.

Transition from neonatal to adult myosin with high ATPase characteristics corresponds to surges in high-energy and glycolytic enzymes. Periasamy et al. (1984) have shown that mRNA transcripts for adult IIA and IIB myosin heavy chains first appear between 5 and 7 days postpartum, which is consistent with the report that the adult isozymes of fast myosin emerge in the EDL between 10 and 15 days of development (Lyons et al., 1983). It is not known, however, whether this indicates coregulation of metabolic and contractile proteins or whether the transformation to high myosin ATPase activity leads to increased rates of energy turnover.

Substrate Availability

The neonate emerges suddenly into an aerobic environment where fatty acids and ketone bodies derived from milk and fat stores become the major source of energy. Total ketone concentrations in the blood are approximately six times higher and free fatty acids three to four times higher during suckling than after weaning (Kimura and Warshaw, 1983). Fibers in the EDL and soleus of suckling rats increase in oxidative capacity, particularly the beta-oxidative enzyme activity of fatty acids, to make use of the greater availability of lipid substrates. For both growth and function, this type of metabolism has the obvious advantage of the high yield of ATP per molecule of substrate.

Shortly after weaning, the profiles of enzymes for oxidation of fatty acids and glucose diverge. In both the EDL and soleus, malate dehydrogenase activity rises precipitously between 21 and 30 days, and remains high or increases further to maturity, while beta-hydroxyacyl coenzyme A (CoA) dehydrogenase activity declines. The increase in capacity for glucose end-oxidation occurs as the animal switches from a diet rich in lipids and poor in carbohydrates during suckling to a carbohydrate-rich, lipid-poor diet at weaning.

Orchestration by Thyroid Hormone

Metabolic enzymes are clearly sensitive to thyroid control (Nemeth et al., in press). Enzymes of various metabolic pathways rise to at least adult levels by 10 days with administration of thyroxin to the newborn (Fig. 14–3). Conversely, normal developmental increases in enzyme activities are inhibited or restricted in hypothyroid animals. The effect of thyroid on beta-hydroxyacyl CoA dehydrogenase activity is unusual in that hyperthyroid animals do not maintain elevated enzyme levels after 10 days. This effect on beta-hydroxyacyl CoA dehydrogenase supports the idea that the role of the thyroid is to accelerate metabolism. Hyperthyroidism presumably accelerates beta-oxidation of excess endogenous fat stores, as it hastens all enzymes to adult levels.

Thyroid hormone is also known to play a significant role in regulating myosin heavy chain gene expression. The hormone inhibits expression of neonatal and slow myosin heavy chains, particularly in the EDL, and stimulates the expression of IIB myosin (Gambke et al., 1983; Butler-Browne et al., 1984; Izumo et al., 1986). The thyroid also stimulates expression of the IIA myosin heavy chain gene in the soleus but inhibits it in the EDL. Thus, the transient surge in thyroid secretion, known to occur between 10 and 25 days, potentially accounts for the induction of IIB myosin heavy chain expression in the EDL, for the transient presence of a significant population of IIA fibers in the soleus, and for the temporary elevation of metabolic enzyme activities in both muscles. The close timing of these events shows that the thyroid regulates both the metabolic and contractile proteins.

In summary, activities of enzymes of the major energy pathways are low in all fibers of prospective fast and future slow muscles at birth, indicating their modest functional capacity. Nevertheless, the prospective fast and slow fiber populations are distinct at birth for levels of enzymes associated with contractile function, and this condition does not appear to be under neural control. Subsequent changes in these enzymes parallel the transition from neonatal to adult fast myosins and closely reflect the timing of energy demands imposed by different patterns of contractile activity. Levels of oxidative enzymes, in

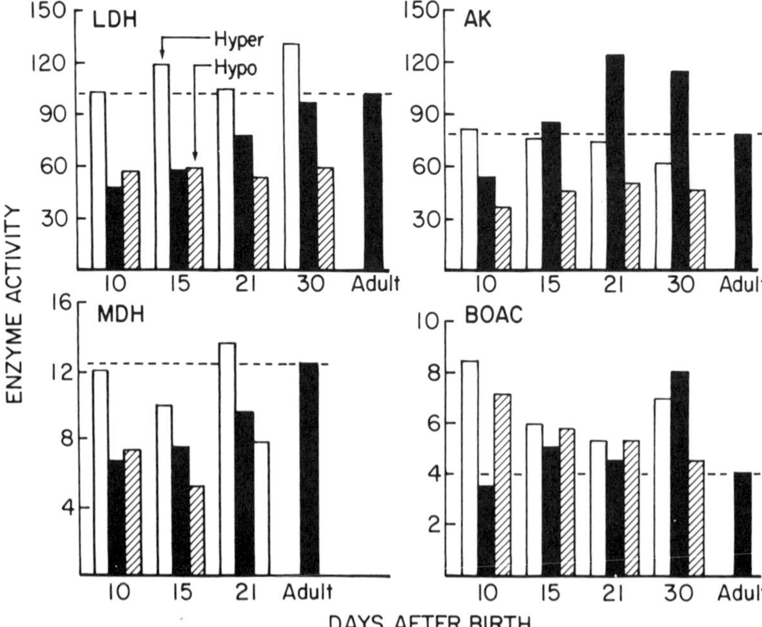

Fig. 14–3. The effect of thyroid hormone on enzymatic phenotype maturation. Average enzyme activities of individual fibers in EDL muscle of hyperthyroid (clear bars) and hypothyroid (hatched bars) rat siblings compared to those of euthyroid (shaded bars) rats of the same postnatal age. Dashed lines indicate the relationship to adult EDL values. Activities and abbreviations are as in Figure 14–1, except for beta-hydroxyacyl CoA dehydrogenase (BOAC). (Modified from Nemeth et al., in press.)

contrast, are similar in prospective fast and slow muscles at birth, and steadily increase and differentiate as the animal adapts to the aerobic extrauterine environment and to dietary changes associated with weaning. Hyperthyroid induction accelerates metabolic and contractile maturation, and hypothyroidism generally inhibits it.

TRANSFORMATIONS IN MATURE MUSCLE

Many cellular processes involved in muscle performance are believed to be under persistent neural control and are capable of changing to meet new functional demands directed by the nervous system. The most common example of muscle plasticity is the response to voluntary exercise.

Endurance Training

Biochemical studies on muscle biopsy specimens from humans have shown that training regimens of low resistance and high repetition, designed to increase endurance, induce large metabolic changes (Holloszy and Booth, 1976; Saltin and Gollnick, 1983). All oxidative systems are elevated, resulting in a greater capacity to oxidize pyruvate, fatty acids, and ketone bodies. Changes in glycolytic enzymes are less pronounced, with the most consistently reported changes being a mild increase in phosphofructokinase activity and a large increase in hexokinase activity. There are, however, conflicting reports on the adaptive response of the glycolyic pathways to endurance, perhaps due to the differences in severity of the exercise stress on glycolysis. Mild exercise does not elicit changes in the glycolytic systems of rat hindlimb muscle, while strenuous treadmill running increases some of them in soleus but not in the white quadriceps (Holloszy, 1967; Baldwin et al., 1973).

The general consensus is that training regimens for either strength or endurance produce no major shifts in the population of slow- and fast-twitch fibers, although, to the extent that metabolic enzymes change, there are shifts in the fast subgroups of FG and FOG. The most likely mechanism is simply an enhanced substrate flux that induces an increase in oxidative capacity.

The cessation of training programs, or detraining, is a sensible approach to testing plasticity in humans to overcome motivational limitations. It is easier to persuade a trained individual to stop training temporarily than to induce a sedentary person to initiate a productive training program. A human detraining study has been undertaken, using single-fiber analysis to make accurate assessments of individual fibers in the vastus lateralis muscle, where enzyme levels vary up to 10-fold (Chi et al., 1983). Before detraining, activities of citrate synthase, malate dehydrogenase, and beta-hydroxyacyl CoA dehydrogenase were substantially higher than in control untrained muscle, and the metabolic differences between fast and slow fibers were small. During detraining, these oxidative enzymes decreased in both fiber types, but far more rapidly and substantially in the fast fibers. Differences in oxidative enzyme activities between fast and slow fibers, reduced in the trained state, were restored by detraining. However, levels in fast fibers remained considerably above untrained levels, even after nearly 3 months of detraining. Activities of lactate dehydrogenase, glycogen phosphorylase, and adenylokinase, on the other hand, increased with detraining, again mainly in the fast fibers. The extent of exercise-induced plasticity is summarized in Figure 14–4 by the enzyme changes during the detraining of a well trained cyclist.

Electrical Stimulation

An extreme adaptive situation can be achieved by chronic electrical stimulation of the motor nerve. Simulation of endurance training by a continuous low-frequency stimulus produces major changes in oxidative and glycolytic energy metabolism in experimental animals. These changes consist of an exceedingly high increase in all oxidative pathways and a concomitant decrease in the activities of glycolytic and high-energy transfer enzymes (Pette et al., 1973; Salmons and Henriksson, 1981; Henriksson et al., 1986). Recent studies employing single-fiber analysis (Buchegger et al., 1984; Chi et al., 1986) have shown that

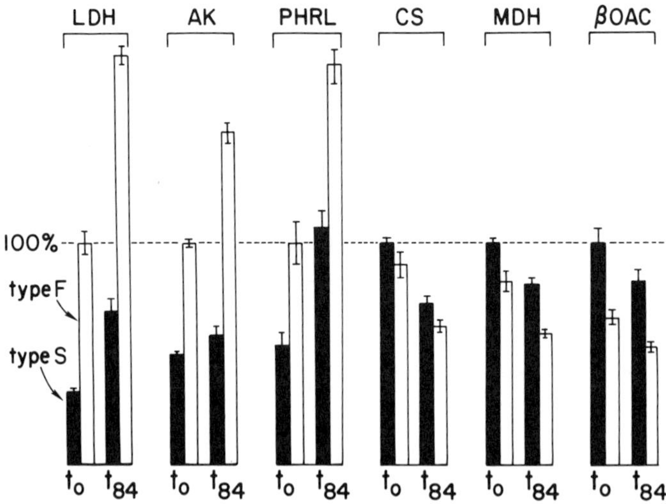

Fig. 14–4. The effect of detraining on enzyme activities of slow and fast fibers of the vastus lateralis muscle of a highly trained cyclist. Activities are expressed as a percentage of the average trained (t) value of the fiber type with the highest value. Activities and abbreviations are as in Figures 14–1 and 14–2, except for glycogen phosphorylase (PHRL) and citrate synthase (CS). (Modified from Chi et al., 1983.)

prolonged stimulation increases oxidative enzyme activities to levels 5- to 14-fold above control levels. Glycogenolytic enzymes fall to 15–20% of the levels in the unstimulated controls.

The metabolic reorganization that takes place as a result of stimulation is illustrated in Figure 14–5. It gives the duration of the stimulus paradigm required for maximal change and the intracellular location for each enzyme. The half-times for maximal change covered a threefold range, with oxidative enzymes averaging 2 weeks and glycolytic enzymes close to 3. The maximal increase for oxidative enzymes ranged from 3- to 14-fold, while the decrease in glycolytic enzymes was 70–90%.

Comparing oxidative and glycolytic capacities, the average 3-oxoacid CoA transferase activity was 160-fold less than the average glycogen phosphorylase activity in unstimulated fast muscle. The stimulation increased this oxidative enzyme to levels higher than those of control fast muscle. Similarly, the ratio of phosphorylase to hexokinase was decreased from a difference of 114-fold to nearly equal values by stimulation.

The large amounts of change produced by electrical stimulation make it possible to examine the mechanisms of adult plasticity. There is strong evidence that fiber transformations are produced by a direct effect on existing fibers and not by a process of regeneration of new fibers (reviewed by Henriksson et al., 1986). The intracellular mechanism almost certainly involves altered synthesis. Decreased mRNA for aldolase, quantitatively similar to the reduction in aldolase activity, was found after 3 weeks of stimulation (Williams et al., 1986). Pette (1984) described how increased synthesis is at least partially

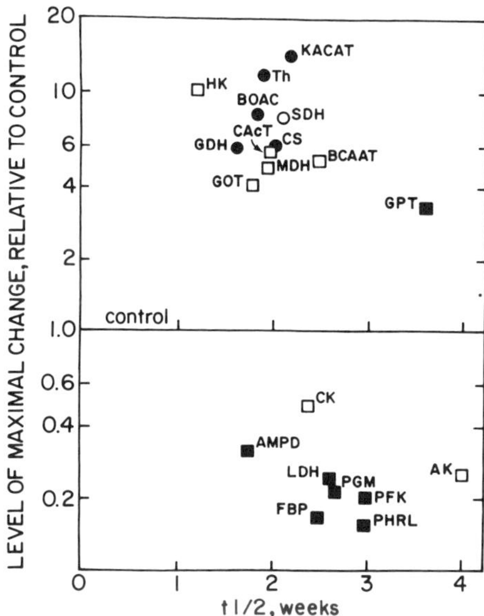

Fig. 14–5. Maximal changes in enzyme activities with low-frequency electrical stimulation of rabbit tibialis anterior muscles. Approximate half-times ($t1/2$) of the changes and the intracellular localization of each enzyme are given: ●, mitochondrial matrix; ○, mitochondrial inner membrane; □, mitochondria and cytosol; ■, cytosol. The localization of KACAT and BCAAT is not well established in skeletal muscle. Abbreviations are as in Figures 14–1 to 14–3, except for adenylate deaminase (AMPD), branched-chain amino acid aminotransferase (BCAAT), carnitine acetyltransferase (CAcT), creatine kinase (CK), fructose 1,6-bisphosphatase (FBP), glutamate dehydrogenase (GDH), aspartate transaminase (GOT), alanine transaminase (GPT), hexokinase (HK), 3-keto acid CoA transferase (KACAT), phosphofructokinase (PFK), phosphoglucomutase (PGM), succinate dehydrogenase (SDH), and thiolase (Th). (Modified with permission from Henriksson et al., 1986.)

responsible for increases in citrate synthase and 3-oxoacid CoA transferase following stimulation.

The metabolic rearrangement induced by stimulation appears to be appropriate for the adaptation to lower energy consumption: The aerobic energy supply increases and the glycolytic capacity needed to fuel intensive short-term power decreases. What, then, does electrical stimulation reveal about the limits of metabolic transformation? Prolonged stimulation of fast muscle increases oxidative enzymes not only to levels above control, but to levels three- to fivefold above normal soleus, the definitive SO muscle, and above cardiac muscle (Table 14–2). Glycolytic enzymes, on the other hand, fall to levels not far above those of soleus. These results illustrate an extreme adaptive potential for adult muscle, and indicate that control levels of fast and slow muscles do not set the absolute limits of plasticity.

Relationship of Metabolism to Other Functional Changes

In a review of the mutable properties of muscle affected by low-frequency stimulation, Pette and Vrbová (1985) note that the intrinsic capacity of the

Table 14–2 Enzyme changes in stimulated fast muscle relative to slow and cardiac muscle.

	Stimulated	Control			
	TA	TA	Soleus	Myocard.	Purkinje
Oxidative enzymes					
MDH	42	8	14	36	19
CS	18	3	4	16	6
BOAC	20	2	6	18	9
HK[a]	2.4	0.2	0.4	1.3	1.6
Glycolytic enzymes					
PFK	6	31	3	6	6
LDH	102	442	52	30	19
PHRL	5	30	4	2	2
GS	0.4	0.5	0.4	0.2	0.3

Source: Data compiled from Henriksson et al. (1986), Chi et al. (1986), and Henry and Loury (1983, 1985).

Note: Enzyme activities are in moles per kilogram of dry weight per hour at 21°C.

Abbreviations are as in Figure 14–1 to 14–5, except for glycogen synthetase (GS), tibialis anterior (TA), and myocardium (Myocard.).

[a]HK is glycolytic but involved in glucose transport into cells.

contractile elements to develop tension does not change. This is consistent with the findings that under normal conditions no difference has been found in maximum tetanic force per cross-sectional area of cat soleus and EDL (Faulkner et al., 1980) or in the force development of glycerol-extracted or mechanically skinned fast- and slow-twitch fibers (Sexton and Gersten, 1967; Donaldson et al., 1978; Lucas et al., 1987). However, this important concept is controversial, as others have reported threefold differences between fast- and slow-twitch fibers (Burke and Tsairis, 1973; see also Chapters 11 and 15, this volume). While conditioned muscle retains its capacity to develop force, the twitch contraction time is increased. Thus, the overall physiological effect of the fast-to-slow transformation is the reduction of fusion frequency.

Structural changes accommodate metabolic needs. The most important change is the reduction in fiber diameter, which serves to limit the diffusion distance for substrates and oxygen. In addition, slow isozymes of myosin and regulatory contractile proteins are expressed; excess sarcoplasmic reticulum for quick release and sequestration of calcium is no longer needed and is, therefore, disassembled; capillary density is increased to facilitate the enhanced substrate and oxygen flux; and mitochondrial volume is increased to provide additional binding surface for the increased concentration of oxidative enzymes (Pette and Vrbová, 1985).

These transformations occur in an orderly sequence (reviewed by Pette and Vrbová, 1985). The earliest changes appear to be the prolonged rise and relaxation times of the twitch contraction, appropriately accompanied by a decrease in the machinery to pump, bind, and sequester calcium. The reduction in contraction time and calcium pumping, in turn, reduces the rate at which ATP is needed to accommodate oxidative metabolism. Finally, enzyme changes are augmented by a shift toward the more fuel-efficient slow myosin isoforms. The extent of completion of this sequence is a function of the strength and duration of the adaptive stimulus, which may account for the incomplete transformations with less strenuous volitional exercises.

Strength Training

Exercise programs designed to increase strength do not simply produce the reverse of endurance-induced responses. High-resistance, low-repetition activities increase the maximum force output of muscle, made possible by an increase in the cross-sectional area of individual fibers. However, strength training programs do not greatly alter mitochondrial or glycolytic enzymes; these appear to be in the range of those exhibited by sedentary subjects (Gollnick et al., 1972; Costill et al., 1979). Concurrent strength and endurance training increases aerobic power but has little effect on muscle strength (Dudley and Fleck, 1987). Thus, oxidative demands are met regardless of force production. A plausible explanation for the limitation on strength by concurrent endurance training is competitive demands on cellular structure. Increased power requires a large cross-sectional area to maximize contractile elements, whereas oxidative capacity requires a short diffusion distance for oxygen and substrates, and therefore a small cross-sectional area.

The Intrinsic Capacity to Change

Many forms of alterations in muscle performance besides growth and exercise affect metabolic capacity—for example, those induced by hormonal modifications, hypoxia, denervation and chordotomy, space travel and other forms of disuse, and a broad range of diseases. The extent of change that can be attributed to neural influences alone has been questioned since Buller et al. (1960) first showed that the contractile and molecular properties that define fiber types are reversed with cross-innervation of fast and slow muscles. There are continued efforts to separate the roles of neural influences and genetic preprogramming in determining muscle phenotype. The experimental results presented in this chapter suggest that preprogrammed nerve–muscle pairing does not preclude the potential impact of environmental influences during neonatal times when the nerve message is minimal, or the overriding influence of nerve on mature muscles when the neural signal becomes strong. The challenge is to use this information to help uncover the nature of the intracellular signals that are responsible for changes in the metabolic and contractile proteins of muscle.

REFERENCES

Baldwin, D. M., Winder, W. W., and Holloszy, J. O. (1973). Glycolytic enzymes in different types of skeletal muscle: Adaptation to exercise. *Am. J. Physiol.* 225, 962–966.

Bárány, M. (1967). ATPase activity of myosin correlated with speed of muscle shortening. *J. Gen. Physiol.* 50 (Suppl, Pt 2), 197–218.

Betto, D. D., Zerbato, E., and Betto, R. (1986). Type 1, 2A, and 2B myosin heavy chain electrophoretic analysis of rat muscle fibers. *Biochem. Biophys. Res. Commun.* 138, 981–987.

Billeter, R., Heizmann, C. W., and Jenny, H. H. (1981). Analysis of myosin light and heavy chain types in single human skeletal muscle fibers. *Eur. J. Biochem.* 116, 389–395.

Brooke, M. H., and Kaiser, K. K. (1970). Three "myosin adenosine triphosphatase" systems: The nature of their pH lability and sulfhydryl dependence. *J. Histochem. Cytochem.* 18, 670–672.

Buchegger, A., Nemeth, P. M., Pette, D., and Reichmann, H. (1984). Effects of chronic stimulation on the metabolic heterogeneity of the fibre population in rabbit tibialis anterior muscle. *J. Physiol.* 350, 109–119.

Buller, J. J., Eccles, J. C., and Eccles, R. M. (1960). Interactions between motoneurones and muscles in respect of the characteristic speeds of their responses. *J. Physiol.* 150, 417–439.

Burke, R. E. (1981). Motor units: Anatomy, physiology and functional organization. In *Handbook of Physiology*, Sect. 1, Part 1: *The Nervous System: Motor Control* (ed. V. B. Brooks). American Physiological Society, Bethesda, Md., pp. 345–422.

Burke, R. E., Levine, D. N., Tsairis, P., and Zajac, F. E., III (1973). Physiological types and histochemical profiles in motor units of the cat gastrocnemius. *J. Physiol.* 234, 723–748.

Burke, R. E., and Tsairis, P. (1973). Anatomy and innervation ratios in motor units of cat gastrocnemius. *J. Physiol.* 234, 749–765.

Butler-Browne, G. S., Herlicoviez, D., and Whalen, R. G. (1984). Effects of hypothyroidism on myosin isozyme transitions in developing rat muscle. *FEBS Lett.* 166, 71–75.

Chi, M. M.-Y., Hintz, C. S., Coyle, E. F., Martin, W. H. III, Ivy, J. L., Nemeth, P. M., Holloszy, J. O., and Lowry, O. H. (1983). Effects of detraining on enzymes of energy metabolism in individual human muscle fibers. *Am. J. Physiol.* 244, (*Cell Physiol.* 13), C276–C287.

Chi, M. M.-Y., Hintz, C. S., Henriksson, J., Salmons, S., Hellendahl, R. P., Park, J. L., Nemeth, P. M., and Lowry, O. H. (1986). Chronic stimulation of mammalian muscle: Enzyme changes in individual fibers. *Am. J. Physiol.* 251 (*Cell Physiol.* 20), C633–C642.

Close, R. (1972). Dynamic properties of mammalian skeletal muscles. *Physiol. Rev.* 52, 129–197.

Costill, D. L., Coyle, E. F., Fink, W., Lesmes, G. R., and Witzmann, F. A. (1979). Adaptations in skeletal muscle following strength training. *J. Appl. Physiol.* 46, 149–154.

Crow, M. T., and Kushmerick, M. J. (1982). Chemical energetics of slow and fast twitch muscles of the mouse. *J. Gen. Physiol.* 79, 149–166.

Dangain, J., Pette, D., and Vrbová, G. (1987) Developmental changes in succinate dehydrogenase activity in muscle fibers from normal and dystrophic mice. *Exp. Neurol.* 95, 224–234.

Donaldson, S., Bolitho, S. K., and Hermansen, L. (1978). Differential direct effects of H^+ on Ca^{2+} activated force in skinned fibres from soleus, cardiac and adductor magnus muscles of rabbits. *Pfluegers Arch.* 376, 55–65.

Dudley, G. A., and Fleck, S. J. (1987). Strength and endurance training: Are they mutually exclusive? *Sports Med.* 4, 79–85.

Essén, B., Jansson, E., Henriksson, J., Taylor, A. W., and Saltin, B. (1975). Metabolic characteristics of fibre types in human skeletal muscle. *Acta Physiol. Scand.* 95, 153–165.

Faulkner, J. A., Niemeyer, J. H., Maxwell, L. C., and White, T. P. (1980). Contractile properties of transplanted extensor digitorum longus muscles of cats. *Am. J. Physiol.* 238 (*Cell Physiol.* 7), C120–C126.

Gambke, B., Lyons, G., Haselgrove, J., Kelly, A., and Rubinstein, N. (1983). Thyroid and neural control of myosin transitions. *FEBS Lett.* 156, 335–339.

Gollnick, P. D., Armstrong, R. B., Saubert, C. W., IV, Piehl, K., and Saltin, B. (1972). Enzyme activity and fiber composition in skeletal muscle of untrained and trained men. *J. Appl. Physiol.* 33, 312–319.

Gollnick, P. D., and Hodgson, D. R. (1986). The identification of fiber types in skeletal muscle: A continual dilemma. *Exerc. Sport Sci. Rev.* 14, 81–104.

Hamm, T. M., Nemeth, P. M., Solanki, L., Gordon, D. A., Reinking, R. M., and Stuart, D. G. (1988). Association between biochemical and physiological properties in single motor units. *Muscle Nerve* 11, 95–104.

Henriksson, J., Chi, M. M.-Y., Hintz, C. S., Young, D. A., Kaiser, K. K., Salmons, S., and Lowry, O. H. (1986). Chronic stimulation of mammalian muscle: Changes in enzymes of six metabolic pathways. *Am. J. Physiol.* 251 (*Cell Physiol.* 20), C614–C632.

Henry, C. H., and Lowry, O. H. (1983). Quantitative histochemistry of canine cardiac Purkinje fibers. *Am. J. Physiol.* 245 (*Heart Circ. Physiol.* 14), H824–H829.

Henry, C. H., and Lowry, O. H. (1985). Enzyme and metabolites of glycogen metabolism in canine cardiac Purkinje fibers. *Am. J. Physiol.* 248 (*Heart Circ. Physiol.* 17), H599–H605.

Hintz, C. S., Chi, M. M.-Y., Fell, R. D., Ivy, J. L., Kaiser, K. K., Lowry, C. V., and Lowry, O. H. (1982). Metabolite changes in individual rat muscle fibers during stimulation. *Am. J. Physiol.* (*Cell Physiol.* 11), C218–C228.

Hintz, C. S., Coyle, E. F., Kaiser, K. K., Chi, M. M.-Y., and Lowry, O. H. (1984). Comparison of muscle fiber typing by quantitative enzyme assays and by myosin ATPase staining. *J. Histochem. Cytochem.* 32, 655–660.

Hintz, C. S., Lowry, C. V., Kaiser, K. K., McKee, D., and Lowry, O. H. (1980). Enzyme levels in individual rat muscle fibers. *Am. J. Physiol.* 239 (*Cell Physiol.* 8), C58–C65.

Holloszy, J. O. (1967). Biochemical adaptations in muscle. Effects of exercise on mitochondrial oxygen uptake and respiratory enzyme activity in skeletal muscle. *J. Biol. Chem.* 242, 2278–2282.

Holloszy, J. O., and Booth, F. W. (1976). Biochemical adaptations to endurance exercise in muscle. *Ann. Rev. Physiol.* 38, 273–291.

Hudlická, O., Pette, D., and Staudte, H. (1973). The relation between blood flow and enzymatic activities of slow and fast muscles during development. *Pfluegers Arch.* 343, 341–356.

Izumo, S., Nadal-Ginard, B., and Mahdavi, V. (1986). All members of the MHC multigene family respond to thyroid hormone in a highly tissue specific manner. *Science* 231, 597–600.

Kelly, A. M., and Rubinstein, N. A. (1980). Why are fetal muscles slow? *Nature* 288, 266–269.

Kimura, R. E., and Warshaw, J. B. (1983). Metabolic adaptations of the fetus and newborn. *J. Pediatr. Gastroenterol. Nutr.* 2 (Suppl 1), S12–S15.

Kuehne, W. (1865). Ueber den Farbstoff der Muskeln. *Arch. Pathol. Anat. Physiol. Klin. Med.* 33, 79–94.

Kugelberg, E. (1976). Adaptive transformation in rat soleus motor units during growth. *J. Neurol. Sci.* 27, 269–289.

Kugelberg, E., and Edström, L. (1968). Differential histochemical effects of muscle contraction on phosphorylase and glycogen in various types of fibres: Relation to fatigue. *J. Neurol. Neurosurg. Psychiatry* 31, 415–423.

Lowry, C. V., Kimmey, J. S., Felder, S., Chi, M. M.-Y., Kaiser, K. K., Passonneau, P. M., Kirk, K. A., and Lowry, O. H. (1978). Enzyme patterns in single human muscle fibers. *J. Biol. Chem.* 253, 8269–8277.

Lowry, O. H., and Passonneau, J. V. (1972). *A Flexible System of Enzymatic Analysis.* Academic Press, New York.

Lucas, S. M., Ruff, R. L., and Binder, M. D. (1967). Specific tension measurements in single soleus and medial gastrocnemius muscle fibers of the cat. *Exp. Neurol.* 95, 142–154.

Lyons, G. E., Haselgrove, J., Kelly, A. M., and Rubinstein, N. (1983). Myosin transitions in developing fast and slow muscles of the rat hindlimb. *Differentiation* 25, 168–175.

Mahdavi, V., Strehler, E. E., Periasamy, M., Wieczorek, D., Izumo, S., and Nadal-Ginard, B. (1986). Sarcomeric myosin heavy chain gene family: Organization and pattern of expression. *Med. Sci. Sports Exerc.* 18, 299–308.

Margreth, A. (1970). Developmental patterns of LDH isozymes in fast and slow muscle of the rat. *Arch. Biochem. Biophys.* 141, 374–377.

Miller, J. B., Crow, M. T., and Stockdale, F. E. (1985). Slow and fast myosin heavy chain content defines three types of myotubes in early muscle cell cultures. *J. Cell Biol.* 101, 1643–1650.

Narusawa, M., Fitzsimons, R., Izumo, S., Nadal-Ginard, B., Rubinstein, N. A., and Kelly, A. M. (1987). Slow myosin in developing rat skeletal muscle. *J. Cell Biol.* 104, 447–459.

Nemeth, P. M., Hofer, H. W., and Pette, D. (1979). Metabolic heterogeneity of muscle fibers classified by myosin ATPase. *Histochemistry* 63, 191–201.

Nemeth, P. M., Norris, B. J., Lowry, O. H., Gordon, D. A., Enoka, R. M., and Stuart, D. G. (1988). Activation of muscle fibers in individual motor units revealed by 2-deoxyglucose-6-phosphate. *J. Neurosci.* 8(11):3959–3966.

Nemeth, P. M., Norris, B. J., Solanki, L., and Kelly, A. M. (in press). Metabolic specialization in fast and slow muscle fibers of the developing rat. *J. Neurosci.*

Nemeth, P., and Pette, D. (1981). Succinate dehydrogenase activity in fibres classified by myosin ATPase in three hindlimb muscles of the rat. *J. Physiol.* 320, 73–80.

Nemeth, P. M., Pette, D., and Vrbová, G. (1981). Comparison of enzymes activities among fibres within defined motor units. *J. Physiol.* 311, 489–495.

Nemeth, P. M., Solanki, L., and Lawrence, J. C., Jr. (1985). Control of enzyme activities in individual myotubes cultured without nerve. *Am. J. Physiol.* 249 (*Cell Physiol.* 18), C313–C317.

Nemeth, P. M., Solanki, L., Gordon, D. A., Hamm, T. M., Reinking, R. M., and Stuart, D. G. (1986). Uniformity of metabolic enzymes within individual motor units. *J. Neurosci.* 6, 892–898.

Nemeth, P. M., and Turk, W. R. (1984). Biochemistry of rat single muscle fibres in newly assembled motor units following nerve crush. *J. Physiol.* 355, 547–555.

Periasamy, M., Wieczorek, D. F., and Nadal-Ginard, B. (1984). Characterization of a developmentally regulated perinatal myosin heavy chain gene expressed in skeletal muscle. *J. Biol. Chem.* 259, 13573–13578.

Peter, J. B., Barnard, R. J., Edgerton, V. R., Gillespie, C. A., and Stemple, K. E.

(1972). Metabolic profiles of three fiber types of skeletal muscle in guinea pigs and rabbits. *Biochemistry* 11, 2627–2633.

Pette, D. (1984). Activity-induced fast to slow transitions in mammalian muscle. *Med. Sci. Sports Exerc.* 16, 517–528.

Pette, D., Smith, M. E., Staudte, H. W., and Vrbová, G. (1973). Effects of long-term electrical stimulation on some contraction and metabolic characteristics of fast rabbit muscles. *Pfluegers Arch.* 338, 257–272.

Pette, D., and Spamer, C. (1986). Metabolic properties of muscle fibers. *Fed. Proc.* 45, 2910–2914.

Pette, D., and Vrbová, G. (1985). Neural control of phenotypic expression in mammalian muscle fibers. *Muscle Nerve* 8, 676–689.

Reiser, P. J., Moss, R. L., Giulian G. G., and Greaser, M. L. (1985). Shortening velocity in single fibers from adult rabbit soleus muscles is correlated with myosin heavy chain composition. *J. Biol. Chem.* 260, 9077–9080.

Salmons, S., and Henriksson, J. (1981). The adaptive response of skeletal muscle to increased use. *Muscle Nerve* 4, 94–105.

Saltin, B., and Gollnick, P. D. (1983). Skeletal muscle adaptability: Significance for metabolism and performance. In *Handbook of Physiology, Sect. 10. Skeletal Muscle* (ed. L. D. Peachey, R. H. Adrian, and S. R. Geiger). American Physiological Society, Bethesda, Md., pp. 555–631.

Schweighoffer, F., Maire, P., Tuil, D., Gautron, S., Daegelen, D., Bachner, L., and Kahn, A. (1986). In vivo developmental modifications of the expression of genes encoding muscle-specific enzymes in rat. *J. Biol. Chem.* 261, 10272–10276.

Sexton, A. W., and Gersten, J. W. (1967). Isometric tension differences in fibers of red and white muscles. *Science* 157, 135–141.

Staron, R. S., and Pette, D. (1986). Correlation between myofibrillar ATPase activity and myosin heavy chain composition in rabbit muscle fibers. *Histochemistry* 86, 19–23.

Stuart, D. G., Binder, M. D., and Enoka, R. M. (1983). Motor unit organization: Application of the quadripartite scheme to human muscle. In *Peripheral Neuropathy* (ed. P. J. Dyck, P. K. Thomas, E. H. Lambert, and R. P. Bunge). Saunders, Philadelphia, pp. 1067–1090.

Vetter, C., Reichmann, H., and Pette, D. (1984). Microphotometric determination of enzyme activities in type grouped fibres of reinnervated rat muscle. *Histochemistry* 80, 347–351.

Vogel, M., and Landmesser, L. (1987). Distribution of fiber types in embryonic chick limb muscle innervated by foreign motorneurons. *Dev. Biol.* 119, 481–495.

Vrbová, G., Navarrete, R., and Lowrie, M. (1985). Matching of muscle properties and motorneuron firing patterns during early stages of development. *J. Exp. Biol.* 115, 113–123.

Whalen, R. B., Sell, S. M., Butler-Browne, G. S., Swartz, K., Bouveret, P., and Pinset-Harstrom, J. (1981). Three myosin heavy-chain isozymes appear sequentially in rat muscle development. *Nature* 292, 805–809.

Wilkinson, R. S., and Lichtman, J. W. (1985). Regular alternation of fiber types in the transversus abdominus muscle of the garter snake. *J. Neurosci.* 5, 2979–2988.

Williams, R. S., Salmons, S., Newsholme, E. A., Kaufman, R. E., and Mellor, J. (1986). Regulation of nuclear and mitochondrial protein expression by contractile activity in skeletal muscle. *J. Biol. Chem.* 261, 376–380.

15

Mechanisms for Respecifying Muscle Properties Following Reinnervation

RICHARD B. STEIN, TESSA GORDON,
AND JOANNE TOTOSY DE ZEPETNEK

When Elwood Henneman and his collaborators first presented the size principle (Henneman et al., 1965a), it was in the restricted context of experiments on the stretch and flexor reflexes in the spinal cord of decerebrate cats. Even at that time, however, they considered two distinct sets of size-related properties. The first involved the inputs to the motoneuron pool, which, together with the intrinsic properties of the cell bodies, led to an orderly pattern of excitability and inhibitability of motor units of differing size (Henneman et al., 1965b). The second related to the output properties of the motor unit (i.e., the force, contractile speed, and fatigue resistance of the muscle fibers innervated by motoneurons of differing size; Henneman and Olson, 1965). These two aspects will be referred to as the size-related "input" properties and "output" properties.

As documented throughout this volume, the orderly recruitment of motor units according to size (input properties) apply to an increasing number of movements over the years, including slow (Milner-Brown et al., 1973) and fast (Desmedt and Godaux, 1978) voluntary movements in normal human subjects. However, the extent of its applicability remains a controversial issue (Enoka and Stuart, 1984; Gustafsson and Pinter, 1985).

The muscle (output) properties can also be demonstrated to follow the size principle after recovery from pressure block (Milner-Brown et al., 1974) or nerve section and resuture (Thomas et al., 1987) of a peripheral nerve. Thus, these output properties can be respecified in the adult in addition to their emergence during normal growth in the neonatal period. This rematching of nerve and muscle properties according to the size principle following regeneration can be studied experimentally in more depth to explore the origins and underlying mechanisms of the output properties that are related to motoneuronal size. This topic forms the basis for the present chapter.

We first showed that the size principle could reemerge following nerve section and resuture of a nerve to a single muscle or closely synergistic muscles in the cat (see Fig. 15–1) (Gordon and Stein, 1982). The reinnervated motor units were indistinguishable from those in control muscles in terms of the force developed and the relations between motor axon size, muscle force, and contractile speed. Histochemically, however, the reinnervated muscles showed the typical type grouping (Fig. 15–2) first described by Karpati and Engel (1968) and Kugelberg et al. (1970). Since a given motoneuron does not reinnervate its original muscle fibers, but supplies many muscle fibers that were previously

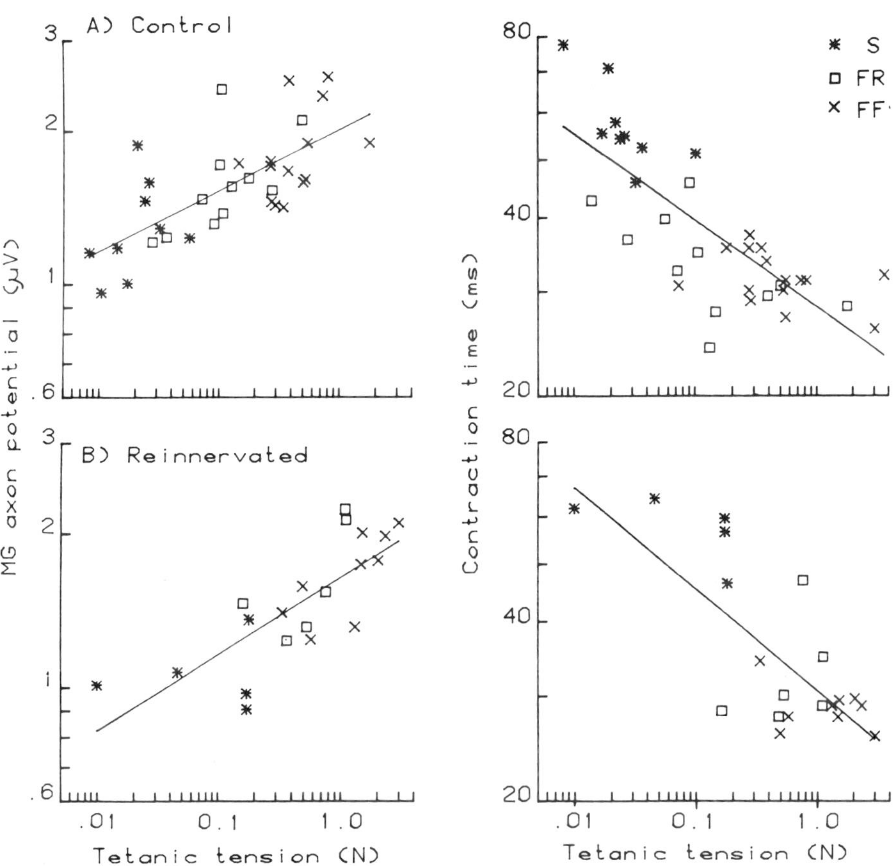

Fig. 15–1. The axon potential recorded extracellularly from a nerve cuff (a measure of motor axon size) is well correlated with the tetanic tension of the muscle unit innervated in control (A) and reinnervated (B) MG muscles of the cat. The contraction time is inversely correlated with the tetanic tension, indicating that large motoneurons innervate fast-contracting muscle fibers. The fatigue resistance of the motor units was measured using the method of Burke (1981). The fast, fatigable (FF) motor units tended to be largest, followed by the fast, fatigue-resistant (FR) and slow (S) units, although there was overlap of units in both control (normal) and reinnervated muscles. All scales are logarithmic. (From Gordon and Stein, 1982.)

A) Normal

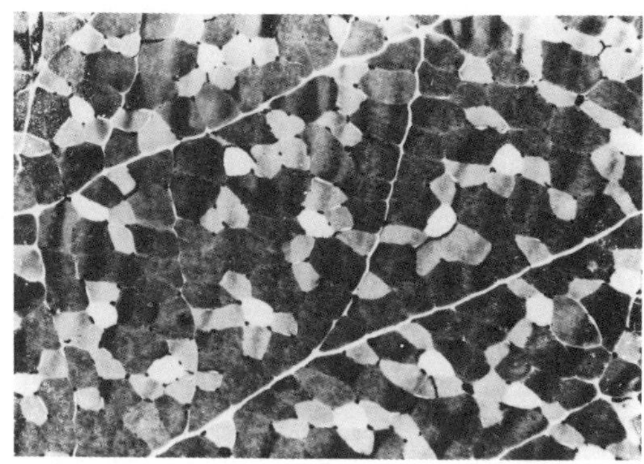

B) Reinnervated

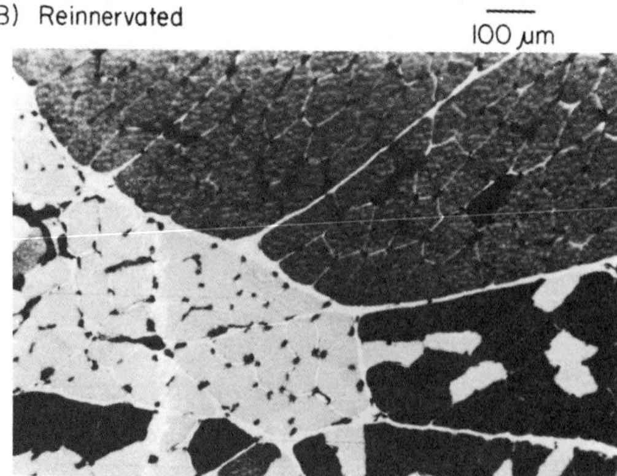

Fig. 15–2. Histochemical profiles from normally innervated (A) and cross-innervated (B) LG muscles of the cat after alkali ATPase staining. Fibers of the same histochemical type are clearly grouped together after cross-innervation. The slow oxidative (SO) fibers (lightly stained) are much larger and more numerous than in the control muscles and are comparable in size to the dark-staining fast glycolytic (FG) and intermediate-staining fast oxidative glycolytic (FOG) fibers. The calibration bar corresponds to 100 μm. (Modified from Gordon et al., 1988.)

of different histochemical types, the question arises as to what is respecified to result in this size matching after reinnervation. Respecification of muscle properties involves contractile force, speed of contraction, and fatigue properties, but in this chapter we concentrate on contractile force alone (see also Chapter 11, this volume).

NORMAL MOTOR UNITS

In reviewing the motor unit properties of cat muscles, Burke (1981) pointed out that the force, F, of a motor unit is the product of three factors:

$$F = NAS \tag{15–1}$$

where N is the number of muscle fibers innervated by the motoneuron (also referred to as the *innervation ratio*), A is the mean cross-sectional area of the muscle fibers, and S is the specific force or intrinsic contractility of the fibers (i.e., the force generated per unit cross-sectional area).

Any combination of these three factors may be responsible for the normal range of forces generated by motor units in a muscle. Various techniques have been applied to determine the relative importance of these factors in normal muscle. Since a variety of results have emerged, we will briefly reanalyze published data on normal muscles before considering the effect of reinnervation. Taking the logarithm of Equation 15–1 gives

$$\log F = \log N + \log A + \log S \qquad (15\text{--}2)$$

so that the effects of the three factors are additive when logarithmic scales are used.

Perhaps the most careful published study is that of Bodine et al. (1987) on units of the cat tibialis anterior muscle. The authors stimulated single motor units to deplete their stores of glycogen, then counted the number of glycogen-depleted muscle fibers in the whole muscle and measured the cross-sectional areas of these fibers. Tabulated data from the 11 units they studied in this way are replotted on logarithmic scales in Figure 15–3. The data are well fitted by straight lines on the logarithmic scales used, so that

$$\log N = m_n \log F + b_n$$
$$\log A = m_a \log F + b_a \qquad (15\text{--}3)$$
$$\log S = m_s \log F + b_s$$

where the m_i are the slopes and the b_i are the intercepts of the fitted lines on these double logarithmic plots. Adding the three parts of Equation 15–3 together will give Equation 15–2 if and only if

$$m_n + m_a + m_s = 1 \qquad (15\text{--}4)$$
$$b_n + b_a + b_s = 0$$

The summation of the intercepts (b_i) to zero is not of particular interest, but the summation of the slopes (m_i) to unity is, since the individual slopes give the relative weighting of each of the three factors in determining the variation in motor unit forces observed.

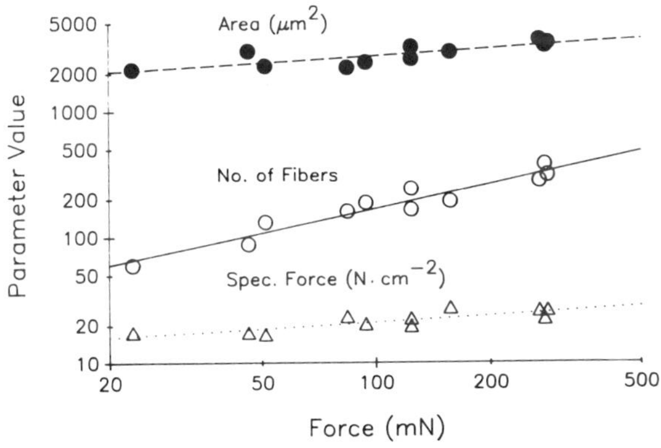

Fig. 15–3. Single-motor units were repeatedly stimulated to deplete their glycogen. The force generated by each motor unit was then compared with the number of fibers innervated, the cross-sectional area of these fibers, and the specific force (intrinsic contractility) of the muscle fibers (obtained from Eq. 15–1). Note that the steepest dependence, as measured by the slopes of the fitted lines (by the method of least mean square error) in this study by Bodine et al. (1987), is on the number of fibers. All scales are logarithmic for reasons described in the text.

From Figure 15–3, it is evident that the dependence of force on the number of muscle fibers in each motor unit is the strongest factor, as pointed out by Bodine et al. (1987), but Equation 15–4 permits this to be quantified. The magnitudes of the three slopes are illustrated in the bar graph of Figure 15–4. Their values are $m_n = 0.64$, $m_a = 0.18$, and $m_s = 0.18$, which means that 64% of the variation in motor unit force is accounted for by variation in the number of fibers innervated and the balance is equally divided between the other two factors.

From preliminary results (Totosy de Zepetnek et al., 1987), using the same techniques in another species (rat instead of cat), quite a different balance was found, as also shown in Figure 15–4. The cross-sectional area is the predominant factor ($m_a = 0.69$) determining force, while the contribution of specific force is negligible ($m_s = 0.01$). The standard errors of the slopes were also calculated for these two studies and are shown on the bar graphs. The values of the two major factors (number of fibers and cross-sectional area) are significantly different between the two studies ($p < 0.02$ using Student's t-test), but the values of the specific force are not.

The results of both of these studies contrast markedly to those of the earlier studies of Burke and his colleagues on cat medial gastrocnemius and those of Dum and his colleagues on cat flexor digitorum longus muscle. The data shown in Figure 15–4 were those tabulated by Burke (1981), who gives references to original published (Burke and Tsairis, 1973; Dum and Kennedy, 1980) and unpublished work. The data from Foehring et al. (1986) and our own work (Gordon et al., 1988) on cat medial gastrocnemius muscle (both studies also shown in Fig. 15–4) are in reasonable agreement with the work from Burke's group.

The results from the last four studies (in which Burke, Dum, Foehring, and Gordon were the first authors) were based on average data for motor unit types. Thus, the forces were measured physiologically in units classified as fast-twitch, fatigable (FF), fast-twitch, fatigue resistant (FR), or slow (S), using the methods described by Burke (1981). Some fast units have intermediate fatigue resistance (FI), but these few units were distributed between the FF and FR categories in each study.

The proportion of each motor unit type measured physiologically can then be compared with the proportion of muscle fibers classified histochemically as fast glycolytic (FG), fast oxidative glycolytic (FOG), and slow oxidative (SO) (Brooke and Kaiser, 1970). The ratio of proportions for corresponding types (e.g., % FG muscle fibers/% FF motor units) is often referred to as the *relative innervation ratio*. The cross-sectional areas can also be measured for each histochemical fiber type and, finally, a relative specific force can be calculated to satisfy Equation 15–1, again assuming a direct correspondance between the motor unit types measured physiologically and the muscle fibers measured histochemically.

This method, with some variations, was applied in each of the four studies cited earlier, data from which are summarized in the middle and lower portions of Figure 15–4. Note that there are only three data points for computing each slope (the values for FF, FR, and S units in these studies), so the standard

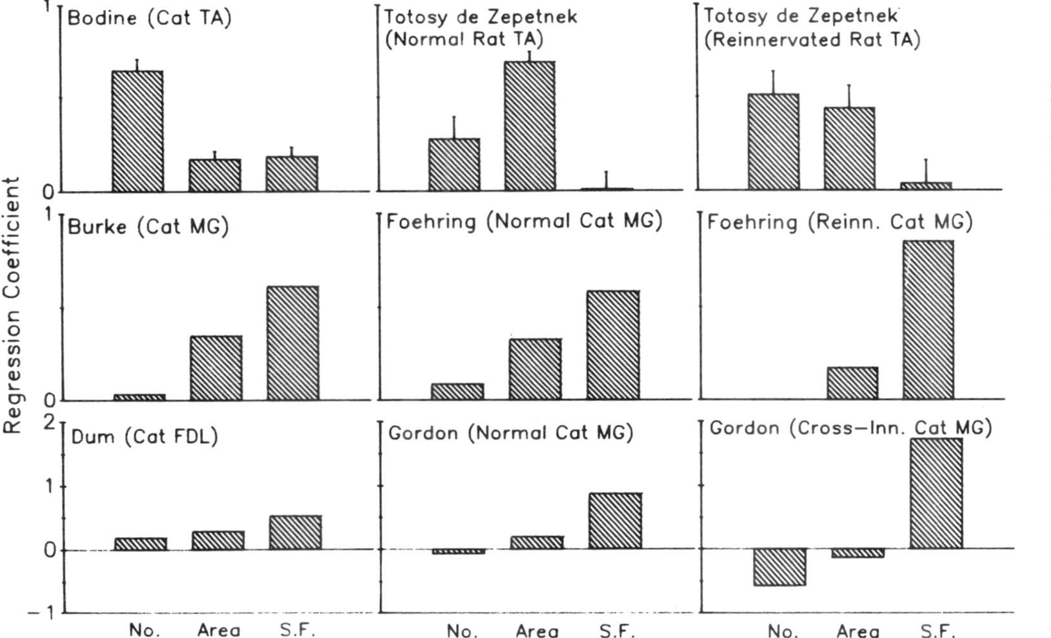

Fig. 15–4. Regression coefficients (the slopes of the lines as shown in Fig. 15–3) are plotted in the form of bar histograms for nine studies, each of which is identified by the name of the first author and the muscle studied. The six studies on the left and in the center of this figure are for normal TA, medial MG, or FDL muscles of the cat or rat. The data on the right are for muscles that were either reinnervated by the same nerve (Totosy de Zepetnek, Foehring) or a foreign nerve (Gordon). The coefficients relate the motor unit force measured physiologically to the number of fibers and the cross-sectional area of the fibers measured histochemically. The specific force (intrinsic contractility of the muscle fibers) was computed from Equation 15–1 for each data set. The coefficients sum to 1.0 for each study, as indicated in Equation 15–4, so the values of the coefficients give the relative dependence of the force output on each of the three factors. In the three studies on the top, single motor units were studied by glycogen depletion of 11 units (Bodine) 6 units (Totosy de Zepetnek, normal) and 9 units (Totosy de Zepetnek, reinnervated). A full discussion of the widely varying results from different studies is given in the text.

errors of the slopes are not shown because they are not meaningful with such a small sample size. Nonetheless, the approximate agreement between the four studies gives some confidence in the data.

Furthermore, if the data for each motor unit type are averaged in the study of Bodine et al. (1987), for example, the same slopes are obtained to within the normal statistical limits, so combining motor unit data of the same type to approximate the whole muscle samples cannot produce the large disparities observed between different studies. Finally, Dr. Burke kindly provided us with his single-unit data on cross-sectional areas, which similarly highlight the importance of this variable in determining overall motor unit force, which is indicated in his averaged data.

MOTOR UNITS AFTER REINNERVATION

The disparity between different studies in the relative weighting of the three factors determining muscle force is even greater when studies on reinnervated muscles are included (right side of Fig. 15–4). In the rat tibialis anterior (Totosy de Zepetnek et al., 1987), the force generated by motor units depends mainly on the number of muscle fibers supplied during reinnervation ($m_n = 0.51$) and on their cross-sectional area ($m_a = 0.44$). However, in the averaged cat motor units of Foehring et al. (1986) and Gordon et al. (1988), the force output of the motor units seems to depend almost completely on intrinsic contractility (*specific tension* in Chapter 11, this volume). In fact, in the data of Gordon et al., in which the muscles were cross-innervated by a foreign nerve, the other two factors went in the opposite direction (i.e., the values of the slopes were negative). The small, slow motor units actually innervated more and larger muscle fibers than many fast motor units (see Fig. 15–2). Note that since the three numbers must add up to 1.0, the presence of negative numbers must be balanced by a positive number that can be greater than 1.0.

DISCUSSION

Why are the results of these various studies so disparate, and what mechanisms might underlie the differences? The study of Bodine et al. (1987) suggests that motor units producing large forces do so mainly because they innervate more muscle fibers. Various possible mechanisms can be imagined to explain how this might come about during development. Nerve fibers that are successful in innervating large numbers of target fibers might receive more of a trophic factor and grow to become larger (Purves, 1986). Alternatively, differences in motoneuron size may occur before innervation (Huizar et al., 1975). Large motoneurons tend to be less excitable because of their greater membrane area, and hence are active less of the time (Hennig and Lømo, 1985). Neuromuscular activity tends to promote the elimination of polyneuronal innervation that occurs in developing and reinnervating muscle (O'Brien et al., 1978). Thus, smaller, more active motoneurons might reduce the number of their terminals on dually innervated muscle fibers more than larger fibers, and thus tend to generate less force.

The effect of muscle fiber area on force is a secondary factor in the units studied by Bodine et al. (1987) but is the primary factor in the normal units of Totosy de Zepetnek et al. (1987). Motor unit force is known to be inversely related to nerve activity (Eerbeek et al., 1984), and greater force is often achieved by increasing the number of thick and thin filaments, which increases the bulk and hence the cross-sectional area of the muscle fibers (Close, 1972; Walsh et al., 1978). Interestingly, in the reinnervated units of Totosy de Zepetnek et al. (1987), the number of fibers is again the major factor determining motor unit force, suggesting that the larger nerve cells are more effective in capturing denervated muscle fibers.

The other studies in Figure 15–4 on normal motor units, in which averaged data from physiological and histochemical measurements were compared, all suggest that the main factor explaining differences in force output is the specific force (i.e., intrinsic contractility of the fibers per cross-sectional area of muscle) of muscle fibers in different motor units. A mechanism to account for a large difference in intrinsic contractility has not been discovered, and a recent study by Lucas et al. (1987) failed to find any difference in intrinsic contractility of single type-identified, isolated, and skinned muscle fibers in cat medial gastrocnemius muscle. Perhaps, single skinned fibers behave quite differently from intact fibers in a whole muscle, but the small differences in specific force between fibers observed by Bodine et al. (1987) and the negligible differences observed by Totosy de Zepetnek et al. (1987) from glycogen-depleted motor units make this argument unlikely.

All the studies that concluded that specific force (intrinsic contractility) was the major factor in determining motor unit force were based on comparisons of histochemical fiber types with physiologically identified fiber types. Physiologically, a somewhat arbitrary division of motor units into fatigable and fatigue-resistant types must be made at some point (typically after 2 min of stimulation). Similarly, a somewhat arbitrary division must be made histochemically in terms of the intensity of particular stains. If these breakpoints do not correspond, i.e., if more fibers belong to FF motor units than stain as fast glycolytic FG muscle fibers and/or fewer fibers belong to the S motor units than stain as SO muscle fibers, then the discrepancies between different studies can be explained. The importance of the differences in specific force would be overestimated in these studies, and the importance of the number of fibers innervated would be underestimated.

CONCLUSIONS

A role for variations in the cross-sectional area of single muscle fibers in determining the range of motor unit forces seems assured. The six studies on normal muscles summarized in Figure 15–4 gave weightings to this factor of between 0.175 and 0.693 (mean, 0.339). The values in all three studies on reinnervated muscles were lower (mean, 0.158), suggesting that fiber area is not as important a factor in reinnervated muscles.

The relative importance of the other two factors (number of muscle fibers and specific force) remains more controversial. The direct measurements, using glycogen depletion in normal and reinnervated muscles, all indicate a major role for variations in fiber number in determining the total force output of normal and reinnervated motor units. The indirect measurements comparing physiological and histochemical classifications all claim a major role for variations in specific force, but possible errors were discussed earlier that may invalidate this approach (see also Chapter 11, this volume). The direct methods find a small or negligible role for variations of specific force in determining the force output of motor units. Finally, if the fatigability of motor units is continuously graded (see Chapter 13, this volume) and the somewhat arbitrary physiological and histochemical divisions do not correspond to each other, the meaningfulness of typing motor units into distinct species may also be questioned. Although by using several properties one can reliably "classify" motor units or motoneurons into distinct types (Zengel et al., 1985), when looking at a single variable (e.g., force) or a pair of variables (e.g., force versus area in Fig. 15–3), one is more struck by the continuous range of values and the goodness of fit for the lines drawn. It may still be useful to refer to different motor unit types in mammalian muscles when considering variables that form discrete groups or to summarize a number of different properties. However, the idea of size as a continuous variable that relates to many input and output properties of motor units, first proposed by Henneman about 25 years ago, remains an important and viable concept.

Acknowledgment

The work described in this chapter was supported in part by grants from the Medical Research Council of Canada, the Muscular Dystrophy Association of Canada, and the Alberta Heritage Foundation for Medical Research.

REFERENCES

Bodine, S. C., Roy, R. R., Eldred, E., and Edgerton, V. R. (1987). Maximal force as a function of anatomical features of motor units in the cat tibialis anterior. *J. Neurophysiol.* 57, 1730–1745.

Brooke, M. H., and Kaiser, K. K. (1970). Muscle fibre types: How many and what kind? *Arch. Neurol.* 23, 309–379.

Burke, R. E. (1981). Motor units: Anatomy, physiology and functional organization. In *Handbook of Physiology.*, Vol. II, Sect. 1.: *The Nervous System* (ed. V. B. Brooks). American Physiological Society, Bethesda, Md., pp. 345–422.

Burke, R. E., and Tsairis, P. (1973). Anatomy and innervation ratios in motor units of cat gastrocnemius. *J. Physiol.* 234, 749–765.

Close, R. I. (1972). Dynamic properties of mammalian skeletal muscles. *Physiol. Rev.* 52, 129–197.

Desmedt, J. E., and Godaux, E. (1978). Ballistic contractions in fast or slow human muscles: Discharge patterns of single motor units. *J. Physiol.* 285, 185–196.

Dum, R. P., and Kennedy, T. T. (1980). Physiological and histochemical characteristics in the cat tibialis anterior and extensor digitorum longus muscles. *J. Neurophysiol.* 4, 837–851.

Eerbeek, O., Kernell, D., and Verhey, B. A. (1984). Effects of fast and slow patterns of tonic long-term stimulation on contractile properties of fast muscle in the cat. *J. Physiol.* 352, 73–90.

Enoka, R. M., and Stuart, D. G. (1984). Henneman's "size principle": Current issues. *Trends Neurosci.* 7, 226–228.

Foehring, R. C., Sypert, G. W., and Munson, J. B. (1986). Properties of self-reinnervated motor units of medial gastrocnemius of cat. I. Long-term reinnervation. *J. Physiol.* 55, 931–946.

Gordon, T., and Stein, R. B. (1982). Reorganization of motor unit properties in reinnervated muscles of the cat. *J. Neurophysiol.* 48, 1175–1190.

Gordon, T., Thomas, C. K., Stein, R. B., and Erdebil, S. (1988). Comparison of physiological and histochemical properties of motor units following cross-reinnervation of antagonistic muscles in the cat hindlimb. *J. Neurophysiol.* 60, 365–378.

Gustafsson, B., and Pinter, M. J. (1985). On factors determining orderly recruitment of motor units: A role for intrinsic membrane properties. *Trends Neurosci.* 8, 431–433.

Henneman, E., and Olson, C. B. (1965). Relations between structure and function in the design of skeletal muscles. *J. Neurophysiol.* 28, 581–598.

Henneman, E., Somjen, G., and Carpenter, D. O. (1965a). Functional significance of cell size in spinal motoneurons. *J. Neurophysiol.* 28, 560–580.

Henneman, E., Somjen, G., and Carpenter, D. O. (1965b). Excitability and inhibitability of motoneurons of different sizes. *J. Neurophysiol.* 28, 599–620.

Hennig, R., and Lømo, T. (1985). Firing patterns of motor units in normal rats. *Nature* 314, 164–166.

Huizar, P., Kuno, M., and Miyata, Y. (1975). Differentiation of motoneurons and skeletal muscles in kittens. *J. Physiol.* 252, 465–479.

Karpati, G., and Engel, W. K. (1968). "Type-grouping" in skeletal muscles after experimental reinnervation. *Neurology* 18, 447–455.

Kugelberg, E., Edström, L., and Abbruzzese, M. (1970). Mapping of motor units in experimentally reinnervated rat muscle. Interpretation of histochemical and atrophic fibre patterns in neurogenic lesions. *J. Neurol. Neurosurg. Psychiatry* 33, 319–329.

Lucas, S. M., Ruff, R. L., and Binder, M. D. (1987). Specific tension measurements in single soleus and medial gastrocnemius muscle fibers of the cat. *Exp. Neurol.* 95, 142–154.

Milner-Brown, H. S., Stein, R. B., and Lee, R. G. (1974). The pattern of recruiting human motor units in neuropathies and motor neurone disease. *J. Neurol. Neurosurg. Psychiatry* 37, 665–669.

Milner-Brown, H. S., Stein, R. B., and Yemm, R. (1973). The orderly recruitment of human motor units during voluntary isometric contractions. *J. Physiol.* 230, 359–370.

O'Brien, R. A. D., Ostberg, A. J. C., and Vrbova, G. (1978). Observations on the elimination of polyneuronal innervation in developing mammalian skeletal muscle. *J. Physiol.* 282, 571–582.

Purves, D. (1986). The trophic theory of neural connections. *Trends Neurosci.* 9, 486–489.

Thomas, C. K., Stein, R. B., Gordon, T., Lee, R. G., and Elleker, M. G. (1987). Patterns of reinnervation and motor unit recruitment in human muscles after complete ulnar and median nerve section and resuture. *J. Neurol. Neurosurg. Psychiatry* 50, 259–268.

Totosy de Zepetnek, J. E., Zung, H. V., and Gordon, T. (1987). Motor unit force, innervation ratio and muscle fiber size in normal and reinnervated muscle. *Soc. Neurosci. Abst.* 13, 874.

Walsh, J. V., Burke, R. E., Rymer, W. Z., and Tsairis, P. (1978). Effect of compensatory hypertrophy studied in individual motor units in medial gastrocnemius muscle of the cat. *J. Neurophysiol.* 41, 496–508.

Zengel, J. E., Reid S. A., Sypert, G. W., and Munson, J. B. (1985). Membrane electrical properties and prediction of motor-unit type of medial gastrocnemius motoneurons in the cat. *J. Neurophysiol.* 53, 1323–1344.

V
SYNAPTIC INPUTS TO MOTONEURONS

16

Synaptic Inputs to Type-Identified Motor Units

JOHN B. MUNSON

There is general agreement that motor units have a usual order of recruitment, i.e., from small to large. There is no universal agreement, however, on small or large *what* (i.e., motoneuron size? motor axon size? muscle unit size?). In his original description of orderly recruitment, Henneman related recruitment order to amplitude of axonal action potential, from which he extrapolated axon size and thence motoneuron size (Henneman, 1957). It was further assumed that motoneuron size, axon size, and muscle unit size were all closely inter-correlated, and thus that recruitment in order of contraction strength would follow from recruitment in order of motoneuron (and axon) size (Henneman et al., 1965).

Assuming that such intercorrelations exist, how could gradations of motoneuron size provide a mechanism for their orderly size-related recruitment (thus provisionally providing recruitment in order of muscle unit contraction strength)? In the specific case of the size-dependent susceptibility of motoneurons to discharge by Ia volleys, Ia afferents were hypothesized to project to *all* homonymous motoneurons in proportion to the size of those motoneurons, thus creating an "equal density" of Ia synapses on the motoneuron surface. Differential synaptic drive could come about through greater specific membrane resistance of small motoneurons or because of greater partial failure of transmission to large motoneurons (reviewed in Henneman and Mendell, 1981).

A test of the hypothesis of 100% frequency of homonymous projection was conducted by Mendell and Henneman (1968, 1971). In this seminal work, the technique later to be known as "spike-triggered averaging" was first described and used to map physiologically the synaptic projections of individual group Ia spindle afferents to individual homonymous motoneurons. As Henneman had predicted (see Chapter 17, this volume), each group Ia afferent generated a detectable excitatory postsynaptic potential (EPSP) in virtually all (~93%) of the homonymous motoneurons. [Homonymous *anatomical* group Ia afferent-to-motoneuron projection frequency, at least within the medial gastrocnemius (MG) motoneuron pool, may be 100%, based on the observation of Nelson et al. (1979) of such projection frequency within hours of acute spinal transection.] In some experiments, the predicted inverse relationship between motor axon conduction velocity and individual EPSP amplitude was also observed (Mendell and Henneman, 1971, Fig. 13).

The view that "The essence of the motoneuron pool . . . is the spectrum of sizes represented in it" (Henneman et al., 1965, p. 577) was not held by all; there existed alternatives to ordering motoneurons simply on the basis of presumed size. The simplest scheme dichotomized motoneurons as fast (type F: brief muscle unit twitch time, fast axon conduction velocity, brief afterhyperpolarization) or slow (type S: parameters reversed from those of type F). The fast category was subsequently refined into three subcategories, which were defined rigorously on the basis of the associated muscle unit's resistance to fatigue: types FF, F(int), and FR (see Chapter 11, this volume). Recruitment was considered to proceed in the order S → FR → F(int) → FF. This recruitment by motor unit type is in part consistent with recruitment by motoneuron size (see Burke et al., 1982). Type S motor units have small, high-resistance motoneurons, slowly conducting axons, and weakly contracting muscle units; type FF motor units have large, low-resistance motoneurons, rapidly conducting axons, and strongly contracting muscle units. However type FR motor units, whose contraction strength and motoneuron properties are intermediate between those of types S and FF, have axon conduction velocities (and thus, presumably, axon sizes) identical to those of type FF units. While recruitment in order of conduction velocity as well as of contraction strength seems the rule for both the all-slow cat soleus muscle and for the type S units of the cat's heterogeneous MG muscle (Bawa, et al., 1984; Zajac and Faden, 1985), recruitment of MG fast units is random for conduction velocity, although orderly for contraction strength (Chapter 5, this volume). This random relationship between axon conduction velocity and contraction strength for motor units with fast conduction velocity (provisional fast motor units) was observed by Henneman and co-workers as well (Wuerker et al., 1965, Fig. 9).

The immediate factors responsible for motoneuron activation include the balance of excitatory and inhibitory synaptic drives and the motoneuron's intrinsic properties (the latter, in part, determine the former). The latter have been discussed in Chapters 9 and 10 of this volume; the present chapter deals with the excitatory and inhibitory synaptic drives upon motoneurons as they relate to the motor unit type of the recipient motoneuron, and thus to their recruitment and activity.

EXCITATORY POSTSYNAPTIC POTENTIALS FROM MUSCLE AFFERENTS

The most commonly studied source of EPSPs in motoneurons is group Ia (muscle spindle) afferents, which make monosynaptic connection with both homonymous and heteronymous motoneurons. Electrical stimulation of a muscle nerve evokes a synchronous volley of group I action potentials and generates a *composite* EPSP. These were found to be larger in the motoneurons of the cat's slow, red soleus, crureus, and caput mediale muscles than in those of their fast, pale synergists (Eccles et al., 1957). This fact was attributed to the "larger group Ia receptiveness" of the motoneurons controlling slow postural muscles. Subsequent authors have categorized individual triceps surae motoneurons (on the basis of muscle unit contractile properties) as slow or fast (Burke, 1967) or as type S, FR, F(int), or FF (Burke et al., 1973) and have confirmed that group I composite monosynaptic EPSPs increase in amplitude according to motoneuron type: FF < F(int) < FR < S. This is true for both homonymous projections (e.g., MG Ia → MG motoneuron; Burke et al., 1976) and heteronymous projections (e.g., LGS → MG; Mayer et al., 1984; Munson et al., 1986). The generality of these findings has been tested by Dum and Kennedy (1980), who examined homonymous EPSPs of the flexor muscle tibialis anterior (an antagonist of the commonly studied triceps surae muscle group), and by Dum et al. (1978), who examined the flexor digitorum longus muscle. The relation of group I composite EPSPs to motor unit type was the same in all systems.

Over the motoneuron pool of the heterogeneous MG muscle, group I composite EPSP amplitude is not only organized in accordance with motor unit type, but is directly correlated with motoneuron input resistance and inversely correlated with axon conduction velocity, contraction strength, and soma size in accordance with a size principle (see the earlier discussion). However these correlations, which are observed over heterogeneous populations, may simply be the result of combining subgroups (i.e., motor unit type groups) with intrinsically different characteristics, since such correlations may or may not be seen *within* the separate motor unit groups (e.g., Fleshman et al., 1981a). It should be pointed out, however, that each of these measured electrical properties of motoneurons is distributed continuously over the entire motoneuron pool (e.g., Zengel et al., 1985).

The amplitude of the composite EPSP measured in a motoneuron derives directly from two factors: the number of afferents generating EPSPs in that motoneuron and the amplitude of the single-fiber EPSP contributed by each afferent (among other factors are nonlinear summation and synchrony of arrival time of afferent action potentials; see Munson et al., 1980). Spike-trigger averaged group Ia EPSPs in triceps surae motoneurons can be analyzed to test the relative contributions of these factors. Table 16–1 compares and combines data from three studies that analyzed projections (EPSP amplitude and projection frequency) of individual MG group Ia afferents to type-identified MG motoneurons.

The agreement among the separate studies (Table 16–1A) is striking, as is that between these combined single-fiber data (Tables 16–1A and 16–1B) and the original such data of Mendell and Henneman (1971): i.e., projection frequencies, 89% vs. 93%, respectively, and mean amplitudes, 109 μV vs. 102 μV. Similar population values were obtained by Scott and Mendell (1976), Watt et al. (1976), and Munson and Sypert (1979).

The agreement between the obtained and calculated values for composite EPSPs (Table 16–1C) is similarly striking. Similar computations (although not by motor unit type) were presented for MG → MG and MG → LG projections by Mendell and Henneman (1971), and for all Ia → motoneuron projections within the triceps surae by Scott and Mendell (1976). These various computed composite EPSP amplitudes agreed quite closely with amplitudes obtained experimentally by Eccles et al. (1957).

Interestingly, an apparent paradox exists within these data. The single-fiber data were obtained from pentobarbital-anesthetized cats with intact spinal cord (but see Mendell and Henneman, 1971). However, the composite MG → MG EPSP data of Burke et al. (1976) and those of Eccles et al. (1957) (who

Table 16–1 Determinants of composite EPSP amplitude[a]

A. Projection frequency (%) of individual MG group Ia afferents to MG motoneurons of each type

Reference	FF	F(int)	FR	S	All
			Motoneuron type		
Harrison and Taylor (1981)	69 (22)	50 (2)	91 (23)	93 (14)	82 (61)
Fleshman et al. (1981a)	87 (97)	100 (15)	97 (61)	94 (50)	92 (223)
Munson et al. (1984)	84 (58)	67 (6)	93 (40)	91 (34)	88 (138)
All	84 (177)	87 (23)	95 (124)	93 (98)	89 (422)

B. Amplitude (µV) of single MG Ia fiber EPSPs in MG motoneurons of each type

Reference	FF	F(int)	FR	S	All
			Motoneuron type		
Harrison and Taylor (1981)	52 (15)	34 (1)	128 (21)	212 (13)	125 (50)
Fleshman et al. (1981a)	71 (85)	115 (15)	118 (59)	179 (47)	112 (206)
Munson et al. (1984)	75 (49)	134 (4)	111 (37)	106 (31)	96 (121)
All	70 (149)	115 (20)	118 (117)	159 (91)	109 (377)

C. Obtained and calculated amplitudes (mV) of homonymous composite EPSPs in MG motoneurons of each type

Source	FF	F(int)	FR	S	All
			Motoneuron type		
Burke et al. (1976)	4.1 (58)	6.7 (10)	7.5 (23)	9.1 (28)	6.2 (119)
Calculated[b]	4.2 (149)	7.1 (20)	8.0 (117)	10.5 (91)	6.9 (377)

[a]Numbers in parentheses are *n*.

[b]Values are calculated on the basis of (71 MG group Ia afferents) [Boyd and Davey, 1968] × (projection frequency to that motoneuron type) × (mean single Ia fiber EPSP amplitude in that motoneuron type).

obtained identical mean values of 6.2 mV) were obtained in cats with acute transection of the spinal cord. In single-fiber experiments, Nelson et al. (1979; see also Mendell and Henneman, 1971) observed that MG Ia $\rightarrow$ MG motoneuron projection frequency increased to 97% and mean EPSP amplitude increased to 313 μV following such transection (cf. Table 16–1). Based upon those values, the predicted mean composite EPSP value following cord transection (calculated as in Table 16–1C) would be 22 mV rather than the observed 6.2 mV. Heteronymous composite EPSPs (LGS afferents to MG motoneurons) may also be unaltered by acute spinal transection: Identical mean values were obtained both for each motor unit type and for the overall motoneuron populations in cats with spinal cord intact (Munson et al., 1986) and with spinal cord acutely transected (Mayer et al., 1984). An attempt to obtain enlarged intratriceps surae composite EPSPs by acute spinal cord transection was unsuccessful (Walmsley & Tracey, 1983; however, see the discussion in Cope et al., 1988).

Thus, while acute spinal transection clearly *may* result in increased amplitude and projection frequency of single-fiber MG EPSPs, it appears not always to be a *sufficient* condition for such increases. For example, enlarged EPSPs were not observed by Watt et al. (1976) following $T_{12}–L_1$ transection (but with chloralose-urethane anesthesia), nor were they observed in the flexor muscle system semitendinosus by Cope et al. (1980b), even though MG EPSPs were enlarged in the same experiments. On the other hand, such augmentation is reported for homonymous soleus projections (Cope et al., 1988). Remarkably, acute spinal transection with an interposed chronic spinal transection also strengthens projections (Cope et al., 1980a), leading these authors to postulate the existence of nonneural factors influencing the functional properties of the Ia afferent–motoneuron synapse. To further complicate the issue, the augmented afferent-to-motoneuron projections are seen only after several hours following the spinal transection, and even then not in all cases (Nelson et al., 1979), which may contribute to the apparently contradictory results.

In any event, the data of Table 16–1A and 16–1B suggest that the larger composite EPSPs in types S and FR motoneurons are due primarily to the unit type-related distribution of amplitudes of the single-fiber EPSPs rather than to their projection frequencies, since the differences in projection frequency are marginal and not systematic. Does this result from differences in the properties of the motoneurons themselves? One such property that might contribute to these differences in single-fiber EPSP amplitude is motoneuron input resistance (e.g., Burke et al., in press), which is known to differ in the same manner as EPSP amplitude among the motor unit types: type S > FR > F(int) > FF (e.g., Fleshman et al., 1981b). Two points from the data of Fleshman et al. (1981a) suggest that factors in addition to motoneuron properties are involved. First, while the *mean* amplitude of single Ia fiber EPSPs increases in the order FF < F(int) < FR < S, *small* EPSPs (i.e., <50 μV) may occur in motoneurons of any type (Fig 16–1). The large amplitude of composite EPSPs in type S motoneurons seems, then, to result from the significant population of *large* (in addition to small) single-fiber EPSPs found almost exclusively in type S motoneurons (>300 μV: Fig. 16–1). Figure 4 of Fleshman et al. (1981a) shows

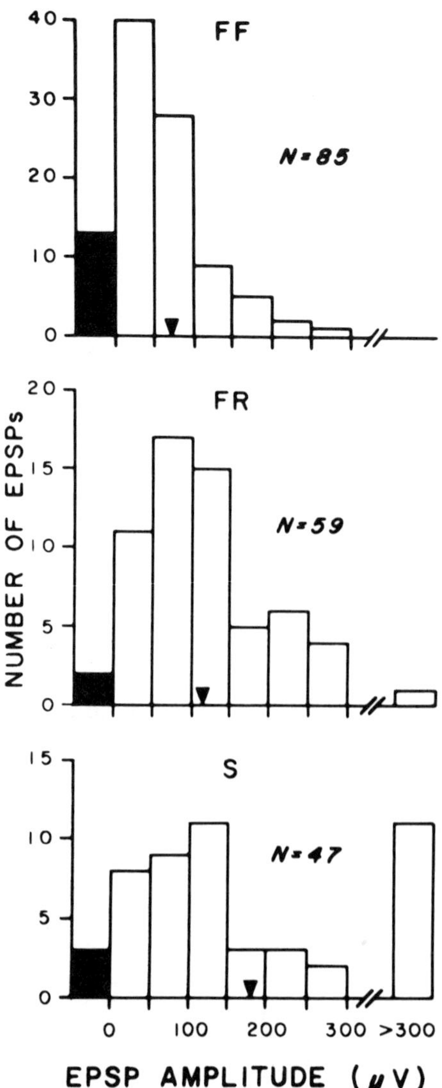

Fig. 16–1. Distributions of EPSP amplitudes for the different motor unit types. Filled bars denote connections where no EPSP was detected. Arrowheads denote means, not including connection failures. Note that small EPSPs (<50 μV) occur in motoneurons of all types, but large EPSPs (>300 μV) are most characteristic of type S motoneurons. (Reproduced from Fleshman et al., 1981a, with permission of the American Physiological Society.)

that the input resistance of those type S motoneurons with large (>300 μV) EPSPs is no different from that of the rest of the type S population; thus, the motoneurons with unusually large EPSPs do not constitute a special population, at least in this regard.

Second, Figure 3 of Fleshman et al. (1981a) shows that in cases where two single-fiber EPSPs were recorded from the same motoneuron, the presence of a small (<40 μV) or a large (>300 μV) EPSP does not predict the amplitude of the second EPSP. Data of Munson et al. (1984, Fig. 4) show that while the group Ia afferents generating the largest EPSPs in motoneurons of each motor unit type are strongly coupled mechanically to those motor units (i.e., are unloaded particularly strongly by their muscle units), such strong unloading occurs as well with afferents generating the smallest EPSPs.

Further evidence against determination of EPSP amplitude solely on the basis of motoneuron electrical properties or size derives from analysis of the amplitude of individual spindle group II afferent-to-motoneuron EPSPs in type-identified MG motoneurons: No differences related to motor unit types were found (mean amplitudes were 23, 19, 31, and 22 μV, respectively, for types FF, F(int), FR, and S: Munson et al., 1982).

Amplitudes of single Ia fiber EPSPs in MG motoneurons, measured in pentobarbital-anesthetized cats with intact spinal cord, cover more than a 50-fold range (<10 μV to >500 μV). Of the properties of motoneurons traditionally measured (e.g., rheobase, input resistance, axon conduction velocity, afterhyperpolarization, and derived values such as time and space constants, capacitance, and soma-dendritic conductance ratio), only rheobase covers such a range (~1 nA to ~40 nA), and their relation is inverse (the lowest rheobase and the largest EPSPs are found in type S motoneurons). What, then, accounts for the range of values of single-fiber (and thus composite) EPSPs and for their differences among the motor unit types?

Burke and colleagues (in press) have attempted to answer this question by labeling with horseradish peroxidase both group Ia afferents and type-identified motoneurons, and then examining the apparent synaptic contacts between them. The electrical properties of the motoneurons were also determined, thus permitting computer modeling of factors that could contribute to the systematic variation in Ia EPSP amplitudes. The authors concluded that the average number of synaptic contacts from Ia afferents to motoneurons did not differ systematically among the motor unit types (mean number, about 9; range, 3–32 for homonymous connections). The type-specific variations in synaptic efficacy are thus attributed to the resulting *density* of such contacts, i.e., greatest on type S and smallest on type FF motoneurons. The range of values for EPSPs generated by different Ia afferents within individual motoneurons is attributed to variations around the average in the number of Ia synapses or to differing probabilities of transmitter release (see also Chapters 10, 17, and 18, this volume).

Recent data have added new dimensions to the determinants of such single-fiber EPSP amplitudes (see Chapters 17 and 18, this volume). In brief, Mendell and colleagues (Chapter 17) have shown that these amplitudes, even at a given afferent-to-motoneuron synapse, are not constant, but vary systematically with the rate and history of activation and differentially according to the properties of the motoneuron. Lüscher and colleagues (Chapter 18) have shown that apparently spontaneous fluctuations occur in functional connectivity from individual group Ia afferents to motoneurons in recordings made over extensive periods.

PRESYNAPTIC INHIBITION OF EXCITATORY POSTSYNAPTIC POTENTIALS

The distribution of presynaptic inhibition to motoneurons of the various types was tested by Zengel et al. (1983). Trains of electrical shocks, as conditioning stimuli, were delivered to the posterior biceps-semitendinosus nerve in order to test their effect on group I composite EPSPs, subsequently evoked by heteronymous muscle nerve stimulation within the triceps surae motoneuron group. Within the MG motor unit group, such conditioning stimulation reduced EPSP amplitude within each motor unit type by the same percentage: 27%. Since unconditioned EPSPs in type S motoneurons were largest, this required that the *absolute* amount of inhibition of their EPSPs (in millivolts) be greatest, with the reverse situation for type FF motoneurons. Comparable results were obtained in the smaller populations of LG and soleus motoneurons. The effect of presynaptic inhibition thus seems to relate to motor unit type only insofar as EPSP amplitude is related to motor unit type.

INHIBITORY POSTSYNAPTIC POTENTIALS

Inhibitory postsynaptic potentials (IPSPs) from several sources have been studied in type-identified motoneurons. However the measurement of IPSPs (and the interpretation of their significance; see the later discussion) is not simple. One problem is the much greater dependence of IPSP amplitude than EPSP amplitude on resting membrane potential, and thus the requirement for optimal recording conditions at least for the former. Another is the fact that the techniques most commonly used to elicit IPSPs require at least disynaptic activation of the inhibitory interneurons, with attendant problems such as an unknown proportion of those interneurons being activated by the stimulus (however, see Jankowska and Roberts, 1972). When activity of interneurons is a factor, considerations such as anesthetics and the condition of the animal are particularly important. In some cases, conditioning stimulation of another system may be used in order to obtain IPSPs reliably (e.g., disynaptic group Ia IPSPs; Hongo et al., 1969).

In spite of these caveats, disynaptic group Ia composite IPSPs have been examined in relation to motor unit type. Burke et al. (1976; see also Burke et al., 1970) recorded such IPSPs, generated by electrical stimulation of tibialis anterior-extensor digitorum longus (TA-EDL) group I muscle afferents in type-identified MG motoneurons. The reciprocal experiment (triceps surae-evoked IPSPs in TA motoneurons) was performed by Dum and Kennedy (1980). Light pentobarbital anesthesia was used, at least in part, by both groups. The former but not the latter group used electrical stimulation of the red nucleus or spinal cord dorsal quadrant as a conditioning stimulus. Perhaps as a consequence, the conditioned postsynaptic potentials (PSPs) of the former study (TA-EDL to gastrocnemius) were about 50% greater in amplitude, on average. However the same patterns were seen by both groups: IPSPs in type S > FR > F(int) > FF. [Note that Nichols (1985) has found that stretch-evoked inhibition between TA and soleus is largely unidirectional, i.e., from TA to soleus.]

Recurrent inhibition was studied by Friedman et al. (1981), who recorded recurrent IPSPs (RIPSPs) in type-identified MG motoneurons following antidromic electrical stimulation of LGS (or MG) motor axons. Their findings concur with those of other studies of synaptic actions on motoneurons: RIPSPs were largest in type S, smallest in type FF, and intermediate in type FR motoneurons. This is in accord with the findings of many previous studies, such as that of Kuno (1959), who found smaller RIPSPs in motoneurons of the pale LG muscle than in the red soleus muscle. The pattern of organization seems to be that large (type FF?) motoneurons are particularly effective in activating the pool of recurrent inhibitory interneurons (Renshaw cells), while small (type S?) motoneurons are the preferred synaptic targets of recurrent inhibition. Evidence for this comes, for example, from Ryall et al. (1972; see also Hultborn et al., 1988b), who found that weak antidromic muscle nerve stimulation (preferentially activating large motor axons) recruits a large proportion of the Renshaw cell pool, while weak orthodromic stimulation (synaptically activating small motoneurons preferentially) recruits only a small fraction of the pool. Anatomical evidence of Cullheim and Kellerth (1978) shows that the number of recurrent collaterals per motoneuron increases in the order type S < FR < FF. The fact that the normally tonically active soleus muscle is silenced during rapidly alternating paw shakes (Smith et al., 1980) has been attributed to recurrent inhibition of the type S motoneurons of soleus by the type F motoneurons of MG and LG.

In a partial departure from the previously described procedures, Hultborn and colleagues (1988a, b) have tested recurrent inhibition in two conditions: with motoneurons at their normal resting potential and again with motoneurons depolarized with a just-subthreshold (i.e., just subrheobase) current injection. At normal resting potential, they found that RIPSPs increased in amplitude in order of motor unit type: type FF < F(int) < FR < S, in agreement with Friedman et al. (1981). They also calculated the resulting outward synaptic current, using the Ohm's law relation (RIPSP/R_N), and found the same order of result at resting potential. When tested near threshold, RIPSPs (voltages) were rank ordered as before, but calculated inhibitory *currents* did not differ among the different motor unit types. The authors attribute these findings to the fact that voltage thresholds may increase in the order type S < FR < FF; thus, the driving potential for inhibitory currents, measured near motoneuron threshold, is greater for type FF than for type FR and for type FR than for type S. The authors argue that the *functional consequences* of recurrent inhibition are thus equal in motoneurons of all types, in spite of the type-specific distribution of RIPSP voltages in motoneurons when measured at resting potential. It should be pointed out, however, that not all authors agree on the magnitude *or even the existence* of systematic differences in voltage threshold among the various motor unit types. This question is addressed in detail by Gustafsson and Pinter (1984; see also Chapter 9, this volume).

This finding raises the question of the functional significance of the type-specifically differential amplitudes of IPSPs from other sources as well (see the earlier discussion). All intracellular studies were conducted with motoneurons at "resting potential," ideally as negative as possible (thus close to E_{IPSP} and far from motoneuron threshold). It is perhaps significant that the *ratios* of mean amplitudes of IPSPs among the various motor unit groups (i.e., type S:FR:FF) are quite similar among the various studies (approximately 3.5:2.5:1), both for homonymous RIPSPs (Friedman et al., 1981; Hultborn et al., 1988a) and for group I disynaptic IPSPs (Burke et al., 1973; Dum and Kennedy, 1980). Thus, to the extent that similar ionic conductances are involved with IPSPs of different origin, the functional consequences of other types of inhibition as well may be dispersed equally among the motor unit types. This would be consistent with the observation of Henneman et al. (1965) that the largest cells are the first to cease firing during activation of the group I afferents in the antagonist muscle, in spite of the fact that such IPSPs (measured at resting potential) are smallest in these largest motoneurons (see also Chapter 10, this volume).

SYNAPTIC INPUTS FROM HIGH-THRESHOLD MUSCLE AND JOINT AFFERENTS

Electrical stimulation of high-threshold (eight or fewer times threshold) joint and muscle afferents produced inhibitory potentials in virtually all motoneurons of the triceps surae motor pool, perhaps slightly larger in slow than in fast motoneurons (Burke et al., 1970). In the antagonist TA muscle, high-threshold muscle afferents generated primarily excitatory polysynaptic potentials in most type FF motoneurons, while the pattern in types FR and type S motoneurons was primarily inhibitory and quite variable (Dum and Kennedy, 1980).

SYNAPTIC INPUTS FROM CUTANEOUS NERVES

Burke and colleagues (Burke et al., 1970, 1973) have examined the polysynaptic PSPs evoked in type-identified motoneurons by electrical stimulation of cutaneous nerves. Typically, these responses consist of two components: a depolarizing followed by a hyperpolarizing potential, with different components predominating in motor units of different types. Single-shock stimulation of the sural nerve, for example, usually generates a PSP consisting primarily of an IPSP in type S motoneurons of the gastrocnemius and soleus muscles. In types FF and FR MG motoneurons, the response usually consists primarily of an EPSP or an EPSP followed by an IPSP. Similar effects were obtained from stimulation of the saphenous nerve. In general, the trend was toward polysynaptic inhibition from cutaneous afferents to type S motoneurons and toward polysynaptic excitation of fast motoneurons of MG. LaBella et al. (1989) have reported IPSPs to predominate in sural-evoked PSPs in all motoneurons of the cat's lateral gastrocnemius and soleus, but unit types were not determined.

A pattern of polysynaptic potentials similar to those in MG was evoked in TA motoneurons by stimulation of the sural nerve (Dum and Kennedy, 1980). Stimulation of the saphenous (and superficial peroneal) nerves, however, produced predominantly excitation in all types of TA motoneurons.

In functional studies of these circuits, Kanda et al. (1977) showed that natural or electrical activation of the sural nerve suppressed activity in the (all-slow) soleus muscle and also in low-threshold (presumably type S) motoneurons of MG, and activated high-threshold (presumably type FR or FF) moto-neurons of MG. Moreover, these effects are in accord with studies on reflex effects of stimulation of the skin on flexor and extensor muscle systems (e.g., Hagbarth, 1952).

SUPRASPINAL INPUTS TO MOTONEURONS

Effects of stimulation of four descending pathways on type-identified moto-neurons have been reported: rubrospinals, vestibulospinals, reticulospinals, and medial longitudinal fasciculus.

Rubrospinal

Trains of electrical stimuli to the contralateral red nucleus produce combina-tions of EPSPs and IPSPs in MG motoneurons (Burke et al., 1970). Similar to PSPs from the sural nerve, these are predominantly excitatory to fast units and predominantly inhibitory to slow units. In addition, such stimulation (or stimulation of the same system in the dorsal spinal quadrant) used as a con-ditioning stimulus greatly augments group Ia disynaptic IPSPs from TA-EDL to MG (Hongo et al., 1969). The amplitudes of the resulting IPSPs are then rank-ordered: type FF < FR < S (Burke et al., 1970, 1973; see also Dum and Kennedy, 1980). The degree of augmentation produced by the rubrospinal con-ditioning stimulation appears not to differ from one motor unit type group to another.

Vestibulospinal

Small monosynaptic EPSPs were recorded in type-identified MG motoneurons following electrical stimulation of the surgically isolated ventral spinal quadrant (presumably containing lateral vestibulospinal tract fibers) by Burke et al. (1973). Amplitudes in the fast motor units were quite similar and were somewhat smaller, on average, than those in type S units.

Reticulospinal

Stimulation of the surgically isolated spinal dorsal quadrant (dorsal columns removed) produces selective suppression of the inhibitory component of PSPs evoked by sural nerve stimulation (Burke et al., 1973). This effect, presumably mediated by the dorsolateral reticulospinal inhibitory system, appears to affect such IPSPs of all motor unit types equally.

Medial Longitudinal Fasciculus

Electrical stimulation of this pathway in the lateral ventral spinal quadrant elic-ited monosynaptic and/or polysynaptic EPSPs in TA motoneurons (Dum and Kennedy, 1980). Like group Ia EPSPs over the same population, these EPSPs were larger in type S than in type FR, and in type FR than type FF motoneurons (although not significantly), but in individual motoneurons, the size of one EPSP did not predict the size of the other.

NET EFFECTS OF SYNAPTIC INPUTS ON MOTONEURON ACTIVITY

It is clear from these and other studies (e.g., Burke, 1968) that the monosynaptic excitatory input from group Ia afferents is distributed broadly to the homonymous and heteronymous motoneuron pools, differentially according to motor unit type, thus biasing the weakly contracting and fatigue-resistant motor units toward or to threshold. Monosynaptic excitatory actions of spindle group II afferents are not differentially distributed, and thus seem to depolarize all unit types equally. It is likely, however, that these latter spindle afferents have powerful multisynaptic actions on motoneurons as well (Cavallari et al., 1987); the unit type-specific effects of these actions remain to be explored.

Net segmental inhibitory actions are still unclear. Presynaptic inhibition is equally effective on group I EPSPs in motoneurons of all types. IPSPs (Ia disynaptic and recurrent), measured at resting potential, are distributed differentially according to unit type. However, because threshold voltage may differ according to motor unit type, such inhibition may be equally effective in motoneurons of all types when those motoneurons are near their firing threshold, an effect due to the differences in the driving potentials then operating.

Cutaneous nerves (sural, saphenous), when stimulated with single shocks, elicit an EPSP–IPSP complex in MG motoneurons. This complex is biased toward excitation in most fast motor units and toward inhibition in most slow motor units. In LG and soleus motor units of all types, these PSPs are strongly inhibitory (LaBella et al., 1989). However, while useful for analytical purposes, single-shock stimulation does not correspond to normal physiological function. Repetitive stimulation of the sural nerve, or its physiological activation by skin pinch, inhibits low-threshold sural and gastrocnemius motoneurons and activates high-threshold motoneurons.

The effects of supraspinal inputs are largely excitatory or disinhibitory, the primary exception among the systems studied being an inhibitory input from the rubrospinal tract to MG type S motoneurons. In addition, conditioning stimulation of the rubrospinal tract augments group Ia disynaptic IPSPs in all MG motoneurons.

BASIS OF SEGMENTAL MOTOR CONTROL: MOTONEURON SIZE OR MOTOR UNIT TYPE?

In 1981, we published an article under the above title (Sypert and Munson, 1981). One conclusion in that article was "that the critical factor controlling motor unit recruitment in heterogeneous muscles is motor unit type" (p. 608). As we had hoped, the article provoked some controversy and stimulated some research (e.g., Bawa et al., 1984). In the intervening years, where have further thought and research on the issues brought us?

We have been particularly influenced by the work of Zajac and Faden (1985; see also Chapter 5, this volume), who demonstrated the great precision with which motor units in heterogeneous muscles are recruited, i.e., without exception, in order of contraction strength. How could a correspondence between the properties of the motoneuron and its synaptic inputs (i.e., factors thought to result in recruitment) come to be matched so precisely to the contraction strength of its muscle unit? In other words, how does a motoneuron "know" the contraction strength of its muscle unit? This becomes all the more remarkable with the appearance of new data concerning the *inconstancy* of properties of components of the ensemble. For example, the properties of the group Ia motoneuron EPSPs are not constant even at a given Ia–motoneuron synapse, but vary with activation rate and history differentially according to the specific afferent–motoneuron connection (see Chapters 17 and 18, this volume). The amplitude of the postspike afterhyperpolarization may *decrease* in a motoneuron as it nears threshold (Jordan and Shefchyk, 1984). Input resistance of a motoneuron may increase as it approaches threshold (Schmidt et al., 1988). Depolarization or hyperpolarization of a motoneuron activates nonlinear processes that alter its properties with time (Ito and Oshima, 1965). The constancy with which recruitment reportedly occurs, i.e., strictly in order of muscle unit contraction strength, seems even more remarkable in the face of the inconstancy of the variables thought to contribute to recruitment.

A second great influence on our thinking has been the finding that when the MG nerve reinnervates a heterogeneous muscle, the original proportions and properties of MG motor units of each type are restored (Foehring et al., 1986, 1987). Thus, the reinnervated muscle fibers acquire contractile (and other) properties that are appropriate for the motor unit type of their newly innervating motoneuron.

Not known at present is the *precision* with which recruitment occurs in respect to contraction strength following reinnervation. We predict that such precision as observed by Zajac and Faden (1985) would not be reestablished even after self-reinnervation, since it is difficult to envision sufficiently precise reestablishment of the innervation ratio, one of the contributors to muscle unit contraction strength (other contributors are muscle fiber cross-sectional area and specific tension: Burke and Tsairis, 1973). Consistent with this, a few very weakly contracting type FF motor units, never seen in normal MG, were found in self-reinnervated MG muscle (Fig. 1 of Foehring et al., 1986).

While the manner in which the correspondence between motoneuron and muscle unit properties is restored following reinnervation is not established, it is likely that contributing factors include the pattern and amount of activity (e.g., Pette and Vrbóva, 1985; Edstrom and Grimby, 1986) imposed upon the diverse muscle fibers by their newly innervating motoneuron. If this is true, then it seems possible that during development as well, motor units within a muscle may constitute, to some extent, a *self-organizing system*. In this case, there need not be a preexisting precise master plan for each motoneuron and each muscle fiber; the plan emerges simply out of use. By virtue of the net ensemble of excitatory and inhibitory inputs, and the inconstant (but lawfully and predictably so) properties of each motoneuron and its inputs, a "usual" order of recruitment must evolve. Certain motoneurons thereby are invariably used more than others in the course of the usual activities. The well-known "plasticity" of muscle can account for the rest: Muscle units that are used more differentiate from those that are used less in such measures as histochemical and contractile properties.

Such a scheme, as described, is clearly simplistic; for example, it ignores the likely role of trophic influences of nerve on muscle. However it may be usefully provocative to consider the reverse of our previous statement, i.e., "the critical factor controlling motor unit type [and thus muscle unit properties] is motor unit recruitment."

Acknowledgment

Work from this laboratory reported in this chapter was supported by grant NS15913, to the author, and by a grant from the Medical Research Service of the Veterans Administration to my friend and colleague George W. Sypert.

REFERENCES

Bawa, P., Binder, M. D., Ruenzel, P., and Henneman, E. (1984). Recruitment order of motoneurons in stretch reflexes is highly correlated with their conduction velocity. *J. Neurophysiol.* 52, 410–420.

Boyd, I. A., and Davey, M. R. (1968). *Composition of Peripheral Nerves.* Livingston, Edinburgh, pp. 1–57.

Burke, R. E. (1967). Motor unit types of cat triceps surae muscle. *J. Physiol. (Lond.)* 193, 141–160.

Burke, R. E. (1968). Firing patterns of gastrocnemius motor units in the decerebrate cat. *J. Physiol. (Lond.)* 196, 631–654.

Burke, R. E., Dum, R. P., Fleshman, J. W., Glenn, L. L., Lev-Tov, A., O'Donovan, M. J., and Pinter, M. J. (1982). An HRP study of the relation between cell size and motor unit type in cat ankle extensor motoneurons. *J. Comp. Neurol.* 209, 17–28.

Burke, R. E., Fleshman, J. W., and Segev, I. (In press). The control of synaptic efficacy: Lessons from the Ia synapse. *J. Physiol. (Paris).*

Burke, R. E., Jankowska, E., and Ten Bruggencate, E. (1970). A comparison of peripheral and central synaptic input to slow and fast twitch motor units of triceps surae. *J. Physiol. (Lond.)* 207, 709–732.

Burke, R. E., Levine, D. N., Tsairis, P., and Zajac, F. E. (1973). Physiological types and histochemical profiles in motor units of the cat gastrocnemius. *J. Physiol. (Lond.)* 234, 723–748.

Burke, R. E., Rymer, W. Z., and Walsh, J. V. (1976). Relative strength of synaptic input from short-latency pathways to motor units of defined type in cat medial gastrocnemius. *J. Neurophysiol.* 39, 447–458.

Burke, R. E., and Tsairis, P. (1973). Anatomy and innervation ratios in motor units of cat gastrocnemius. *J. Physiol. (Lond.)* 234, 749–765.

Cavallari, P., Edgley, S. A., and Jankowska, E. (1987). Post-synaptic actions of mid-lumbar interneurones on motoneurones of hind-limb muscles in the cat. *J. Physiol. (Lond.)* 389, 675–689.

Cope, T. C., Hickman, K. R., and Botterman, B. R. (1988). Acute effects of spinal transection on EPSPs produced by single homonymous Ia fibers in soleus α-motoneurons in the cat. *J. Neurophysiol.* 60, 1678–1694.

Cope, T. C., Nelson, S. G., and Mendell, L. M. (1980a). Factors outside neuraxis mediate "acute" increase in EPSP amplitude caudal to spinal cord transection. *J. Neurophysiol.* 44, 174–183.

Cope, T. C., Nelson, S. G., and Mendell, L. M. (1980b). Selectivity in synaptic changes caudal to acute spinal cord transection. *Neurosci. Lett.* 20, 289–294.

Cullheim, S., and Kellerth, J.-O. (1978). A morphological study of the axons and recurrent axon collaterals of cat α-motoneurons supplying different functional types of muscle units. *J. Physiol. (Lond.)* 281, 301–313.

Dum, R. P., Burke, R. E., and Hodgson, J. A. (1978). Analysis of the motor unit population in cat flexor digitorum longus (FDL) muscle. *Soc. Neurosci. Abstr.* 4, 294.

Dum, R. P., and Kennedy, T. T. (1980). Synaptic organization of defined motor-unit types in cat tibialis anterior. *J. Neurophysiol.* 43, 1631–1644.

Eccles, J. C., Eccles, R. M., and Lundberg, A. (1957) The convergence of monosynaptic excitatory afferents on to many different species of alpha motoneurons. *J. Physiol. (Lond.)* 137, 22–50.

Edstrom, L., and Grimby, L. (1986). Effect of exercise on the motor unit. *Muscle Nerve* 9, 104–126.

Fleshman, J. W., Munson, J. B., and Sypert, G. W., (1981a). The homonymous projection of individual group Ia fibers to physiologically characterized medial gastrocnemius motoneurons in the cat. *J. Neurophysiol.* 46, 1339–1348

Fleshman, J. W., Munson, J. B., Sypert, G. W., and Friedman, W. A. (1981b). Rheobase, input resistance and motor-unit type in medial gastrocnemius motoneurons in the cat. *J. Neurophysiol.* 46, 1326–1338.

Foehring, R. C., Sypert, G. W., and Munson, J. B. (1986). Properties of self-reinnervated motor units of medial gastrocnemius of cat. I. Long-term reinnervation. *J. Neurophysiol.* 55, 931–946.

Foehring, R. C., Sypert, G. W., and Munson, J. B. (1987). Motor-unit properties following cross-innervation of cat lateral gastrocnemius and soleus muscles with medial gastrocnemius nerve. I. Influence of motoneurons on muscle. *J. Neurophysiol.* 57, 1210–1226.

Friedman, W. A., Sypert, G. W., Munson, J. B., and Fleshman, J. W. (1981). Recurrent inhibition in type-identified motoneurons. *J. Neurophysiol.* 46, 1349–1359.

Gustafsson, B., and Pinter, M. J. (1984). An investigation of threshold properties among cat spinal α-motoneurones. *J. Physiol. (Lond.)* 357, 453–483.

Hagbarth, K.-E. (1952). Excitatory and inhibitory skin areas for flexor and extensor motoneurones. *Acta Physiol. Scand.* Suppl 94, 1–58.

Harrison, P. J., and Taylor, A. (1981). Individual excitatory post-synaptic potentials due to muscle spindle Ia afferents in cat triceps surae motoneurones. *J. Physiol. (Lond.)* 312, 455–470.

Henneman, E. (1957). Relation between size of neurons and their susceptibility to discharge. *Science* 126, 1345–1346.

Henneman, E., and Mendell, L. M. (1981). Functional organization of motoneuron pool and its inputs. In *Handbook of Physiology*, Vol. I, Sect. 1, Part 2: *The Nervous System. Cellular Biology of Neurons* (ed. E. R. Kandel). American Physiological Society, Bethesda, Md., pp. 423–507.

Henneman, E., Somjen, G., and Carpenter, D. O. (1965). Functional significance of cell size in spinal motoneurons. *J. Neurophysiol.* 28, 560–580.

Hongo, T., Jankowska, E., and Lundberg, A. (1969). The rubrospinal tract. II. Facilitation of interneuronal transmission in reflex paths to motoneurones. *Exp. Brain Res.* 7, 365–391.

Hultborn, H., Katz, R., and Mackel, R. (1988a). Distribution of recurrent inhibition within a motor nucleus. II. Amount of recurrent inhibition in motoneurones to fast and slow units. *Acta Physiol. Scand.* 134, 363–374.

Hultborn, H., Lipski, J., Mackel, R., and Wigstrom, H. (1988b). Distribution of recurrent inhibition within a motor nucleus. I. Contribution from slow and fast motor units to the excitation of Renshaw cells. *Acta Physiol. Scand.* 134, 347–361.

Ito, M., and Oshima, T. (1965). Electrical behaviour of the motoneurone membrane during intracellularly applied current steps. *J. Physiol. (Lond.)* 180, 607–635.

Jankowska, E., and Roberts, W. (1972). Synaptic action of single interneurones mediating reciprocal Ia inhibition of motoneurones. *J. Physiol. (Lond.)* 222, 623–642.

Jordan, L. M., and Shefchyk, S. J. (1984). Does the afterhyperpolarization control alpha motoneurone firing during locomotion? *Soc. Neurosci. Abstr.* 10, 633.

Kanda, K., Burke, R. E., and Walmsley, B. (1977). Differential control of fast and slow twitch motor units in the decerebrate cat. *Exp. Brain Res.* 29, 57–74.

Kuno, M. (1959). Excitability following antidromic activation in spinal motoneurones supplying red muscle. *J. Physiol. (Lond.)* 149, 374–393.

LaBella, L. A., Kehler, J. P., and McCrea, D. A. (1989). A differential synaptic input to the motor nuclei of triceps surae from the caudal and lateral cutaneous sural nerves. *J. Neurophysiol.* 61, 291–301.

Mayer, R. F., Burke, R. E., Toop, J., Walmsley, B., and Hodgson, J. A. (1984). The effect of spinal cord transection on motor units in cat medial gastrocnemius muscle. *Muscle Nerve* 7, 23–31.

Mendell, L. M., and Henneman, E. (1968). Terminals of single Ia fibers: Distribution within a pool of 300 homonymous motor neurons *Science* 160, 96–98.

Mendell, L. M., and Henneman, E. (1971). Terminals of single Ia fibers: Location, density, and distribution within a pool of 300 homonymous motoneurons. *J. Neurophysiol.* 34, 171–187.

Munson, J. B., Fleshman, J. W., and Sypert, G. W. (1980). Properties of single fiber spindle group II EPSPs in triceps surae motoneurons. *J. Neurophysiol.* 44, 713–725.

Munson, J. B., Fleshman, J. W., Zengel, J. E., and Sypert, G. W. (1984). Synaptic and mechanical coupling between type-identified motor units and individual spindle afferents of medial gastrocnemius muscle of the cat. *J. Neurophysiol.* 51, 1268–1283.

Munson, J. B., Foehring, R. C., Lofton, S. A., Zengel, J. E., and Sypert, G. W. (1986). Plasticity of medial gastrocnemius motor units following cordotomy in the cat. *J. Neurophysiol.* 55, 619–634.

Munson, J. B., and Sypert, G. W. (1979). Properties of single fibre EPSPs in triceps surae motoneurones. *J. Physiol.* 196, 329–342.

Munson, J. B., Sypert, G. W., Zengel, J. E., Lofton, S. A., and Fleshman, J. W. (1982). Monosynaptic projections of individual spindle group II afferents to type-identified medial gastrocnemius motoneurons in the cat. *J. Neurophysiol.* 48, 1164–1174.

Nelson, S. G., Collatos, T. C., Niechaj, A., and Mendell, L. M. (1979). Immediate increase in Ia-motoneuron synaptic transmission caudal to spinal cord transection. *J. Neurophysiol.* 42, 655–664.

Nichols, T. R. (1985). Mechanical analysis of "antagonogenic" reflex action in decerebrate cats. *Soc. Neurosci. Abstr.* 11, 213.

Pette, D., and Vrbóva, G. (1985). Neural control of phenotypic expression in mammalian muscle fibers. *Muscle Nerve* 8, 676–689.

Ryall, R. W., Piercey, M. F., Polosa, C., and Goldfarb, J. (1972). Excitation of Renshaw cells in relation to orthodromic and antidromic excitation of motoneurons. *J. Neurophysiol.* 35, 137–148.

Schmidt, B. J., Meyers, D. E. R., Fleshman, J. W., Tokuriki, M., and Burke, R. E. (1988). Phasic modulation of short latency cutaneous excitation in flexor digitorum longus motoneurons during fictive locomotion. *Exp. Brain Res.* 71, 568–578.

Scott, J. G., and Mendell, L. M. (1976). Individual EPSPs produced by single triceps surae Ia afferent fibers in homonymous and heteronymous motoneurons. *J. Neurophysiol.* 39, 679–692.

Smith, J. L., Betts, B., Edgerton, V. R., and Zernicke, R. F. (1980). Rapid ankle extension during paw shakes: Selective recruitment of fast ankle extensors. *J. Neurophysiol.* 43, 612–620.

Sypert, G. W., and Munson, J. B. (1981). Basis of segmental motor control: Motoneuron size or motor unit type? *Neurosurgery* 8, 608–621.

Walmsley, B., and Tracey, D. J. (1983). The effect of transection and cold block of the spinal cord on synaptic transmission between Ia afferents and motoneurons. *Neuroscience* 9, 445–451.

Watt, D. G. D., Stauffer, E. K., Taylor, A., Reinking, R. M., and Stuart, D. G. (1976). Analysis of muscle receptor connections by spike-triggered averaging. 1. Spindle primary and tendon organ afferents. *J. Neurophysiol.* 39, 1375–1392.

Wuerker, R. B., McPhedran, A. M., and Henneman, E. (1965). Properties of motor units in a heterogeneous pale muscle (M. gastrocnemius) of the cat. *J. Neurophysiol.* 28, 85–99.

Zajac, F. E., and Faden, J. S. (1985). Relationship among recruitment order, axonal conduction velocity, and muscle-unit properties of type-identified motor units in cat plantaris muscle. *J. Neurophysiol.* 53, 1303–1322.

Zengel, J. E., Reid, S. A., Sypert, G. W., and Munson, J. B. (1983). Presynaptic inhibition, EPSP amplitude, and motor-unit type in triceps surae motoneurons in the cat. *J. Neurophysiol.* 49, 922–931.

Zengel, J. E., Reid, S. A., Sypert, G. W., and Munson, J. B. (1985). Membrane electrical properties and prediction of motor-unit type of medial gastrocnemius motoneurons in the cat. *J. Neurophysiol.* 53, 1323–1344.

17

How Are Ia Synapses Distributed on Spinal Motoneurons to Permit Orderly Recruitment?

LORNE M. MENDELL, WILLIAM F. COLLINS III,
AND H. RICHARD KOERBER

The finding that motoneurons are recruited in an orderly manner (Henneman et al., 1965a, 1965b; reviewed in Henneman and Mendell, 1981) has important implications beyond how the motoneuron pool functions to generate motor output. In their original reports describing the size principle, Henneman and co-workers hypothesized that differences in the properties of the motoneurons themselves were likely responsible for their different susceptibility to excitation and inhibition according to size. They suggested that small motoneurons would be expected to have larger values of input resistance, which would cause them to develop larger synaptic potentials in response to a given synaptic input, and this, in turn, would make them most excitable in the motor pool. However, this theory had additional requirements concerning the arrangement of synaptic inputs to the pool, requirements stated explicitly by Henneman et al. (1965b, p. 618 with permission):

> . . . . the properties of the motoneurons themselves dictate the order of recruitment and inhibition. In reaching this conclusion, however, we do not imply that the input is unimportant.
>
> Cell size can only determine the firing order in a group of cells if the excitatory drive impinging on each cell is of equal intensity relative to all other cells. We do not know how this equalization of input is achieved for cells of different size. An arrangement whereby each cell in a pool has an equal density of endings from a particular afferent system might result in equal synaptic drive for each cell. Whatever the organization may be, the laws governing the distribution of terminals to motoneurons must be very stringent to ensure adherence to the size principle under a wide variety of inputs.

In a speculative vein, we infer that the number and arrangement of endings on motoneurons is precisely regulated so that input from each afferent system is apportioned among all the cells of the pool.

Thus, from the very beginning of the studies to determine how motoneurons achieved different reflex thresholds, the distribution of input to them has played a prominent role. Although a very large number of input fiber types converge on motoneurons, most studies have been concerned with inputs from group Ia fibers. The reasons for this are:

1. Group Ia fibers innervate the stretch-sensitive muscle spindles in the periphery and, as such, represent the afferent limb of the functionally important stretch reflex.
2. Group Ia fibers make monosynaptic connections on alpha-motoneurons, so it is not necessary to account for the effects of intercalated interneurons in evaluating the measured strength of the projection.
3. Group Ia fibers are easy to activate physiologically or electrically and can be stimulated selectively.

Earlier work had revealed that the population of group Ia fibers produces monosynaptic excitatory postsynaptic potentials (EPSPs) in virtually every (homonymous) motoneuron supplying the same muscle (Eccles et al., 1957). It had also been reported that these population EPSPs are largest, on average, in motoneurons supplying postural muscles (e.g., soleus) that were known to have lower thresholds for reflex activation than other ankle extensors such as medial and lateral gastrocnemius (MG and LG). Although this suggested that the size principle was explained, at least in part, by a more powerful synaptic drive to motoneurons of lower reflex threshold, the way in which this was achieved remained uncertain at that time. Three principal explanations were possible:

1. A greater percentage of afferents might converge on smaller, more excitable motoneurons, or
2. Each individual afferent might evoke larger EPSPs, on average, in smaller, more excitable motoneurons, or
3. Some combination of both of these might occur.

PROJECTION OF SINGLE Ia AFFERENTS TO MOTONEURONS

The development of procedures to study the synaptic effects produced by single afferents has revealed that the major factor determining differences in the strength of group Ia projections (i.e., the level of depolarization produced by activation of the entire population of Ia afferents) to motoneurons of different threshold in the pool is the amplitude of the EPSP produced by individual afferents rather than the amount of convergence from group Ia fibers onto alpha-motoneurons. The procedure that has proven most useful in these studies is spike-triggered averaging. This originated in Henneman's laboratory (Mendell and Henneman,

1968, 1971) as an attempt to gain additional understanding of the distribution of input to motoneurons in terms of the issues raised in the 1965 paper quoted above.

The cat MG muscle contains about 60 muscle spindles, and thus is supplied by an equal number of group Ia fibers. These afferent fibers, as a population, project to about 300 alpha-motoneurons that innervate the MG muscle. A number of measures have been used to assign a motoneuron's putative position in the recruitment hierarchy. These include axonal conduction velocity (recruitment order—small to large [size principle]: Mendell and Henneman, 1971; Bawa et al., 1984), motor unit type (recruitment order—S, $\rightarrow$ FR, $\rightarrow$ FF: Burke, 1981; Fleshman et al., 1981b), motoneuron rheobase (recruitment order—small rheobase to large rheobase: Fleshman et al., 1981b), and tension output of the associated motor unit (recruitment order—small tension output to large tension output: Harrison and Taylor, 1981). Recent findings indicate that the latter may be the best index (Zajac and Faden, 1985; see also Chapter 5, this volume). It has been found that each MG Ia afferent distributes terminals to virtually all homonymous alpha-motoneurons, regardless of recruitability, as measured by these methods (Mendell and Henneman, 1971; Scott and Mendell, 1976; Watt et al., 1976; Nelson and Mendell, 1978; Fleshman et al., 1981a; Harrison and Taylor, 1981). The actual Ia projection percentages reported range from about 80% up to 100%, depending in part on the preparation (projections are higher in spinal preparations than in intact anesthetized ones: Nelson et al., 1979). In studies reporting percentages less than 100%, the evidence for greater convergence on putative low-threshold motoneurons, as measured by axonal conduction velocity or rheobase, is not definitive (compare Fleshman et al., 1981a, with Lüscher et al., 1984). However, the fact that projections can be 100% in preparations made acutely spinal (Nelson et al., 1979) indicates that afferent–motoneuron pairs not exhibiting synaptic connectivity in intact preparations may indeed have the anatomical substrate underlying synaptic connectivity but that such synapses are for some reason nonfunctional (Redman and Walmsley, 1983; Henneman et al., 1984). This line of reasoning emphasizes that the differences between motoneurons of low and high reflex threshold is not likely to reside in the tendency of individual group Ia afferents to synapse preferentially on low-threshold motoneurons.

EPSP PEAK AMPLITUDE DIFFERENCES AND RECRUITMENT ORDER

These same studies revealed consistent differences in the amplitude of EPSPs evoked in different populations of alpha-motoneurons supplying a given muscle. Putative low-threshold motoneurons reliably generate EPSPs of larger peak amplitude in response to stimulation of single afferent fibers than putative high-threshold motoneurons (Mendell and Henneman, 1971; Fleshman et al., 1981b; Harrison and Taylor, 1981; Collins et al., 1988). Since there is evidence that the distribution of voltage thresholds of motoneurons is similar for the different constituents of the pool (Pinter et al., 1983), it follows that the recruitment threshold differences are achieved by systematically different amounts of depolarization of the motoneurons in a pool. Thus, the extensive series of studies carried out in the 15 years since the introduction of the spike-triggered averaging technique repeatedly confirmed the importance of differences in EPSP amplitude in the determination of differences in recruitment order.

The mechanisms responsible for these systematic differences in EPSP amplitudes among motoneurons of different threshold have attracted much attention (see Chapters 2 and 10, this volume). In the original reports from the Henneman laboratory (Henneman et al., 1965a, 1965b), it was suggested that EPSPs might be larger, on average, in small motoneurons (whose size was assumed to be proportional to their axonal conduction velocity) because the higher input resistance of their soma-dendritic membrane (Kernell, 1966; Burke, 1968). This larger resistance, now recognized to be due to both the smaller surface area of the membrane (Burke et al., 1982; Ulfhake and Kellerth, 1982; Gustafsson and Pinter, 1984) and the higher specific resistance of these cells (Kernell and Zwaagstra, 1981; Burke et al., 1982; Gustafsson and Pinter, 1984), would cause a unit synaptic current to produce a larger voltage drop across the membrane, thereby generating a larger EPSP. The analogy was drawn to the neuromuscular junction, where Katz and Thesleff (1957) had previously demonstrated a positive correlation between amplitude of the endplate potential and muscle fiber input resistance. Direct relationships have been demonstrated between the amplitude of composite group Ia fiber EPSPs and motoneuron input resistance (Burke, 1968; Dum and Kennedy, 1980). The amplitude of single-fiber EPSPs sampled in motoneurons over the entire motoneuron pool is also directly correlated with input resistance, although weakly, and within unit type (S, FR, FF) there is no relationship between single-fiber peak EPSP amplitude and motoneuron input resistance (Fleshman et al., 1981a). Thus, motoneuron input resistance reflecting differences in size and specific membrane resistance may be a partial determinant of EPSP amplitude (see Chapter 10, this volume), but other factors are also likely to play an important role, as discussed later.

Others have suggested, on theoretical grounds, that the motoneuron property more likely to be responsible for EPSP amplitude is input capacitance, because the synaptic current time course is much briefer than the time constant of the motoneuron (100 μs vs. 5 ms), and the principal component of such brief currents would be likely to flow through the capacitance of the membrane (Gage, 1976; see the discussion in Munson et al., 1982). However, this would not alter the conclusion that the peak amplitude of the EPSP is determined by cell size, since whole cell capacitance is largest in large cells and, according to Coulomb's law ($V = Q/C$), would cause EPSPs to be larger in small cells. Nonetheless, these considerations raise another complication, namely, that the duration of synaptic current is an important determinant of EPSP amplitude (Rall, 1967; Redman, 1973; Gage, 1976), and this might obscure any relationship related to motoneuron size. Another consideration is that Ia synapses are located on motoneuron dendrites at variable distances from the spike initiation site (Conradi, 1969; Jack et al., 1971); cable properties of the dendrites (Rall, 1967; Redman, 1973) would be expected to distort the relationship of

EPSP amplitude to motoneuron size. Thus, it is clear that although peak amplitude differences among the motoneurons of different threshold were determined in part by the properties of the motoneurons themselves, other factors were likely to be important (see Chapters 9 and 10, this volume).

HIGH-FREQUENCY ACTIVITY IN SPINDLE AFFERENTS

Spike-triggered averaging relies on passive muscle stretch to activate afferent group Ia fibers. The typical firing pattern under such conditions is a relatively steady discharge with a frequency of 20–40 Hz. However, recordings in moving animals reveal that spindles discharge in bursts of high frequency (up to 500 Hz) that are time locked with phases of the step (Prochazka et al., 1976; Loeb and Duysens, 1979). This pattern is very different from the regular low-frequency discharge used to study synaptic function with spike-triggered averaging. Two major new issues are raised by such studies that relate to the main theme of this discussion on the distribution of input to elements of the motoneuron pool:

1. High-frequency bursts in single afferent fibers imply the possibility of temporal summation of successively generated EPSPs in target motoneurons (Calvin, 1972).
2. Synaptic transmission during high-frequency stimulation has been shown not to be constant in response to the successive stimuli of the burst (Curtis and Eccles, 1960; Honig et al., 1983).

Both of these nonlinearities would alter the effective synaptically generated depolarizing drive to the target motoneurons. Variation in these factors, if nonuniform, could radically alter our notion of how the distribution of group Ia input to motoneurons is instrumental in achieving orderly recruitment of motoneurons. However, in order to study these phenomena, it is necessary to adopt techniques that routinely permit activation of single group Ia fibers at physiologically high frequencies. Because high frequencies of spindle afferent discharge cannot be achieved with passive stretch, electrical stimulation of single afferents is required.

We have carried out numerous studies with simultaneous impalements of a group Ia afferent and a target homonymous alpha-motoneuron (Honig et al., 1983; Collins et al., 1984; Davis et al., 1985; Collins et al., 1986). Impalement of two such neurons, identified by responses to stimulation of the peripheral nerve and, in the case of the afferent, by a pause in firing during isometric contraction of the muscle, yields an afferent–motoneuron pair with a high probability of being synaptically coupled. Thus, when the Ia fiber is stimulated by depolarizing pulses passed through the microelectrode, one generally records EPSPs in the impaled motoneuron. This has permitted us to examine transmission at different synapses under conditions that are more nearly equivalent to physiological, at least with regard to discharge rate and pattern.

EFFECTS OF TEMPORAL SUMMATION

Ranking connections using values of EPSP peak amplitude obtained under conditions of low-frequency stimulation (as in a spike-triggered averaging experiment) does not provide an assessment that is valid under all conditions. A comparison of the results obtained at two representative connections is displayed in Figure 17–1. At each connection, the Ia fiber was stimulated at 18 Hz and the EPSP was averaged over 1024 trials. Note the difference in peak amplitude of the two EPSPs (Fig. 17–1A). Then the afferent fiber was activated with a burst of 32 stimuli at 167 Hz. The bursts were repeated every 2 sec and the response of 128 such bursts were averaged, using direct coupled recording. This permitted calculation of the average depolarization of the motoneuron, measured arbitrarily over the first 15 responses, which is expressed as a horizontal line superimposed on the burst response. The height of the line above the baseline denotes the value of the mean response, calculated as the time integral of the voltage divided by the time over which the integral was carried out. The major result is clear from inspection of the results at the two connections. Ranking the efficacy of connections according to EPSP peak amplitude yields a result quite different from that obtained by ranking according to mean depolarization. This comparison is demonstrated at 13 connections studied in this way (Fig. 17–1B). Although peak value and mean value were highly correlated, it is evident in this sample that the correlation was by no means perfect.

One factor responsible for the departure from perfect agreement between peak and mean EPSP amplitude is the variation in EPSP half-width, which was positively correlated with the ratio mean EPSP/peak EPSP (Fig. 17–1C). This is not surprising in view of the expectation that temporal summation would be more prominent at connections with long half-widths (Calvin, 1972). However, other factors also play a role, notably the degree to which EPSP amplitude changes during the burst (see the following discussion). EPSPs increasing in amplitude during the burst elevate mean EPSP amplitude, but only if the half-width is large enough to cause temporal summation at that frequency of stimulation. The opposite is true at connections where EPSPs depress during the high-frequency stimulation (Fig. 17–1D). We noted that plotting mean EPSP/peak EPSP as a function of the product of half-width and depression/facilitation resulted in a relationship with a much higher correlation than that found using either variable alone (Fig. 17–1E).

It is now known that EPSPs in high resistance, low-threshold motoneurons exhibit the largest half-widths, on average (Fleshman et al., 1981a), in part because of the longer time constant in such cells (Zengel et al., 1985). Half-width values in high-threshold motoneurons (type FF) average 3.33 ms compared to 3.99 ms for type FR and 4.51 ms for type S (Table 2 in Fleshman et al., 1981a). These differences, although small, would become significant in determining the mean depolarization produced by afferent firing frequencies greater than 200 Hz. However, (low-threshold) motoneurons with larger EPSP half-widths would be expected to exhibit more depression of the successive

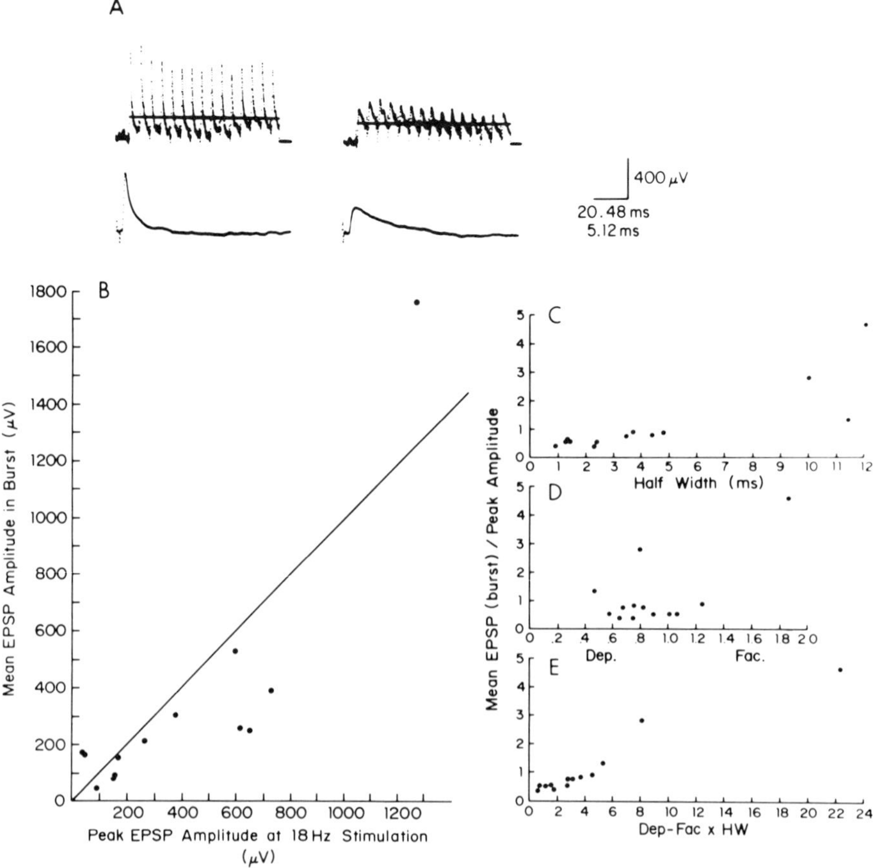

Fig. 17–1. Dependence of temporal summation on EPSP half-width and degree of depression or facilitation of EPSP amplitude during the burst. (A) EPSPs at two connections: below is the EPSP averaged after 1024 stimuli to the single Ia fiber at 18 Hz; above is the depolarization produced by a 167-Hz burst of 15 shocks to the same Ia fiber, with the resultant EPSPs averaged in register ($EPSP_1$, $EPSP_2$, ... , $EPSP_{15}$). Mean level of depolarization during the burst is indicated by the height of the horizontal line superimposed on the burst. Note the similarity in the mean depolarization despite large differences in the peak depolarization produced by low-frequency stimulation. (B) Plot of mean EPSP during the burst versus amplitude of the peak EPSP elicited by single-shock stimulation at 18 Hz. Note that as the amplitude of the peak EPSP increases, the amplitude of the mean EPSP during the burst increases. The diagonal line is a reference for mean EPSP = peak EPSP. (C) Plot of mean EPSP (burst)/peak EPSP (single shock) as a function of EPSP half-width demonstrating that the disparity between mean and peak amplitudes increases with half-width. (D) Plot of mean EPSP (burst)/peak EPSP (single shock) as a function of changes in EPSP amplitude during the burst. Values of the abcissa below 1.0 indicate depression, i.e., ($EPSP_{15}/EPSP_1$) < 1.0. Values above 1.0 indicate facilitation. Note two clusters of points that, by comparison with Figure 17–1C, is due to differences in the half-widths of the EPSPs. (E) Using an index that combines half-width with the amount of facilitation or depression improves the predictability of the mean EPSP (burst)/peak EPSP. (Collins and Mendell, unpublished data.)

EPSPs during the burst (Collins et al., 1984; see the following discussion), and this would tend to counteract the effects of increased half-width. This would reduce differences in the mean depolarization anticipated as a result of variation in half-width. This leads to the prediction that differences in functional input to the different motoneurons in the pool tend to be minimized in the sense that connections (to small motoneurons) whose EPSPs are large and long-lasting tend to undergo less mean depolarization than anticipated, while those (to large motoneurons) whose EPSPs are small and shorter-lasting tend to undergo more. This tendency toward "equalization" of input to motoneurons *during* high-frequency activity is taken up below.

A recent body of experimental data (Kirkwood and Sears, 1982; Fetz and Gustafsson, 1983; Cope et al., 1987) indicates that the first derivative of the rising phase of the EPSP is an important determinant of spike initiation in a motoneuron. Because of differences in motoneuron time constant, one would anticipate that high-threshold motoneurons (short time constant) would have faster rising EPSPs, and so the role of this factor would be greater in such motoneurons. Thus, the low-threshold motoneurons would reach firing threshold based primarily on the magnitude of depolarizing drive, while the high-threshold constituents of the pool would have a relative advantage in reaching threshold due to their fast rising EPSPs. This might be necessary in order for them to discharge despite their relatively small level of depolarizing drive.

AMPLITUDE MODULATION OF EPSP AMPLITUDE

As noted previously, EPSP amplitude is not constant during the response to high-frequency stimulation. In our experiments designed to analyze the extent to which EPSP amplitude is modulated under these conditions (Honig et al., 1983; Collins et al., 1984; Davis et al., 1985; Collins et al., 1986), we have noted that EPSP peak amplitude can vary by factors as high as 5. These changes take place over the course of a high-frequency burst during which EPSP amplitude can either increase (i.e., facilitation) or decrease (i.e., depression). In addition, for several seconds after high-frequency activity, even in a single afferent fiber, there is a period of enhanced transmission (i.e., posttetanic potentiation). The changes during and after a high-frequency burst are correlated (Davis et al., 1985; Collins et al., 1986, 1988). This finding, to be summarized in more detail later, challenges the notion that EPSP peak amplitude, or any other parameter such as area (Barrett and Crill, 1974), measured under conditions of low-frequency stimulation, is an accurate index of the efficacy of the synapse under all stimulus conditions. Our results, to be summarized, indicate that potentiation acts to support the orderly recruitment of motoneurons, but that other aspects of EPSP amplitude modulation seem designed to "correct" for some of the necessary but undesirable consequences of temporal summation. These considerations necessitate refinement of the proposition advanced by Henneman et al. (1965) that inputs are equally distributed to motoneurons of a pool.

The details of these modulation patterns have been established using short bursts of high-frequency stimulation (32 shocks at 167 Hz delivered every 2 sec (see Fig. 17–2A). During the response to high-frequency stimulation, large EPSPs, which tend to be generated in motoneurons of low rheobase (Collins et al., 1988), generally exhibit depression (i.e., become progressively smaller), at least for the initial stimuli in the burst. Conversely, small EPSPs, which tend to be generated in high-rheobase motoneurons (Collins et al., 1988), tend to exhibit facilitation during the high-frequency burst. Examples of these extremes are displayed in Figure 17–2B. Connections with intermediate-amplitude EPSPs can either depress or facilitate moderately, although at many such connections there is little modulation of EPSP amplitude. Modulation of EPSP amplitude at 43 connections studied in this way is shown in Figure 17–2C as a function of EPSP amplitude and in Figure 17–2D as a function of motoneuron rheobase, which is a measure of the motoneuron's putative position in the recruitment hierarchy (see earlier). The modulation displayed on these graphs is total modulation, which consists of a facilitation/depression process during the burst (Collins et al., 1984), as well as the potentiation process after each burst that increases the amplitude of the initial EPSP in the burst (see the following description and Collins et al., 1988). Both facilitation/depression and potentiation are measured with respect to the EPSP generated at that connection during low-frequency (18-Hz) stimulation. It is clear that negative modulation (decrease in EPSP amplitude during the burst) is greatest in motoneurons that are at the low end of the recruitment scale, i.e., low values of rheobase, whereas positive modulation occurs in motoneurons at the high end of the recruitment scale.

Potentiation following a high-frequency burst reaches its peak 100–150 ms after the end of the burst and then falls off relatively slowly (Davis et al., 1985). The peak magnitude of the potentiation, as well as its time course, differ according to the amplitude of the EPSP and the rheobase of the motoneuron. Small EPSPs generated in large-rheobase motoneurons tend to exhibit the largest values of peak potentiation (i.e., 100–150 ms after the burst), but the potentiation at these connections tends to decay most rapidly. This conclusion has been reached because potentiation 2 sec after the end of the burst is *smaller* at these connections than at connections on motoneurons of small rheobase with large EPSPs. In other words, the distribution of potentiation across the constituents of the motoneuron pool undergoes a reversal between the period of peak potentiation (largest in high-rheobase motoneurons) and 2 sec later when potentiation is largest in low-rheobase motoneurons. The consequence of this arrangement is that synapses on low-threshold motoneurons exhibit the greatest amount of potentiation (measured at 2 sec, the interburst interval) and the largest amount of depression, and so the EPSPs produced in these motoneurons display the most negative modulation during the high-frequency burst (Fig. 17–2D). Conversely, EPSPs in high-threshold motoneurons exhibit relatively little potentiation 2 sec after the previous burst, and facilitation during the burst, and so the peak EPSP amplitude modulation is positive.

One important corollary of this potentiation time course already mentioned implicitly is that averaging the EPSPs in register (i.e., each first EPSP, each second, and so on) in response to identical bursts of stimulation delivered every 2 sec means, in effect, that the first averaged EPSP in the burst (i.e., in Fig. 17–2) is a measure of potentiation at 2 sec. The subsequent EPSPs in the burst

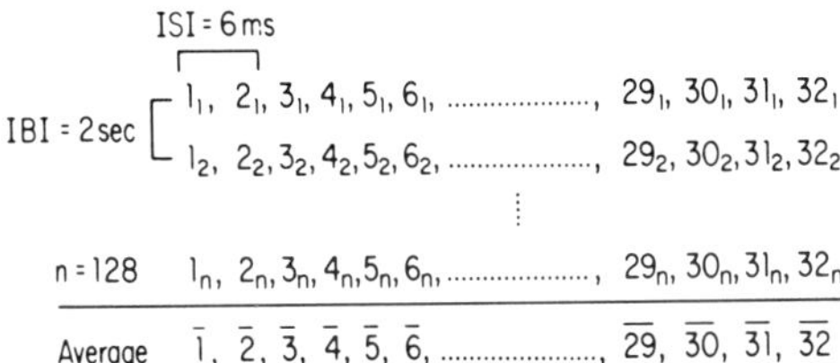

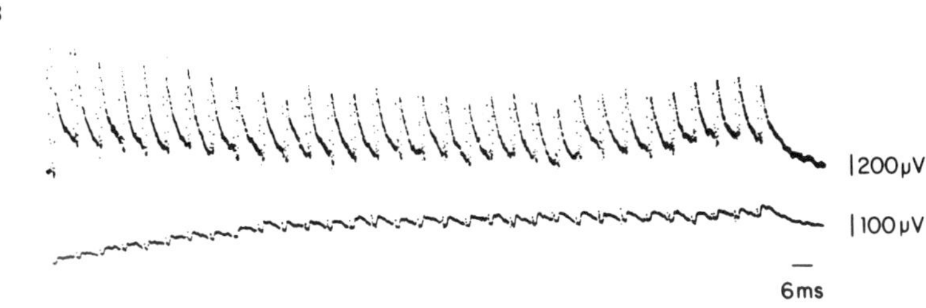

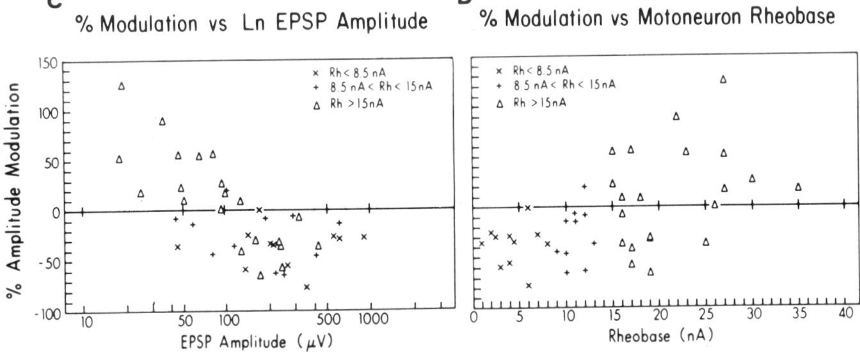

Fig. 17–2. (A) Typical paradigm used to demonstrate differences in modulation of peak EPSP amplitude at different Ia/motoneuron connections. (B) Examples of two extremes of the amplitude modulation. (C) Plot of amplitude modulation as a function of log EPSP amplitude. Modulation defined as $100\{1 - [EPSP_{30} + EPSP_{31}/2EPSP_1]\}$. Note that facilitation (modulation >1) is dominant for small EPSPs, whereas depression is dominant for large EPSPs. (D) Plot of amplitude modulation as a function of motoneuron rheobase. Note the tendency toward facilitation in high-rheobase (putative high-threshold) motoneurons and depression in low-threshold ones. (A and B from Collins et al., 1984; C and D from Collins et al., 1988, with permission.)

are not potentiated to any significant extent, since potentiation cannot be maintained during high frequency stimulation (Davis et al., 1987).

The differences in amplitude modulation of synaptic transmission at different connections have been confirmed under more realistic conditions using a frequency modulated burst derived from a hindlimb extensor muscle spindle recorded in an animal walking on a treadmill (Collins et al., 1986). At burst intervals of 800 ms, which is the step interval for this particular treadmill speed, potentiation of the initial EPSP in the burst was largest at connections on low-rheobase motoneurons. This distribution of potentiation is similar to that observed 2 sec after high-frequency bursts of a single frequency. The important point to be made here is that the connections exhibiting the greatest amount of potentiation of the initial EPSP in the burst are those that generate the largest EPSPs. They are evoked in low-rheobase motoneurons, which are those expected to have the lowest reflex thresholds for recruitment. Thus, the potentiation mechanism supports the orderly pattern of recruitment (Fig. 17–3).

We have interpreted the facilitation/depression pattern during the high-frequency burst as tending to limit the amount of temporal summation in the low-rheobase motoneurons generating the largest EPSPs while enhancing it in high-rheobase motoneurons producing the smallest EPSPs (Fig. 17–3). The former may be necessary because the large EPSPs, when temporally summated, would bring the motoneuron too far above threshold (recalling that EPSPs generated in low-rheobase motoneurons tend to be larger and to have longer half-widths, on average, than those in high-rheobase motoneurons), making it insensitive to any inhibitory input. Similarly, the summation of small EPSPs in high-rheobase motoneurons would be enhanced by facilitation and would make them far more able to affect motoneuron activity. Such a mechanism might be particularly significant in the case of the very small monosynaptic EPSPs produced in homonymous motoneurons by the action of spindle group II afferent fibers (Stauffer et al., 1976; Munson et al., 1982).

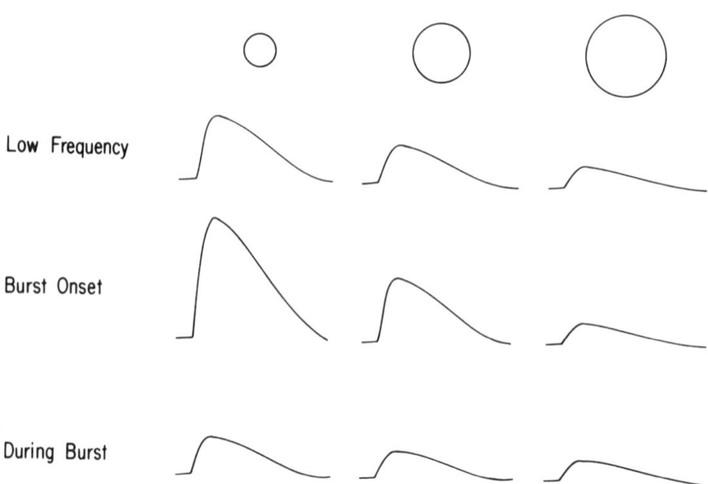

Fig. 17–3. Simulation of relative differences in EPSP amplitude at connections on three motoneurons (small, medium, and large) during different phases of the high-frequency burst. The top row is a drawing of the EPSPs produced by single-shock stimulation at low frequency. Note that the EPSP amplitude is largest in small motoneurons and smallest in large motoneurons. At burst onset, these differences are exaggerated as a consequence of the distribution of PTP produced by the burst associated with the previous step cycle. During the high-frequency burst, EPSP amplitude differences are reduced because of systematic differences in the distribution of facilitation/depression at connections on these motoneurons.

INTRINSIC DIFFERENCES IN Ia–MOTONEURON CONNECTIONS

One implication of these differences in amplitude modulation of EPSPs according to EPSP amplitude and motoneuron rheobase (or resistance) is that the amplitude of an EPSP is determined by factors beyond those related to cell size (see the earlier discussion) and the number of boutons or release sites given off by a single presynaptic Ia fiber to an alpha-motoneuron. The reason for this assertion is that these structural factors would not lead to the prediction that large EPSPs (on motoneurons of low rheobase) should depress, while small EPSPs (on motoneurons of high rheobase) should facilitate. Thus, it would appear likely that there is an intrinsic difference in the synapses on motoneurons of putatively different threshold (i.e., low and high rheobase). From the perspective of equalization of input on the different motoneurons in the pool as part of the strategy to achieve orderly recruitment (Henneman et al., 1965b), it appears that physiological factors related to susceptibility to potentiation and facilitation/depression play important roles.

The precise biophysical mechanisms responsible for these physiological differences are not known at present. It is generally assumed that high-frequency stimulation brings into play two competing presynaptic mechanisms that have opposite effects on EPSP amplitude (reviewed in Martin, 1977; see the discussion in Collins et al., 1984). One of these is accumulation of residual Ca^{2+}, which would be expected to increase the amplitude of successive EPSPs, i.e., cause facilitation. The second mechanism is depletion of transmitter, which would be expected to cause depression of later EPSPs in a burst. The relative strength of these two effects at any given connection would determine whether a given connection exhibits facilitation or depression. Such a scheme has been suggested to operate at the neuromuscular junction, where the synapse can be converted from one type to the other by altering the amount of Ca^{2+} in the extracellular fluid (see the discussion in Collins et al., 1984).

The important implication of these conclusions is that connections on low- and high-rheobase motoneurons differ in their physiology. According to this scheme, synapses on small motoneurons might release more transmitter per impulse, which would make them more susceptible to depression. At these connections on low-threshold motoneurons, transmitter depletion would more than counterbalance the facilitation due to residual Ca^{2+}, whereas at connections on high-threshold motoneurons (high rheobase), facilitation would predominate because transmitter depletion is minimal. However, it should be kept in mind that we have no direct evidence for such a mechanism at Ia–motoneuron connections, although there is evidence for differences at the ultrastructural level between boutons at facilitating and depressing synapses elsewhere in the central nervous system (Bower and Haberly, 1986). It is also possible that the differences among these connections reside at the postsynaptic receptor rather than at, or in addition to, the presynaptic terminals.

The connections examined in these studies generally involve different afferent–motoneuron pairs. However, it is known from earlier studies that each Ia afferent diverges to form synapses with virtually all motoneurons supplying a given muscle (reviewed in Henneman and Mendell, 1981). Thus, it follows that the connections made by a given afferent on low- and high-rheobase motoneurons should differ in their response to repetitive stimulation. Recent studies from this laboratory (Mendell et al., 1986) have demonstrated this (Fig. 17–4B). Single-group Ia fibers were impaled in the cell body, where impalements can be maintained much longer than in the dorsal root axon (where the penetrations of the sensory neuron had been made in previous work), and the connections made by the same axon to several motoneurons were studied. It was found that some connections exhibit considerably more EPSP depression than others made by the same Ia axon. Similar findings were made when examining the composite EPSPs produced in medial gastrocnemius motoneurons by stimulation of the heteronymous lateral gastrocnemius-soleus muscle nerve at supramaximal strength for group Ia fibers (Fig. 17–4A). The facilitation/ depression behavior observed in response to whole nerve stimulation tends to be similar to that noted in response to stimulation of the single fiber. These findings taken together suggest that the motoneuron determines the facilitation/ depression behavior, and that the synapses made by individual afferents differ according to the motoneuron on which they synapse. The locus (loci) of these differences (pre- and/or postsynaptic) is (are) not known (see earlier), although we tend to favor the presynaptic site by analogy with the neuromuscular junction (see the discussion in Collins et al., 1984).

HOW ARE Ia SYNAPSES DISTRIBUTED BY MOTONEURONS TO PERMIT ORDERLY RECRUITMENT?

There has been considerable speculation on how input is distributed in order to achieve orderly recruitment. As pointed out at the beginning of this chapter, the original view of Henneman et al. (1965b) was that the density of Ia terminals is the same on small and large motoneurons (Fig. 17–5A). However, it was pointed out that equal density of terminals on small and large motoneurons would imply a smaller *number* of Ia terminals on small motoneurons, which would cancel the advantage such neurons enjoyed as a result of their larger input resistance (see the review by Burke, 1981). Thus, it was suggested that the *numbers* of boutons provided by a given group Ia afferent to motoneurons of low and high threshold were identical. The then available physiological evidence, as well as more recently reported anatomical findings (Burke et al., 1982), indicate that low-threshold neurons are systematically smaller than high-threshold motoneurons. Thus, for numbers of terminals to be equal on these cells, synaptic density would have to be higher on the small (low-threshold) motoneurons (Burke, 1981; Stein and Bertoldi, 1981; Fig. 17–5B). However, since the size principle seemed to operate for all reflex inputs to motoneurons (reviewed in Henneman and Mendell, 1981), this would require an appreciably higher density (number/unit area) of boutons on small than on large motoneurons. Early ultrastructural evidence suggested that this was not the case (Conradi, 1969).

Further physiological studies of inputs to alpha-motoneurons revealed some

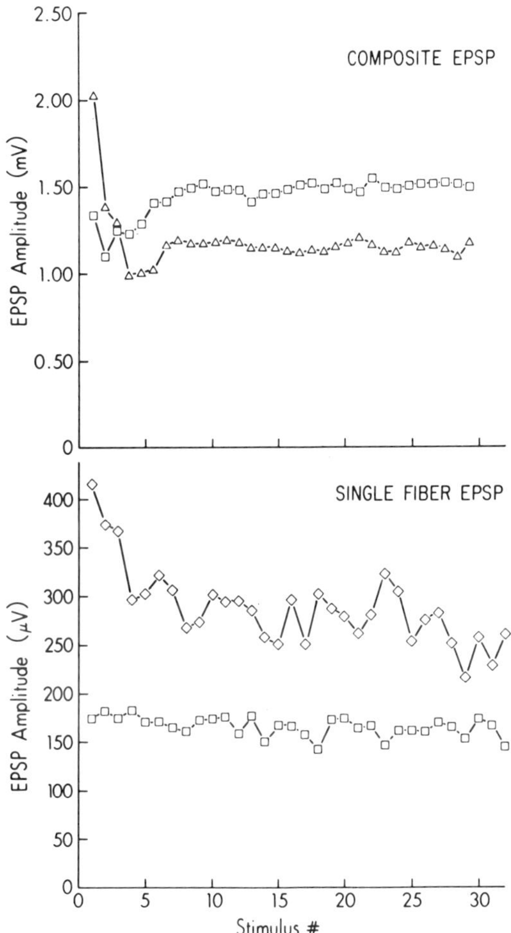

Fig. 17–4. (A) Differences in the facilitation/depression properties of composite EPSPs produced by supramaximal stimulation of the LGS nerve in (heteronymous) MG motoneurons in the same preparation. Note that the last EPSP in the burst is smaller than the first in one case and larger than the first in the other. (B) Single-MG Ia fiber stimulation with recording from two different homonymous motoneurons. Note the different modulation patterns evoked by the terminals of the same afferent terminating on two different motoneurons. The initial, transient depression in amplitude of the composite EPSPs below steady-state levels is characteristic of the results obtained with whole nerve stimulation and is probably due to the presence of an inhibitory process (group Ib, II) that is unable to follow high-frequency stimulation. Such depression is never noted after single-fiber stimulation. (Koerber and Mendell, unpublished data.)

heterogeneity in the ranking of input magnitude in putatively low- and high-recruitment threshold motoneurons. It was found that multisynaptic excitatory inputs from the sural nerve to MG motoneurons were distributed such that the largest EPSPs were evoked in high-threshold rather than low-threshold motoneurons (reviewed in Burke, 1981). Thus, the total density of inputs on alpha-motoneurons might be equal despite the higher density of Ia inputs (Fig. 17–5B) because of the correspondingly lower density of other inputs.

Some recent anatomical data derived from reconstructions of filled identified Ia fibers and their target motoneurons suggest that the number of boutons does not vary systematically on low- and high-threshold motoneurons (Glenn et al., 1982; Burke et al., in press), although the results are at present too fragmentary to permit more than tentative conclusions on this matter. There has also been the suggestion from Henneman's laboratory (Lüscher et al., 1979) that even if the numbers of boutons on low- and high-threshold motoneurons are equal, many of them are inactive, and that these unused boutons are disproportionately concentrated on high-threshold (high-rheobase) motoneurons

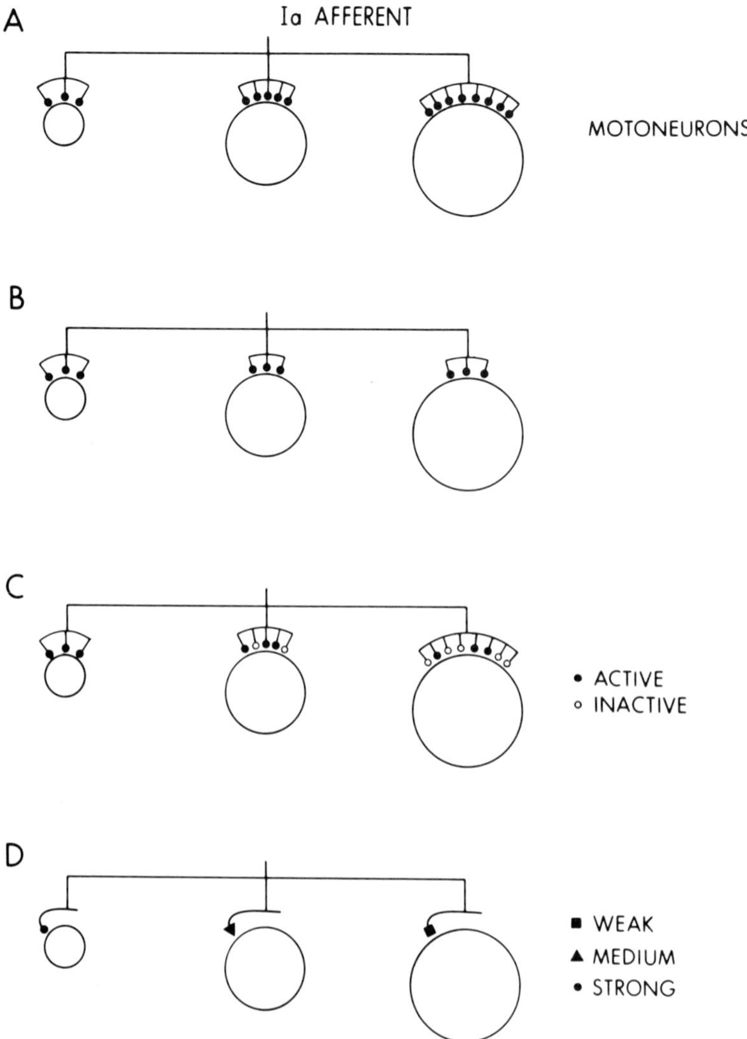

Fig. 17–5. Schemata to account for larger single-fiber EPSPs in small motoneurons. (A) Original hypothesis advanced by Henneman et al. (1965) that *density* of Ia terminals is equal on all motoneurons in the pool. This implies that the *number* of terminals increases in parallel with the surface area of the motoneurons. (B) Burke's concept of the arrangement of Ia terminals on motoneurons in the pool. *Numbers* of terminals are equal on large and small motoneurons implying that *density* of the terminals decreases as surface area increases. (C) Hypothesis advanced by Lüscher et al. suggesting that anatomical *density* of terminals is equal on small and large motoneurons (as in A), but that a smaller proportion is activated on large motoneurons, resulting in decreasing density of *active* terminals on larger motoneurons (as in B). (D) Conclusion reached by Collins et al. (1984) that the synapses on motoneurons in the pool differ physiologically such that those on small motoneurons are stronger, e.g., release more transmitter per impulse (or have a higher probability of release) on average than those on large motoneurons. This hypothesis would help account for the larger single-fiber EPSPs in small motoneurons, regardless of the anatomical arrangement of Ia boutons on the different motoneurons in the pool. Such a scheme could operate in parallel with any of the anatomical arrangements described, and so the number or density of terminals is not specified.

(Fig. 17–5C). These assertions derive from studies of posttetanic potentiation that have demonstrated that peak potentiation is systematically larger on high threshold motoneurons than on low-threshold ones (Lev Tov et al., 1983; Lüscher et al., 1983; Davis et al., 1985). The conclusion that this is due to recruitment of greater numbers of inactive boutons, either uninvaded (Lüscher et al., 1983) or unable to release transmitter (Jack et al., 1981) during low-frequency stimulation, is tenable, although the cause could as easily be related to intrinsic differences among the synapses on low- and high-threshold motoneurons. Connections that facilitate the most might, in addition to exhibiting less depletion of transmitter, also have enhanced residual Ca^{2+}, permitting higher levels of peak potentiation (see also Pawson and Grinnell, 1983). Thus, one would expect that connections that facilitate the most during high-frequency stimulation would exhibit the greatest amount of peak potentiation, and this has been observed (Davis et al., 1985). These data indicate that synapses on low- and high-threshold motoneurons are different physiologically (Fig. 17–5D), with the former being "strong" synapses (i.e., more transmitter release/release site) and the latter "weak." These properties act to fine-tune the connections made by the same Ia afferent to the heterogeneous motoneurons in the pool in order to ensure that the conditions necessary for orderly recruitment do not prevent the distribution of appropriate levels of excitatory drive to the pool during subsequent high-frequency activity.

CONCLUSION

The original papers on the size principle were important not only in describing the phenomenology in a way that motivated research workers to examine the general applicability of this rule, but also by setting down the conditions that might be necessary for such a scheme to operate. Early emphasis was on the properties of motoneurons that would permit orderly recruitment. It is now abundantly clear that there also exist systematic physiological differences among Ia synapses on alpha-motoneurons that help to ensure that the hundreds of cells in the pool function as an integrated unit to control the output of the target muscle.

Acknowledgment

This research was supported by grants RO1 NS16996 and PO1 NS14899 (L.M.M.), RO1 NS24206 (W.F.C.), and RO1 NS 23275 (H.R.K.). LMM was the recipient of a Javits Neuroscience Investigator Award.

REFERENCES

Barrett, J. N., and Crill, W. E. (1974). Influence of dendritic location and membrane properties on the effectiveness of synapses in cat motoneurones. *J. Physiol.* (*Lond.*) 239, 325–345.

Bawa, P., Binder, M. D., Ruenzel, P., and Henneman, E. (1984). Recruitment order of motoneurons in stretch reflexes is highly correlated with their axonal conduction velocity. *J. Neurophysiol.* 52, 410–420.

Bower, J. M., and Haberly, L. B. (1986). Facilitating and nonfacilitating synapses on pyramidal cells: A correlation between physiology and morphology. *Proc. Natl. Acad. Sci. USA* 83, 115–119.

Burke, R. E. (1968). Group Ia synaptic input to fast and slow twitch motor units of cat triceps surae. *J. Physiol. (Lond.)* 196, 605–630.

Burke, R. E. (1981). Motor units: Anatomy, physiology, and functional organization. In *Handbook of Physiology,* Vol. II, Sect. 1, Part 1: *The Nervous System. Motor Control* (ed.). American Physiological Society, Bethesda, Md., pp. 345–422.

Burke, R. E., Dum, R. P., Fleshman, J. W., Glenn, L. L., Lev Tov, A., O'Donovan, M. J., and Pinter, M. J. (1982). An HRP study of the relation between cell size and motor unit type in cat ankle extensor motoneurons. *J. Comp. Neurol.* 209, 17–28.

Burke, R. E., Fleshman, J. W., and Segev, I. (In press). The control of synaptic efficacy: Lessons from the Ia synapse. *J. Physiol. (Paris).*

Calvin, W. H. (1972). Synaptic potential summation and repetitive firing mechanisms: Input–output theory for the recruitment of neurons into epileptic bursting firing patterns. *Brain Res.* 39, 71–94.

Collins, W. F., III, Davis, B. M., and Mendell, L. M. (1988). Amplitude modulation of EPSPs in motoneurons in response to a frequency modulated trains in single Ia afferent fibers. *J. Neurosci.* 6, 1463–1468.

Collins, W. F., III, Davis, B. M., and Mendell, L. M. (1986). Modulation of EPSP amplitude during high frequency stimulation depends on the correlation between potentiation, depression and facilitation. *Brain Res.* 442, 161–165.

Collins, W. F., III, Honig, M. G., and Mendell, L. M. (1984). Heterogeneity of group Ia synapses on homonymous α-motoneurons as revealed by high frequency stimulation of Ia afferent fibers. *J. Neurophysiol.* 52, 980–993.

Conradi, S. (1969). Ultrastructure of dorsal root boutons on lumbosacral motoneurons of the adult cat. *Acta. Physiol. Scand.* 332 (Suppl), 49–64.

Cope, T. C., Fetz, E. E., and Matsumura, M. (1987). Cross-correlation assessment of synaptic strength of single Ia fibre connections with triceps surae motoneurons in cats. *J. Physiol. (Lond.)* 390, 161–188.

Curtis, D. R., and Eccles, J. C. (1960). Synaptic action during and after repetitive stimulation. *J. Physiol. (Lond.)* 150, 374–398.

Davis, B. M., Collins, W. F., III, and Mendell, L. M. (1985). Potentiation of transmission at Ia–motoneuron connections induced by repeated short bursts of afferent activity. *J. Neurophysiol.* 54, 1541–1552.

Davis, B. M., Druzinsky, R. E., and Mendell, L. M. (1987). Distribution of potentiation following short high frequency bursts to motoneurons of different rheobase. *Exp. Brain Res.* 65, 639–648.

Dum, R. P., and Kennedy, T. T. (1980). Synaptic organization of defined motor-unit types in cat tibialis anterior. *J. Neurophysiol.* 43, 1631–1644.

Eccles, J. C., Eccles, R. M., and Lundberg, A. (1957). The convergence of monosynaptic excitatory afferents on to many different species of alpha motoneurones. *J. Physiol. (Lond.)* 137, 22–50.

Fetz, E. E., and Gustafsson, B. G. (1983). Relation between shapes and post-synaptic potentials and changes in firing probabilities of cat motoneurons. *J. Physiol. (Lond.)* 341, 387–410.

Fleshman, J. W., Munson, J. B., Sypert, G. W. (1981a). Homonymous projection of individual group Ia fibers to physiologically characterized medial gastrocnemius motoneurons in the cat. *J. Neurophysiol.* 46, 1339–1348.

Fleshman, J. W., Munson, J. B., Sypert, G. W., and Friedman, W. A. (1981b). Rheobase, input resistance and motor unit type in medial gastrocnemius motoneurons in the cat. *J. Neurophysiol.* 46, 1326–1338.

Gage, P. W. (1976). Generation of end-plate potentials. *Physiol Rev.* 56, 177–247.

Glenn, L. L., Burke, R. E., Fleshman, J. W., and Lev-Tov, A. (1982). Estimates of electrotonic distance of group Ia contacts of cat α-motoneurons: An HRP morphological study. *Neurosci. Abstr.* 8, 944.

Gustafsson, B., and Pinter, M. J. (1984). Relations among passive electrical properties of lumbar α-motoneurons of the cat. *J. Physiol. (Lond.)* 356, 401–431.

Harrison, P.J., and Taylor, A. (1981). Individual excitatory post-synaptic potentials due to muscle spindle Ia afferents in cat triceps surae motoneurones. *J. Physiol. (Lond.)* 312, 455–470.

Henneman, E., Lüscher, H. -R., and Mathis, J. (1984). Simultaneously active and inactive synapses of single Ia fibers on cat spinal motoneurons. *J. Physiol. (Lond.)* 352, 147–161.

Henneman, E., and Mendell, L. M. (1981). Functional organization of the motoneuron pool and its inputs. In *Handbook of Physiology*, Vol. II, Sect. 1, Part 1: *The Nervous System, Motor Control.* (ed. J. M. Brookhart and V. B. Mountcastle). American Physiological Society, Bethesda, Md., pp. 423–507.

Henneman, E., Somjen, G. G., and Carpenter, D. O. (1965a). Functional significance of cell size in spinal motoneurons. *J. Neurophysiol.* 28, 560–580.

Henneman, E., Somjen, G. G., and Carpenter, D. O., (1965b). Excitability and inhibitability of motoneurons of different sizes. *J. Neurophysiol.* 28, 599–620.

Honig, M., Collins, W. F., III, and Mendell, L. M. (1983). α-Motoneuron EPSPs exhibit different frequency sensitivities to single Ia-afferent fiber stimulation. *J. Neurophysiol.* 49, 886–901.

Jack, J. J. B., Miller, S., Porter, R., and Redman, S. J. (1971). The time course of minimal excitatory post-synaptic potentials evoked in spinal motoneurons by group Ia afferent fibers. *J. Physiol.* 215, 353–380.

Jack, J. J. B., Redman, S. J., and Wong, K. (1981). The components of synaptic potentials evoked in spinal motoneurons by group Ia afferent fibers. *J. Physiol. (Lond.)* 215, 65–96.

Katz, B., and Thesleff, S. (1957). On the factors which determine the amplitude of the miniature end plate potential. *J. Physiol. (Lond.)* 137, 267–278.

Kernell, D. (1966). Input resistance, electrical excitability and size of ventral horn cells in cat spinal cord. *Science* 152, 1637–1640.

Kernell, D., and Zwaagstra, B. (1981). Input conductance, axonal conduction velocity and cell size among hindlimb motoneurones of the cat. *Brain Res.* 204, 311–326.

Kirkwood, P. A., and Sears, T. A. (1982). The effects of single afferent impulses on the firing probability of firing of external intercostal motoneurons in the cat. *J. Physiol. (Lond.)* 322, 315–336.

Lev-Tov, A., Pinter, M. J., and Burke, R. E. (1983). Post-tetanic potentiation of group Ia EPSPs: Possible mechanisms for differential distribution among medical gastrocnemius motoneurons. *J. Neurophysiol.* 50, 379–398.

Loeb, G. E., and Duysens, J. (1979). Activity patterns in individual hindlimb primary and secondary muscle spindle afferents during normal movements in unrestrained cats. *J. Neurophysiol.* 43, 968–985.

Lüscher, H.-R., Mathis, J., and Henneman, E. (1984). Wiring diagrams of functional connectivity in monosynaptic reflex arcs of the spinal cord. *Neurosci. Lett.* 45, 217–222.

Lüscher, H.-R., Ruenzel, P., Fetz, E., and Henneman, E. (1979). Postsynaptic population potentials recorded from ventral roots perfused with isotonic sucrose: Connections of groups Ia and II spindle afferent fibers with large populations of motoneurons. *J. Neurophysiol.* 42, 1146–1164.

Lüscher, H.-R. Ruenzel, P., and Henneman, E. (1979). How the size of motoneurons determines their susceptibility to discharge. *Nature (Lond.)* 282, 859–861.

Lüscher, H.-R., Ruenzel, P., and Henneman, E. (1983). Composite EPSPs in motoneurons of different sizes before and during PTP: Implications for transmission failure and its relief in Ia projections. *J. Neurophysiol.* 49, 269–289.

Martin, A. R. (1977). Junctional transmission. II. Presynaptic mechanisms. In *Handbook of Physiology*, Vol. I, Sect. 1 *The Nervous System*. American Physiological Society, Bethesda, Md., pp. 329–356.

Mendell, L. M., and Henneman, E. (1968). Terminals of single Ia fibers: Distribution within a pool of 300 homonymous motoneurons. *Science* 160, 96–98.

Mendell, L. M., and Henneman, E. (1971). Terminals of single Ia fibers: Location, density and distribution within a pool of 300 homonymous motoneurons. *J. Neurophysiol.* 34, 171–187.

Mendell, L. M., Koerber, H. R., Druzinsky, R. E., Davis, B. M., and Collins, W. F., III. (1986). Analysis of functional differentiation of muscle spindle afferent/motoneuron synapses. *Neurosci. Abst.* 12, p. 247.

Munson, J. B., Fleshman, J. W., and Sypert, G. W. (1980). Properties of single fiber group II EPSPs in triceps sural motoneurons. *J. Neurophysiol.* 44, 713–725.

Munson, J. B., Sypert, G. W., Zengel, J. E., Lofton, S. A., and Fleshman, J. W. (1982). Monosynaptic projections of individual spindle group II afferents to type-identified medial gastrocremius motoneurons in the cat. *J. Neurophysiol.* 48, 1164–1174.

Nelson, S. G., Collatos, T. C., Niechaj, A., and Mendell, L. M. (1979). Immediate increase in Ia-motoneuron synaptic transmission caudal to spinal cord transection. *J. Neurophysiol.* 42, 655–664.

Nelson, S. G., and Mendell, L. M. (1978). Projection of single knee flexor Ia fibers to homonymous and heteronymous motoneurons. *J. Neurophysiol.* 42, 778–787.

Pawson, P. A., and Grinnell, A. D. (1983). Posttetanic potentiation in strong and weak neuromuscular junctions: Physiological differences caused by differential Ca^{2+}-influx. *Brain Res.* 323, 311–315.

Pinter, M. J., Curtis, R. L., and Hosko, M. J. (1983). Voltage threshold and excitability among variously sized cat hindlimb motoneurons. *J. Neurophysiol.* 50, 644–657.

Prochazka, A., Westerman, R. A., and Ziccone, S. P. (1976). Discharge of single hindlimb afferents in the freely moving cat. *J. Neurophysiol.* 39, 1090–1104.

Rall, W. (1967). Distinguishing theoretical synaptic potentials computed for different soma-dendritic distributions of synaptic input. *J. Neurophysiol.* 30, 1138–1168.

Redman, S. J. (1973). The attenuation of passively propagating dendritic potentials in a motoneurone cable model. *J. Physiol. (Lond.)* 234, 637–664.

Redman, S. J., and Walmsley, B. (1983). Amplitude fluctuations in synaptic potentials evoked in cat spinal motoneurones at identified group Ia synapses. *J. Physiol. (Lond.)* 343, 135–145.

Scott, J. G., and Mendell, L. M. (1976). Individual EPSPs produced by single triceps surae Ia afferents in homonymous and heteronymous motoneurons. *J. Neurophysiol.* 39, 679–692.

Stauffer, E. K., Watt, D. G. D., Taylor, A., Reinking, R. M., and Stuart, D. G. (1976). Analysis of muscle receptor connections by spike triggered averaging. 2. Spindle group II afferents. *J. Neurophysiol.* 39, 1393–1402.

Stein, R. B., and Bertoldi, R. (1981). The size principle: A synthesis of neurophysiological data. In *Motor Unit Types, Recruitment and Plasticity in Health and Disease, Progress in Clinical Neurophysiology,* (ed. J. E. Desmedt). Karger, Basel, 85–96.

Sypert, G. W., Fleshman, J. W., and Munson, J. B. (1980). Comparison of monosynaptic actions of medial gastrocnemius group Ia and group II muscle spindle afferents triceps surae motoneurons. *J. Neurophysiol.* 44, 726–738.

Ulfhake, B., and Kellerth, J.-O. (1982). Does α-motoneuron size correlate with motor unit type in cat triceps surae? *Brain Res.* 251, 201–209.

Watt, D. G. D., Stauffer, E. K., Taylor, A., Reinking, R. M., and Stuart, D. G. (1976). Analysis of muscle receptor connections by spike-triggered averaging. I. Spindle primary and tendon organ afferents. *J. Neurophysiol.* 39, 1375–1392.

Zajac, F. E., and Faden, J. S. (1985). Relationship among recruitment order, axonal conduction velocity, and muscle–unit properties of type-identified motor units in cat plantaris muscle. *J. Neurophysiol.* 53, 1303–1322.

Zengel, J. E., Reid, S. A., Sypert, G. W., and Munson, J. B. (1985). Membrane electrical properties and prediction of motor-unit type of medial gastrocnemius motoneurons in the bat. *J. Neurophysiol.* 53, 1323–1344.

18

Transmission Failure and Its Relief in the Spinal Monosynaptic Reflex Arc

HANS-R. LÜSCHER

The orderly, size-related recruitment of motor units in the tonic stretch reflex results from the cooperative action of large populations of neurons. Intimate interrelations between various pre- and postsynaptic factors guarantee the coherent action of the motoneuron pool. The contribution of each factor to this collective action is not well understood (see Chapters 9 and 10, this volume), but it is recognized that the widespread connections of the muscle spindle afferent fibers with each member of the pool are of great importance in understanding how the motoneuron pool operates as a functional entity to regulate tension in a single muscle (Chapter 17, this volume). The question of how input is functionally distributed within the motoneuron pool is not a purely anatomical one. Although presumed anatomical connections between single Ia fibers and homonymous motoneurons can always be found when the two cells are injected intracellularly with horseradish peroxidase (R. E. Burke, personal communication), functional connectivity, as determined by the presence or absence of single-fiber excitatory postsynaptic potentials (EPSPs) is, in general, less than 100% (Scott and Mendell, 1976; Clamann et al., 1985). Moreover, spinal cord transection leads to an immediate increase in functional projections from single Ia fibers to homonymous motoneurons (Nelson et al., 1979). These observations suggest that synaptic transmission may fail completely in the projection of Ia fibers to homonymous motoneurons and that this failure may be relieved by spinal cord transection. Since synaptic contact systems between Ia fibers and motoneurons consists of several boutons (for references, see Brown, 1981), each of these boutons must fail to release transmitter in response to an afferent impulse. If, on the other hand, only a fraction of the boutons making up a synaptic contact system fails to release transmitter, the contact system would still be recognized as functional.

This chapter presents evidence from different sources to support the concept of transmission failure and its relief in the spinal monosynaptic reflex arc of the cat under different experimental conditions. Since transmission failure leading to silent or ineffective synapses bears on any hypothesis of central synaptic transmission, the chapter begins with a short review of the current concepts of synaptic transmission at the Ia–motoneuron junction.

Terminology

Depending on the technique employed to record EPSPs, different types of responses can be distinguished, for which the following terms will be used:

1. *Unit EPSP:* The all-or-none synaptic potential resulting from the release of one quantum of transmitter.
2. *Single-fiber EPSP:* The synaptic potential elicited by a single afferent impulse or the spike-triggered average of many afferent impulses in the same afferent fiber. It consists of a variable number of unit EPSPs. "Individual EPSP" has been used as a synonym.
3. *Composite EPSP:* The synaptic potential produced in a motoneuron by synchronous activation of many or all Ia fibers of a muscle nerve. It represents the sum of many single-fiber EPSPs. This term is synonymous with "aggregate EPSPs," which has been used as well.

CURRENT CONCEPTS OF TRANSMITTER RELEASE AT Ia SYNAPSES

The early concepts of synaptic transmission at the Ia–motoneuron junction derived from theories established through extensive work at the neuromuscular junction. When depressed by low extracellular calcium, the amplitude distribution of the fluctuating endplate potential can be described by Poisson's law (Del Castillo and Katz, 1954). This suggests that the evoked endplate potential is composed of an integral number of equal units called "quanta." The basic assumption of the quantum hypothesis is that transmitter is stored in the presynaptic terminals in a large number (n) of preformed packets. Each packet, or quantum, is released with a certain probability (p) from the presynaptic ending upon depolarization by an action potential. The number of quanta released by a nerve impulse is determined by chance and varies from trial to trial. The mean number of quanta released per action potential (m, mean quantal content) is given by

$$m = n \cdot p \qquad (18-1)$$

The mean amplitude of the evoked potential ($\bar{E}_1$) is then given by

$$\bar{E}_1 = m \cdot v_1 \qquad (18-2)$$

v_1 being the unit amplitude evoked by the release of one quantum of transmitter. The applicability of Poisson statistics to this process implies that a very large number of quanta are available at the junction, each with a very low probability of responding to an action potential. The probability (p_x) that an endplate potential is made up of 1, 2, 3, ..., x quanta is given by

$$p_x = e^{-m} \cdot m^x / x! \tag{18-3}$$

Kuno (1964a) was the first to apply this basic concept, initially worked out at the neuromuscular junction, to central synaptic transmission at the Ia–motoneuron junction. To reproduce his analysis it might be useful to redefine the relevant parameters in terms of the different EPSPs defined earlier as follows:

v_1 = amplitude of unit EPSP.

$\bar{E}_1$ = amplitude of single-fiber EPSP.

E = $\bar{E}_1 \cdot F$ = amplitude of composite EPSP,

where F is the number of stimulated afferent fibers converging on the motoneuron under study.

It is not possible to measure v_1 reliably in motoneurons because spontaneous unit EPSPs cannot be related to the synaptic junction eliciting the evoked EPSP. In addition, both the number of quanta (n) and the release probability (p) of each quantum are unknown. Consequently neither Equation 18–1 nor Equation 18–2 can be used to calculate m. If the number of stimuli delivered to a single Ia fiber is N, then the number of occurrences of single-fiber EPSPs in which x quanta are released (N_x) is predicted by

$$N_x = N \cdot \frac{m^x}{x!} \cdot e^{-m} \tag{18-4}$$

For $x = 0$, which means that an afferent impulse fails to release a quantum of transmitter, the number of failures (N_o) will be $N_o = N \cdot e^{-m}$, or

$$m = \log_e \frac{N}{N_o} \tag{18-5}$$

Failures to release a quantum of transmitter in the statistical definition of Equation 18–5 should not be confused with transmission failure, discussed later, which will be used to define synapses with a release probability of $p = 0$ under certain conditions.

With Equation 18–5, the range of m obtained was 0.63 to 5.4 (Kuno, 1964a). The predicted distribution of the EPSP amplitude was then calculated from Equation 18–4. To allow for noise and the possibility of variance in the unit EPSP amplitude, a Gaussian curve was added by trial and error to find the curve yielding the best fit to the experimentally observed amplitude distribution. The amplitude distribution of EPSPs was in good agreement with Poisson's law for small m ($m < 3$). For larger m the Poisson equation failed to predict the observed amplitude distribution. The amplitude of the unit EPSP calculated from evoked responses with m less than 3 was in the range of 0.12 to 0.24 mV. Since Kuno stimulated small strands of the muscle nerve, m may have been a function of the number of Ia fibers stimulated. Using the spike-triggered averaging technique, which ensures that true single-fiber EPSPs are analysed, Mendell and Weiner (1976) demonstrated that in 22 out of 33 cases the EPSP amplitude distributions satisfied Poisson's law. From the remaining 11, 6 satisfied the binomial predictions. For the 22 connections following Poisson's law, the mean unit amplitude v_1 was calculated to be 0.92 mV and the mean quantal content m to be 1.7. Although the authors pointed out that differences in the amplitude of single-fiber EPSPs are related to differences in m, while the unit amplitude v_1 remains the same for all Ia synapses, no attempt was made to relate m to structural differences in the junctions, e.g., to the number of boutons given off by an individual Ia fiber to a single motoneuron.

The advent of the technique of intracellular staining of afferent fibers and motoneurons with horseradish peroxidase (HRP) (for references, see Brown, 1981) opened a window to the structural complexity of the Ia–motoneuron junction. With this new insight, the temptation to give the different statistical parameters a physical meaning arose. In addition, because neither the Poisson nor the binomial model of quantal transmitter release could satisfactorily predict all the experimental data, new analytical procedures were sought without any a priori assumptions about the type of distribution that the amplitude fluctuations might follow. This was a very important step, because it was not known whether every synaptic bouton had homogeneous release properties.

The analysis of the fluctuating amplitude of Ia single-fiber EPSPs is made difficult by high noise contamination. Redman and his group developed analytical procedures to remove the noise from the recorded EPSPs in order to uncover the true fluctuations of the uncontaminated EPSP. The technique used was deconvolution (Edwards et al., 1976a, 1976b; Wong and Redman, 1980). The assumptions required to perform this analysis are that (1) the mechanisms generating the noise are statistically independent of those causing the fluctuations in the true EPSP, and that (2) noise and signal add linearly. Recently, however, these assumptions have been questioned, since some nonlinear interaction between Ia single-fiber EPSPs and background synaptic noise has been demonstrated (Solodkin et al., 1987). In order to use the deconvolution technique, it must be possible to estimate the noise distribution directly from the records. This implicitly assumes that the noise is the same in the presence or absence of an EPSP. Given these assumptions, the measured EPSP can be considered as the sum, y, of the true EPSP signal, s, and the noise, n. In reality y, s, and n are random variables, having probability density functions $Y(v)$, $S(v)$, and $N(v)$, respectively. It can be shown that Y is the convolution of S with N; i.e.,

$$Y(v) = \int_{-\infty}^{\infty} S(v - x)N(x)dx \qquad (18–6)$$

In theory, this equation may be solved directly, because the product of the Fourier transforms of two functions is equal to the Fourier transform of the convolution of the two functions. Thus, taking the Fourier transforms of Equation 18–7, which is a shorthand representation of Equation 18–6, the noise-free function S can be found by taking the inverse Fourier transform of the quotient spectrum (Eq. 17–8).

$$Y = S \otimes N \tag{18-7}$$

$$F(Y) = F(S \otimes N) = F(S) \cdot F(N)$$

$$F(S) = \frac{F(Y)}{F(N)} \tag{18-8}$$

$$S = F^{-1}\left[\frac{F(Y)}{F(N)}\right]$$

The symbol $\otimes$ denotes the convolution operation, F is the Fourier transform operator, and F^{-1} is the inverse Fourier transform operator.

In practice, however, this deterministic solution cannot be used, because $Y(v)$ and $N(v)$ are probability density functions or histograms estimated from experimental data that, due to finite sampling, show considerable statistical variation. Thus, performing the spectral division of Equation (18–8) results in high-frequency components; when the inverse Fourier transform of the quotient spectrum is taken, additional peaks that may completely mask the true responses appear (Harvey, 1984).

There are several practical approaches to the deconvolution problem. The detailed techniques have been described elsewhere (Edwards et al., 1976a, 1976b; Wong and Redman, 1980). In general, it is assumed that the noise-free probability density function represents a series of δ-functions; the number, size, and position of such functions are then to be found. If the measured noise is Gaussian with zero mean, then the distribution of the measured parameters of the EPSPs (charge transfer or peak voltage) can also be considered as a finite mixture of normal distributions (Ling and Tolhurst, 1983), as given by

$$f(x; \Theta) = \frac{p_1}{\sigma_1\sqrt{2\pi}} \cdot e^{-(x-\mu_1)^2/2\sigma_1^2} + \frac{p_2}{\sigma_2\sqrt{2\pi}} \cdot e^{-(x-\mu_2)^2/2\sigma_2^2}$$

$$+ \ldots + \frac{p_c}{\sigma_c\sqrt{2\pi}} \cdot e^{-(x-\mu_c)^2/2\sigma_c^2} \tag{18-9}$$

or simply

$$f(x; \Theta) = \sum_{k=1}^{c} p_k g_k(x; \mu_k, \sigma_k^2) \tag{18-10}$$

where

$$c = \text{number of components}$$
$$g_k = \text{Gaussian distribution}$$
$$p_k = \text{membership probability that an observation } x_i \text{ belongs to the } k\text{th}$$
$$\text{discrete component}$$
$$\mu_k = \text{mean of the } k\text{th component}$$
$$\sigma_k^2 = \text{variance of the noise}$$
$$\Theta = \text{parameter vector}$$

The following two obvious constraints are to be applied to this function:

$$0 \leq p_k \leq 1 \tag{18-11}$$

$$p_1 + p_2 + \ldots + p_c = 1 \tag{18-12}$$

The parameters of the normal mixture distribution of Equation 18–8 can be estimated by finding the maximum of the following likelihood function:

$$L(x_i; \mu_k, \sigma_k^2, p_k) = \prod_{i=1}^{n} \sum_{k=1}^{c} p_k \frac{1}{\sigma_k \sqrt{2\pi}} \cdot e^{(x_i - \mu_k)^2 / 2\sigma_k^2} \qquad (18\text{–}13)$$

where n equals the number of measured data points. This function is a maximum when our guess of what μ_k, p_k, and σ_k^2 are corresponds best to the distribution of the measured x_i. To find the maximum likelihood, the estimation maximization algorithm of Dempster et al. (1977) can be used. The advantage of this procedure is that the algorithm can be applied to the raw data without grouping them first into a histogram. We have carried out a Monte Carlo study to evaluate empirically the performance of the maximum likelihood estimator to predict the means and membership probabilities for mixtures of normal distributions (Clamann and Lüscher, 1985; Lüscher and Clamann, 1985). Since the variance of the noise can be determined reliably in the experiment, this parameter was not free for estimation. From these simulation experiments we concluded that (1) the parameters of normal mixture distributions can reliably be estimated as long as $|\mu_1 - \mu_2| \geq 1.2\sigma$; (2) the procedure can correct for faulty initial assumptions about the number of components by merging two components or giving the excess component a membership probability close to zero; (3) the estimator had no local maxima in the parameter space tested; and (4) the precision of the estimation procedure deteriorates with decreasing sample size (a sample size of 1024 is appropriate).

Two examples of the results obtained with this procedure are illustrated in Figure 18–1A to 18–1H. A total of 1024 EPSPs elicited by impulses in single Ia fibers were sampled and stored in computer memory. Four of these single-fiber EPSPs are illustrated in Fig. 18–1A. The average (Fig. 18–1B) and the variance (not shown) time courses of the EPSPs were calculated. Each single-fiber EPSP amplitude was determined by averaging a short period straddling the peak. The noise voltage was calculated from a period of the same length proceeding the EPSP. The probability density function of the noise (Fig. 18–1C) was calculated and checked for normal distribution by means of the χ^2-test. Mean and standard deviation of the noise were -4.1 μV and 74.9 μV, respectively. Figure 18–1D illustrates the probability density function of peak voltage of the EPSP still contaminated by noise. The noise-free probability density function of the EPSP amplitude in Figure 18–1E indicates that this single-fiber EPSP fluctuated among three discrete peak voltages with the following probabilities: $p_1 = 0.57$, $p_2 = 0.37$, and $p_3 = 0.06$.

The three peak voltages are 134, 142, and 249 μV. The three curves (solid lines) are Gaussian distributions with the same standard deviations as the corresponding noise distribution and means equal to the discrete peak voltages. The amplitudes are scaled according to the membership probabilities of each component. The dashed line represents the sum of the three normal distributions. A similar example is illustrated in Figure 18–1H to 18–1F. The peak voltages of the discrete components are 241, 372, and 511 μV, and their respective probabilities are 0.31, 0.59 and 0.10. These results may be used to search for integer behavior of the EPSP fluctuation. For the two examples il-

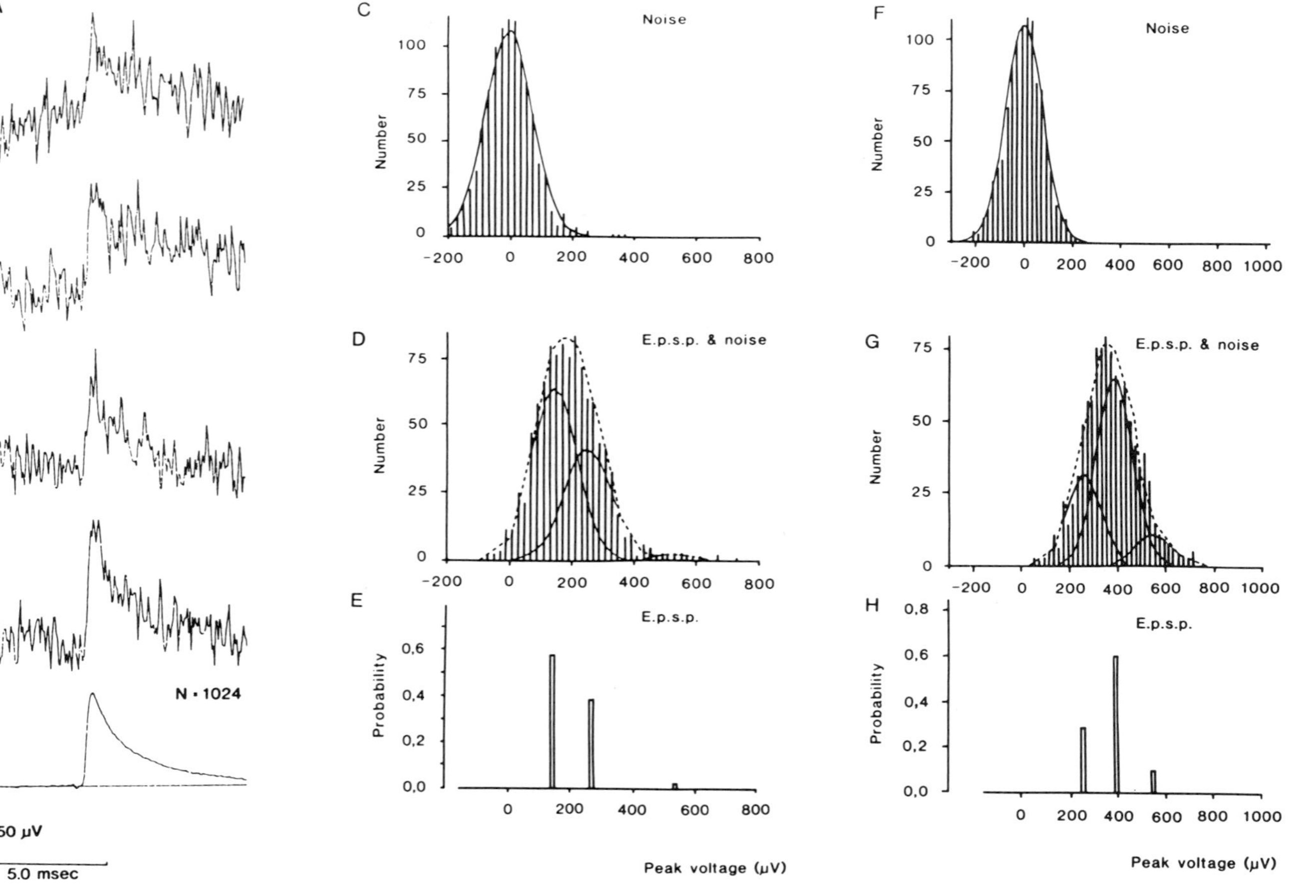

334
A
B
N = 1024
250 µV
5.0 msec
C
Noise
Number
100
75
50
25
0
-200
0
200
400
600
800
D
E.p.s.p. & noise
Number
75
50
25
0
-200
0
200
400
600
800
E
E.p.s.p.
Probability
0,6
0,4
0,2
0,0
0
200
400
600
800
Peak voltage (µV)
F
Noise
Number
100
75
50
25
0
-200
0
200
400
600
800
1000
G
E.p.s.p. & noise
Number
75
50
25
0
-200
0
200
400
600
800
1000
H
E.p.s.p.
Probability
0,8
0,6
0,4
0,2
0,0
0
200
400
600
800
1000
Peak voltage (µV)

lustrated, the increments in peak voltages are 241 (or approximately 2×120.5), 131, and 139 μV and 134, 142, and 259 (or approximately 2×129)μV. The average amplitude of this incremental EPSP was found to be 124 ± 24.7 μV($n = 22$). A similar but somewhat smaller value for the mean incremental voltage has been reported by Jack et al. (1981a), using a different deconvolution procedure. Three out of 19 EPSPs that we analyzed showed single entries in the noise-free amplitude distribution, and no variance above baseline variance could be detected during these EPSPs. This confirms previous results by Jack et al. (1981a). In addition, these authors were able to demonstrate that the component synaptic potential did not fluctuate in amplitude.

The results presented earlier and those of others (Edwards et al., 1976a; 1976b, Hirst et al., 1981; Jack et al., 1981a, 1981b) suggest that the incremental EPSP represents the unit EPSP. It further suggests that this unit EPSP reflects the all-or-nothing action of a single synaptic bouton and that the probability of releasing one quantum of transmitter varies at each bouton within a single Ia–motoneuron contact system. Some or all boutons within a terminal system may have a release probability as high as $p = 1.0$, as demonstrated by the occurrence of single entries in the noise-free amplitude distribution (Jack et al., 1981a; Lüscher and Clamann, unpublished results). An interesting and not yet published observation can be seen in Figure 18–1E. The increment between the second and last entries is approximately twice the increment between the first and second entries. This suggests that two boutons or release sites are coupled in terms of release probabilities.

It must be noted here that this concept of synaptic transmission at the Ia–motoneuron junction is not universally accepted, and it has been challenged by observations made at other central synapses (Korn et al., 1982). The discrepancies arose mostly from observations made at an inhibitory synapse on the teleost Mauthner cell. The amplitude fluctuations of these IPSPs could be described satisfactorily by a simple binomial model. Furthermore, the strong correlation of the binomial parameter n with the number of synaptic boutons impinging on the Mauthner cell gave strong support for the binomial model (Korn et al., 1981). On the other hand, similar experiments at the Ia–motoneuron junction showed that the number of components of the noise-free amplitude distribution was sometimes considerably smaller than the number of

---

Fig. 18–1. Noise removal procedure for uncovering the distribution of the EPSP amplitude fluctuations. (A) Four successive single-fiber EPSPs recorded from an MG motoneuron elicited by single stretch-evoked impulses in an MG Ia fiber. (B) The averaged EPSP waveform of 1024 responses illustrated in (A). (C) Histogram of 1024 noise records. The superimposed Gaussian curve has the same mean (-4.1 μV) and standard deviation (74.9 μV) as the histogram. (D) Histogram of 1024 measured EPSP peak voltages contaminated with noise. (E) Means and membership probabilities estimated by the maximum likelihood estimator for finite mixtures of normal distributions. The result indicates that the noise-free EPSP fluctuated among three discrete peak voltages, with the probabilities of each peak as indicated. The three normal distributions and their sum (dashed line) underlying the EPSP and noise distribution are illustrated in (D). (F–H) A second example of the noise removal procedure. (F) Noise histogram ($n = 1024$) with superimposed Gaussian curve (mean, -1.7 μV; standard deviation 75.5 μV). (G) Histogram ($n = 1024$) of measured EPSP peak voltages contaminated with noise. (H) Deconvolution leads to three entries in the histogram indicating that the noise-free EPSP fluctuated among three discrete peak voltages. (From Lüscher and Clamann, unpublished results.)

synaptic boutons in the histological data obtained by reconstructing HRP-filled Ia terminal arborizations (Redman and Walmsely, 1983). Therefore, it was necessary to postulate that a fraction of boutons within a single terminal arborization are silent at the rate of stimulation used and that the other boutons release transmitter with a relatively high probability. The correct interpretation of the results of Redman and Walmsely is important because they suggest the possibility of transmission failure at central synapses and because they rule out both the Poisson and the binomial model of transmitter release. It seems that the conflicting results and interpretations stem entirely from the different procedures used for noise removal. If the same set of data is analyzed by both methods, the binomial model predicts the number of histologically identified synapses correctly, whereas the deconvolution method has to postulate silent synapses (Korn and Faber, 1987). The concept of transmission failure or silent synapses is potentially important not only for understanding the coherent action of the motoneuron pool but also for many other aspects of nervous control. It seems worthwhile to search for additional and more direct evidence of silent or ineffective synapses.

EVIDENCE FOR TRANSMISSION FAILURE IN WHOLE SYNAPTIC CONTACT SYSTEMS

Using the spike-triggered averaging technique, Nelson et al. (1979) reported an immediate increase in the projection frequency of Ia fibers caudal to spinal cord transection in the anesthetized cat. In cats with an intact spinal cord, Ia fibers project to about 80% of all homonymous motoneurons. In cats whose spinal cords had been severed at the thoracic level T_{13}, the average proportion of the homonymous motoneurons contacted by single Ia fibers rose to approximately 100%. Since these changes took place immediately after spinal cord transection, the authors concluded that the increase in the projection frequency indicates a functional change in previously ineffective synapses rather than the outgrowth of new synaptic connections. Since Ia fibers contact motoneurons with a number of synaptic boutons at different sites (Brown and Fyffe, 1981; Glenn et al., 1982), this observation clearly indicates that the whole set of boutons making up a particular contact system can be silent or ineffective and that all or some of them can become functional after spinal cord transection. One can only speculate about the mechanism of the activation of the silent synapses. Loss of presynaptic inhibition is a likely explanation (Fujimori et al., 1966).

Using an enhanced spike-triggered averaging technique (Lüscher et al., 1983a), we analyzed large quantities of data on the functioning connections between single Ia fibers or group II spindle-afferent fibers and homonymous motoneurons in individual experiments (Clamann et al., 1985). Connectivity matrices, such as the one illustrated in Figure 18–2A, were constructed from these data and revealed that the formation of connectivity follows certain rules.

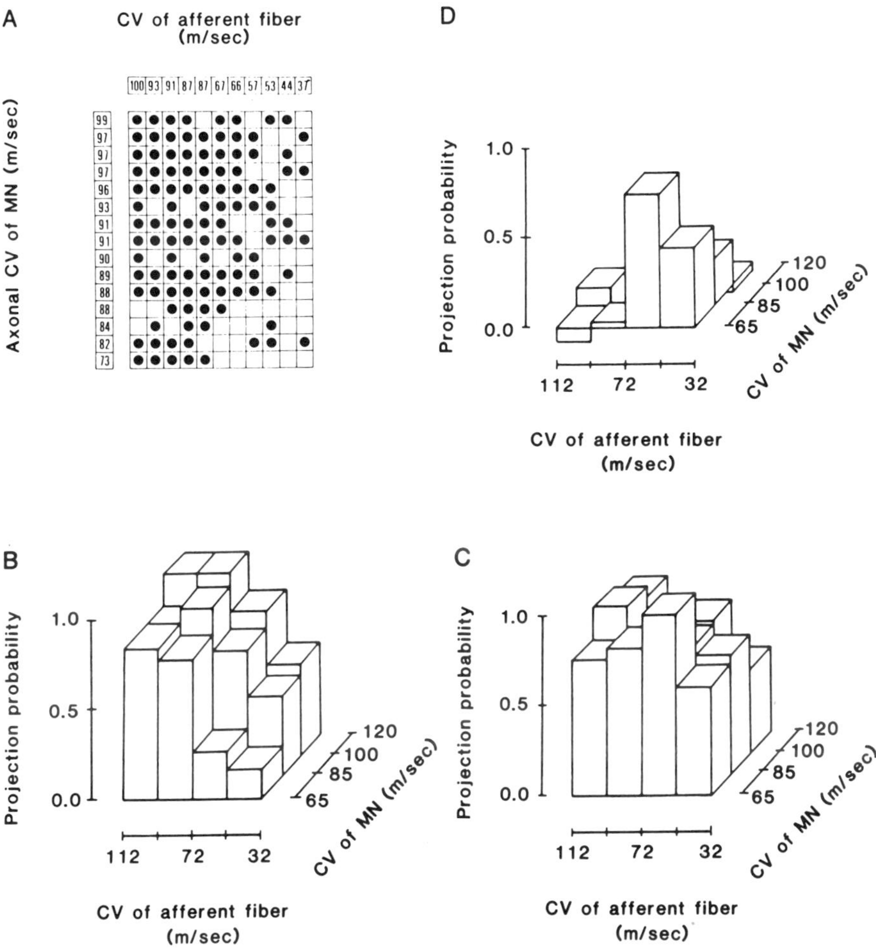

Fig. 18–2. Activation of ineffective connections after acute spinal cord transection. (A) Connectivity matrix based on 165 connections studied in a single experiment. Each dot represents an active contact system between a muscle spindle afferent fiber and a motoneuron, as revealed by spike-triggered averaging. Open squares symbolize the absence of a functional connection. The afferent fibers are arranged from left to right in order of decreasing conduction velocity. Motoneurons are listed from top to bottom in order of decreasing axonal conduction velocity (after Clamann et al., 1985). (B) Three-dimensional histogram illustrating how the probability of functional connections in pooled data from four cats with intact spinal cords (212 connections) varied with the axonal conduction velocity (cv) of the motoneuron and afferent fiber. (C) Same histogram as in (B), but from six experiments (278 connections) in which the spinal cord was transected prior to recording. (D) The difference between the histograms in (B) and (C) illustrates the increased projection probability after spinal cord transection. (From Lüscher and Mathis, unpublished results.)

In this illustration, the existence of functional connections between individual afferent fibers and motoneurons is indicated by dots and the absence of such connections by blank spaces. The 11 afferent fibers are arranged from left to right in order of decreasing conduction velocity. The 15 motoneurons to which they projected are listed from top to bottom, again in order of decreasing axonal conduction velocity. The distribution pattern of the dots clearly shows that far more functional connections exist in the upper left-hand corner of the matrix than in the lower right-hand corner. Thus, a large afferent fiber has a higher probability of making functional connections than a small afferent fiber. On the other hand, large motoneurons seem to have a higher probability of receiving functional connections than small motoneurons. However, even the largest fiber, with a conduction velocity of 100 m/sec, did not make functional connections with two motoneurons. This incomplete projection pattern is surprising, since when HRP is injected into single Ia fibers and homonymous motoneurons, evidence of presumed anatomical connections between the two neurons can always be found (R. E. Burke, personal communication). This suggests that failure to resolve a functional connection by means of spike-triggered averaging does not necessarily mean that no anatomical connections exist.

Even though large numbers of synaptic contact systems could be studied in single experiments, the great variability among the individual experiments sometimes obscured clear connectivity patterns between the afferent fibers and the motoneurons. In order to work out these connectivity patterns more clearly and to strengthen further the observation that functional connectivity depends on both, the size of the motoneurons and the size of the afferent fibers, data from 212 analyzed connections in four experiments were pooled and are represented in a three-dimensional histogram (Fig. 18–2B). The combined influence of these two variables (motoneuron conduction velocity, CV, and afferent fiber CV) is represented in the 12 histogram bins. Motoneurons with axonal conduction velocities in the range of 65–84 m/sec had projection probabilities that increased progressively with increasing conduction velocity of the afferent fibers. A similar trend, but with a less even progression, is apparent in the two groups of motoneurons with more rapidly conducting axons. The influence of motoneuron size on projection probability can be seen for all groups of afferent fibers, although this influence is more prominent in group II than in the Ia range. Projection probability also depends on the topographical relationship between the craniocaudal location of the motoneuron and the entry point of the afferent fiber into the spinal cord (Clamann et al., 1985; Lüscher and Vardar, 1989). In the particular experiments used to compile Figure 18–2B, the motoneurons were relatively close together (maximal craniocaudal separation approximately 2 mm); this topographic factor was therefore ignored.

Figure 18–2C, a similar three-dimensional histogram was constructed from 278 connections studied in six experiments. In all of these experiments, the spinal cord was transected at the level of T_{13} 2–4 hr prior to recording. Figure 18–2D plots the difference between the projection probability found in preparations with the spinal cord intact (Fig. 18–2B) and the projection probability found in the animals with an acutely transected spinal cord (Fig. 18–2C). An increase in the projection probabilities, especially from small afferent fibers to small motoneurons, can be seen. The influence of afferent fiber size and motoneuron size on functional connectivity seen in the intact animal is almost lost. The increase in the projection probability of small afferent fibers to small motoneurons was accompanied by the appearance of small EPSPs. At the same time, the EPSPs elicited by large afferent fibers, probably those that had already been active in the preparation with an intact spinal cord, increased in amplitude by a moderate amount. In contrast to the observation made by Nelson et al. (1979), very large EPSPs have never been observed.

The formation of new functional connections immediately after spinal cord transection suggests that they were already present anatomically but were rendered ineffective by some still unknown mechanisms. It seems unlikely that this increase in projection probability was due to any rapid growth process leading to collateral sprouting (Liu and Chambers, 1958; Murray and Goldberger, 1974). We conclude that transmission failures occur throughout particular anatomical synaptic contact systems and that some of these transmission failures are probably relieved immediately after spinal cord transection. The immediacy of the observed changes in the projection probability suggests that a possible mechanism for the relief of transmission failure is associated with a neural process, e.g., loss of presynaptic inhibition from more cranial input (Fujimori et al., 1966). The novel finding that the observed transmission failures are related to the size of the afferent fibers, as well as to the size of the motoneurons, might give some clues to the site where transmission failure is most likely to occur in the muscle spindle afferent projections to motoneurons.

In the presence of 4-aminopyridine (4-AP), excitatory synaptic potentials recorded from spinal motoneurons increase in amplitude (Jankowska et al., 1977). The augmented transmission was found to be due to an increase in the probability of transmitter release at each bouton, including some boutons that, before application of 4-AP, did not release transmitter at all (Jack et al., 1981b). There was no indication of an increase in the unit EPSP amplitude. In addition, when the control EPSP consisted of a single component, it did not increase in amplitude following 4-AP administration. In similar experiments, we observed the appearance of a single-fiber EPSP from a previously inactive connection between an Ia fiber and a motoneuron after intravenous administration of 4-AP (Lüscher and Clamann, unpublished observation). Trace 1 in Figure 18–3A is a spike-triggered average of intracellularly recorded synaptic noise prior to 4-AP administration. At this level of resolution, no EPSP could be detected. During the slow infusion of the 4-AP solution (1 mg/kg), a small EPSP developed (Fig. 18–3A, trace 2). Five minutes later, the EPSP rose to an amplitude of 124 μV (Fig. 18–3A, trace 3).

When the fluctuation analysis described under "Current Concepts of Transmitter Release at Ia Synapses" was applied to these EPSPs before, during, and after 4-AP infusion, it was found that the appearance of an EPSP, and the increase in EPSP magnitude were due first to the appearance of new components and later to alteration of the probability of occurrence of such components. Traces 1–3 of Figure 18–3B illustrate the corresponding histograms of the peak voltages of these EPSPs after noise removal. This example clearly demonstrates that a whole Ia–motoneuron contact system, consisting of at least four synaptic boutons, may be subject to transmission failure and that this failure can be relieved by 4-AP.

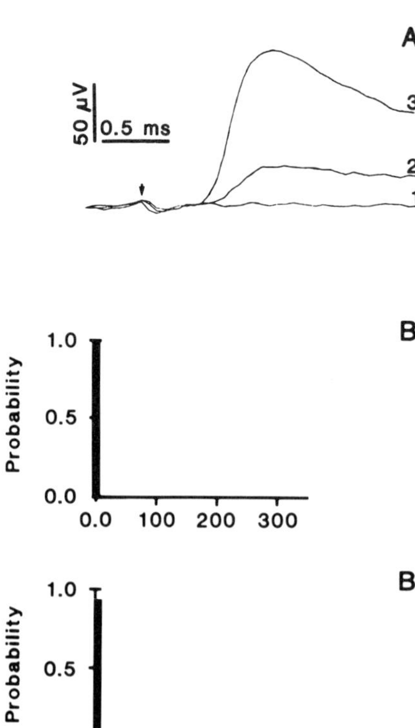

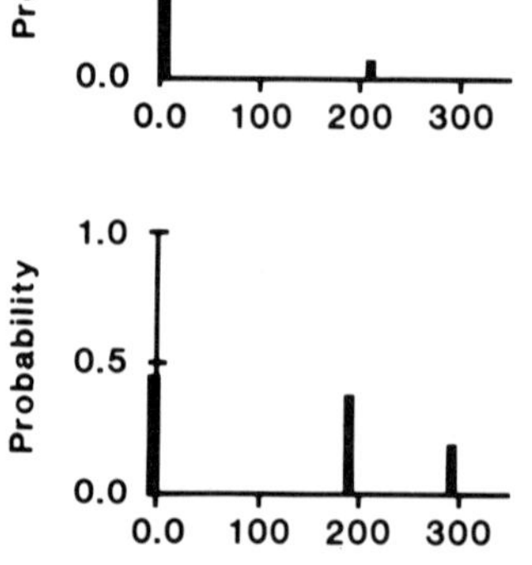

Fig. 18–3. Activation of a "silent" contact system by 4-AP. (A1) Spike-triggered average ($n = 1024$) of intracellularly recorded synaptic noise prior to 4-AP injection. No EPSP could be detected. (A2) EPSP recorded during 4-AP injection. (A3) EPSP 5 min after 4-AP injection. (B1–B3) Results of the deconvolution procedure for the three traces in (A). (B1) The presumed peak voltage was zero μV, with the same standard deviation as the noise records. (B2) During 4-AP injection the EPSP fluctuated between two discrete peak voltages, with the probabilities as indicated. (B3) A third discrete EPSP component appeared 5 min after administration of 4-AP. The results indicate that 4-AP can uncover silent connections. The presynaptic spike (arrow) was always present but became wider with 4-AP. (From Lüscher and Clamann, unpublished results.)

TRANSMISSION FAILURE AT INDIVIDUAL SYNAPTIC BOUTONS

The experiments described in the previous section provide convincing evidence for complete transmission failure at whole synaptic contact systems between muscle spindle afferent fibers and motoneurons. It is therefore conceivable that subsets of boutons within a terminal arborization impinging on motoneurons may fail intermittently or over a longer time period. This section reviews some evidence for the coexistence of active and inactive synapses in the terminal arborizations of Ia fibers.

The possibility of activating or silencing synaptic boutons would provide the central nervous system with a means of modulating synaptic transmission over a wide range. Kuno was the first to note that the augmentation of the

EPSP during posttetanic potentiation (PTP) was due to an increase in the probability of occurrence of unit EPSPs without changes in the size of the unit EPSP itself (Kuno, 1964b). He also realized that some EPSPs could not be potentiated at all. The same difficulties in demonstrating PTP in single-fiber EPSPs was encountered by Edwards et al. (1976b). Of nine EPSPs studied, four showed no evidence of PTP. This difficulty in demonstrating PTP in single-fiber EPSPs is a surprise because PTP can always be seen in composite EPSPs (Curtis and Eccles, 1960; Lüscher et al., 1983b). Using the technique of noise removal by deconvolution, Hirst et al. (1981) analyzed an EPSP that fluctuated between zero amplitude and a component at 90 μV under control conditions. During PTP, the entry at zero amplitude disappeared from the histogram, the probability of the component at 90 μV increased, and a new component at 190 μV appeared. Again, the authors also observed EPSPs without any fluctuation in peak amplitude before PTP that also did not potentiate after the tetanus. These results are consistent with the hypothesis that the amplitude of the unit EPSP (i.e., the magnitude of the synaptic potential generated at a single bouton) does not fluctuate from trial to trial (Edwards et al., 1976a; Jack et al., 1981a). PTP, when it occurs, results from a decrease in the probability of failure to release transmitter from single boutons and to the recruiting of previously silent synapses. If all boutons in a contact system are releasing transmitter with a probability of $p = 1$ (i.e., EPSPs without a fluctuating peak amplitude), no potentiation following a tetanus can be expected. The observation that these particular EPSPs do not potentiate and the fact that the amplitude of the unit EPSP does not change during PTP are strong arguments for the all-or-nothing behavior of the release mechanism at single boutons.

The same arguments can be applied to explain the potentiated EPSP amplitude after administration of 4-AP. These experiments, together with the observation that the number of fluctuating EPSP components may be considerably smaller than the number of histologically identified synaptic boutons (Redman and Walmsely, 1983), strongly support the hypothesis that a single afferent impulse from an Ia fiber does not necessarily activate all of the synapses that the fiber gives off to a motoneuron, but may repeatedly fail to activate some boutons while consistently activating others.

It is possible to infer the location of active boutons on the somatodendritic tree from the time course of the single-fiber EPSPs (Rall, 1967). In particular, synapses given off by a single Ia fiber to more than one discrete site on the somatodendritic tree would produce EPSPs with composite decay time courses, as first reported by Mendell and Henneman (1971) and illustrated in Figure 18–4A. Synapses clustered in a single restricted area would produce EPSPs with simple decay time courses. Using these criteria, the presence of previously ineffective or silent synapses can be recognized by the shape changes of EPSPs when they become active (Henneman et al., 1984).

In Figure 18–4B, one single-fiber EPSP is illustrated that was recorded from a spinal motoneuron in the anesthetized cat together with nine others that are not shown. The EPSP had a slow rate of rise and a simple decay time course (arrowhead in Fig. 18–4B1). The shape index locates the synaptic site at a distal dendrite (Fig. 18–4C■). The shape of this EPSP (elicited by the

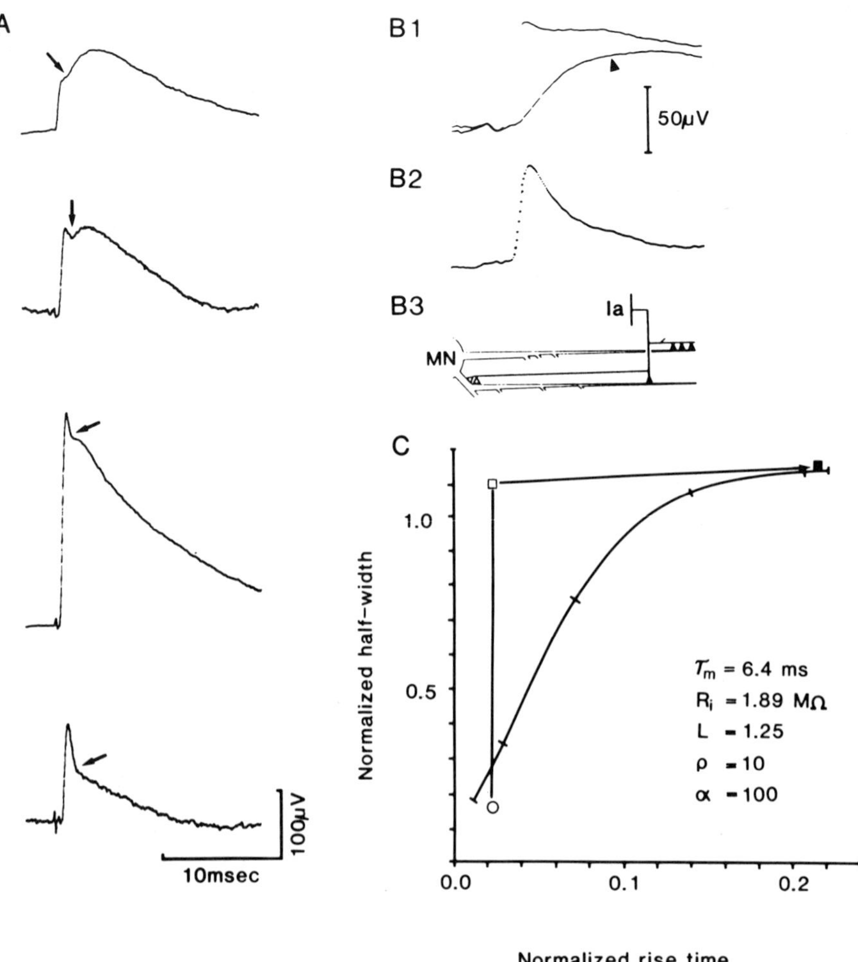

Fig. 18–4. Spontaneous relief of ineffective boutons. (A) Four examples of single-fiber EPSPs with clear breaks in the rising and falling phases indicating that they were evoked by synapses on widely different locations on the somatodendritic tree. (From Lüscher and Clamann, unpublished observation.) (B1) An example of an individual EPSP that changed its shape and amplitude spontaneously. During the first recording period, the EPSP had a slow rate of rise (arrowhead). During the second recording period, the EPSP elicited by the same Ia fiber had a fast rise time and a composite decay time course, an illustrated in the uppermost trace. (B2) Subtraction of the EPSP recorded initially from those obtained later resulted in an EPSP with a fast rise time and a simple time course. (C) Theoretical shape index curve for the motoneuron from which the EPSPs in (B1) was recorded. The shape index of the EPSP recorded first is indicated by ■. The half-width of the EPSP recorded during the second period is much too long for its rise time (□). The shape index of the EPSP obtained by subtraction is indicated by ○. These results suggest that during the first recording period, the EPSP was evoked by boutons located at a distal dendrite. During the second recording period, additional boutons were recruited close to the soma that had been ineffective during the first recording period (B3). It cannot be decided from this experiment whether one or several boutons are involved at each synaptic site. (After Henneman et al., 1984.)

same afferent fiber in the same motoneuron) changed spontaneously when recorded 40 min later. It exhibited a very fast rise time and a clearly composite decay time course, suggesting that synaptic transmission was no longer restricted to a limited area on the somatodendritic tree. Compared to the theoretical shape index curve, the half-width of this EPSP is much too long for its rise time (Fig. 18–4C□). When the EPSP recorded first was subtracted from the EPSP recorded later, the waveform shown in Fig. 18–4B2 was obtained. This potential, with a single peak and a simple decay time course, indicated that the later recorded EPSP was composed of two subcomponents generated at two different dendritic locations. The shape index of the fast-rising subcomponent fits the theoretical shape index curve well and locates the site of transmission at or close to the soma (Figure 18–4C○). Five of the EPSPs recorded simultaneously from the same motoneuron changed their shape or amplitude between the two recording periods, while five others remained exactly the same, suggesting that postsynaptic factors probably cannot be responsible for the observed changes. A possible explanation for the observed changes is illustrated in Figure 18–4B3. The Ia fiber may contact the motoneuron at two different sites on the motoneuron surface. One site, located at a distal dendrite, was active during the first recording period, while the second site, located at or close to the soma, was silent. During the second recording period, the boutons at the soma were releasing transmitter as well. It cannot be decided whether one or more boutons are involved at each synaptic site. Possible mechanisms leading to silent synapses will be discussed in a later section.

HOW MANY BOUTONS ARE SILENT?

An answer to this question can only be obtained by comparing the EPSP fluctuation patterns with the histologically identified group Ia synapse evoking the EPSP. For the cat spinal cord, only four Ia–motoneuron junctions have been studied in this particular way (Redman and Walmsely, 1983). In two cases, the number of physiologically identified components corresponded exactly to the number of histologically identified boutons. In a third case, eight morphologically identified synapses evoked a single EPSP component. Since the EPSP component was about twice the amplitude of a unit EPSP, it was suggested that synaptic transmission occurred at two boutons only, with a release probability of $p = 1.0$, and that the remainder were ineffective or silent. In a fourth case, five synaptic boutons evoked an EPSP consisting of three components. Two boutons in this contact system were probably silent. Because some boutons might have more than one release site (Fyffe and Light, 1984), the number of silent synapses might be higher than the preceding results might suggest.

Similar experiments have been carried out in mice spinal cord–dorsal root ganglia coculture (Pun et al., 1986). These authors reported the coexistence of active and inactive synapses in these terminal arborizations and stated that the proportion of inactive synapses might be as high as 80%.

From these results, one might postulate that synaptic boutons connecting Ia fibers to motoneurons exist in three subpopulations with regard to their release probabilities. One subpopulation has a release probability of $p = 1.0$. A second subpopulation has a release probability of $p < 1.0$. The release probability is probably not uniform throughout this subpopulation. A third subpopulation is ineffective, having a release probability of $p = 0$. This functional distinction does not imply that a particular bouton may always belong to the same subpopulation. In particular, boutons having a release probability of $p = 0$ may become active under certain conditions, such as during PTP, administration of 4–AP, or spinal cord transection. The possibility that synaptic boutons might be recruited and silenced again may provide the monosynaptic reflex arc with a broad range for modulating synaptic strength.

POSSIBLE MECHANISMS OF TRANSMISSION FAILURE AND ITS RELIEF

Transmission failure and its relief, as described in this chapter, refers only to the functional masking of existing contacts or the unmasking of such connections, spontaneously or by different interventions. Sprouting of afferent fibers or the opening of polysynaptic pathways that are normally inhibited has not been considered. This narrow definition of transmission failure does not leave much room for possible mechanisms.

As to the site where transmission failure might most likely occur, two hypotheses prevail. First, transmission failure might reflect a very low intrinsic release probability at individual synaptic endings, or at all endings within a single contact system in the case of complete transmission failure (Jack et al., 1981a). Second, failure of the action potential to invade and activate all the synaptic endings given off by a terminal arborization might lead to ineffective synapses (Edwards et al., 1976b; Lüscher et al., 1979, 1983b). With regard to the second hypothesis, axonal branch points and other axon inhomogeneities like boutons en passant can be regions of low safety for impulse propagation due to increased electrical load (Goldstein and Rall, 1964; Ramón et al., 1975). Branch point failures have been observed in the motor axons of various animals (Krnjević and Miledi, 1959; Parnas, 1972; Hatt and Smith, 1976) and in the central nervous system of the leech, conduction block accounts for silent synapses (Macagno et al., 1987). At present, however, a direct demonstration that conduction block leads to silent synapses in the monosynaptic spinal reflex arc of cats is still missing. The absence of detectable latency fluctuations in the components of single-fiber EPSPs has been used as an argument against the branch point failure hypothesis (Jack et al., 1981a; but see Cope and Mendell, 1982). On the other hand, if a low safety factor in the release probability itself is responsible for transmission failure at the various synapses, it is difficult to explain how the size of the afferent fiber and the architecture of the motoneurons affect release characteristics from the synaptic endings in a systematic way, as our finding would imply. The available evidence is not sufficient to tip the balance in favor of either of the two hypotheses just presented.

Whatever explanation for transmission failure turns out to be correct, the very existence of transmission failure and its relief clearly indicate that functional connectivity is by no means a fixed entity, but reflects a highly state-dependent process.

IMPLICATIONS OF TRANSMISSION FAILURE AND ITS RELIEF IN THE MONOSYNAPTIC REFLEX ARC

The motoneuron pool always exerts its action as a collective entity. Unquestionably, the connectivity pattern between afferent fibers and motoneurons is important for the coherent function of the motoneuron pool. The different analyses reviewed in this chapter indicate very strongly that connectivity is not fixed or "hard wired." Connectivity can be modulated over a wide range by the functional state of the nervous system. Existent but inactive connections can be recruited and already functional connections can increase their efficacy. The extent to which this modulation can take place may depend on the size of the participating neural elements. Transmission failure and its relief, whatever their cause, are not distributed randomly, but according to organizational principles that account for the size-related functional connectivity pattern (Clamann et al., 1985). It is only at the level of the individual contact systems that the relation between the formation of connectivity and the functional state it expresses displays an apparently random behavior within the constraints given by the architecture and size of the afferent fiber and motoneuron (Clamann et al., 1985; Lüscher and Vardar, 1989). The behavior of the motoneuron pool as a system, however, is largely deterministic, as expressed in the nearly invariant rank order in which motoneurons are activated (Henneman et al., 1965). The organizational principles responsible for the transformation of the probabilistic input at the level of the single afferent–motoneuron contact system to the deterministic output at the level of the whole motoneuron pool are still not known. One important factor in this transformation is probably transmission failure.

Acknowledgments

The author wishes to express his admiration and gratitude to Dr. Elwood Henneman for his continued encouragement and help in the past and in ongoing research projects. The original work was supported by grants from the Swiss National Science Foundations (3.308-00.82 and 3.265-0.85).

REFERENCES

Brown, A. G. (1981). *Organization in the Spinal Cord*. Springer Verlag, Heidelberg.

Brown, A. G., and Fyffe, R. E. W. (1981). Direct observations on the contacts made between Ia afferent fibres and alpha-motoneurones in the cat's lumbosacral spinal cord. *J. Physiol.* 313, 121–140.

Clamann, H. P., Henneman, E., Lüscher, H.-R., and Mathis, J. (1985). Structural and topographical influences on functional connectivity in spinal monosynaptic reflex arcs in the cat. *J. Physiol.* 358, 483–507.

Clamann, H. P., and Lüscher, H.-R. (1985). Quantal analysis at Ia–motoneurone junction. *Experientia* 41, 827.

Cope, T. C., and Mendell, L. M. (1982). Parallel fluctuations of EPSP amplitude and rise time with latency at single Ia-fiber–motoneuron connections in cat. *J. Neurophysiol.* 47, 455–468.

Curtis, D. R., and Eccles, J. C. (1960). Synaptic action during and after repetitive stimulation. *J. Physiol.* 150, 374–398.

Del Castillo, J., and Katz, B. (1954). Quantal components of the end-plate potential. *J. Physiol.* 124, 560–573.

Dempster, A. P., Laird, N. M., and Rubin, D. B. (1977). Maximum likelihood from incomplete data via the EM algorithm. *J. R. Statist. Soc. B* 39, 1–21.

Edwards, F. R., Redman, S. J., and Walmsley, B. (1976a). Statistical fluctuations in charge transfer at Ia synapses on spinal motoneurones. *J. Physiol.* 259, 665–688.

Edwards, F. R., Redman, S. J., and Walmsley, B. (1976b). Non-quantal fluctuations and transmission failures in charge transfer at Ia synapses on spinal motoneurones. *J. Physiol.* 259, 689–704.

Fujimori, B., Kato, M., Matsushima, S., Mori, S., and Shimamura, M. (1966). Studies on the mechanism of spasticity following spinal hemisection in the cat. In *Muscular Afferents and Motor Control* (ed. R. Granit). Wiley, New York, pp. 397–413.

Fyffe, R. E. W., and Light, A. R. (1984). The ultrastructure of group Ia afferent fiber synapses in the lumbrosacral spinal cord of the cat. *Brain Res.* 300, 201–209.

Glenn, L. L., Burke, R. E., Fleshman, J. W., and Lev-Tov, A. (1982). Estimates of electrotonic distance of group Ia contacts on cat α-motoneurons. *Neurosci. Abstr.* 8, 248.1.

Goldstein, S. S., and Rall, W. (1964). Changes of action potential shape and velocity for changing core conduction geometry. *Biophys. J.* 14, 731–757.

Harvey, D. J. (1984). Methods to improve resolution of recordings of electrical potentials from neurones. MSc thesis, Imperial College, London.

Hatt, H., and Smith, D. O. (1976). Synaptic depression related to presynaptic axon conduction block. *J. Physiol.* 259, 367–393.

Henneman, E., Lüscher, H.-R., and Mathis, J. (1984). Simultaneously active and inactive synapses of single Ia fibres on cat spinal motoneurones. *J. Physiol.* 352, 147–161.

Henneman, E., Somjen, G., and Carpenter, D. O. (1965). Functional significance of cell size in spinal motoneurons. *J. Neurophysiol.* 28, 560–580.

Hirst, G. D. S., Redman, S. J., and Wong, K. (1981). Post-tetanic potentiation and facilitation of synaptic potentials evoked in cat spinal motoneurones. *J. Physiol.* 321, 97–109.

Jack, J. J. B., Redman, S. J., and Wong, K. (1981a). The component of synaptic potentials evoked in cat spinal motoneurones by impulses in single group Ia afferents. *J. Physiol.* 321, 65–96.

Jack, J. J. B., Redman, S. J., and Wong, K. (1981b). Modifications to synaptic transmission at group Ia synapses on cat spinal motoneurones by 4-aminopyridine. *J. Physiol.* 321, 111–126.

Jankowska, E., Lundberg, A., Rudomin, P., and Sykova, E. (1977). Effects of 4-aminopyridine on transmission at excitatory and inhibitory synapses in the spinal cord. *Brain Res.* 136, 387–392.

Korn, H., and Faber, D. S. (1987). Regulation and significance of probabilistic release mechanisms at central synapses. In *Synaptic Function* (Ed. G. M. Edelman, W. E. Gall, and W. M. Cowan). Wiley, New York, pp. 57–108.

Korn, H., Mallet, A., Triller, A., and Faber D. S. (1982). Transmission at a central synapse. II. Quantal description of release with a physical correlate for binomial *n*. *J. Neurophysiol.* 48, 679-707.

Korn, H., Triller, A., Mallet, A., and Faber, D. S. (1981). Fluctuating responses at a central synapse: *n* of binomial fit predicts number of stained presynaptic boutons. *Science* 213, 898–901.

Krnjević, K., and Miledi, R. (1959). Presynaptic failure of neuromuscular propagation in rats. *J. Physiol.* 149, 1–22.

Kuno, M. (1964a). Quantal components of excitatory synaptic potentials in spinal motoneurones. *J. Physiol.* 175, 81–99.

Kuno, M. (1964b). Mechanisms of facilitation and depression of the excitatory synaptic potential in spinal motoneurones. *J. Physiol.* 175, 100–112.

Ling, L., and Tolhurst, D. J. (1983). Recovering the parameters of finite mixtures of normal distributions from a noisy record: An empirical comparison of different estimating procedures. *J. Neurosci. Methods* 8, 309–333.

Liu, C. N., and Chambers, W. W. (1958). Intraspinal sprouting of dorsal root axons. *Arch. Neurol. Psychiatry* 79, 46–61.

Lüscher, H.-R., and Clamann, H. P. (1985). The recovery of parameters of finite mixtures of normal distributions from a noisy record and its application to the quantal analysis at central synapses. *Experientia* 41, 831.

Lüscher, H.-R., Mathis, J., and Schaffner, H. (1983a). A dual time-voltage window discriminator for multiunit nerve spike decomposition. *J. Neurosci. Methods* 7, 99–105.

Lüscher, H.-R., Ruenzel, P., and Henneman, E. (1979). How the size of motoneurones determines their susceptibility to discharge. *Nature* 282, 859–861.

Lüscher, H.-R., Ruenzel, P., and Henneman, E. (1983b). Composite EPSPs in motoneurons of different sizes before and during PTP: Implications for transmission failure and its relief in Ia projections. *J. Neurophysiol.* 49, 269–289.

Lüscher, H.-R., and Vardar, U. (1989). A comparison of homonymous and heteronymous connectivity in the spinal monosynaptic reflex arc of the cat. *Exp. Brain Res.* 74, 480–492.

Macagno, E. R., Muller, K. J., and Pitman, R. M. (1987). Conduction block silences parts of a chemical synapse in the leech central nervous system. *J. Physiol.* 387, 649–664.

Mendell, L. M., and Henneman, E. (1971). Terminals of single Ia fibers: Location, density and distribution within a pool of 300 homonymous motoneurons. *J. Neurophysiol.* 34, 171–187.

Mendell, L. M., and Weiner, R. (1976). Analysis of pairs of individual Ia-EPSPs in single motoneurones. *J. Physiol.* 255, 81–104.

Murray, M., and Goldberger, M. (1974). Restitution of function and collateral sprouting in the cat spinal cord: The partially hemisected animal. *J. Comp. Neurol.* 158, 19–36.

Nelson, S. G., Collatos, T. C., Niechaj, A., and Mendell, L. H. (1979). Immediate increase in Ia-motoneuron synaptic transmission caudal to spinal cord transection. *J. Neurophysiol.* 42, 655–664.

Parnas, I. (1972). Differential block at high frequency of branches of a single axon, innervating two muscles. *J. Neurophysiol.* 35, 903–914.

Pun, R. Y., Neale, E. A., Guthrie, P. B., and Nelson, P. G. (1986). Active and inactive central synapses in cell culture. *J. Neurophysiol.* 56, 1242–1256.

Rall, W. (1967). Distinguishing theoretical synaptic potentials computed for different soma-dendritic distributions of synaptic input. *J. Neurophysiol.* 30, 1138–1168.

Ramon, F., Joyner, R. W., and More, J. W. (1975). Propagation of action potentials in inhomogeneous axon regions. *Fed. Proc.* 34, 1357–1363.

Redman, S., and Walmsley, B. (1983). Amplitude fluctuations in synaptic potentials evoked in cat spinal motoneurones at identified group Ia synapses. *J. Physiol.* 343, 135–145.

Scott, J. G., and Mendell, L. M. (1976). Individual EPSPs produced by single triceps surae Ia afferent fibers in homonymous and heteronymous motoneurons. *J. Neurophysiol.* 39, 679–692.

Solodkin, M., Ruiz de Leon, O., Zamora, L., Jimenez, I., Collins, W. F., III, Mendell, L., and Rudomin, P. (1987). Non-linear interaction between background synaptic noise and Ia single fiber EPSPs evoked in spinal motoneurons. *Soc. Neurosci. Abstr.* 13, 1697.

Wong, K., and Redman, S. (1980). The recovery of a random variable from a noisy record with application to the study of fluctuations in synaptic potentials. *J. Neurosci. Methods* 2, 389–409.

19

Presynaptic Control of Synaptic Effectiveness of Muscle Spindle and Tendon Organ Afferents in the Mammalian Spinal Cord

P. RUDOMIN

In 1957 Frank and Fuortes tested the effects of a stimulus train applied to the posterior biceps and semitendinosus (PBSt) nerve on the monosynaptic Ia excitatory postsynaptic potentials (EPSPs) elicited in extensor motoneurons. They found that the Ia EPSPs could be depressed without associated changes in the membrane potential or in the antidromic action potentials of the motoneuron. Frank and Fuortes suggested that the depression of the monosynaptic Ia EPSPs was due to presynaptic inhibition. Later on, Frank (1959) proposed an alternative explanation for the depression of the Ia EPSPs, namely, that the inhibition was postsynaptic and was exerted directly on the motoneuron distal dendrites (remote dendritic inhibition) close to the synapses of Ia fibers.

It should be noted that this is a negative definition of presynaptic inhibition because it is based on the lack of changes in electrical properties of the motoneuron during the EPSP depression. Nevertheless, the proposal of presynaptic control mechanisms was a very important conceptual contribution because it implied that afferent fibers were not passive conveyors of action potentials, but rather that conduction of impulses along the terminal arborizations of the afferent fibers and/or transmitter release could be subjected to a central control. This would allow, at least in principle, a selective control of neuronal responses to synaptic inputs. In contrast, postsynaptic inhibition would affect responses to all excitatory inputs acting on the soma and proximal dendrites.

This chapter reviews some issues related to presynaptic inhibition and primary afferent depolarization of muscle afferents in mammals. It is not comprehensive, but rather represents my own interests in the field. Several other reviews may be consulted for additional information (Schmidt, 1971; Burke and Rudomin, 1977; Levy, 1977; Nicoll and Alger, 1979; Redman, 1979; Baldissera et al., 1982; Davidoff and Hackman, 1984).

PRESYNAPTIC VERSUS POSTSYNAPTIC INHIBITION

Remote dendritic inhibition and presynaptic inhibition have been regarded by several investigators as mutually exclusive (Green and Kellerth, 1966; Eide et al., 1968; Granit, 1968), and attempts have been made to evaluate the relative contributions of these two inhibitory mechanisms to the depression of the Ia EPSPs. These have included analysis of the effects of electrical stimulation of sensory nerves on (1) motoneuron input resistance (Eide et al., 1968), (2) motoneuron repetitive firing produced by intracellularly injected currents (Green and Kellerth, 1966; Kellerth, 1968; Cook and Cangiano, 1972), and (3) the amplitude and time course of monosynaptic EPSPs produced in the same motoneuron by the activation of Ia and vestibulo-spinal fibers (Eide et al., 1968; Rudomin et al., 1975b). The outcome of these studies is that in some cases, particularly when using weak stimulation of nerves from flexor muscles, depression of Ia EPSPs can be produced without measureable postsynaptic changes, and that this depression is rather selective, since it occurs without affecting the monosynaptic EPSPs evoked in the same motoneuron by other (vestibulospinal) pathways (Eide et al., 1968; Rudomin et al., 1975b). More recently, using brief pulses to measure the passive properties of motoneurons, Carlen et al. (1980) have concluded that there is always a conductance increase in the motoneuron distal dendrites, even with the weakest conditioning volleys, and have suggested that postsynaptic inhibition is primarily responsible for the depression of the Ia EPSPs. However, it was never determined if *all* of the depression could in fact be accounted for by postsynaptic inhibitory changes (see also McCrea and Carlen, 1983).

Most of the work on presynaptic inhibition has been performed by applying electrical stimulation of variable strength to segmental nerves and supraspinal structures. It could be argued that these stimuli are, to some extent, artificial because the high degree of synchrony from electrical stimulation provides strong spatial and temporal summation, and may activate interneuronal pathways not involved during more physiological activation of the peripheral receptors.

In 1964, Granit et al. analyzed the effects produced during slow stretch of several flexor and extensor muscles on the monosynaptic EPSPs recorded from popliteal, hamstring, and peroneal motoneurons. Pulling a muscle at another joint decreased the EPSPs without hyperpolarizing the motoneuron. However, since the discharge set up by transmembrane stimulation *always* underwent a reduction, the authors concluded that the inhibitory effects were largely, it not wholly, postsynaptic.

On the other hand, Devanandan et al. (1965) found that monosynaptic reflexes and Ia EPSPs elicited in motoneurons of extensor muscles of the ankle or of a flexor muscle of the foot were depressed by stretching the flexor muscles of the knee or the ankle over a time course of about 120–140 ms, the peak being at about 30 ms. Muscle stretch produced some changes in membrane potential of the motoneuron, but these were small and short-lasting, and, according to the investigators, did not account for depression of the EPSP and the monosynaptic reflex. Since Ia EPSPs were depressed without changing their time course, and since the depression could not be abolished by strychnine, the authors concluded that depression of the Ia EPSPs elicited under their experimental conditions was not due to postsynaptic inhibition, but rather to presynaptic inhibition.

Kellerth and Szumski (1966a, 1966b) studied the pharmacological behavior of the inhibitory potentials produced in hindlimb motoneurons by muscle stretch and by electrical stimulation of the afferent nerves of these muscles. They identified two types of inhibitory postsynaptic potentials (IPSPs) generated in the postsynaptic membrane with different sensitivities to strychnine and picrotoxin. The strychnine-resistant as well as the picrotoxin-sensitive IPSPs recorded from motoneurons were found to have characteristics similar to those described for presynaptic inhibition: They had the same duration as the dorsal root potentials (DRPs), a putative sign of presynaptic inhibition (see the later discussion), and both depressed the Ia EPSPs without affecting their time course. However, in no case was a postsynaptic inhibition found to be resistant to both strychnine and picrotoxin, and in strychninized cats, the remaining postsynaptic inhibitions were always abolished by picrotoxin.

It thus seems that muscle stretch is indeed able to depress Ia EPSPs while it depolarizes the Ia fiber terminals and produces IPSPs in motoneurons that last about as long as primary afferent depolarization. These inhibitory potentials are strychnine resistant and picrotoxin sensitive, as expected for GABAergically mediated actions (see the later discussion).

EVIDENCE SUPPORTING THE EXISTENCE OF PRESYNAPTIC INHIBITION

One of the strongest arguments that has been used to rule out any contribution of remote postsynaptic inhibitory changes has been the finding that Ia EPSP depression occurs virtually without changing the time course of the synaptic potential (Eccles et al., 1962c; Eide et al., 1968; Rudomin et al., 1975b). According to Rall's compartmental model (1967, 1970), the falling phase of the Ia EPSP is a very sensitive index of the conductance associated with synaptic potentials generated in the motoneuron distal dendrites. It has been argued that if the synaptic components generated on the distal dendrites were depressed by some postsynaptic conductances, this should produce EPSPs with a faster falling phase (Eide et al., 1968; Cook and Cangiano, 1972; Pottala et al., 1973; Rudomin et al., 1975b; Lev Tov et al., 1983). However, according to Carlen et al. (1980), if the Ia EPSP is generated wholly at a remote site and the conditioning conductance increases also take place nearby, little change in the decay of the EPSP would be expected, since the decay would depend primarily on the characteristics of the centripetal and perisomatic time constants. To account for presynaptic depression of the Ia EPSP without changes in its falling phase, it seems necessary to postulate that transmitter release in all Ia terminals is reduced to the *same extent* by the conditioning volleys, which seems difficult to sustain. Alternatively, it is possible that the depression of the Ia EPSP results from conduction blockade in the intraspinal arborizations of the afferent fibers (Howland ct al., 1955). At present, there is no experimental evidence to distinguish between these two possibilities.

Direct evidence supporting the existence of presynaptic mechanisms responsible for the depression of the Ia EPSPs is scarce. In 1964 Kuno showed that PBSt conditioning volleys increased the number of failures of the monosynaptic EPSPs produced by stimulation of *single* Ia afferent fibers. Since the unitary EPSPs were not changed by the conditioning stimuli, he concluded that the Ia EPSP depression was due to reduction in the mean quantal content of the transmitter released at the Ia fiber terminals. Seen in retrospect, Kuno's findings can be explained either by a reduction in the amount of transmitter released by the action potential (see, for example, Dudel and Kuffler, 1961) or by conduction failure in the intraspinal arborizations of the Ia afferent fibers (Howland et al., 1955), but they certainly support the existence of a presynaptic mechanism controlling the synaptic efficacy of muscle spindle afferents.

More recently, Clements et al. (1987) have reanalyzed this problem and measured the fluctuations of single-fiber Ia EPSPs, using deconvolution techniques. They found that after conditioning stimulation, larger discrete EPSP amplitudes became less probable, while smaller discrete amplitudes became more probable, as expected for presynaptic inhibition. Their calculations were based on the fact that ongoing synaptic noise and evoked Ia EPSPs add linearly. However, it must be pointed out that Solodkin et al. (1987) have shown recently that smaller Ia EPSP components can be also obtained in model neurons by assuming nonlinear interaction between background and evoked EPSPs, which means that similar results could probably be obtained if the interactions were only postsynaptic.

PRESYNAPTIC INHIBITION AND MOTONEURON TYPE

The size of the Ia EPSPs produced in various types of motoneurons appears to be related to motoneuron size, which in turn is related to the contractile properties of the muscle fibers they innervate (Burke, 1981; Henneman and Mendell, 1981; see also Chapters 16, 17, and 18, this volume). There is also evidence that the strength of recurrent inhibition and the Ia antagonistic inhibition vary with motoneuron size and motor unit type (Dum and Kennedy, 1980; Friedman et al., 1981). Hence, it seems adequate to ask whether or not presynaptic inhibition has any relation to these functional parameters. Zengel et al. (1983) have analyzed this problem in the triceps surae motoneurons in the cat. They measured motoneuron rheobase, input resistance, and axonal conduction velocity, and motoneurons were classified on the basis of the mechanical responses of their motor units. In confirmation of previous studies, the mean Ia EPSP amplitude differed among the major medial gastrocnemius (MG) motor unit types, increasing on the average as one proceeds from fast-twitch, fast-fatiguing (FF), to fast-twitch, fatigue-resistant (FR), to slow-twitch, fatigue-resistant (S). That is FF < FR < S (see Burke, 1981).

Presynaptic inhibition of EPSPs was produced by standardized trains of conditioning volleys in the PBSt nerve (see Eccles et al., 1962b). When the magnitude of the presynaptic inhibition was expressed as percent inhibition, there was no relation between presynaptic inhibition and either motor unit type or EPSP amplitude. However, when presynaptic inhibition was expressed as absolute inhibition (in millivolts), the magnitude of the inhibition was highly correlated with EPSP amplitude, both across the entire triceps surae population (MG, lateral gastrocnemius [LG], and soleus) and within each muscle population. This correlation was also significant within the FF and FR MG motor unit population. These results suggest that EPSP amplitude, and not motor unit type, is the major determinant of the magnitude of presynaptic inhibition. However, because of the effect of motor unit type on EPSP amplitude, the net effect is that presynaptic inhibition increases in the order FF < FR < S.

PRIMARY AFFERENT DEPOLARIZATION (PAD): THE CAUSE OF PRESYNAPTIC INHIBITION

Independent evidence that conditioning volleys to sensory nerves have indeed some action on afferent fibers has been obtained by studying the changes in membrane potential of the intraspinal arborizations of the afferent fibers themselves. Initially, this was done by recording the potential changes elicited in the central ends of the dorsal roots (Barron and Matthews, 1938; Eccles and Malcolm, 1946; Lloyd and McIntyre, 1949). Stimulation of muscle and cutaneous nerves produced a slow negative potential in the dorsal roots (DRP) that was explained as the electrotonic recording of a depolarization elicited at the central terminals of the afferent fibers (Barron and Matthews, 1938). Additional support for this interpretation was provided later by showing that during the DRP the intraspinal terminals of the afferent fibers increase their excitability with a similar time course (Wall, 1958; Eccles et al. 1962b). Some examples of threshold changes of the intraspinal terminals of Ia and Ib afferent fibers produced by segmental and supraspinal conditioning volleys are illustrated in Figures 19–2H, 19–3E and H, 19–4A and C, and 19–5A to C. In addition, it has been possible to record the transmembrane potential changes from afferent fibers in the dorsal columns (Eccles et al., 1962b, 1963a; Jankowska et al., 1981c; Jiménez et al., 1988). These measurements show very clearly that afferent fibers are indeed depolarized following stimulation of sensory nerves (see Fig. 19–1E, G, and H). In most cases, stimulation of group I fibers of flexor muscles produces a small positive extracellular field that increases in size following impalement of the afferent fiber (as in Fig. 19–1E),

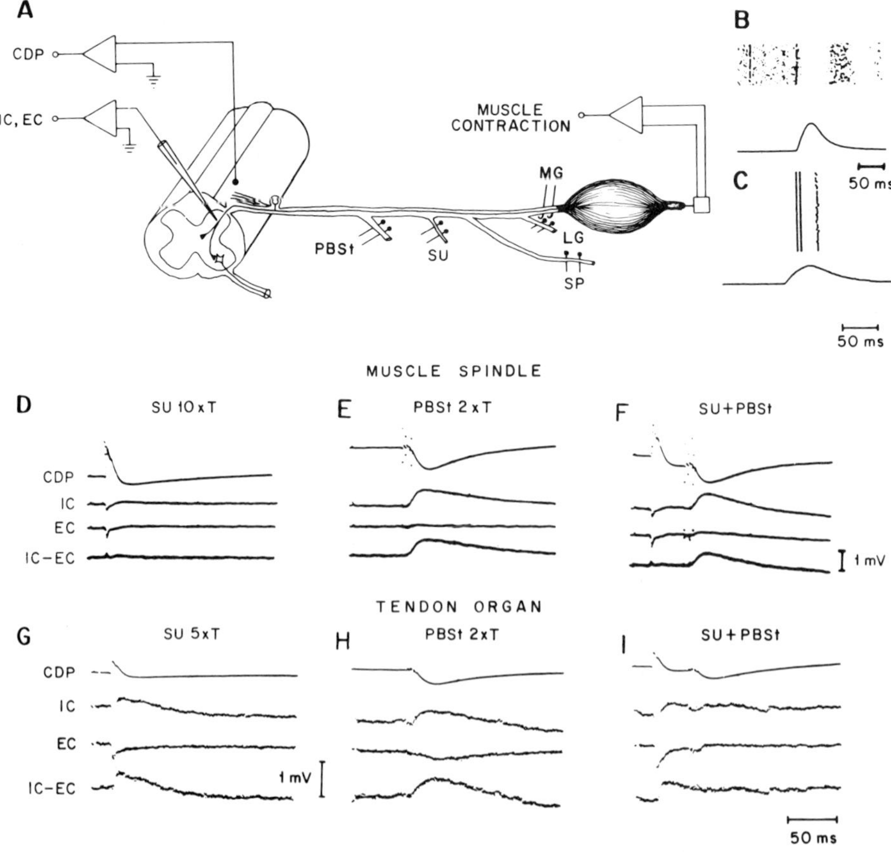

Fig. 19–1. PAD of functionally identified Ia and Ib fibers. (A) Diagram of the experimental method. All afferent nerves in the hindlimb were sectioned, except for the MG, which was left connected with the muscle. Once an afferent fiber was impaled, the muscle was stretched and the MG nerve stimulated with single pulses at 1 Hz. (B) and (C) show the dot display of the activity of two afferent fibers following electrical stimulation of the MG nerve to produce a muscle twitch (low trace). Note the silent period of the afferent discharge in (B) and the increased activity at peak tension for the fiber in (C), as expected for muscle spindles and tendon organs, respectively. (D–I) Membrane potential changes produced in two different afferent fibers following a single pulse to the SU nerve, a train of three pulses at 300 Hz to the PBSt nerve, and the combined stimulation of both (SU + PBSt) at the indicated strengths ($\times T$). Traces show, from above down, the averaged responses of the incoming volleys recorded at the cord dorsum (CDP; negativity upward), the intrafiber (IC) and extracellular (EC) recordings, the latter obtained after withdrawing the recording micropipette from the afferent fiber (positivity upward) and the transmembrane potential (IC-EC). All records are averages of 64 responses taken at 3-sec intervals. (D–F) Data taken from the fiber identified in (B) as from a muscle spindle conducting at 94 m/s. (G–I) Records taken from the fiber identified in (C) as from a tendon organ conducting at 60.2 m/s. Note in (D) that SU stimulation produced no transmembrane potential changes in the spindle afferent fiber but, as shown in (F), inhibited the PAD produced by PBSt stimulation. The tendon organ afferent was instead depolarized by stimulation of the SU nerve (G), which also inhibited the PAD produced by PBSt stimulation (I). (Modified from Jiménez et al., 1988; reproduced with permission of *Experimental Brain Research*.)

354

which means that the recordings of the PAD were made far from the terminal arborizations of the fiber where the PAD appeared to be generated. In a very few cases (Fig. 19–1H), it has been possible to impale the fiber in sites where the extracellular field is negative, that is, at sites closer to the region of active depolarization. The time course of the intracellularly recorded PAD parallels that of the DRPs and of the excitability increases produced by the same inputs (see Burke and Rudomin, 1977).

Soon after the discovery of PAD, it was suggested that this phenomenon was associated with inhibition of neuronal activity in the spinal cord, but it was not until 1962 that Eccles et al., (1962c) postulated that PAD was in fact the cause of presynaptic inhibition. At first, it seems somewhat strange that depolarization of afferent terminals leads to inhibition instead of excitation. However, it is possible that excessive depolarization blocks conduction along the intraspinal arborizations of afferent fibers, thus preventing transmitter release from the terminals (Howland et al., 1955). Eccles (1964) suggested instead that the amplitude of the action potentials conducted in the terminal arborizations of the afferent fibers is reduced during PAD, and that this produces a concomitant decrease in transmitter release. There have been other proposals to explain presynaptic inhibition. It has been suggested that PAD is generated by activation of axo-axonic GABAergic synapses of interneurons with afferent fibers (Eccles, 1961; Eccles et al., 1963a; Rudomin et al., 1981, 1983; Curtis and Lodge, 1982). In such case, the conductance increase in the intraspinal arborizations of the afferent fibers produced by GABA may prevent conduction of action potentials into the very fine terminals (see Dudel, 1963) and decrease transmitter release. Alternatively, GABA could reduce the inward calcium currents occurring during the action potential as well as transmitter release (Dunlap and Fischbach, 1981).

The experimental analysis of the mechanisms involved in the generation of PAD has been limited because, as mentioned before, the depolarization appears to occur in the intraspinal terminals of the afferent fibers, whereas impalements are usually made far away in the dorsal columns and dorsal horn, where afferent fibers are relatively coarse. Although at present it is difficult to decide which is the ultimate mechanism producing the presynaptic inhibition, it is clear that PAD is *closely* associated *with this inhibitory process* (Eccles et al., 1962b, 1962c), and the former can be used as a reliable indicator of the occurrence of the latter (however, see Peng and Frank, 1987).

THE ORIGIN OF PAD

To the extent that PAD is the cause of presynaptic inhibition, disclosure of the mechanisms involved in its generation is required to understand the nature of presynaptic inhibition. Three hypotheses have been proposed to account for PAD. The evidence supporting each of them has been discussed in detail elsewhere (Burke and Rudomin, 1977; Levy, 1977; Nicoll and Alger, 1979; Davidoff and Hackman, 1984). New information will be emphasized.

1. PAD is due to electrical fields generated by interneurons: This proposal was made more than 50 years ago (Gasser and Graham, 1933; Eccles and Malcolm, 1946; Lloyd and McIntyre, 1949). It assumes that the intraspinal fields that are recorded at the same time as the DRPs arise from current flowing in interneurons and that afferent fibers are depolarized by these currents. Electrical interaction between motoneurons and between motoneurons and afferent fibers does occur in the mammalian spinal cord, but usually it does not outlast the duration of the action potential elicited in the motoneurons (Nelson, 1969; Decima and Goldberg, 1970). There is also evidence of electrical coupling between afferent fibers and motoneurons in the frog spinal cord, where antidromic activation of motoneurons produces a short-latency depolarization in the afferent fibers lasting no more than several milliseconds, in contrast to the hundreds of milliseconds for PAD (Grinnell, 1970; Galindo and Rudomin, 1978; Shapovalov and Shiriaev, 1978; Alvarez-Leefmans et al., 1979).

Glusman and Rudomin (1974) performed a series of investigations to test whether PAD arises from current flowing in interneurons. In the frog spinal cord, PAD can be evoked by stimulation of either sensory nerves or the motoneuron axons. In both cases, PAD appears to be mediated by interneurons. The hypothesis that afferent fibers are depolarized by current flow implies that these fibers are *passive detectors* of the current flow elicited elsewhere. Glusman and Rudomin (1974) observed that no PAD-related currents were produced by ventral root stimulation after the dorsal roots were sectioned and the afferent fibers allowed to degenerate, even though antidromic invasion of motoneurons was not impaired. They conclued that PAD was not due to the electrical fields generated by interneurons, but to current generated by the depolarized afferent fibers.

2. PAD is due to extracellular accumulation of potassium ions: This proposal was made in 1938 by Barron and Matthews to explain the origin of the DRPs, but it was not until the discovery of potassium-sensitive resins that it became possible to measure the intraspinal changes in the extracellular concentration of potassium ions resulting from high-frequency stimulation of mixed nerves and of dorsal roots (Krnjevic and Morris, 1972, 1974, 1975; Somjen and Lothman, 1974; Kriz et al., 1975; Lothman and Somjen, 1975).Under these conditions, extracellular potassium increased from a baseline value of 3 mM up to 15 mM during repetitive stimulation. These changes were largest in the dorsal horn but were also of appreciable magnitude in the intermediate nucleus and in the ventral horn. Although they were significantly slower than the simultaneously recorded DRPs, it was postulated that most, if not all, of the PAD was due to potassium accumulation (Kriz et al., 1975; Vyklicky et al., 1975; see also Sykova, 1981, 1983). The slower time course of the potassium transients was explained as being due to an artificially increased diffusional space around the potassium-sensitive electrode tip.

Other investigators have proposed instead that potassium accumulation plays a minor role in the generation of PAD. Somjen and Lothman (1974) recorded from glial cells in the spinal cord of the cat and showed that their membrane potential closely paralleled the changes in extracellular potassium, whereas DRPs were always faster, and suggested that PAD was not primarily due to potassium accumulation. Equivalent findings are now available in the frog spinal cord, where it has been shown that antidromic stimulation of ventral roots, unlike stimulation of dorsal roots, produces PAD without associated changes in the membrane potential of glial cells or in extracellular potassium (Nicoll, 1979). In the cat, Bruggencate et al. (1974) have shown, in addition, that the pharmacological behavior of DRPs and potassium accumulation is not the same. DRPs produced by volleys to sensory nerves are increased by pentobarbital and reduced by picrotoxin, whereas the extracellular concentration of potassium ions is affected in the opposite direction by these drugs. The authors also showed that the DRPs produced by stimulation of group Ia fibers are inhibited by conditioning stimulation of cutaneous nerves (see also Lund et al., 1965, and Rudomin et al., 1983), even though stimulation of the latter increases the extracellular concentration of potassium.

Rudomin et al. (1981) have provided evidence to support the specificity of the PAD mechanisms, which argues to some extent against the view that presynaptic depolarization is mediated by potassium accumulation. In their experiments, stimulation of group I fibers from flexor muscles or intraspinal microstimulation (used to activate the last-order interneurons mediating the PAD; see Jankowska et al., 1981c) reduced the intraspinal threshold of group Ia fibers without affecting the threshold of vestibulospinal and rubrospinal fibers ending close to the Ia fibers in the motor and intermediate nuclei (Figs. 19–2B, C, H, and I). Repetitive stimulation of cutaneous nerves produced a small, slow reduction in the activation threshold of rubrospinal fibers (Fig. 19–2C) and of group Ia fibers ending close to each other in the intermediate nucleus but had no effects on the threshold of Ia and vestibulospinal fibers ending in the motor nucleus.

The changes in the threshold of the rubrospinal fibers produced by stimulation of cutaneous afferents (Fig. 19–2C) were initially interpreted as evidence for the existence of specific pathways depolarizing rubrospinal terminals (Rudomin and Jankowska, 1981). However, it was shown later that iontophoretic application of GABA reduces the intraspinal threshold of the group Ia fiber terminals (as expected if this were the transmitter mediating PAD; see Figure 19–2J and the later discussion), but increases the threshold of rubrospinal and vestibulo-spinal fibers (Fig. 19–2E, F; see also Curtis and Malik, 1984; Curtis, et al., 1984). In view of this, Rudomin et al. (1981) concluded that the depolarization of the rubrospinal fibers produced by cutaneous volleys was not GABAergic, but most likely due to potassium accumulated in the dorsal horn as a consequence of the repetitive stimulation of the cutaneous nerves.

Taken together, the preceding evidence suggests that in the mammalian spinal cord the PAD has a dual origin. However, the relative contributions of specific (synaptic) and nonspecific (potassium) components in the generation of PAD in identified types of afferent fibers have not been documented with detail. More recently, Jiménez et al. (1984) analyzed the possible correlation of the intraspinal threshold changes of single Ia fibers with the potassium transients produced at the *same site* by stimulation of group I muscle and cutaneous nerves. It was shown that stimulation of group I fibers from flexor muscles could depolarize group Ia fibers from extensor muscles very effectively *without*

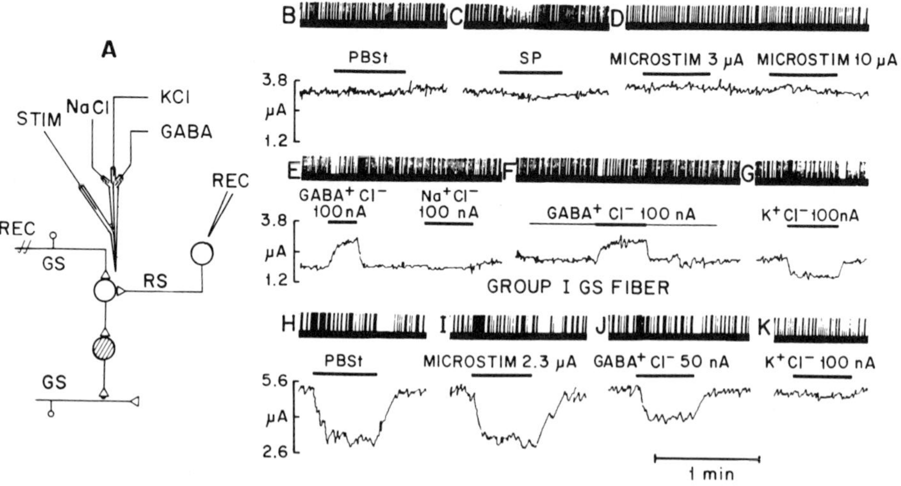

Fig. 19–2. Comparative effects of GABA, sensory nerve stimulation, and intraspinal microstimulation on the threshold of single rubrospinal and group I gastrocnemius afferent fibers. A three-barrel microelectrode array was placed in the intermediate nucleus for GABA, KCl, and NaCl iontophoresis, as indicated in (A). A single micropipette was glued to this array in order to pass current to test the threshold changes of a single rubrospinal (B–G) and a single group I GS fiber (H–K) ending in close proximity, as well as for intraspinal microstimulation. All tests were performed with the microelectrode array placed in a fixed position (2.35 mm from the cord surface). Antidromic responses of single units were recorded from the red nucleus and from the GS nerve, as indicated in (A). The low traces in B–K show the current required for antidromic activation of the fiber with a constant probability (set to 0.5). This was done automatically by means of a digital computer that generated a stimulating pulse once per second. The pulse of stimulating current was integrated, and the resulting value was maintained until the next cycle to have a continuous trace. With this method, PAD was detected as a reduction in the fiber's activation threshold. Upper traces show the window discriminator output, which generated a pulse of 5 V when there was antidromic firing and of 2 V when there was no firing. GABA was applied iontophoretically by passing current between the GABA and the NaCl electrode (indicated by the GABA⁺Cl⁻ label; reversed current is indicated by the Na⁺Cl⁻ label). Strength and duration of current flow are indicated above the current trace. In (F) the fine bar indicates additional injection of a small retaining balanced current (5 nA) passed through the GABA and NaCl electrode. Injection of K⁺Cl⁻ (100 nA) reduced the firing threshold of the rubrospinal (RS) fiber, but not that of the GS fiber. The PBSt stimulus was a train of three shocks at 300 Hz, maximal for group I, and superficial peroneus (SP), one shock two times threshold. Intraspinal microstimulation was applied through the same electrode used for threshold determination and was of three shocks at 300 Hz, 0.5 ms duration. These stimuli were applied 25 ms before the test pulse. Note that PBSt nerve stimulation and intraspinal microstimulation reduced the threshold of the group I fiber but had no effects on the threshold of the RS fiber. Note also that although GABA iontophoresis reduced the threshold on the group I fiber, it had the opposite effect on the RS fiber. (Modified from Rudomin et al., 1980, 1981; reproduced with permission of *Brain Research*.)

significantly increasing the concentration of extracellular potassium at the site of threshold testing. On the other hand, repetitive stimulation of cutaneous nerves produced a much smaller PAD in the same Ia fiber, even though the potassium transients were severalfold larger (Fig. 19–3). These observations suggested that extracellular accumulation of potassium plays a secondary role in the generation of the PAD of Ia fibers produced by stimulation of group I fibers from flexor nerves. Similar results have been obtained with cutaneous fibers (Jiménez et al. 1987), where it has been shown that low-intensity, low-frequency trains applied to cutaneous nerves, and particularly to the red nucleus and brain stem reticular formation, may produce PAD of single cutaneous fibers without significant accumulation of potassium ions at the site of termination of these fibers in the dorsal horn.

The functional role of the potassium-induced depolarization remains to be elucidated. One possibility is that the extracellular concentration of this ion is related to the overall level of interneuronal activity in a given spinal cord region and acts as a triggering signal for other functionally relevant processes such as the release of endorphins, peptides, and/or neuromodulators (Jessel and Iver-

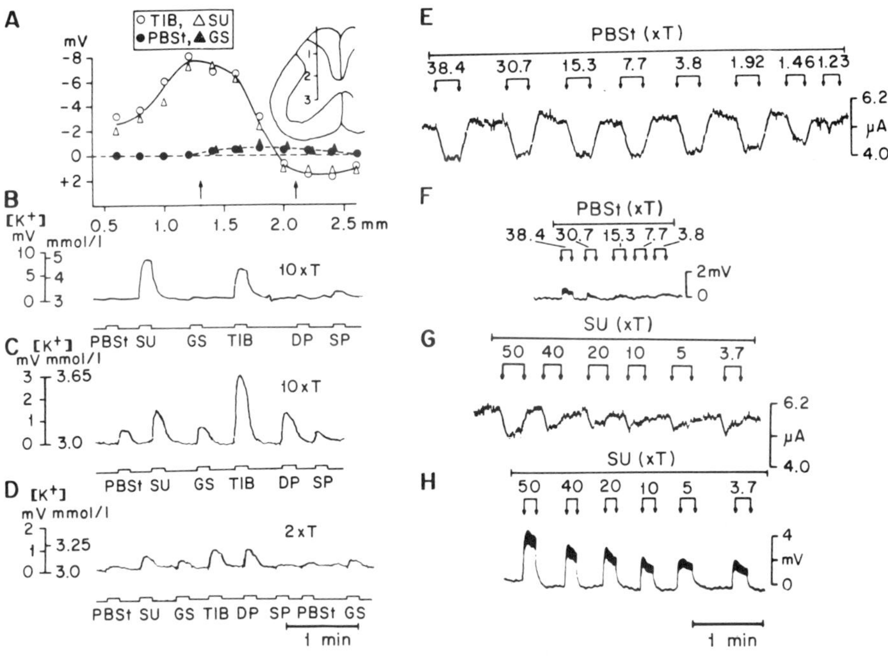

Fig. 19–3. Lack of correlation between potassium transients and PAD of group Ia gastrocnemius fibers in the spinal cord. (A) Peak amplitude distribution within the spinal cord of postsynaptic focal potentials produced by single shock (2 × T) stimulation of various sensory nerves, as indicated. Insert shows the electrode track within the spinal cord. (B–D) Changes in the concentration of extracellular potassium ([K⁺]) produced by 100-Hz trains to several hindlimb nerves with 10 × T and 2 × T strengths. Records in (B) were obtained at a depth of 1.3 mm, and records in (C) and (D) at 2.1 mm, as indicated by the arrows in (A). Note that largest increases in [K⁺] were obtained following stimulation of cutaneous (SU and SP) and mixed nerves (tibialis posterior, TIB) as compared with muscle nerves (PBSt, GS, and deep peroneus, DP), even when the recording electrode was within the intermediate nucleus and the stimulus strength was of 2 × T. (E–H) Threshold changes of a single Ia GS fiber and associated negative DC shifts produced by graded stimulation of the PBSt and SU nerve. (E, G) Records of intraspinal current required to maintain constant antidromic firing. (F, H) Records of negative DC shifts made at the same site as that of threshold testing (2.1-mm depth). Stimuli were trains of 100 Hz at indicated strengths. Note that stimulation of the PBSt nerve with a strength as low as 1.92 × T reduced the threshold of the fiber almost maximally without producing significant negative DC shifts (which are proportional to the potassium signal), whereas stimulation of the SU nerve produced large negative DC shifts but a much smaller threshold reduction. (Modified from Jiménez et al., 1983, 1984; reproduced with permission of *Brain Research* and the *Journal of Neurophysiology*.)

sen, 1977; Hajek and Sykova, 1981), which in turn may affect synaptic transmission in a more enduring manner. Alternatively, as in the retina (Pentreath and Kai-Kai, 1982), potassium accumulation could be a signal that modifies the metabolism of glia and neurons in order to keep up with increased neuronal activity.

3. *The axo-axonic hypothesis:* The possibility that PAD arises from activation of interneurons making axo-axonic, presumably GABAergic, synapses with afferent fibers was proposed for the first time by Eccles in 1961 (see also Eccles et al., 1963c). Considerable pharmacological work has since been carried out to test this hypothesis. This work has been extensively reviewed (Burke and Rudomin, 1977; Levy, 1977; Nicoll and Alger, 1979; Davidoff and Hackman, 1984) and will only be summarized here. Muscle and cutaneous afferent fibers are depolarized by iontophoretic application of GABA (as in Fig. 19–2J), and this effect is antagonized by picrotoxin and bicuculline (Gmelin, 1976, 1978; Rudomin et al., 1981; Curtis and Lodge, 1982; Curtis et al., 1982, 1984; Gmelin and Zimmermann, 1984), suggesting the existence of GABA-type A receptors in the terminals of the afferent fibers. Semicarbazide-induced depletion of GABA reduces DRPs and the long-lasting inhibition of monosynaptic reflexes attributed to presynaptic inhibition (Banna and Jabbur, 1971; Bell and Anderson, 1972). In the frog spinal cord, inhibitors of GABA transaminase, a major degradative enzyme for GABA, increase the DRPs and the associated excitability increases of afferent terminals, as well as the concentration of GABA within the cord (Davidoff et al., 1973). Determinations of GABA in the spinal cord have shown that this amino acid is found in higher concentrations in the dorsal part of the dorsal horn than in the ventral horn (Ljungdahl and Hokfelt, 1973; Miyata and Otsuka, 1972), the location of presumed synapses generating PAD in cutaneous afferents (Jankowska et al., 1981c; see also Rethelyi, 1984a; Ribeiro da Silva and Coimbra, 1980).

Since it has not been possible to impale the fine terminals of the afferent fibers, where PAD is generated (Eccles et al., 1963c), many studies have been done to analyze the action of GABA on spinal ganglion cells, assuming that the changes seen there also occur in the intraspinal arborizations of these neurons. GABA has been shown to produce depolarization (De Groat, 1972; De Groat et al., 1972; Deschenes et al., 1976; Desarmenien et al., 1984a, 1984b), mostly by increasing the conductance to chloride ions (Gallagher et al., 1978; Gallagher and Shinnick-Gallagher, 1983), which in the frog appear to be more concentrated inside than outside of the fiber because of the existence of an inward chloride pump (Alvarez-Leefmans et al., 1988). Also, it is now known that GABA may block the inward calcium currents activated during the action potential via activation of $GABA_B$ receptors, and it has been suggested that this action, rather than the depolarization per se, accounts for the inhibition of transmitter release (Dunlap and Fischbach, 1981; Peng and Frank, 1987).

Whereas electrophysiological and pharmacological evidence supporting the role of GABA in PAD is very suggestive, ultrastructural evidence documenting the existence of axo-axonic synapses of GABAergic interneurons with *functionally identified* afferent fibers is still scarce (see the reviews by Rethelyi, 1984a, 1984b). Following Eccles' proposal in 1961, Gray (1962) described axo-axonic synapses in the dorsal horn, but the identity of the involved neuronal elements and of the target afferent fibers was not established. Similarly, Conradi (1969) described P boutons presynaptic to M boutons synapsing with motoneurons that were assumed to be from Ia fibers, but this was not proven. McLaughlin et al. (1975) and Barber et al. (1978) used immunohistochemical labeling of glutamic acid decarboxylase (GAD), the enzyme mediating the synthesis of GABA from glutamic acid, and demonstrated in the rat the existence of small axon terminals containing GAD that make axo-axonic contacts with afferent boutons of unknown origin.

Studies made with functionally identified cutaneous afferent fibers have indicated that horseradish peroxidase (HRP)-labeled G-2 hair follicle afferent fibers (Ralston, 1981), as well as type I slowly adapting mechanoreceptors and Pacinian corpuscle afferent fibers in cat lamina IV (Egger et al., 1981), receive axo-axonic synapses from ovoid vesicle-containing axon endings. Similar findings have been reported with D hair follicle receptors in lamina III (Rethelyi et al., 1982). In the intermediate nucleus terminal boutons of Ia muscle, spindle afferent fibers in lamina VI synapse with somata and large dendritic shafts. They frequently receive axo-axonic contacts from small axon terminals containing flattened synaptic vescicles (Maxwell and Bannatyne, 1983). In the motor nucleus, Fyffe and Light (1984) have shown axo-axonic contacts of interneurons with identified Ia afferent fibers. According to these investigators, some of the P boutons also made synapses with motoneurons, suggesting the existence of common interneurons mediating pre- and postsynaptic inhibition (see the later discussion). Ia fiber terminals in Clarke's column are also subjected to PAD (Jankowska and Padel, 1984), and it has been shown that they receive axo-axonic synapses from interneurons (Rethelyi, 1970; Conradi et al., 1983; Walmsley et al., 1987).

The use of GABA antibodies has revealed the presence of GABAergic terminals in the spinal cord, many in contact with motoneuron proximal dendrites (Holstege and Nuñez-Cardozo, 1987). Some of these axons also make axo-axonic synapses onto the central terminals of synaptic glomeruli (De la Roza et al., 1987). However, further work seems necessary to establish the existence of axo-axonic synapses with specific types of target afferent fibers and motoneurons. This requires electrophysiological identification of the neurons producing PAD (see the later discussion).

Demonstration of axo-axonic synapses on afferent fibers is a necessary but not a sufficient condition to prove that they do in fact mediate PAD. It is also important to show that fibers *not subjected* to presynaptic control mechanisms of the type of PAD are *devoid* of axo-axonic synapses on their intraspinal terminations. In the frog spinal cord, Glusman and Rudomin (1974) have shown that fibers descending in the dorsolateral column that make monosynaptic connections with motoneurons are not depolarized following repetitive stimulation of dorsal roots. Ultrastructural studies on spinal cords hemisected at the level of the brachial plexus have shown, in addition, that synaptic boutons from (degenerated) descending fibers contact lumbar motoneurons in areas largely devoid of nearby boutons (Glusman et al., 1976). In the cat, rubrospinal axons are not depolarized by stimulation of group I flexor fibers (Rudomin et al.,

1981; Curtis and Malik, 1984). The terminal arborizations of these fibers have also failed to exhibit axo-axonic synapses both in the cat (Kostyuk and Skibo, 1975; Hanaway and Smith, 1978; Shinoda et al., 1982) and in the opossum (Goode and Sreesai, 1978).

NEURONAL PATHWAYS MEDIATING THE PAD OF GROUP I FIBERS

Since the discovery of the dorsal root potentials, there has been great interest in defining the types of afferent fibers involved in their generation. In some muscle nerves, such as the PBSt, group Ia and group Ib fibers have different electrical thresholds and conduction velocities, and it has been possible, by means of graded stimulation, to activate the group Ia fibers selectively or to stimulate the whole range of group I fibers (see Fig. 19–5E; Bradley and Eccles, 1953; Eccles et al., 1962b, 1963a). By using this procedure, it has become clear that, although Ia fibers produce DRPs, group Ib and cutaneous fibers are more effective (Eccles et al., 1962b, 1963a). DRPs have also been obtained by stimulation of the red nucleus (Hongo et al., 1972), vestibular nucleus (Cook et al., 1969), bulbar reticular formation (Carpenter et al., 1963; Lundberg and Vyklicky, 1966), motor cortex (Lundberg, 1964) and raphe nuclei (Proudfit et al., 1980).

Interactions between DRPs of various origins have been used to derive information pertaining to the organization of the neuronal pathways mediating PAD. In a recent study, Brink et al. (1984) analyzed the interactions between the DRPs elicited by activation of afferent fibers of various origins. They found spatial facilitation when testing interaction between DRPs produced by stimulation of Ia afferents, whether from flexors or extensors; from Ib afferents, whether from flexors or extensors; and from flexor Ib and extensor Ia afferents. However, they found no indications of common pathways from extensor Ib and any Ia afferents under conditions that proved effective in other combinations. These studies led to the suggestion that some neuronal pathways are used to modulate transmission via Ia afferents independently of their muscle origin, and that the same may hold true for extensor and flexor Ib afferents. Brink et al. also concluded that the minimal number of distinct neuronal populations subserving PAD of group I afferents may vary from two to six.

Studies on the intraspinal threshold changes of afferent fibers have provided direct information on the target afferent fibers subjected to PAD. Although there is a considerable overlap in the threshold and conduction velocities of group Ia and Ib fibers (Bradley and Eccles, 1953; Coppin et al., 1969), it is now fairly well established that stimulation of group Ia and particularly group Ib fibers produces PAD in group Ia fibers of both flexors and extensors (see Fig. 19–4A and 19–5A; see also Eccles et al., 1962b; Rudomin et al., 1981, 1983). Cutaneous volleys do not appear to produce PAD in group Ia fibers under normal circumstances, but in the lightly anesthetized or decerebrate cat they may increase the threshold of group Ia fibers for antidromic activation, probably because of inhibition exerted on the interneurons mediating the PAD,

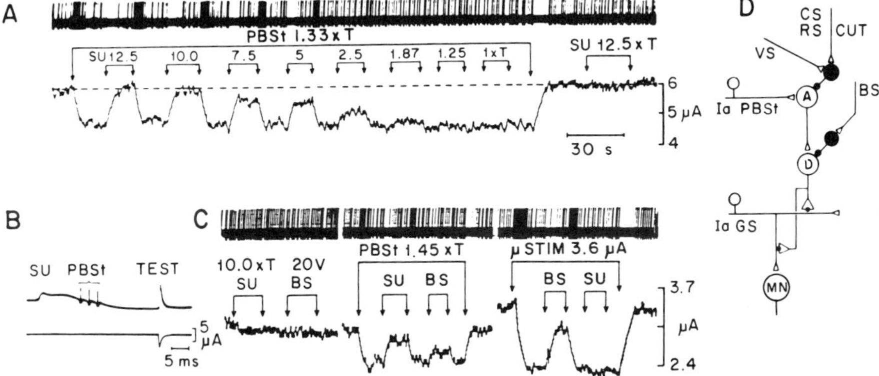

Fig. 19–4. Sites of action of segmental and supraspinal inputs on the pathways mediating the PAD of Ia fibers. The upper trace in (A) and (C) shows the penwriter recording of the window discriminator output following the occurrence of the antidromic spike of a single Ia afferent fiber, and the lower trace gives the theshold current necessary to maintain constant firing. (A) The SU-induced inhibition of the PAD of Ia fibers. A conditioning train was given once per second to the PBSt nerve (three pulses at 280 Hz applied 23 ms before the test pulse). This reduced the threshold of the Ia fiber, which was maintained low throughout the whole period of PBSt stimulation, as indicated. Conditioning stimulation of SU nerve [see (B) for pulse timing] reversed the effects produced by PBSt stimulation. The amount of inhibition varied with the strength of the SU stimulus. (C) Data from another Ia fiber taken from a preparation with the contralateral spinal cord hemisected at the thoracic level. SU and brain stem (BS) stimulation had no effect on the resting threshold of the fiber but were able to reverse the effects produced by a conditioning train to the PBSt nerve. Intraspinal microstimulation (μstim) also reduced the threshold of the fiber; this effect was reversed by BS but not by SU stimulation. PBSt stimulation was a train at 400 Hz applied 33 ms before the test pulse. The SU stimulus was a single pulse and the BS stimulus a train of eight pulses at 600 Hz, both applied 53 ms before the excitability testing pulse at the indicated strengths. The BS stimulating electrode was placed 3 mm rostral to the obex, 2 mm lateral at a depth of 5.5 mm depth. The intraspinal microstimulation was one pulse of 3.6 μA, applied 3.3 ms before the test pulse to produce a monosynaptic PAD. (D) The sites of action of segmental and descending inputs along the pathway mediating the PAD derived from all observations. Excitatory synapses are indicated by open triangles, inhibitory synapses by filled triangles, and axo-axonic synapses by triangles and a dot. CUT, cutaneous fibers; CS, corticospinal fibers; MN, motoneurons; RS, rubrospinal fibers; BS, reticulospinal fibers; VS, vestibulospinal fibers. (Modified from Rudomin et al., 1983; reproduced with permission of the *Journal of Neurophysiology*.)

since they also inhibit the PAD elicited by group I flexors (Figs. 19–4A and 19–5A; see Lund et al., 1965; Rudomin et al., 1974, 1983, 1986). Inhibition of the PAD of group Ia fibers is also produced following stimulation of the red nucleus (Hongo et al., 1972), brain stem reticular formation (Figs. 19–4C and 19–5A), and pyramidal tract (Rudomin et al., 1983, 1986). However, stimulation of the vestibular nucleus produces PAD of Ia fibers (Cook et al., 1969; Rudomin et al., 1986).

Until recently, it was accepted that group Ib fibers had a PAD pattern different from that documented for Ia fibers, since they appeared to be depolarized by group Ib and by cutaneous fibers (Fig. 19–5B; see also Eccles et al., 1963a; Rudomin et al., 1983; Brink et al., 1984), as well as by rubrospinal (Fig. 19–4E), corticospinal, reticulospinal (Fig. 19–5B), and vestibulospinal fibers (Fig. 19–5B and Lundberg, 1964; Rudomin et al., 1983). However,

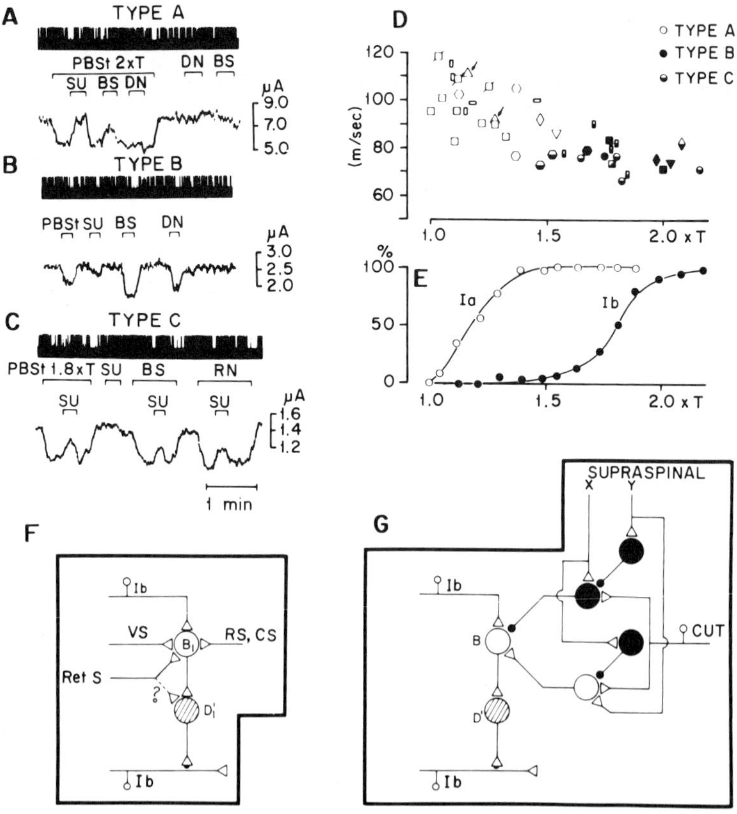

Fig. 19–5. Patterns of PAD in group I fibers. The threshold changes of the intraspinal terminals of group I PBSt afferent fibers produced during stimulation of sensory nerves and supraspinal nuclei can be grouped in three different types, as illustrated in (A), (B), and (C). In type A fibers, SU and BS stimulation produce no changes in the resting threshold of the fiber but are nevertheless able to reduce the PAD produced by stimulation of group I flexors. Stimulation of Deiter's nucleus (DN) produces PAD in some fibers. Type B fibers show PAD produced by both SU and supraspinal stimulation. Type C fibers are depolarized both by PBSt and by supraspinal but not SU stimulation, which instead inhibits the PAD elicited both by group I flexor and by RN and BS stimulation. (D) Peripheral threshold versus conduction velocity of single group I fibers. The peripheral threshold was determined in each case by colliding the antidromic spike with an orthodromic volley elicited in the same nerve. Open symbols indicate fibers with a type A PAD pattern; filled and half-filled symbols, fibers with type B and C PAD patterns, respectively. Each symbol denotes fibers tested in the same experiment. Squares are from fibers tested in the same experiment used to construct graph (E), which gives the relative amplitudes of the Ia and Ib components of the afferent volley produced by graded stimulation of the PBSt nerve. The abcissa in (D) and (E) gives the stimulus strength relative to that of the most excitable fibers in the nerve. Note that in this particular case, stimuli of $1.4 \times T$ strength already produced maximal Ia volleys. The threshold for the Ib volley was between 1.4 and $1.5 \times T$; maximal values were obtained with stimuli of about $2.2 \times T$. (F) Diagram showing the possible sites of action of supraspinal inputs on the interneurons mediating the PAD of Ib fibers. In this diagram, reticulospinal fibers are shown to have excitatory connections with first-order interneurons because in some Ib fibers (type C) the PAD produced by them is inhibited by cutaneous stimulation. However, with available information, it cannot be excluded that reticulospinal fibers also have connections with last-order interneurons. (G) The neuronal arrangement that explains the dual action of cutaneous inputs on the PAD of group Ib fibers. Facilitation or inhibition of the PAD by cutaneous volleys depends on the relative balance in the activity of supraspinal fibers (x and y) with reciprocal connections on spinal interneurons. CUT, cutaneous fibers; CS, corticospinal; RS, rubrospinal; VS, vestibulospinal; RetS, reticulospinal fibers. (Modified from Rudomin et al., 1986; reproduced with permission of the *Journal of Neurophysiology*.)

Rudomin et al. (1983) found a set of group I gastrocnemius fibers in which the PAD induced by group I volleys in flexors was inhibited by cutaneous volleys, whereas brain stem stimulation produced PAD (Fig. 19–5C). Initially, it was assumed that these were Ia fibers and that brain stem stimulation coactivated descending fibers with excitatory connections on the PAD-mediating pathways (e.g., vestibulospinal). A more detailed investigation of the threshold changes produced in single PBSt nerve fibers suggested instead that fibers with this "mixed" PAD pattern were not Ia but most likely Ib (see Fig. 19–5D and 19–5E and Rudomin et al., 1986). Recording of the transmembrane potential changes produced in afferent fibers following stimulation of sensory nerves has in general confirmed the results obtained from the analysis of the intraspinal threshold changes of single group I fibers (Eccles et al., 1962b, 1963a; Brink et al., 1984).

Intrafiber recordings made from afferents left in continuity with the MG muscle allow functional identification of the fibers as being from either muscle spindles or tendon organs, according to their responses to muscle stretch and contraction (see Figs. 19–1A, 19–1B, and 19–1C). With this approach, it has been possible to establish that in some Ib fibers cutaneous volleys produce no PAD, but are nevertheless able to inhibit the PAD generated either by activation of group I fibers or by stimulation of the red nucleus (Jiménez et al., 1988). Since rubrospinal terminals are not subjected to presynaptic control (Rudomin et al., 1981; Curtis and Malik, 1984), it can be concluded that cutaneous volleys also inhibit transmission along the pathways mediating the PAD of some Ib fibers. At present, it is not clear if the excitatory and inhibitory actions of cutaneous fibers on the pathways mediating the PAD of Ib fibers are exerted on the same or on different fibers. In the latter case, expression of excitatory or inhibitory actions may depend on the balance of descending inputs acting at the segmental level, as illustrated in Fig. 19–5G (see Rudomin et al., 1986, for further discussion).

SITES OF ACTION OF SEGMENTAL AND DESCENDING INPUTS ON THE PAD PATHWAYS

Disclosure of the sites of action of segmental and descending inputs on the segmental pathways producing the PAD is important in order to understand the functional role that presynaptic inhibition may play in motor performance, as well as for the proper identification of the interneurons mediating the PAD. Recent estimates of the shortest latency of the PAD produced by intraspinal microstimulation (Jankowska et al., 1981c) have given values as short as 0.6 to 0.8 ms, consistent with a monosynaptic delay, as expected if this procedure were to activate the last-order interneurons mediating the PAD. Since the shortest latency of the PAD produced by stimulation of group I fibers was found to vary between 1.7 and 2.0 ms, it was concluded that the shortest pathways had at least two interposed interneurons. Rudomin et al. (1983) showed, in addition, that stimulation of cutaneous afferents may inhibit the PAD of GS Ia fibers produced by group Ia flexors without affecting the monosynaptic PAD produced in the same fibers by intraspinal microstimulation, whereas brain stem stimulation may inhibit the PAD produced by both procedures (Fig. 19–4C). These observations suggested to them that cutaneous and reticulospinal inhibitory inputs were acting *at different sites* along the pathways mediating the PAD of Ia fibers. Since cutaneous inputs do not appear to depolarize Ia fibers (Figs. 19–1D and 19–4A; see Lund et al., 1965; Rudomin et al., 1983), it was concluded that they inhibit transmission at the level of the first-order interneurons in the PAD pathway. The reticulospinal fibers would instead inhibit the second (last)-order interneurons in the same pathway, as indicated in Fig. 19–4D (see also Rudomin et al., 1983). Using similar tests, it has been established that rubrospinal and corticospinal fibers exert their inhibitory actions on the first-order interneurons mediating the PAD of the Ia fibers. Vestibulospinal fibers have instead excitatory actions that are exerted on the first-order interneurons, as shown in Fig. 19–4D (see Rudomin et al., 1986).

The situation with Ib afferent fibers is completely different. All of them appear to be depolarized by rubrospinal, reticulospinal, corticospinal, and vestibulospinal fibers (see Figs. 19–5B and 19–5C; see also Rudomin et al., 1986). The PAD produced by these inputs, as well as the PAD that cutaneous nerves produce in a fraction of Ib fibers (Rudomin et al., 1986) has been shown to add linearly or to occlude with the monosynaptic PAD produced by intraspinal stimulation, as expected if both procedures activated common sets of interneurons, as indicated in Fig. 19–1F (see Rudomin et al., 1983). The simplest way to explain the preceding findings has been to assume that *different last-order interneurons* mediate the PAD of Ia and Ib fibers. It thus appears that the relative balance of the Ia versus the Ib input reaching the spinal cord may be controlled presynaptically by the central nervous system. Some of the functional consequences of such a differential control of presynaptic inhibition are discussed at the end of this chapter.

IDENTIFICATION OF THE INTERNEURONS MEDIATING THE PAD OF GROUP I AFFERENT FIBERS

More than 25 years ago, Eccles et al. (1962a) recorded the activity of some spinal interneurons that they assumed were mediating the PAD of group I fibers. These interneurons responded with monosynaptic latencies to stimulation of group I muscle afferents and were assumed to be first-order cells in the PAD pathways. Eccles et al. also postulated that last-order cells in these pathways made synaptic contacts with the central terminals of Ia fibers in the motor nucleus, and probably also with Ib and cutaneous afferents and with other flexor reflex afferents. Later, Lucas and Willis (1974) found interneurons in the intermediate nucleus activated primarily by group Ib fibers and suggested that some of them could participate in the Ib-mediated presynaptic inhibition. Subsequent studies of Jankowska et al. (1981b), Brink et al. (1983), and Harrison and Jankowska (1985a, 1985b) indicated that many of the Ib-activated interneurons in the intermediate nucleus mediate nonreciprocal inhibition of motoneurons. However, it was not clear whether these interneurons mediated only postsynaptic inhibitory actions on motoneurons or whether they were also shared by pathways producing presynaptic inhibition of afferent fibers.

Studies on the PAD patterns of identified muscle afferents have provided valuable information on the activation patterns expected for the interneurons mediating the PAD of Ia and Ib fibers. However, finding interneurons with these response patterns is not sufficient evidence to ensure that they do in fact mediate the PAD. It is also necessary to show they have the proper connections with the target afferent fibers. Using the spike-triggered averaging techniques developed by Mendell and Henneman (1971), Solodkin et al. (1984) and Rudomin et al. (1987) have investigated the possible connections of single interneurons in the intermediate nucleus with motoneurons and afferent fibers (Fig. 19–6A). Sucrose gap recordings of ventral root potentials have been used as indicators of membrane potential changes occurring in populations of motoneurons (see Fig. 19–6B, 19–6C, and Lüscher et al., 1979; Brink et al., 1983) and dorsal root potentials as indicators of PAD (Eccles et al., 1963a). With this approach, Rudomin et al. (1987) have documented the existence of five different functional groups of intermediate nucleus interneurons responding to group I and/or group II muscle afferents and to relatively low-threshold (<2.5 xT) cutaneous afferents, which can be grouped into two broad classes, depending on their connections with afferent fibers and motoneurons.

The first class of interneurons (types A and B) was antidromically activated from the Clarke's column. Their action potentials were time-locked with inhibitory potentials in the ventral roots (iVRPs) without associated DRPs (Fig. 19–6D). The onset latencies of the iVRPs associated with activity of these interneurons varied between 1.7 and 3.1 ms, and it was assumed that the iVRPs with the shortest latencies were produced by the activation of interneurons with direct inhibitory connections with motoneurons. These interneurons could therefore be the same last-order interneurons assumed by Jankowska and collaborators to mediate the nonreciprocal postsynaptic inhibition of motoneurons (Jankowska et al., 1981b; Harrison and Jankowska, 1985a, 1985b).

The second class of interneurons (types C, D, and E) was not antidromically activated from the Clarke's column. Their action potentials were time-locked with iVRPs, as well as with negative dorsal root potentials (nDRPs; see Fig. 19–6E), both with similar onset latencies varying between 1.7 and 6.1 ms. The interneurons whose activity was associated with the shortest-latency iVRPs and nDRPs were assumed to be common last-order interneurons mediating PAD as well as postsynaptic inhibition of motoneurons. Since these interneurons responded both to group I muscle and to intermediate-threshold cutaneous afferents, it seems very likely that they mediated the PAD of group Ib fibers (Fig. 19–6F).

In this second class, there were a couple of interneurons that responded to group I muscle but not to cutaneous afferents (type E). These neurons were initially considered as interposed in the pathways mediating the PAD of group Ia fibers and postsynaptic inhibition of motoneurons (Solodkin et al., 1984). However, in view of the recent finding that stimulation of cutaneous nerves

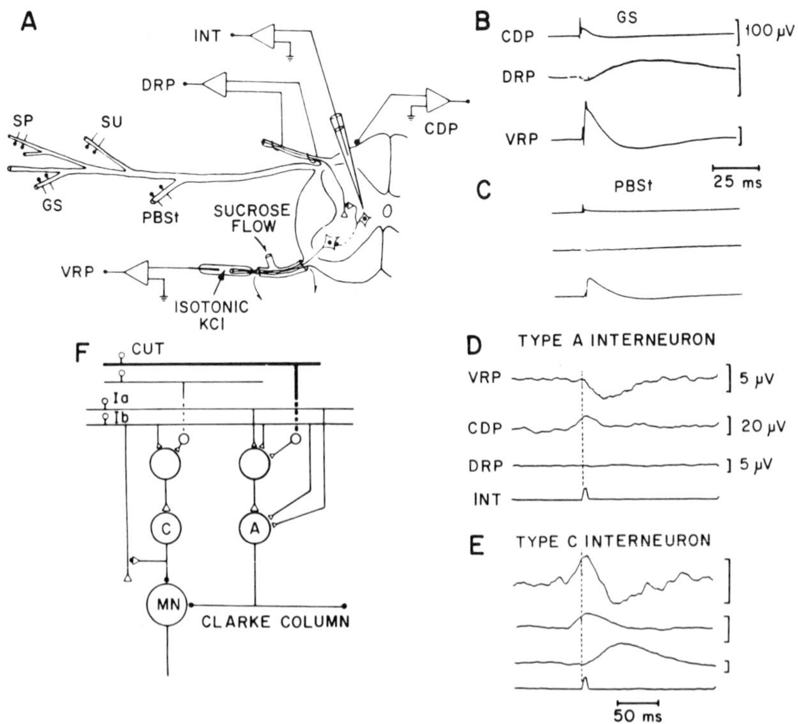

Fig. 19–6. Synaptic actions of intermediate nucleus interneurons on afferent fibers and motoneurons. Diagram of the experimental method. Interneuronal activity was extracellularly recorded by means of a glass micropipette filled with sodium glutamate (to increase interneuronal activity) introduced into the intermediate nucleus region of the spinal cord (INT). Potentials were simultaneously recorded from the cord dorsum (CDP), dorsal roots (DRP), and ventral roots (VRP), the latter by means of the sucrose gap technique. Dorsal and ventral root potentials are electrotonic recordings of synaptic potentials generated in afferent fibers and motoneurons, respectively. (B) and (C) show the averaged responses ($n = 64$ at 1 Hz) produced by electrical stimulation of the GS and PBSt nerves with single shocks of 2.0 and $1.5 \times T$ strength, respectively. Note that stimulation of the GS nerve produced a slow negativity in the dorsal root (DRP) and an EPSP with superposed spikes followed by a IPSP in the ventral root. With this intensity, PBSt nerve stimulation produced only a monosynaptic EPSP in the ventral root, but stimuli of 2 $\times T$ strength produced large DRPs. (D) and (E) show the averaged potentials obtained when using the "spontaneous" spike potentials of the interneuron to trigger the averager. Pretrigger facilities allow examination of time-locked events occurring before the interneuronal (reference) spike. The lowest trace shows the window discriminator pulse produced by the interneuron action potentials, whose onset time is indicated by the vertical lines. Averages were derived from 400 and 512 events, respectively. (D) shows that the activity of a type A interneuron was time-locked to inhibitory potentials in the ventral root (VRP) but not to DRPs. (E) Activity of a type C interneuron associated with negative DRPs as well as with inhibitory VRPs, the latter preceded by a slow EPSP. Note in (D) and (E) the appearance of a slow negativity in the cord dorsum associated with the interneuronal activation. The slow EPSP preceding the IPSP has been interpreted as being due to the activation of interneurons, with common inputs to the reference interneuron and to the motoneuron (see Rudomin et al., 1987, for further discussion). (F) Diagram of the possible connections of type A and type C interneurons. MN, motoneurons. Dotted lines are pathways that may have interposed interneurons. For cutaneous afferents, thick lines represent the lowest-threshold fibers. (Modified from Rudomin et al., 1987; reproduced with permission of the *Journal of Neurophysiology*.)

may also inhibit the PAD in a fraction of group Ib fibers (Figs. 19–5C and 19–5D; see Rudomin et al., 1986; Jiménez et al., 1988), these interneurons could instead have mediated the PAD of Ib fibers. Nevertheless, it should be pointed out that, quite recently, Fyffe and Light (1984) have seen in the spinal cord P boutons synapsing with terminal boutons of Ia fibers as well as with motoneuron dendrites, so it is not unlikely that last-order interneurons mediating PAD of Ia fibers will also be found to have direct inhibitory connections with motoneurons. Some of the implications of finding common interneurons mediating pre- and postsynaptic inhibition are considered in the next section.

SOME FUNCTIONAL IMPLICATIONS

Considering the information presented in previous sections, it seems now fairly well established that the synaptic effectiveness of muscle and cutaneous afferents can be controlled by specific sets of interneurons making axo-axonic synapses with the afferent fiber terminals in the spinal cord. This presynaptic control has been conceived by most investigators as a powerful mechanism of inhibition of synaptic transmission (Eccles et al., 1962c; Eccles, 1964; Schmidt, 1971). However, it must be pointed out that presynaptic inhibition, like postsynaptic excitatory and inhibitory actions, has no unique functional role. These are basic control mechanisms, and their relative potency and functional role will depend on the particular neuronal circuits in which they are utilized.

In the cutaneous fiber system, PAD seems to be modality specific, and it has been suggested that it increases spatial discrimination and limits surplus excitation (Janig et al., 1968a, 1968b; Schmidt, 1971). PAD of muscle afferents does not appear to be organized as a feedback system since (1) Ia fiber terminals are presynaptically depolarized by other Ia and also by Ib fibers Eccles et al., 1962b, 1963a; Rudomin et al., 1983; Brink et al., 1984); (2) Ib fibers are depolarized mostly by other Ib fibers (Eccles et al., 1963a; Brink et al., 1984); and (3) cutaneous inputs inhibit the PAD of Ia fibers (Lund et al., 1965; Rudomin et al., 1974, 1986; Jiménez et al., 1988) and have a dual action on the PAD of Ib fibers (Rudomin et al., 1986; Jiménez et al., 1988). Nevertheless, it is extremely interesting that reticulospinal, rubrospinal, and corticospinal fibers do have *opposing actions* on Ia and Ib fibers: They inhibit the PAD of Ia fibers and produce PAD in Ib fibers (Rudomin et al., 1986; Jiménez et al., 1988). This feature, together with the finding that different last-order interneurons possibly mediate the PAD of Ia and Ib fibers (Rudomin et al., 1983), could be the basis of a control mechanism used to emphasize information arising either from the muscle spindles or from the tendon organs, and thus have the system working under position-feedback or tension-feedback conditions. This selectivity would be very difficult to achieve by means of postsynaptic control mechanisms because Ia and Ib inputs have extensive convergence onto second-order interneurons (Czarkowska et al., 1981; Jankowska et al., 1981a).

The possibility that some last-order interneurons are common to pathways mediating pre- and postsynaptic inhibition (Solodkin et al., 1984; Rudomin et al., 1987) indicates that these two inhibitory control mechanisms are not mutually exclusive, as implied by previous investigations, and fully explains the strychnine-resistant, picrotoxin-sensitive postsynaptic inhibition described by Kellerth and Szumski (1966a, 1966b). This does not mean, of course, that there are no private pathways for presynaptic inhibition of Ia or Ib fibers, but this issue remains open for future investigations.

It might appear redundant that presynaptic inhibition of Ia and Ib fibers occurs together with postsynaptic inhibition of motoneurons, particularly in the case of Ia fibers. However, it should be recalled that the interneurons mediating pre- and postsynaptic inhibition are premotor inhibitory interneurons in their own right, primarily involved in the execution of descending motor commands (Fig. 19–6F). Several investigators have shown that descending fiber systems such as the rubrospinal and the vestibulospinal (and probably others as well) are able to control the synaptic efficacy of the intraspinal terminals of afferent fibers (see Lundberg, 1964; Rudomin et al., 1983, 1986), although they themselves are not subjected to presynaptic control mechanisms (Eide et al., 1968; Rudomin et al., 1975b, 1981; Curtis and Malik, 1984; Curtis et al., 1984). Therefore, these descending commands will have a "priority status" compared with afferent inputs. Once a descending command is started (for example, during the initiation of ballistic and/or goal-oriented movements), some motoneurons will be excited and others will be inhibited. Whenever the inhibition is mediated via the common interneurons mediating PAD and postsynaptic inhibition, the synaptic efficacy of the afferent inputs will be reduced at the time of the descending postsynaptic inhibition, thus preventing sensory information from interfering with the descending motor commands. On the other hand, whenever the inhibition is produced by interneurons mediating the nonreciprocal inhibition (Jankowska et al., 1981b; Brink et al., 1983; Harrison and Jankowska, 1985a, 1985b), the sensory information is not prevented from reaching the spinal cord, since these interneurons have no connections with the pathways producing PAD (Rudomin et al., 1987).

At present, information on the discharge patterns of the various types of spinal interneurons during performance of specific motor tasks is not available. This is clearly necessary to understand the role played by the various classes of interneurons in sensorimotor integration. In this context, the observations recently made by Hultborn et al. (1987a, 1987b) are very encouraging. These authors have developed a method that allows indirect estimation of the amount of presynaptic inhibition present in the Ia fibers making monosynaptic connections with motoneurons, and they have used this method to explore in humans the changes in the effectiveness of Ia fibers during the voluntary activation of specific sets of muscles. Their results suggest that the Ia afferent fibers synapsing with the activated motoneurons have a background presynaptic inhibition that is *decreased* during voluntary contraction, whereas presynaptic inhibition exerted on Ia fibers connected with motoneurons of muscles not involved in this contraction is *increased*. They have proposed that this differential presynaptic inhibition is mediated by different sets of interneurons subjected to supraspinal control. The decrease in the presynaptic inhibition would allow Ia activity to contribute to excitation of voluntarily activated motoneurons, and the increased presynaptic inhibition would prevent activation of unrelated motoneurons, thus increasing motor contrast.

Besides being involved in inhibitory control of synaptic transmission, the pathways producing PAD of afferent fibers could serve other functions as well. Rudomin and Dutton (1969a) have shown that a constant stimulus to the Ia gastrocnemius afferent fibers produces monosynaptic reflexes of varying amplitudes, that these fluctuations occur simultaneously in many motoneurons (that is, they are correlated), and that conditioning stimulation of group I fibers in flexor nerves may *reduce these correlated fluctuations* (Rudomin et al., 1969; Rudomin and Madrid, 1972). In subsequent studies, they demonstrated that the excitability fluctuations of populations of Ia fibers ending in the motor nucleus were also correlated and that these fluctuations could be decreased by the same stimuli that reduced the fluctuations of the monosynaptic reflexes (Rudomin et al., 1974). They concluded that the fluctuations of the monosynaptic reflexes were introduced presynaptically via the interneurons mediating the PAD of the Ia fibers (Rudomin and Dutton, 1969b). Recording of Ia monosynaptic EPSPs in motoneuron pairs belonging to the same motor nucleus supported this view, since the Ia EPSPs showed correlated fluctuations that were also reduced by conditioning volleys to group I PBSt afferents (Rudomin et al., 1975a).

The existence of presynaptic control mechanisms acting simultaneously on a significant number of afferent fibers implies that the information transmitted by a given set of Ia fibers is not completely independent of the information transmitted by another set. This implies that the information arising in the periphery will be *transformed* before its arrival to the second-order cells. Clearly, this is not a desirable situation if the Ia afferents participate in feedback control mechanisms. Furthermore, the correlated membrane potential fluctuations imposed on Ia fiber terminals via the PAD mediating interneurons are not really redundant information reflecting events occurring in the periphery, since the PAD mediating interneurons also receive inputs of supraspinal origin. At present, the functional role of the correlated membrane potential fluctuations that are introduced presynaptically into the afferent fibers has not been elucidated. It is possible that high correlation is required for presynaptic inhibition to act as a "gating" control mechanism simultaneously affecting transmitter release of a substantial number of afferent fibers (Rudomin et al., 1975a, 1987). Alternatively, the PAD mediating interneurons may, by introducing correlated membrane potential fluctuations on the afferent fibers, erase the information transmitted through some groups of afferent fibers but not through others (Rudomin et al., 1975b). Obviously, to test these proposals, it will be necessary to record activity from identified last-order interneurons mediating the PAD of Ia and Ib fibers in unrestrained animals during the execution of specific motor tasks. This is clearly a very challenging task, but we must recognize that defining connectivities between spinal interneurons in the anesthetized or decerebrated preparation gives only a restricted view of the complexity of the neuronal circuits associated with a given reflex pathway. Interneurons must be considered as nodal points of converging and diverging information. Their functional connectivities will depend on the balance of excitatory and inhibitory influences received by the network at a given moment, and this in turn will depend on the specific motor or sensory task to be executed.

Acknowledgment

I would like to thank Dr. Lorne Mendell for his valuable comments on the manuscript. This work was partly supported by NIH grant NS-09196 and CONACYT grant PCEXCCNA 41739 and by Sistema Nacional de Investigadores, México.

REFERENCES

Alvarez-Leefmans, J. F., de Santis, A., and Miledi, R. (1979). Effects of some divalent ions on synaptic transmission in frog spinal neurons. *J. Physiol. (Lond.)* 294, 387–406.

Alvarez-Leefmans, J. F., Gamino, F. J., Giraldez, S. M., and Nogueron, I. (1988). Intracellular chloride regulation in amphibian dorsal root ganglion neurones studied with ion-selective microelectrodes. *J. Physiol. (Lond.)* 406, 225–246.

Baldissera, F., Hultborn, H., and Illert, M. (1982). Integration in spinal neuronal Systems. In V. B. Brooks (ed.): *Handbook of Physiology*, Vol. II, Sect. 1, Part 1: *The Nervous System. Motor Control.* American Physiological Society, Bethesda, Md., pp. 509–595.

Banna, N. R., and Jabbur, S. J. (1971). The effects of depleting GABA on cuneate presynaptic inhibition. *Brain Res.* 33, 530–532.

Barber, R. P., Vaugh, J. E., Saito, K., McLaughlin, B. J., and Roberts, E. (1978). GABAergic terminals are presynaptic to primary afferent terminals in the substantia gelatinosa of the rat spinal cord. *Brain Res.* 141, 35–55.

Barron, D. H., and Matthews, B. H. C. (1938). The interpretation of potential changes in the spinal cord. *J. Physiol. (Lond.)* 92, 276–321.

Bell, J. A., and Anderson, E. G. (1972). The influence of semicarbazide induced depletion of gama-aminobutyric acid on presynaptic inhibition. *Brain Res.* 43, 161–169.

Bradley, K., and Eccles, J. C. (1953). Analysis of the fast afferent impulses from thigh muscles. *J. Physiol. (Lond.)* 122, 462–473.

Brink, E., Harrison, P. J., Jankowska, E., McCrea, D., and Skoog, B. (1983). Postsynaptic potentials in a population of motoneurones following activity of single interneurones in the cat. *J. Physiol. (Lond.)* 343, 341–359.

Brink, E., Jankowska, E., and Skoog, B. (1984). Convergence onto interneurons subserving primary afferent depolarization of group I afferents. *J. Neurophysiol.* 51, 432–449.

Bruggencate, G. T., Lux, H. D., and Liebl, L. (1974). Possible relationships between extracellular potassium activity and presynaptic inhibition in the spinal cord of the cat. *Pflugers Arch.* 349, 301–317.

Burke, R. E. (1981). Motor units: Anatomy, physiology and functional organization. In The Nervous System. Vol. II, Sect. 1: *Handbook of Physiology.* (ed. V. B. Brooks). *American Physiological Society,* Bethesda, Md., pp. 345–422.

Burke, R. E., and Rudomin, P. (1977). Spinal neurons and synapses. In *Handbook of Physiology*, Vol. I, Sect. 1: *The Nervous System* (ed. E. R. Kandel). American Physiological Society, Bethesda, Md., 877–944.

Carlen, P. L., Werman, R., and Yaari, Y. (1980). Post-synaptic conductance increase associated with presynaptic inhibition in cat lumbar motoneurones. *J. Physiol. (Lond.)* 298, 539–556.

Carpenter, D., Engberg, I., and Lundberg, A. (1963). Primary afferent depolarization evoked from the brain stem and the cerebellum. *Arch. Ital. Biol.* 104, 73–83.

Clements, J. D., Forsythe, I. D., and Redman, S. J. (1987). Presynaptic inhibition of synaptic potentials evoked in cat spinal motoneurones by impulses in single group Ia axons. *J. Physiol. (Lond.)* 383, 153–169.

Conradi, S. (1969). On motoneuron synaptology in adult cats. *Acta Physiol. Scand.* 332 (Suppl), 5, 115.

Conradi, S., Cullheim, S., Gollvik, L., and Kellerth, J. O. (1983). Electron microscopic observations on the synaptic contacts of group Ia muscle spindle afferents in the cat lumbosacral spinal cord. *Brain Res.* 265, 35–39.

Cook, W. A., and Cangiano, A. (1972). Presynaptic and postsynaptic inhibition of spinal motoneurons. *J. Neurophysiol.* 35, 389–403.

Cook, W. A., Cangiano, A., and Pompeiano, O. (1969). Dorsal root potentials in the lumbar cord evoked from the vestibular systems. *Arch. Ital. Biol.* 107, 275–295.

Coppin, C. M. L., Jack, J. J. B., and McIntyre, A. (1969). Properties of group I afferent fibres from semitendinosus muscle in the cat. *J. Physiol. (Lond.)* 203, 45–46P.

Curtis, D. R., Headley, P. M., and Lodge, D. R. (1984). Depolarization of feline primary afferent fibers by acidic amino acids. *J. Physiol. (Lond.)* 351, 461–472.

Curtis, D. R., and Lodge, D. R. (1982). The depolarization of feline ventral horn group Ia spinal afferent terminations by GABA. *Brain Res.* 46, 215–233.

Curtis, D. R., Lodge, D., Bornstein, J. C., Peet, M. J., and Leah, J. D. (1982). The dual effects of GABA and related amino acids on the electrical threshold of ventral horn group Ia afferent terminations in the cat. *Exp. Brain Res.* 48, 387–400.

Curtis, D. R., and Malik, R. (1984). The effect of GABA on lumbar terminations of rubospinal neurons in the cat spinal cord. *Proc. R. Soc. Lond. B* 223, 25–33.

Curtis, D. R., Wilson, V. J., and Malik, R. (1984). The effect of GABA on the terminations of vestibulospinal neurons in the cat spinal cord. *Brain Res.* 295, 372–375.

Czarkowska, J., Jankowska, E., and Sybirska, E. (1981). Common interneurones in reflex pathways from group Ia and Ib afferents from knee flexors and extensors in the cat. *J. Physiol. (Lond.)* 310, 367–380.

Davidoff, R. A., Grayson, V., and Adair, R. (1973). GABA-transaminase inhibitors and presynaptic inhibition in the amphibian spinal cord. *Am. J. Physiol.* 224, 1230–1234.

Davidoff, R. A., and Hackman, J. C. (1984). Spinal inhibition. In *Handbook of the Spinal Cord.* (ed. R. A. Davidoff). Dekker, Basel, pp. 385–459.

De Groat, W. C. (1972). GABA depolarization of a sensory ganglion. Antagonism by picrotoxin and bicuculline. *Brain Res.* 38, 429–432.

De Groat, W. C., Lalley, P. M., and Saum, W. R. (1972). Depolarization of dorsal root ganglia in the cat by GABA and related aminoacids: Antagonism by picrotoxin and bicuculline. *Brain Res.* 44, 273–277.

Decima, E. E., and Goldberg, J. L. (1970). Centrifugal dorsal root discharges induced by motoneurone activation. *J. Physiol. (Lond.)* 207, 103–118.

De la Roza, C., Gorcs, T. J., and Priestley, J. V. (1987). GABA immunoreactive neurones in the rat spinal cord and spinal trigeminal nucleus. *Neuroscience* 22, S792.

Desarmenien, M., Feltz, P., Occhipinti, G., Santangelo, F., and Schlichter, R. (1984a). Coexistence of GABAa and GABAb receptors on A-delta and C primary afferents. *Br. J. Pharmacol.* 81, 327–333.

Desarmenien, M., Santangelo, F., Loeffer, J. P., and Feltz, P. (1984b). Comparative study of GABA-mediated depolarizations of lumbar Ad and C primary afferent neurones of the rat. *Exp. Brain Res.* 54, 521–528.

Deschenes, M., Feltz, P., and Lamour, Y. (1976). A model for an estimate in vivo of the ionic basis of presynaptic inhibition: An intracellular analysis of the GABA-induced depolarization in rat dorsal root ganglia. *Brain Res.* 118, 486–493.

Devanandan, M. S., Eccles, R. M., and Yokota, T. (1965). Muscle stretch and the presynaptic inhibition of the group Ia pathway to motoneurons. *J. Physiol. (Lond.)* 179, 430–441.

Dudel, J. (1963). Presynaptic inhibition of the excitatory nerve terminal in the neuromuscular junction of the crayfish. *Pflugers Arch.* 277, 537–557.

Dudel, J., and Kuffler, S. W. (1961). Presynaptic inhibition at the crayfish neuromuscular junction. *J. Physiol. (Lond.)* 155, 543–562.

Dum, R. P., and Kennedy, T. T. (1980). Synaptic organization of defined motor-unit types in cat tibialis anterior. *J. Neurophysiol.* 43, 1631–1644.

Dunlap, K., and Fischbach, G. D. (1981). Neurotransmitters decrease the calcium conductance activated by depolarization of embryonic chick sensory neurons. *J. Physiol. (Lond.)* 317, 519–535.

Eccles, J. C. (1961). The mechanism of synaptic transmission. *Ergeb. Physiol.* 51, 299–430.

Eccles, J. C. (1964). *The Physiology of Synapses.* Springer Verlag, New York.

Eccles, J. C., Kostyuk, P. G., and Schmidt, R. F. (1962a). Central pathways responsible for depolarization of primary afferent fibres. *J. Physiol. (Lond.)* 161, 237–257.

Eccles, J. C., Magni, F., and Willis, W. D. (1962b). Depolarization of central terminals of group I afferent fibers from muscle. *J. Physiol. (Lond.)* 160, 62–93.

Eccles, J. C., and Malcolm, J. L. (1946). Dorsal root potentials of the spinal cord. *J. Neurophysiol.* 9, 139–160.

Eccles, J. C., Schmidt, R. F., and Willis, W. D. (1962c). Presynaptic inhibition of the spinal monosynaptic reflex pathway. *J. Physiol. (Lond.)* 161, 282–297.

Eccles, J. C., Schmidt, R. F., and Willis, W. D. (1963a). Depolarization of central terminals of group Ib afferent fibers from muscle. *J. Neurophysiol.* 26, 1–27.

Eccles, J. C., Schmidt, R. F., and Willis, W. D. (1963b). Pharmacological studies on presynaptic inhibition. *J. Physiol. (Lond.)* 168, 500–530.

Eccles, J. C., Schmidt, R. F., and Willis, W. D. (1963c). The location and the mode of action of the presynaptic inhibitory pathways on group I afferent fibers from muscle. *J. Neurophysiol.* 26, 506–522.

Egger, M. D., Freeman, N. C. G., Malamed, S. M., Masarachia, P., and Prosohansky, E. (1981). Electron microscopic observations of functionally identified afferent fibers in cat spinal cord. *Brain Res.* 207, 157–162.

Eide, E., Jurna, I., and Lundberg, A. (1968). Conductance measurements from motoneurons during presynaptic inhibition. In *Structure and Function of Inhibitory Neuronal Mechanisms* (ed. C. Von Euler, A. Skoglund, and U. Soderberg). Pergamon Press, New York, pp. 215–219.

Frank, K. (1959). Basic mechanisms of synaptic transmission in the central nervous system. *Inst. Radio Eng. Trans. Med. Electron.* 6, 85–88.

Frank, K., and Fuortes, M. G. F. (1957). Presynaptic and postsynaptic inhibition of monosynaptic reflexes. *Fed. Proc.* 16, 39–40.

Friedman, W. A., Sypert, G. W., Munson, J. B., and Fleshman, J. W. (1981). Recurrent inhibition of type-identified motoneurons. *J. Neurophysiol.* 46, 1349–1359.

Fyffe, R. E. W., and Light, A. R. (1984). The ultrastructure of group Ia afferent fibre synapses in the lumbosacral spinal cord of the cat. *Brain Res.* 300, 201–209.

Galindo, J., and Rudomin, P. (1978). The effects of gallamine on field and dorsal root potentials produced by antidromic stimulation of motor fibres in the frog spinal cord. *Exp. Brain Res.* 32, 135–150.

Gallagher, J. P., Higashi, H., and Nishi, S. (1978). Characterization and ionic basis of GABA-induced depolarization recorded in vitro from rat primary neurons. *J. Physiol. (Lond.)* 275, 263–282.

Gallagher, J. P., and Shinnick-Gallagher, P. (1983). Electrophysiological characteristics of GABA-receptor complexes. In *GABA Receptors* (ed. S. Enna). Humana Press, 25–65.

Gasser, H., and Graham, H. T. (1933). Potentials produced in the spinal cord by stimulation of the dorsal roots. *Am. J. Physiol.* 103, 303–320.

Glusman, S., and Rudomin, P. (1974). Presynaptic modulation of synaptic effectiveness of afferent and ventrolateral tract fibers in the frog spinal cord. *Exp. Neurol.* 45, 474–490.

Glusman, S., Vazquez-Nin, H., and Rudomin, P. (1976). Ultrastructural observations in the frog spinal cord in relation to primary afferent depolarization. *Neurosci. Lett.* 2, 137–145.

Gmelin, G. W. (1976). Effects of electrophoretically applied GABA and bicuculline on presynaptic inhibition in the spinal cord of mammalia. *Pflugers Arch.* 362, R31.

Gmelin, G. W. (1978). Electrophoretic studies on presynaptic inhibition in the mammalian spinal cord. In *Iontophoresis and Transmitter Mechanisms in the Mammalian Central Nervous System* (ed. R. W. Ryall and J. E. Kelly). Elsevier/North Holland, Amsterdam, pp. 267–269.

Gmelin, G. W., and Zimmermann, M. (1984). Effects of γ-aminobutyrate and bicuculline on primary afferent depolarization of cutaneous fibres in the cat spinal cord. *Neuroscience* 10, 869–874.

Goode, G. E., and Sreesai, M. (1978). An electron microscopic study of rubospinal projections to the lumbar spinal cord of the opossum. *Brain Res.* 143, 61–70.

Granit, R. (1968). The case for presynaptic inhibition by synapses on the terminals of motoneurons. In *Structure and Function of Inhibitory Neuronal Mechanisms* (ed. C. Von Euler, S. Skoglund, and U. Soderberg). Pergamon Press, New York, pp. 183–195.

Granit, R. Kellerth, J. O., and Williams, T. D. (1964). Intracellular aspects of stimulating motoneurones by muscle sketch. *J. Physiol. (Lond.)* 174, 435–452.

Gray, E. G. (1962). A morphological basis for presynaptic inhibition? *Nature* 193, 82–83.

Green, D. G., and Kellerth, J. O. (1966). Postsynaptic versus presynaptic inhibition in antagonistic stretch reflexes. *Science* 152, 1097–1099.

Grinnell, A. D. (1970). Electrical interaction between antidromically stimulated frog motoneurones and dorsal root afferents: Enhancement by gallamine and TEA. *J. Physiol. (Lond.)* 210, 17–43.

Hajek, I., and Sykova, E. (1981). Potassium-induced decrease of enkephalin binding in the frog spinal cord. *Physiol. Bohemoslov* 30, 428–429.

Hanaway, J., and Smith, J. M. (1978). Fine structure of the rubrospinal terminals in the cervical cord of the cat. *J. Neurol. Sci.* 39, 31–36.

Harrison, P. J., and Jankowska, E. (1985a). Organization of input to the interneurones mediating group I non-reciprocal inhibition of motoneurones in the cat. *J. Physiol. (Lond.)* 361, 403–418.

Harrison, P. J., and Jankowska, E. (1985b). Sources of input to interneurones mediating group I non-reciprocal inhibition of motoneurones in the cat. *J. Physiol. (Lond.)* 361, 379–401.

Henneman, E., and Mendell, L. M. (1981). Functional organization of motoneuron pool and its inputs. In *Handbook of Physiology. The Nervous System,* Vol. II. (ed. V. B. Brooks). American Physiological Society, Bethesda, Md., pp. 423–507.

Holstege, J. C., and Núñez-Cardozo, B. (1987). Ultrastructural identification of GABAergic terminals in rat lumbar motoneuronal cell groups. *Neuroscience* 22, S794.

Hongo, T., Jankowska, E., and Lundberg, A. (1972). The rubrospinal tract. III. Effects on primary afferent terminals. *Exp. Brain Res.* 15, 39–53.

Howland, B., Lettvin, J. Y., McCulloch, W. S., Pitts, W., and Wall, P. D. (1955). Reflex inhibition by dorsal root interaction. *J. Neurophysiol.* 18, 1–17.

Hultborn, H., Meunier, S., Pierrot-Deseilligny, E., and Shindo, M. (1987b). Changes in presynaptic inhibition of Ia fibres at the onset of voluntary contraction in man. *J. Physiol. (Lond.)* 389, 757–772.

Hultborn, H., Meunier, S., Pierrot-Deseilligny E., and Shindo, M. (1987b). Changes in presynaptic inhibition of Ia fibres at the onset of voluntary contraction in man. *J. Physiol. (Lond.)* 389, 757–772.

Janig, W., Schmidt, F. R., and Zimmermann, M. (1968a). Single unit responses and the total afferent outflow from the cat's foot pad upon mechanical stimulation. *Exp. Brain Res.* 6, 100–115.

Janig, W., Schmidt, F. R., and Zimmermann, M. (1968b). Two specific feedback pathways to the central afferent terminals of phasic and tonic mechanoreceptors. *Exp. Brain Res.* 6, 116–129.

Jankowska, E., Johannison, T., and Lipski, J. (1981a). Common interneurones in reflex pathways from group Ia and Ib afferents of ankle extensors in the cat. *J. Physiol. (Lond.)* 310, 381–402.

Jankowska, E., McCrea, D., and Mackel, R. (1981b). Pattern of "non-reciprocal" inhibition of motoneurones by impulses in group Ia muscle spindle afferents. *J. Physiol. (Lond.)* 316, 393–409.

Jankowska, E., McCrea, D., Rudomin, P., and Sykova, E. (1981c). Observations on neuronal pathways subserving primary afferent depolarization. *J. Neurophysiol.* 46, 506–516.

Jankowska, E., and Padel, Y. (1984). On the origin of presynaptic depolarization of group I muscle afferents in Clarke's column in the cat. *Brain Res.* 295, 195–201.

Jessel, T. M., and Iversen, L. L. (1977). Opiate analgesics inhibit substance P release from rat trigeminal nucleus. *Nature* 268, 549–551.

Jiménez, I., Rudomin, P., and Solodkin, M. (1987). Mechanisms involved in the depolarization of cutaneous afferents produced by segmental and descending inputs in the cat spinal cord. *Exp. Brain Res.* 69, 195–207.

Jiménez, I., Rudomin, P., and Solodkin, M. (1988). PAD patterns of physiologically identified afferent fibres from the medial gastrocnemius muscle. *Exp. Brain Res.* 71, 643–657.

Jiménez, I., Rudomin, P., Solodkin, M., and Vyklicky, L. (1983). Specific and potassium components in the depolarization of the Ia afferents in the spinal cord of the cat. *Brain Res.* 272, 179–184.

Jiménez, I., Rudomin, P., Solodkin, M., and Vyklicky, L. (1984). Specific and non-specific mechanisms involved in generation of PAD of group Ia afferents in cat spinal cord. *J. Neurophysiol.* 52, 921–940.

Kellerth, J. O. (1968). Aspects on the relative significance of pre- and postsynaptic inhibition in the spinal cord. In *Structure and Function of Inhibitory Neuronal Mechanisms* (ed. C. Von Euler, S. Skoglund, and U. Soderberg). Pergamon Press, New York, pp. 197–212.

Kellerth, J. O., and Szumski, A. J. (1966a). Two types of stretch-activated post-synaptic inhibitions in spinal motoneurones as differentiated by strychnine. *Acta Physiol. Scand.* 66, 133–145.

Kellerth, J. O., and Szumsky, A. J. (1966b). Effects of picrotoxin on stretch activated postsynaptic inhibition in spinal motoneurons. *Acta Physiol. Scand.* 66, 146–156.

Kostyuk, P. G., and Skibo, G. G. (1975). An electron microscopic analysis of rubrospinal tract termination in the spinal cord of the cat. *Brain Res.* 85, 511–516.

Kriz, N., Sykova, E., and Vyklicky, L. (1975). Extracellular potassium changes in the spinal cord of the cat and their relation to slow potentials, active transport and impulse transmission. *J. Physiol. (Lond.)* 249, 167–182.

Krnjevic, K., and Morris, M. E. (1972). Extracellular K^+ activity and slow potential changes in spinal cord and medulla. *Can. J. Physiol. Pharmacol.* 50, 1214–1217.

Krnjevic, K., and Morris, M. E. (1974). Extracellular accumulation of K^+ evoked by activity of primary afferent fibers in the cuneate nucleus and dorsal horn of cats. *Can. J. Physiol. Pharmacol.* 52, 852–871.

Krnjevic, K., and Morris, M. E. (1975). Correlation between focal potentials and K^+ potentials evoked by primary afferent activity. *Can. J. Physiol. Pharmacol.* 53, 912–922.

Kuno, M. (1964). Mechanisms of facilitation and depression of the excitatory synaptic potential in spinal motoneurones. *J. Physiol. (Lond.)* 175, 100–112.

Lev-Tov, A., Fleshman, J. W., and Burke, R. E. (1983). Primary afferent depolarization and presynaptic inhibition of monosynaptic group Ia EPSPs during post-tetanic potentiation. *J. Neurophysiol.* 50, 413–427.

Levy, R. A. (1977). Role of GABA in primary afferent depolarization. *Prog. Neurobiol.* 9, 211–267.

Ljungdahl, A., and Hokfelt, T. (1973). Autoradiographic uptake patterns of 3H GABA and 3H glycine in central nervous tissues with special reference to the cat spinal cord. *Brain Res.* 62, 587–595.

Lloyd, D. P. C., and McIntyre, A. K. (1949). On the origins of dorsal root potentials. *J. Gen. Physiol.* 32, 409–443.

Lothman, E. W., and Somjen, G. G. (1975). Extracellular potassium activity, intracellular and extracellular potential responses in the spinal cord. *J. Physiol. (Lond.)* 252, 115–136.

Lucas, M. E., and Willis, W. D. (1974). Identification of muscle afferents which activate interneurons in the intermediate nucleus. *J. Neurophysiol.* 37, 282–293.

Lund, S., Lundberg, A., and Vyklicky, L. (1965). Inhibitory action from the flexor reflex afferents on transmission to Ia afferents. *Acta Physiol. Scand.* 64, 345–355.

Lundberg, A. (1964). Supraspinal control of transmission in reflex paths to motoneurons and primary afferents. In *Physiology of Spinal Neurons* (ed. J. C. Eccles and J. P. Schade). Elsevier, Amsterdam, pp. 197–219.

Lundberg, A., and Vyklicky, L. (1966). Inhibition of transmission to primary afferents by electrical stimulation of the brainstem. *Arch. Ital. Biol.* 104, 86–97.

Lüscher, H. R., Ruenzel, P., Fetz, E., and Henneman, E. (1979). Postsynaptic population potentials recorded from ventral roots perfused with isotonic sucrose: Connections of groups Ia and II spindle afferent fibers with large populations of motoneurons. *J. Neurophysiol.* 42, 1146–1164.

Maxwell, D. J., and Bannatyne, B. A. (1983). Ultrastructure of muscle spindle afferent terminations in lamina VI of the cat spinal cord. *Brain Res.* 288, 297–301.

McCrea, D. A., and Carlen, P. L. (1983). Minimal or no post-synaptic conductance changes during presynaptic inhibition in chloralose anesthetized cats. *Proc. Soc. Neurosci.* 9, 881.

McLaughlin, B. J., Barber, R., Saito, K., Roberts, E., and Wu, J. Y. (1975). Immunocytochemical localization of glutamate decarboxylase in rat spinal cord. *J. Comp. Neurol.* 164, 305–322.

Mendell, L. M., and Henneman, E. (1971). Terminals of single Ia fibers: Location, density and distribution within a pool of 300 homonymous motoneurons. *J. Neurophysiol.* 34, 171–187.

Miyata, Y., and Otsuka, M. (1972). Distribution of gama-aminobutyric acid in cat spinal cord and the alteration produced by local ischemia. *J. Neurochem.* 19, 1833–1834.

Nelson, P. G. (1966). Interaction between spinal motoneurons of the cat. *J. Neurophysiol.* 29, 275–287.

Nicoll, R. A. (1979). Dorsal root potentials and changes in extracellular potassium in the spinal cord of the frog. *J. Physiol. (Lond.)* 290, 113–127.

Nicoll, R. A., and Alger, B. E. (1979). Presynaptic inhibition: Transmitter and ionic mechanisms. *Int. Rev. Neurobiol.* 21, 217–258.

Peng, Y. Y., and Frank, E. (1987). Activation of GABA b receptors induces presynaptic inhibition at muscle spindle afferent–motoneuron synapses in the frog spinal cord. *Proc. Soc. Neurosci.* 13, 1352.

Pentreath, V. W., and Kai-Kai, M. A. (1982). Significance of the potassium signal from neurones to glial cells. *Nature* 295, 59–61.

Pottala, E. W., Colburn, T. R., and Humphrey, A. (1973). A dendritic compartment model neuron. *Inst. Elect. Electron. Eng. Trans. Biomed. Eng.* 20, 132–139.

Proudfit, H. K., Larson, A. A., and Anderson, E. G. (1980). The role of GABA and serotonin in the mediation of raphe-evoked spinal cord dorsal root potentials. *Brain Res.* 195, 149–165.

Rall, W. (1967). Distinguishing theoretical synaptic potentials computed from different soma-dendritic distributions of synaptic input. *J. Neurophysiol.* 30, 1138–1168.

Rall, W. (1970). Cable properties and effects of synaptic location. In *Excitatory Synaptic Mechanisms* (ed. P. Andersen and J. K. S. Jansen). Universitetsforlaget, Oslo, pp. 175–187.

Ralston, H. J. (1981). The synaptic organization of the macaque dorsal horn. In *Spinal Cord Sensation* (ed. A. G. Brown and M. Rethelyi). Scottish Academic Press, Edinburgh, pp. 13–21.

Redman, S. (1979). Junctional mechanisms at group Ia synapses. *Prog. Neurobiol.* 12, 33–83.

Rethelyi, M. (1970). Ultrastructural synaptology of Clarke's column. *Exp. Brain Res.* 11, 159–174.

Rethelyi, M. (1984a). Synaptic connectivity in the dorsal horn. In *Handbook of the Spinal Cord* (ed. R. A. Davidoff). Dekker, Basel, pp. 137–177.

Rethelyi, M. (1984b). Types of synaptic connections in the core of the spinal gray matter. In *Handbook of the Spinal Cord* (ed. R. A. Davidoff). Dekker, Basel, pp. 179–198.

Rethelyi, M., Light, A., and Perl, E. R. (1982). Synaptic complexes formed by functionally defined primary afferent units with fine myelinated fibers. *J. Comp. Neurol.* 207, 381–393.

Ribeiro da Silva, A., and Coimbra, A. (1980). Neuronal uptake of 3H GABA and 3H glycine in laminae I–II (substantia gelatinosa Rolandi) of the rat spinal cord. An autoradiographic study. *Brain Res.* 188, 449–464.

Rudomin, P., Burke, R. E., Núñez, R., Madrid, J., and Dutton, H. (1975a). Control by presynaptic correlation: A mechanism affecting information transmission from Ia fibers to motoneurons. *J. Neurophysiol.* 38, 267–284.

Rudomin, P., and Dutton, H. (1969a). Effects of conditioning afferent volleys on variability of monosynaptic responses of extensor motoneurons. *J. Neurophysiol.* 32, 130–157.

Rudomin, P., and Dutton, H. (1969b). Effects of muscle and cutaneous afferent volleys on excitability fluctuations in Ia terminals. *J. Neurophysiol.* 32, 158–169.

Rudomin, P., Dutton, H., and Muñoz-Martinez, J. (1969). Changes in correlation between monosynaptic reflexes produced by conditioning afferent volleys. *J. Neurophysiol.* 32, 759–772.

Rudomin, P., Engberg, I., Jankowska, E., and Jiménez, I. (1980). Evidence of two different mechanisms involved in the generation of presynaptic depolarization of afferent and rubrospinal fibers in the cat spinal cord. *Brain Res.* 189, 256–261.

Rudomin, P., Engberg, I., and Jiménez, I. (1981). Mechanisms involved in presynaptic depolarization of group I and rubrospinal fibers in cat spinal cord. *J. Neurophysiol.* 46, 532–548.

Rudomin, P., and Jankowska, E. (1981). Presynaptic depolarization of terminals of rubrospinal tract fibers in intermediate nucleus of cat spinal cord. *J. Neurophysiol.* 46, 517–531.

Rudomin, P., Jiménez, I., Solodkin, M., and Dueñas, S. (1983). Sites of action of segmental and descending control of transmission on pathways mediating PAD of Ia and Ib afferent fibers in cat spinal cord. *J. Neurophysiol.* 50, 743–769.

Rudomin, P., and Madrid, J. (1972). Changes in correlation between monosynaptic reflexes and in information transmission produced by conditioning volleys to cutaneous nerves. *J. Neurophysiol.* 35, 44–64.

Rudomin, P., Núñez, R., and Madrid, J. (1975b). Modulation of synaptic effectiveness of Ia and descending fibers in the cat spinal cord. *J. Neurophysiol.* 38, 1181–1195.

Rudomin, P., Núñez, R., Madrid, J., and Burke, R. E. (1974). Primary afferent hyperpolarization and presynaptic facilitation of Ia afferent terminals induced by large cutaneous afferents. *J. Neurophysiol.* 37, 413–429.

Rudomin, P., Solodkin, M., and Jiménez, I. (1986). PAD and PAH response patterns of group Ia and Ib fibers to cutaneous and descending inputs in the cat spinal cord. *J. Neurophysiol.* 56, 987–1006.

Rudomin, P., Solodkin, M., and Jiménez, I. (1987). Synaptic potentials of primary afferent fibers and motoneurons evoked by single intermediate nucleus interneurons in the cat spinal cord. *J. Neurophysiol.* 57, 1288–1313.

Schmidt, R. F. (1971). Presynaptic inhibition in the vertebrate central nervous system. *Ergeb. Physiol.* 63, 20–101.

Shapovalov, A. I., and Shiriaev, B. I. (1978). Electrical coupling between primary afferents and amphibian motoneurons. *Exp. Brain Res.* 33, 299–312.

Shinoda, Y., Yokota, J.-I., and Futami, T. (1982). Morphology of physiologically identified rubrospinal axons in the spinal cord of the cat. *Brain Res.* 242, 321–325.

Solodkin, M., Jiménez, I., and Rudomin, P. (1984). Identification of common interneurons mediating pre- and postsynaptic inhibition in the cat spinal cord. *Science* 224, 1453–1456.

Solodkin, M., Ruiz de León, O., Zamora, L., Jiménez, I., Collins, L. M., III, Mendell, L. M., and Rudomin, P. (1987). Non-linear interaction between background synaptic noise and Ia single fiber EPSPs evoked in spinal motoneurons. *Proc. Soc. Neurosci.* 13, 1687.

Somjen, G. G., and Lothman, E. W. (1974). Potassium, sustained focal potentials shifts and dorsal root potentials of the mammalian spinal cord. *Brain Res.* 69; 153–157.

Sykova, E. (1981). K^+ changes in the extracellular space of the spinal cord and their physiological role. *J. Exp. Physiol.* 95, 93–109.

Sykova, E. (1983). Extracellular K^+ accumulation in the central nervous system. *Prog. Biophys. Mol. Biol.* 42, 135–189.

Vyklicky, L., Sykova, E., and Kriz, N. (1975). Slow potentials induced by changes of extracellular potassium in the spinal cord of the cat. *Brain Res.* 87, 77–80.

Vyklicky, L., Sykova, E., Kriz, N., and Ujec, E., (1972). Post-stimulation changes of extracellular potassium concentration in the spinal cord of the rat. *Brain Res.* 45, 608–611.

Wall, P. D. (1958). Excitability changes in afferent fibre terminations and their relation to slow potentials. *J. Physiol.* (*Lond.*) 142, 1–21.

Walmsley, B., Wieniawa-Narkiewicz, E., and Nicol, M. J. (1987). Ultrastructural evidence related to presynaptic inhibition of primary muscle afferents in Clarke's column of the cat. *J. Neurosci.* 7, 236–243.

Zengel, J. E., Reid, S. A., Sypert, G. W., and Munson, J. B. (1983). Presynaptic inhibition, EPSP amplitude and motor-unit type in triceps surae motoneurons in the cat. *J. Neurophysiol.* 49, 922–931.

20

Functional Properties of Primate Corticomotoneuronal Cells: Comparisons with Spindle Afferents and Motor Units

E. E. FETZ AND P. D. CHENEY

A causal explanation of the neural mechanisms that generate active movement will ultimately require quantitative information on the connectivity and response properties of the mediating neurons. In their studies of the functional organization of Ia afferent fiber connections to motoneurons, Elwood Henneman and colleagues substantially advanced our understanding of this model system and, at the same time, pioneered techniques that have helped to elucidate the organization of other inputs to motoneurons. In particular, the spike-triggered averaging (STA) technique has been used to document the effects of single-fiber inputs to motoneurons (Mendell and Henneman, 1971; Fetz et al., 1979; Kirkwood and Sears, 1980; Cope, et al., 1987; see also Chapters 16, 17, and 18, this volume). In their landmark paper, Mendell and Henneman (1971) first demonstrated the elegance and power of STA to document the postsynaptic effects of single neurons: they found that Ia afferent fibers produce unitary excitatory postsynaptic potentials (EPSPs) in motoneurons with a remarkable variety of shapes and sizes; moreover, a single afferent typically distributes terminals to most homonymous and many heteronymous motoneurons. In an analogous fashion, STA of electromyographic (EMG) activity has been used in awake, behaving monkeys to identify particular motor cortex cells that have correlational links with coactivated forelimb muscles (Fetz and Cheney, 1978, 1980; Muir and Lemon, 1983; Buys et al., 1986). These so-called corticomotoneuronal (CM) cells produce post-spike facilitation of muscle activity with a time course suggesting that they make a monosynaptic connection with motoneurons. As a direct synaptic input to motoneurons, CM cells provide an interesting comparison with the segmental monosynaptic input from Ia afferent fibers. Moreover, as the final output from motor cortex, the CM cells can also be compared in many ways with another spinal analogue, the segmental motoneurons.

DISTRIBUTION OF POSTSPIKE EFFECTS OF CM CELLS

The sequence of events mediating the postspike facilitation of EMG is illustrated in Figure 20–1. The action potentials of a premotor input cell produce monosynaptic EPSPs, which in turn increase the firing probability of the target motoneuron. The effects of unitary EPSPs on motoneuron firing probability were documented for Ia EPSPs by Cope et al. (1987). In cat lumbar motoneurons, the single-fiber EPSPs were documented by STA of membrane potential first with the motoneuron at rest. Then the motoneuron was made to fire rhythmically by current injection, and the Ia spikes and motoneuron firing were cross-correlated. As illustrated by the correlogram in Figure 20–1, single-fiber EPSPs produced an increase in motoneuron firing probability during their rising phase. The peak of the cross-correlogram between the afferent and the

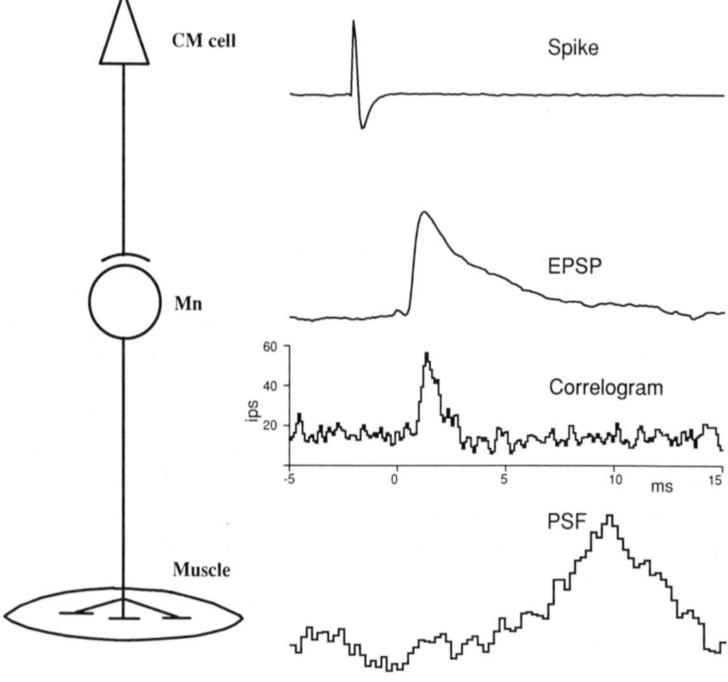

Fig. 20–1.   Events mediating postspike effects of the CM cell. A monosynaptic CM connection produces an EPSP and increases the motoneuron firing probability, represented here by STA of an Ia EPSP and its associated correlogram (from Cope et al., 1987). The STA of a multiunit EMG produces postspike facilitation (PSF), representing the contribution of all facilitated motor units.

motoneuron had a shape that was largely proportional to the derivative of the EPSP and a peak area (above baseline) that was proportional to the EPSP amplitude.

The postspike facilitation of multiunit EMG would represent the contributions of many motor units. The contribution of a single motor unit to the STA would be its postspike correlogram peak convolved with the motor unit potential. In comparison to correlograms with single motoneurons, STA of EMG activity is less quantitative, but is more effective in detecting the existence of a connection because it sums the contributions of all the facilitated motor units, and the contribution of each unit to the rectified EMG is proportional to the size of its motor unit potential. A major advantage of using STA of muscle activity in behaving animals is that one can also document the normal response properties of these cells and their targets during voluntary movements. The functional interpretation of these responses becomes more meaningful when combined with such evidence of a correlational linkage.

The typical experimental situation is illustrated in Figure 20–2: the monkey makes ramp-and-hold wrist movements against an elastic load, and holds in a force zone for over a second to provide a steady level of tonic EMG activity. The action potentials of cortical cells that are modulated with the task are used to trigger averages of rectified EMG activity. Consistent postspike effects typically appear in the STA after several thousand triggers. By averaging the activity of multiple muscles simultaneously, STA has shown that single CM cells usually facilitate motor units in several synergistic muscles. About half of the CM cells facilitate only one of the six recorded muscles, and the remainder facilitate two, three, and up to all six muscles. On average, about 30–40% of the recorded coactivated muscles are clearly facilitated (Fetz and Cheney, 1980; Buys et al., 1986). These distributed effects are analogous to the divergent effects of a single Ia afferent fiber in motoneurons of heteronymous synergists as well as homonymous muscle.

Mendell and Henneman (1971) found that a single Ia afferent distributes terminals to virtually all motoneurons of the homonymous muscle. The analogous projection of single CM cells to multiple motor units *within* a muscle remains to be thoroughly documented, but some relevant evidence to date suggests that CM cells facilitate most of the motor units of their target muscles. The first evidence was based on the effects evoked by single intracortical stimuli, which produce poststimulus facilitation of EMG in stimulus-triggered averages. When multiple motor units were isolated within a muscle, cortical microstimuli of minimal intensities tended to facilitate all the recorded motor units of the muscle, including units exhibiting every type of firing pattern (Palmer and Fetz, 1985b). More recently, Mantel and Lemon (1987) cross-correlated the activity of CM cells and motor units and found that most of the motor units were facilitated by single CM cells. Thus, CM cells are likely to exert divergent effects on most, if not all, motor units of a facilitated target muscle, much like Ia afferent fibers.

In addition to their excitatory effects on motoneurons of their target muscles, both Ia afferent fibers and CM cells may exert *inhibitory effects* on antagonists of the target muscles. In the case of Ia afferents, a powerful

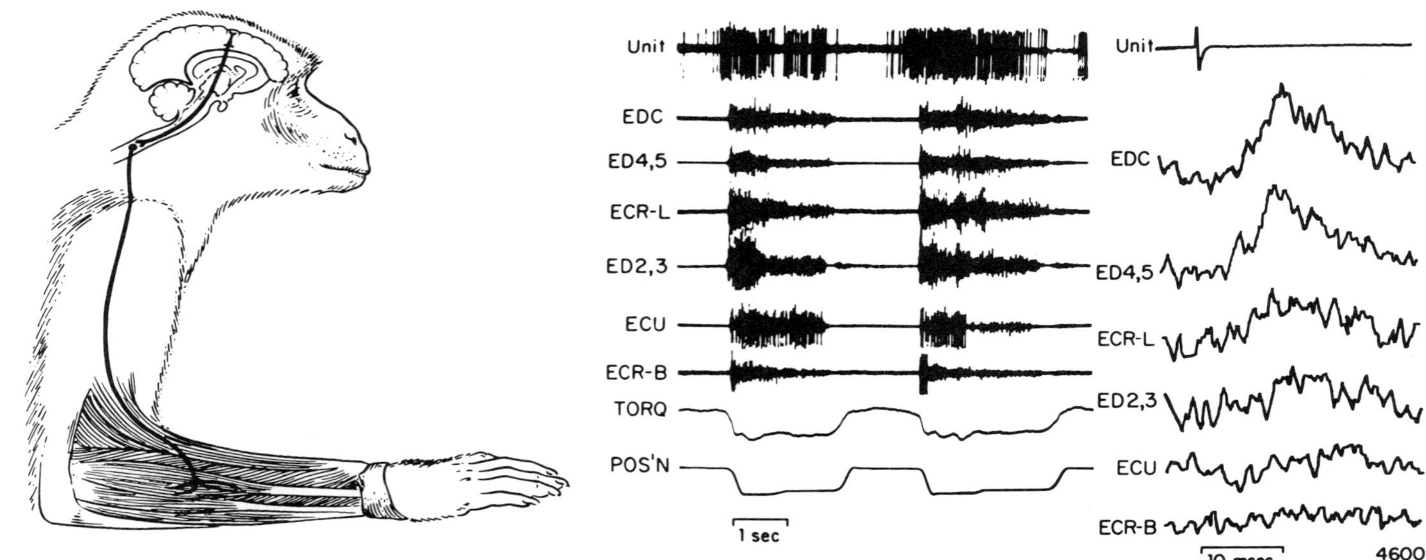

Fig. 20–2. *Left*: schematic diagram of a CM cell connected to a motoneuron of an extensor wrist muscle. *Middle*: responses of an extension-related CM cell during wrist movements against an elastic load with coactivated extensor muscles of the wrist (ECR-L; ECR-B; ECU) and the digits (EDC; ED4, 5; ED2, 3). *Right*: STAs of rectified EMG showing postspike facilitation in several target muscles. (Redrawn from Fetz and Cheney, 1978.)

reciprocal inhibition is mediated by the Ia inhibitory interneuron, which also receives monosynaptic input from corticospinal cells in the monkey (Jankowska et al., 1975). Experiments designed to test the effect of CM cells on antagonists of their target muscles have revealed reciprocal inhibition. Single intracortical microstimuli delivered at the site of CM cells typically produce poststimulus facilitation in the cell's target muscles. When delivered during the phase of movement in which the antagonists of the target muscles were active, these stimuli produced reciprocal inhibition on antagonists from about one-third of the cortical sites (Cheney et al., 1985). The postspike effects of *single* CM cells on antagonists of their target muscles are more difficult to document with STA, since the cells and antagonists are normally activated reciprocally. However, by activating CM cells with glutamate during the phase of movement in which they would normally be inactive, Kasser and Cheney (1985) showed that about one-third of the extensor-related CM cells inhibited flexor muscles, and one-sixth of the flexor CM cells produced reciprocal inhibition of extensor muscles. An example of such a reciprocal CM cell is illustrated in Figure 20–3. The averages at the top show the postspike and poststimulus effects on the forelimb muscles, illustrating facilitation of extensors and inhibition of flexors.

RESPONSE PROPERTIES OF CM CELLS: COMPARISON WITH MOTOR UNITS

In addition to elucidating the organization of divergent output effects on different target muscles, chronic recording experiments have provided new information on the *response patterns* of CM cells under normal behavioral conditions. Monkeys performed ramp-and-hold wrist movements, which were designed to reveal the relation of cell activity to phasic change in force as well as tonic sustained force. During this task, the response patterns of CM cells fell into four categories (Cheney and Fetz, 1980). The predominant cell type (half of the CM cells) exhibited a phasic-tonic discharge pattern, consisting of a phasic burst of activity at the onset of movement, followed by tonic discharge during the static hold period (Fig. 20–4). The next most frequent type (28%) was the tonic CM cell, with constant firing during the static hold period. For both types, the tonic activity was proportional to the amount of isometric force that the animal exerted. The remaining two categories of CM cells were those that showed a gradually increasing level of activity during the hold period, either with or without a preceding phasic burst of activity at the onset of movement.

The response patterns of CM cells can be contrasted with those of motor units in the agonist muscles (Palmer and Fetz, 1985a). Under similar behavioral conditions, forelimb motor units showed four types of response patterns: phasic-tonic (23%), tonic (33%), phasic (5%), and decrementing (39%). The possibility of preferential correlational links between particular types of CM cells and motor units remains to be investigated.

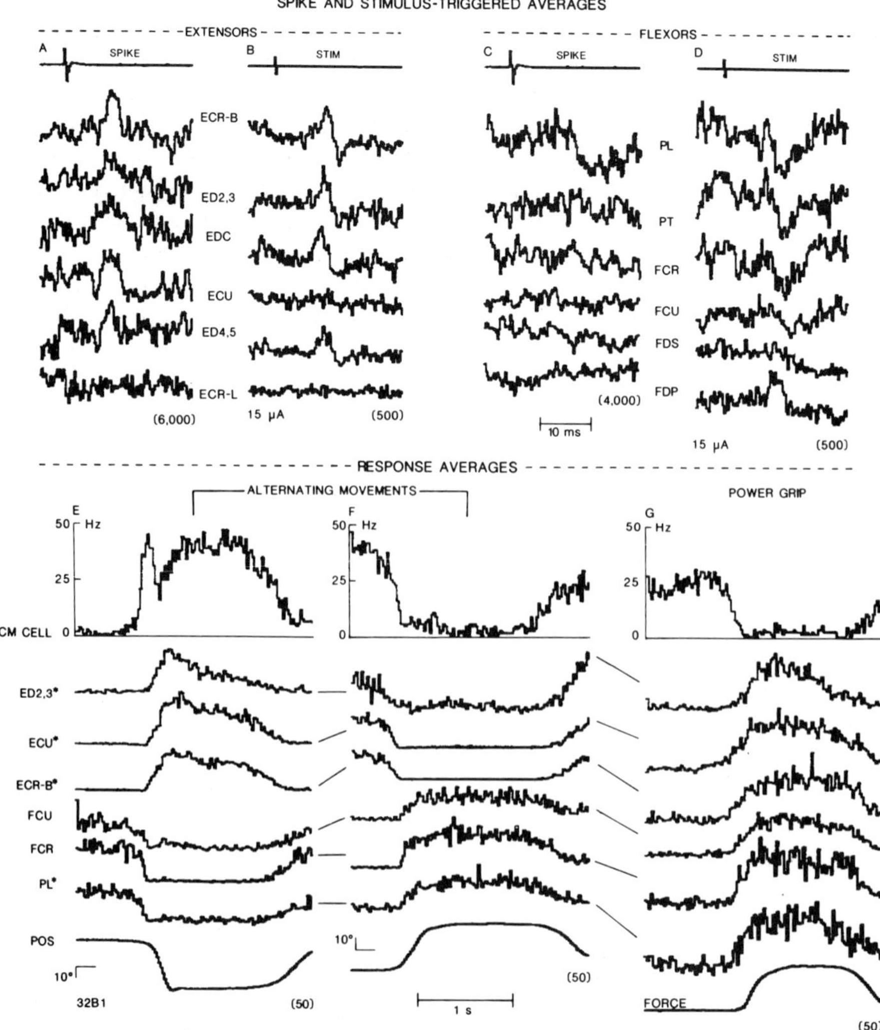

Fig. 20–3. Postspike effects of a reciprocal CM cell and its responses during alternating wrist movements and power grip. Top records show reciprocal correlational linkages of the cell: postspike facilitation of extensor muscles (A) and postspike suppression of flexors (C). These reciprocal output effects are further demonstrated by similar patterns of poststimulus effects in averages triggered from single-pulse microstimuli (15 μa) delivered at the site of this CM cell (B, D). Response averages at the bottom show that the CM cell was coactivated with its target muscles during alternating wrist movements (E, F). The cell was suppressed during cocontraction of extensors and flexors in the power grip (G). Target muscles are indicated by asterisks. In this and subsequent figures, the numbers in parentheses indicate the number of events averaged. (From Cheney et al., 1985.)

As would be expected, the tonic discharge of both CM cells and motor units is an increasing function of the amount of static force that the monkey exerts. However, there is a clear difference in the recruitment properties of CM cells and motor units as a function of active force. In accordance with Henne-

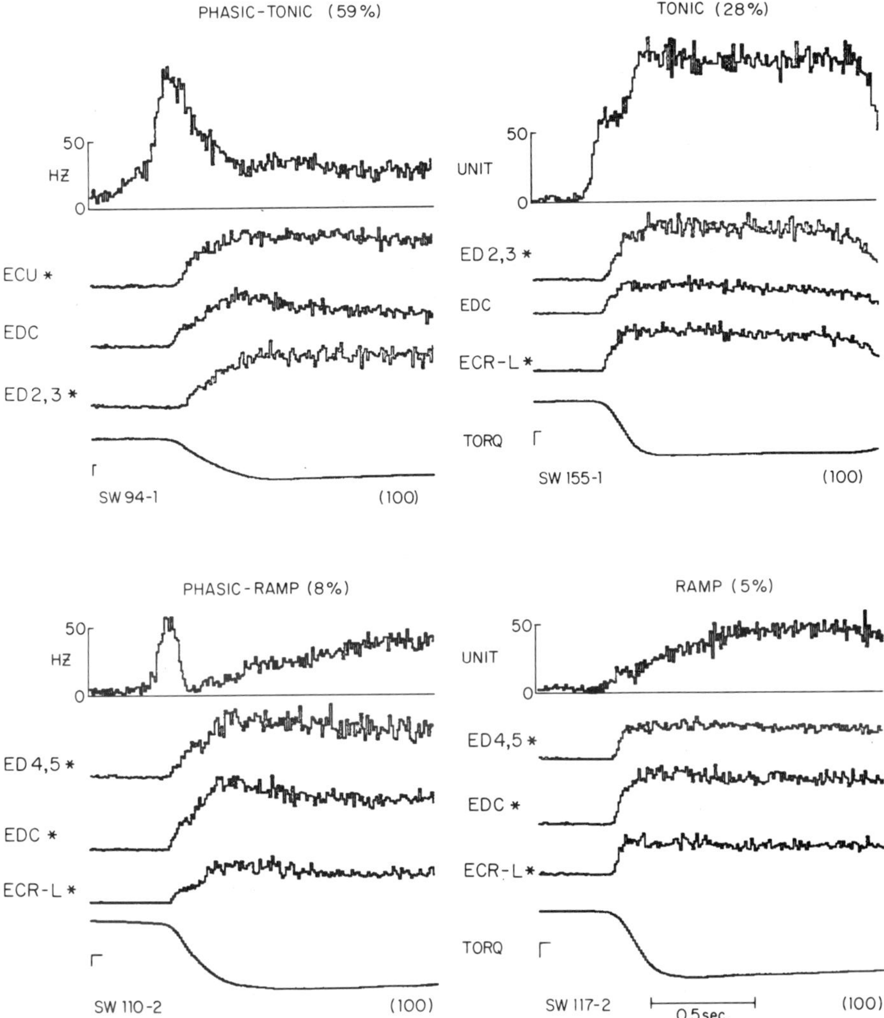

Fig. 20–4. Response patterns of CM cells and target muscles during generation of isometric ramp-and-hold torque responses. Each set shows the time histogram of CM cell activity, averages of rectified EMG (target muscles indicated by asterisk), and isometric torque. (From Cheney and Fetz, 1980.)

man's size principle, different motor units were found to be recruited into sustained activity over a range of static force levels (Palmer and Fetz, 1985a). In contrast, almost all the CM cells were active even at the lowest force levels and increased their discharge rate as a function of increasing force (Cheney and Fetz, 1980). At the upper range of forces, the CM cells tended to reach higher firing rates than the motor units, whose rates typically saturated.

Although CM cells seem to have a lower recruitment level than their target motor units, this applies specifically to well-controlled movements. CM cells are much more active during finely controlled movements than during rapid or forceful movements, despite the fact that the latter involve greater activity in their target muscles. For example, Muir and Lemon (1983) found that CM cells were strongly modulated during a precision grip task performed with the thumb and forefinger, but, paradoxically, were less active during a power grip. Similarly, our monkeys[1] CM cells fired intensely during the ramp-and-hold tracking task, but were curiously inactive during rapid ballistic shaking of the wrist manipulandum (Cheney and Fetz, 1980). Schieber and Thach (1985) also noted that many motor cortex cells, as well as spindle afferents, exhibited enhanced activity during a precisely controlled slow tracking task. This suggests that different input systems may be preferentially recruited to activate motoneurons during different types of movements.

An example of such a dissociation between a CM cell and its target muscles is illustrated in Figure 20–3. This CM cell fired strongly in association with its facilitated extensor muscles when the monkey performed alternating ramp-and-hold movements (bottom left). However, when the monkey performed a power grip that involved coactivation of flexor and extensor muscles, this cell became entirely inactive (bottom right). In this case, the cell's inhibitory effect on the flexor muscles (top right) may provide a rationale: this postspike suppression would be inappropriate during a response that requires coactivation of the flexor muscles. Indeed, CM cells that produced reciprocal inhibition of antagonists were more likely to decrease their activity during cocontraction of flexors and extensors than CM cells that only facilitated their target muscles (Kasser and Cheney, 1983). It seems noteworthy that during cocontraction of antagonist muscles the nervous system appears to circumvent this inappropriate inhibition by turning off the reciprocal CM cells rather than by the plausible alternative of suppressing the mediating inhibitory interneuron.

CENTRAL VERSUS PERIPHERAL CONTROL OF MOTONEURONS

The function of CM cells, as well as of other descending pathways, is commonly considered to be quite different from the function of monosynaptic input from Ia afferents. The anatomical location of supraspinal versus peripheral afferents suggests the obvious functional distinction, namely, that descending tracts provide pathways for voluntary activation of motor units, while peripheral input provides a feedback system for stabilizing muscle force in the face of changing loads. This functional dichotomy is based on the idea that CM cells are under central control during voluntary movement, whereas muscle afferents are driven predominantly by peripheral stimuli. In light of accumulating evidence, this model is now considered simplistic. In addition to being activated by peripheral events, the Ia afferents may be affected by centrally originating input via gamma bias on the spindle. This gamma bias provides a potent pathway for control of spindle activity from central sources. The remarkable experiments of Schieber and Thach (1985) suggest that Ia afferents are intensely active for finely controlled, slow tracking movements.

Similarly, CM cells are not only activated by central input (which accounts

for their activity prior to voluntary movement), but are also responsive to peripheral input from proprioceptors and cutaneous afferents. One function of this
peripheral input is demonstrated by experiments in which active movements
are perturbed by load changes. Stretch of an active muscle evokes responses
in Ia afferents that produce a segmental reflex that helps to counteract the
lengthening. This well-known myotatic stretch reflex is manifest in the early
M1 EMG response following muscle stretch. The M1 is followed at longer
latencies by an M2 response, sometimes called the "functional stretch reflex"
(see Desmedt, 1978, for reviews). Phillips (1969) initially proposed that pyramidal tract neurons may function in a transcortical stretch reflex analogous
to the segmental stretch reflex. Indeed, CM cells have been shown to contribute
to M2 (Cheney and Fetz, 1984). However, there is an important difference in
the responses evoked by transcortical and peripheral pathways. While Ia afferents are activated by passive stretch of their parent muscle and are inacti-
vated by passive shortening of their parent muscle, many CM cells are activated
by *both* types of movements. This bidirectional excitation of many CM cells

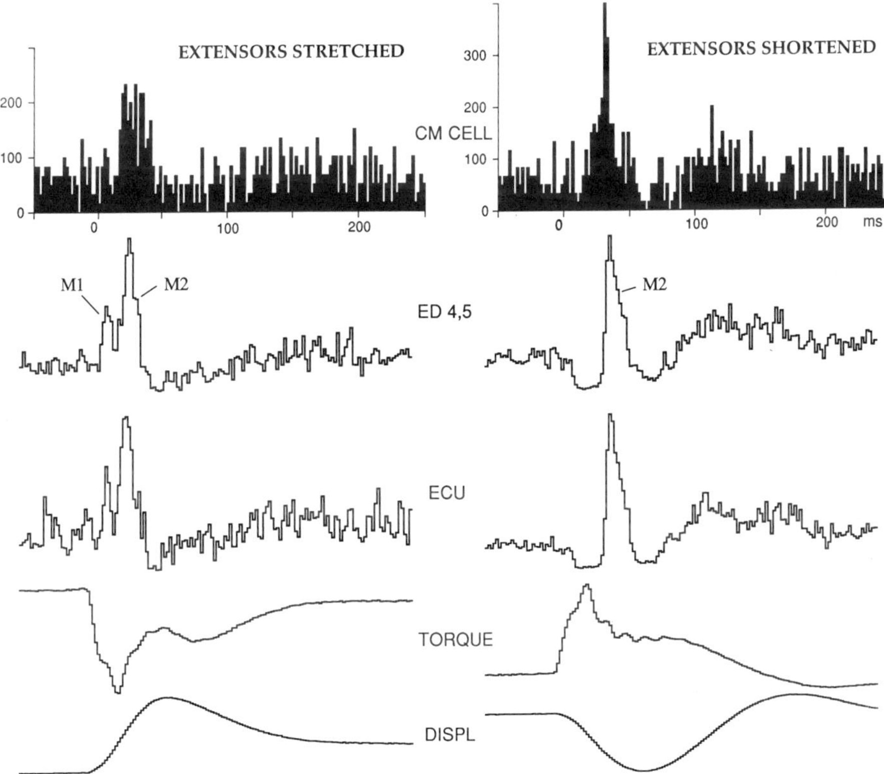

Fig. 20–5. Response of extensor CM cell and extensor muscles to brief perturbations applied
during active wrist extension. This cell, like half of the CM cells, responded ubiquitously to
perturbations that either stretched (left) or shortened (right) its target muscles. Note that in contrast
to the reciprocal M1 response, the later M2 response was bidirectional, like the response of the
CM cell.

(about half) might seem paradoxical but is in fact consistent with the observed coactivation of flexors and extensors during the functional stretch reflex. Figure 20–5 illustrates the responses of such a CM cell and its target muscle to brief load changes imposed while a monkey exerts a steady force. The initial M1 response appears only with perturbations that stretch the active muscle (left), but the later M2 response is evoked by both flexion and extension perturbations of the wrist. This bidirectional response in CM cells and muscles also serves to stabilize movements, but unlike the reciprocal stretch reflex that specifically counteracts the perturbation, such coactivation of flexors and extensors stiffens the joint. This stiffening response serves to stabilize the joint against subsequent perturbations. The involvement of motor cortex in this stabilizing reflex could provide an effective mechanism for its central modulation.

CONCLUDING COMMENTS

To summarize the points of comparison between CM cells and Ia fibers, the organization of their terminal connections appears quite analogous: Both send divergent terminals to multiple muscles, and probably most of the motoneurons in their target muscles. A distributed connection to all motoneurons of the target pool would be consistent with the recruitment of motoneurons in order of size (Henneman and Mendell, 1981). In addition, many CM cells, like Ia afferents, produce reciprocal inhibition in antagonists of their target muscles; indeed, this inhibition may be mediated by the same Ia inhibitory interneuron. Both CM cells and Ia afferents are subject to central as well as peripheral input. However, their responses to load perturbations indicate that Ia afferents mediate a stretch reflex that specifically counteracts change in muscle length, while CM cells mediate a cocontraction of flexors and extensors that stiffens the joint.

Comparisons between the responses of CM cells and motoneurons show that the CM cells are considerably more active at low levels of force. While CM cells are recruited before their target motor units during fine movements, the latter are more active than CM cells during rapid forceful movements. The ability to make these comparisons owes much to the pioneering work of Elwood Henneman and his colleagues, which provided essential information on the properties of motoneurons and Ia fibers; future work on quantitative analysis of other inputs to motoneurons will continue to employ the techniques they pioneered to investigate this model system.

Acknowledgment

This work was supported in part by NIH grants NS 12542, RR 00166, and NS 5082.

REFERENCES

Buys, E. R., Lemon, R. N., Mantel, G. W. B., and Muir, R. B. (1986). Selective facilitation of different hand muscles by single corticospinal neurones in the conscious monkey. *J. Physiol. (Lond.)* 381, 529–549.

Cheney, P. D., and Fetz, E. E. (1980). Functional classes of primate corticomotoneuronal cells and their relation to active force. *J. Neurophysiol.* 44, 773–791.

Cheney, P. D., and Fetz, E. E. (1984). Corticomotoneuronal cells contribute to long-latency stretch reflexes in the rhesus monkey. *J. Physiol. (Lond.)* 349, 249–272.

Cheney, P. D., and Fetz, E. E. (1985). Comparable patterns of muscle facilitation evoked by individual corticomotoneuronal (CM) cells and by single intracortical microstimuli in primates: Evidence for functional groups of CM cells. *J. Neurophysiol.* 53, 786–804.

Cheney, P. D., Fetz, E. E., and Palmer, S. S. (1985). Patterns of facilitation and suppression of antagonist forelimb muscles from motor cortex sites in the awake monkey. *J. Neurophysiol.* 53, 805–820.

Cheney, P. D., Kasser, R. J., and Fetz, E. E. (1985). Motor and sensory properties of primate corticomotoneuronal cells *Exp. Brain Res.* Suppl. 10, 211–231.

Cope, T. C., Fetz E. E., and Matsumura, M. (1987). Cross-correlation assessment of the synaptic strength of single Ia fibre connections with lumbar motoneurones in the cat. *J. Physiol. (Lond.)* 390, 161–188.

Desmedt, J. E. (ed.) (1978). *Cerebral Motor Control in Man: Long Loop Mechanisms.* Karger, New York.

Fetz, E. E., and Cheney, P. D. (1978). Muscle fields of primate corticomotoneuronal cells. *J. Physiol. (Paris)* 74, 239–245.

Fetz, E. E., and Cheney, P. D. (1980). Postspike facilitation of forelimb muscle activity by primate corticomotoneuronal cells. *J. Neurophysiol.* 44, 751–772.

Fetz, E., Henneman, E., Mendell, L., Stein, R. B., and Stuart, D. G. (1979). Properties of single cells in vertebrate motor systems revealed by spike-triggered averaging. In *Summaries of Symposia. Society for Neuroscience, 8th Annual Meeting.* Brain Information Services, pp. 11–32.

Henneman, E., and Mendell, L. M. (1981). Functional organization of the motoneuron pool and its inputs. In *Handbook of Physiology,* Vol. II, Part 1 (ed. V. B. Brooks). American Physiological Society, Bethesda, Md., pp. 423–507.

Jankowska, E., Padel, Y., and Tanaka, P. (1975). Disynaptic inhibition of spinal motoneurones from the motor cortex in the monkey. *J. Physiol. (Lond.)* 258, 467–487.

Kasser, R. J., and Cheney, P. D. (1983). Motor cortical mechanisms mediating reciprocal activation and co-activation of forearm flexor and extensor muscles in the primate. *Soc. Neurosci. Abst.* 9, 492.

Kasser, R. J., and Cheney, P. D. (1985). Characteristics of corticomotoneuronal postspike facilitation and reciprocal suppression of EMG activity in the monkey. *J. Neurophysiol.* 53, 959–978.

Kirkwood, P. A., and Sears, T. A., (1980). The measurement of synaptic connections in the mammalian nervous system by means of spike triggered averaging. In *Spinal and Supraspinal Mechanisms of Voluntary Motor Control and Locomotion,* Vol. 8. *Progress in Clinical Neurophysiology* (ed. J. E. Desmedt). Basel, Karger, pp. 44–71.

Mantel, G. W. H., and Lemon, R. N. (1987). Cross-correlation reveals facilitation of single motor units in thenar muscles by single corticospinal neurons in the conscious monkey. *Neurosci. Lett.* 77, 113–118.

Mendell, L. M., and Henneman, E. (1971). Terminals of single Ia fibers: Location, density and distribution within a pool of 300 homonymous motoneurons *J. Neurophysiol.* 34, 171–187.

Muir, R. B., and Lemon, R. N. (1983). Corticospinal neurons with a special role in precision grip. *Brain Res.* 261, 312–316.

Palmer, S. S., and Fetz, E. E. (1985a). Discharge properties of primate forearm motor units during isometric muscle activity. *J. Neurophysiol.* 54, 1178–1193.

Palmer, S. S., and Fetz, E. E. (1985b). Effects of single intracortical microstimuli in motor cortex on activity of identified forearm motor units in behaving monkeys. *J. Neurophysiol.* 54, 1194–1212.

Phillips, C. G. (1969). Motor apparatus of the baboon's hand. *Proc. R. Soc. B* 173, 141–174.

Schieber, M. A., and Thach, W. T. (1985). Trained slow tracking II. Bidirectional discharge patterns of cerebellar nuclear, motor cortex, and spindle afferent neurons. *J. Neurophysiol.* 54, 1228–1270.

Index